Indian Academy of Pediatrics
Presidential Action Plan 2006
Pediatric Hematology–Oncology Chapter

Reference Manual
for
National Training Project

Practical Pediatric Hematology

Second Edition

Editor
Anupam Sachdeva

Associate Editor
SP Yadav
National Coordinator
National Training Project - Practical Pediatric Hematology

National Advisory Committee

SC Arya *(Delhi)*

VP Choudhury *(Delhi)*

SK Sood *(Delhi)*

Panna Choudhury *(Delhi)*

MR Lokeshwar *(Mumbai)*

Bharat Agarwal *(Mumbai)*

Z Currimbhoy *(Mumbai)*

Mamta Manglani *(Mumbai)*

Rashmi Dalvi *(Mumbai)*

RK Marwaha *(Chandigarh)*

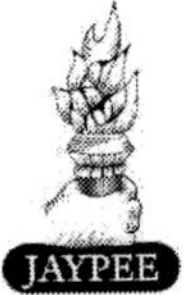

JAYPEE BROTHERS MEDICAL PUBLISHERS
The Health Sciences Publisher
New Delhi | London

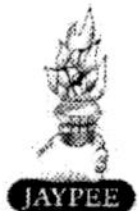

Jaypee Brothers Medical Publishers (P) Ltd.

Headquarters
EMCA House
23/23-B, Ansari Road, Daryaganj
New Delhi 110 002, India
Landline: +91-11-23272143, +91-11-23272703
+91-11-23282021, +91-11-23245672
E-mail: jaypee@jaypeebrothers.com

Corporate Office
Jaypee Brothers Medical Publishers (P) Ltd.
4838/24, Ansari Road, Daryaganj
New Delhi 110 002, India
Phone: +91-11-43574357
Fax: +91-11-43574314
E-mail: jaypee@jaypeebrothers.com

Overseas Office
JP Medical Ltd.
83, Victoria Street, London
SW1H 0HW (UK)
Phone: +44-20 3170 8910
E-mail: info@jpmedpub.com

EU GPSR Authorised Representative
Logos Europe, 9 rue Nicolas Poussin
17000, La Rochelle, France
Phone: +33 (0) 6 67 93 73 78
E-mail: Contact@logoseurope.eu

Website: www.jaypeebrothers.com
Website: www.jaypeedigital.com

Inquiries for bulk sales may be solicited at: jaypee@jaypeebrothers.com

Practical Pediatric Hematology

First Edition: 2006
Second Edition: **2012,** Reprint: 2025

ISBN 978-93-5025-921-4

Printed in India

Indian Academy of Pediatrics
Presidential Action Plan 2006
Pediatric Hematology–Oncology Chapter

Indian Academy of Pediatrics
Presidential Action Plan 2006
Pediatric Hematology–Oncology Chapter

The Executive Board of Central IAP 2005

Indian Academy of Pediatrics
Presidential Action Plan 2006
Pediatric Hematology–Oncology Chapter

Dedicated to

The stalwarts of Pediatric Hematology
in our Country

Contributors

Anshul Gupta MD
Department of Pediatric Hematology and Oncology and Bone Marrow Transplantation
Rajiv Gandhi Cancer Institute and Research Centre
Delhi, India

Anupam Sachdeva
Director
Pediatric Hematology and Oncology and Bone Marrow Transplantation
Chairman
Department of Academics and Convenor Research
Sir Ganga Ram Hospital
New Delhi, India

AP Dubey
Professor-Director and Head
Department of Pediatrics
Sir Ganga Ram Hospital
New Delhi, India

Archana Kumar
Professor
Department of Pediatrics
Chhatrapati Shahuji Maharaj Medical University
Lucknow, Uttar Pradesh, India

Arun Soni
Consultant Neonatologist
Institute for Child Health
Sir Ganga Ram Hospital
New Delhi, India

ATK Rau
Pediatric Hematologist and Oncologist
Professor and Head
Department of Pediatrics
MS Ramaiah Medical College
Bengaluru, Karnataka, India
atkrau@gmail.com

Bharat R Agarwal
Consultant Pediatric
Head
Department of Hematology and Oncology
BJ Wadia Hospital
Mumbai, Maharashtra, India

Biju George DM
Professor
Department of Hematology
Christian Medical College
Vellore, Tamil Nadu, India

Deepak Bansal MD DNB
Additional Professor
Hematology/Oncology Unit
Advanced Pediatric Center
Postgraduate Institute of Medical Education and Research, Chandigarh, India
deepakritu@yahoo.com

Dhiren Gupta
Consultant Pediatric Intensive Care Unit Institute of Child Health
Sir Ganga Ram Hospital
New Delhi, India

Gauri Kapoor
Department of Pediatric Hematology and Oncology and Bone Marrow Transplantation
Rajiv Gandhi Cancer Institute and Research Centre
Delhi, India

Himani Manchanda
Fellow in Pediatric Hematology and Oncology
Institute of Child Health
Sir Ganga Ram Hospital
New Delhi, India

IC Verma
Center of Medical Genetics
Sir Ganga Ram Hospital
New Delhi, India

Jagdish Chandra
Director, Professor
Department of Pediatrics
Lady Hardinge Medical College
Kalawati Saran Children's Hospital
New Delhi, India

Leni Mathew MD
Professor
Department of Pediatrics
Christian Medical College
Vellore, Tamil Nadu, India

LS Arya MD DCH
Senior Consultant
Indraprastha Apollo Hospital
Sarita Vihar
New Delhi, India

Mammen Chandy MD FRACP FRCPA FRCP
Director
Tata Medical Center
Kolkata, West Bengal, India

MB Agarwal
Consultant Hematologist
Bombay Hospital
Mumbai, Maharashtra, India

Mir Sadaqat Hassan Zafar
Fellow in Hematology
Sir Ganga Ram Hospital
New Delhi, India

Mohammed Ramzan
Fellow in Pediatric Hematology and Oncology
Institute of Child Health
Sir Ganga Ram Hospital
New Delhi, India

MR Lokeshwar
Consultant, Pediatrician
Lilavati Hospital
Mumbai, Maharashtra, India

Neha Rastogi
Fellow in Pediatric Hematology and Oncology
Institute of Child Health
Sir Ganga Ram Hospital
New Delhi, India

Nirmalya Roy Moulik
Senior Resident
Department of Pediatrics
Chhatrapati Shahuji Maharaj Medical University
Lucknow, Uttar Pradesh, India

Nitin K Shah
Consultant Pediatrician
PD Hinduja Hospital, Mumbai
Hon. Hematologist Oncologist
BJ Wadia Hospital for Children
Mumbai, Maharashtra, India
President
Indian Academy of Pediatrics, 2006
Fellow
Indian Society of Hematology and Transfusion Medicine

Nivedita Dhingra
Fellow in Pediatric Hematology and Oncology
Institute of Child Health
Sir Ganga Ram Hospital
New Delhi, India

Panna Choudhury
Consultant Pediatrician and President
IAP 2009
New Delhi, India

R Parakh
Chairman
Division of Peripheral Vascular and Endovascular Sciences
Medanta-The Medicity
Gurgaon, Haryana, India

RK Marwaha
Professor of Pediatric Hematology and Oncology
Advanced Pediatric Center
Postgraduate Institute of Medical Education and Research
Chandigarh, India
rammarwaha1@rediffmail.com

R Saxena
Professor and Head
Department of Hematology
All India Institute of Medical Sciences
New Delhi, India

Roma Kumar
Clinical Psychologist
Institute of Child Health
Sir Ganga Ram Hospital
New Delhi, India

Sachin Thakur
Consultant Neonatologist
USA

Samridh Nagar
Consultant Neonatologist
Australia

Shirish Kumar
Consultant Hematologist
Geneva, Switzerland

Shruti Patil
Assistant Professor
Department of Pediatrics
MS Ramaiah Medical College
Bengaluru, Karnataka, India

SP Yadav
Consultant Pediatric Hematologist and Oncologist
Department of Pediatrics
Institute of Child Health
Sir Ganga Ram Hospital
New Delhi, India

Sunil Gomber
Professor of Pediatrics
University College of Medical Sciences and
Guru Teg Bahadur Hospital
New Delhi, India

Sunil Narain
Consultant Pediatrician
New Delhi, India

Trupti Dongre
Consultant Pediatrician
Mumbai, Maharashtra, India

Ushma Singh
Fellow in Pediatric Hematology and Oncology
and Bone Marrow Transplantation
Institute of Child Health
Sir Ganga Ram Hospital
New Delhi, India

Vaishnavi Reddy
Center of Medical Genetics
Sir Ganga Ram Hospital
New Delhi, India

Vasant Chinnabhandar
Fellow in Pediatric Hematology and Oncology
Institute of Child Health
Sir Ganga Ram Hospital
New Delhi, India

Vikas Dua
Fellow in Pediatric Hematology and Oncology
Institute of Child Health
Sir Ganga Ram Hospital
New Delhi, India

Vikram Mathews
Professor of Hematology
Christian Medical College
Vellore, Tamil Nadu, India

Vinita Jain
Consultant
Pediatrician Aastha Medical Center
New Delhi, India

VP Choudhary
Ex-Professor and Head
Hematology
All India Institute of Medical Sciences
Consultant Hematologist
Sunflag Hospital
Faridabad, Haryana, India

From the President, IAP 2006

Dear Colleagues

Evidence-based medicine is the need of the hour. Every pediatrician strives for perfection in his or her practice. While the avenue to learn decrease after one leaves the medical school, the science keeps on evolving. It is impossible to keep pace with what is happening in the field of pediatrics in general and hence the need to specialize is now felt even by the pediatricians. It is still some time before some centers would start providing a postgraduate diploma or degree in various pediatric subspecialties. The only avenue left for learning a specialty then is through regular updates and seminars.

Keeping this in mind, Indian Academy of Pediatrics (IAP) has envisaged starting specialty training under its plan of action 2006. IAP-Pediatric Hematology and Oncology (PHO) Chapter is the first to respond to the call of IAP by starting this year the IAP PHO Training in Hematology. After the grand success of the Pediatric Oncology training workshops, the need to start similar program in Pediatric Hematology was felt by many. This combined with the enthusiasm and hard work put in by Dr Anupam Sachdeva, Dr Bharat R Agarwal and their team has resulted in this dream come true in the form of these workshops. The whole concept is well thought, well conceived, well planned and well executed. The case-based discussion while teaching the skills and the hands on experience are two unique features of this workshop. The icing on the cake is the beautiful and picturesque manual for the delegates to carry back home. I am sure that the manual will be a good desk companion for the delegates while solving the mysteries of Pediatric Hematology cases.

I am sure that the delegates will be better empowered to deal with pediatric hematology cases after attending the workshop. Please do give your feedback so that we can improve on the quality from time to time.

Nitin K Shah
President IAP 2006

From the Chairman, Pediatric Hematology–Oncology Chapter, IAP

Dear Colleagues

These are exciting times for Pediatric Hematology and Oncology. Major advances during the past decade in the field have enhanced our understanding and significantly influenced the management and outcome of many of these chronic and fatal diseases affecting children. Achieving the gold standard of care for children patients should be our goal. Given the realistic situation under which we function, and due to the major sociocultural and economic hurdles this ideal may seem a utopian goal. Nevertheless, I strongly believe that we can achieve together much more than we alone can do. There are many novel adaptations that we could adopt in our clinic practice and management guidelines that would benefit a large chunk of patients. Training, I think, is the cornerstone for this progress!

The PHO Chapter of IAP has been in the forefront of IAP activities leading in many ways—publication on anemia in children, pediatric hematology and oncology; parent education booklet on ALL, hemophilia, thalassemia; publishing management guidelines on sickle cell disease, ITP, blood component therapy national training programs on pediatric oncology; publication of PHO newsletter; promoting subspecialty fellowship training; preparing teaching slide sets on CD; Pediatric Hematology and Oncology, website—*phoindia.org*, etc.

Training in Practical Pediatric Hematology (NTP-PPH) is the latest venture of PHO chapter program for training in practical pediatric hematology will be kicked off in January 2006 at Gurgaon, Haryana, India. This will be a 2 days course in *intensive practical* training for pediatricians and postgraduates. The launch of this program has been *a dream come true* for many of us who have waited for long to make this happen. This unique idea and process of training pediatricians in practical aspects of Pediatric Hematology will instantly raise the standards of care provided to children suffering with hematological disorders throughout the country.

I take this opportunity to thank Dr Nitin K Shah, President IAP 2006, to adopt this program under the IAP Action Plan 2006 and provide us this important platform to spread our message with very wide visibility also acknowledge the massive contributions of our dynamic honorary secretary and the National Co-ordinator of NTP-PPH, Dr Anupam Sachdeva.

Hope you enjoy reading this interesting manual and send us your feedback for its improvement in the future.

Bharat R Agarwal
Chairman
PHO Chapter of IAP and Head
Department of Pediatric Hematology and Oncology
BJ Wadia Hospital for Children
Parel, Mumbai, Maharashtra, India

Preface to the Second Edition

It has been nearly six years since the first edition. There have been major advances in our knowledge. Not only this, a lot of new diagnostic tests are available across the country and this has made it possible for us to deal with hematological problems in a better way. During the last six years, we have held innumerable workshops and trained a lot of pediatricians in hematology. Richer with that experience we have modified the current edition. This book now is well illustrated and has many pictures and diagrams. We hope that this will be of use not only to the postgraduates of pediatrics but also will be of immense use to a general pediatrician as a ready-reckoner to be kept on his desk.

Anupam Sachdeva
SP Yadav

Preface to the First Edition

After the roaring success of the training project in *Practical Pediatric Oncology,* there was a desire in everyone of us that we need to put together a similar course for pediatric hematology. A two-day workshop was organized on 6th and 7th April 2002 in which experts from across the country participated and a training program was formulated. A reference manual was to be prepared and a standard set of slides were to be made.

After a gestation of nearly three years, we bring to you the 1st edition of the *Manual on Pediatric Hematology*.

I gratefully acknowledge the constant advice and active contribution of our President Dr Bharat R Agarwal. I also would like to acknowledge the contribution of various experts without whose patience and work this manual would not have been possible.

We hope that this manual and the workshops will go a long way in improving the standard of care in hematological disorders of children in our country.

I would also like to acknowledge the contribution of Dr Nitin K Shah, President IAP 2006 who has been instrumental in giving the program a large platform by making it a part of the Presidential Action Plan 2006.

I also would like to acknowledge the contribution of Dr Anil Handoo, Dr Nitin Shah, Dr MR Lokeshwar, Dr Mamta Manglani, Dr Amita Mahajan and Dr Deepak Bansal, for parting with their clinical photographs for the manual.

Anupam Sachdeva
Editor

January 2006

Contents

Plate 1

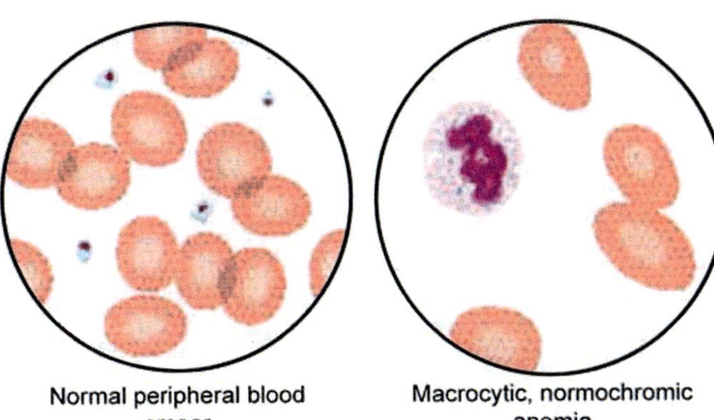

Fig. 1.1: Peripheral smear macrocytic anemia

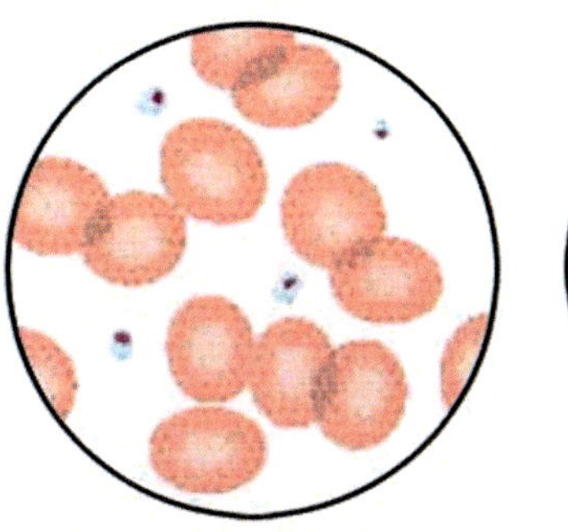

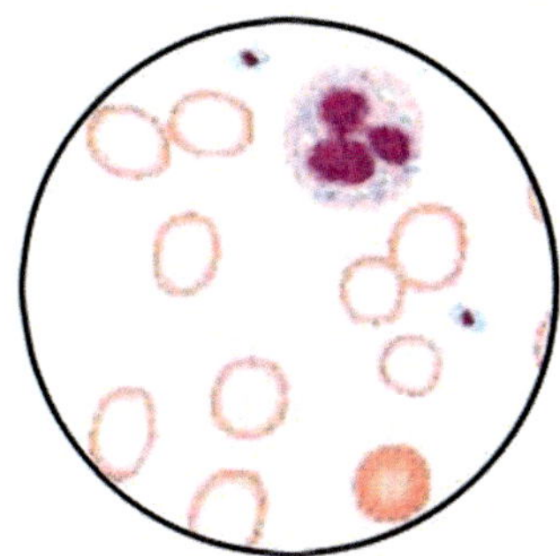

Fig. 1.2: Peripheral smear of microcytic hypochromic anemia

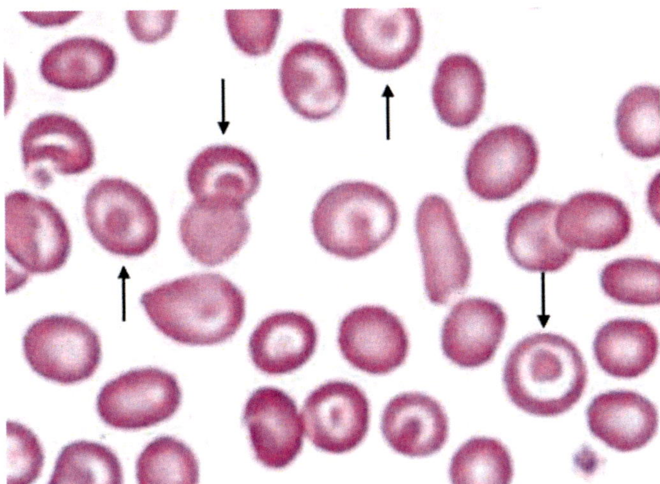

Fig. 1.3: Target cells

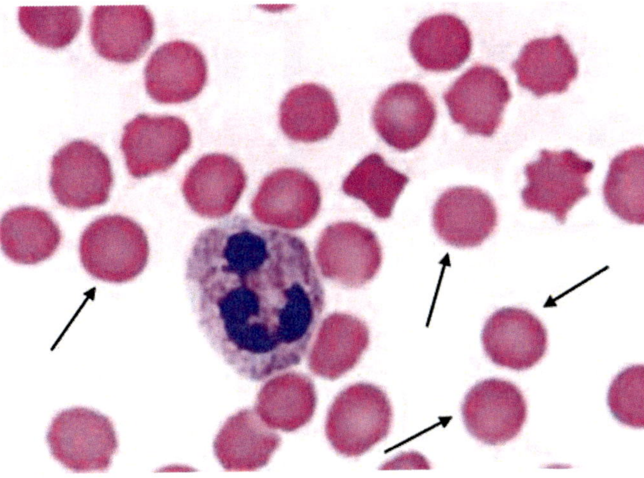

Fig. 1.4: Spherocytes

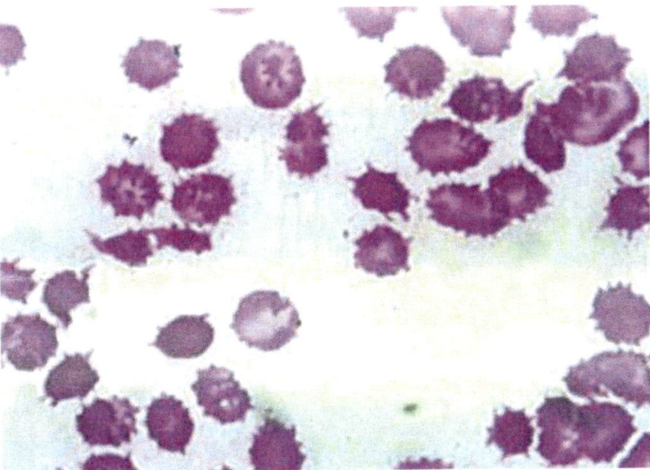

Fig. 1.5: Acanthocytes

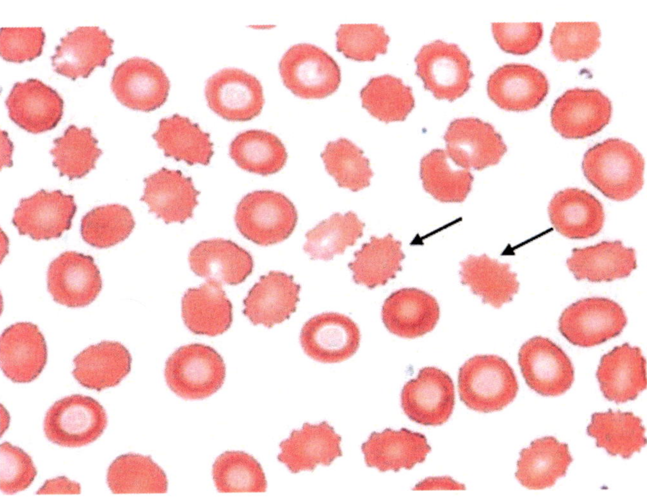

Fig. 1.6: Echinocytes

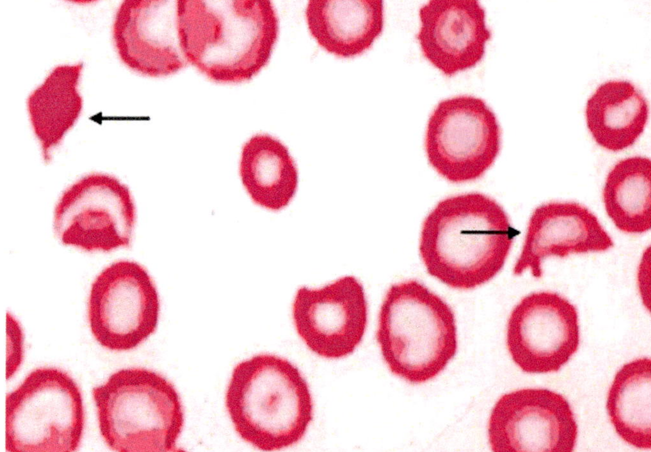

Fig. 1.7: Schistocytes

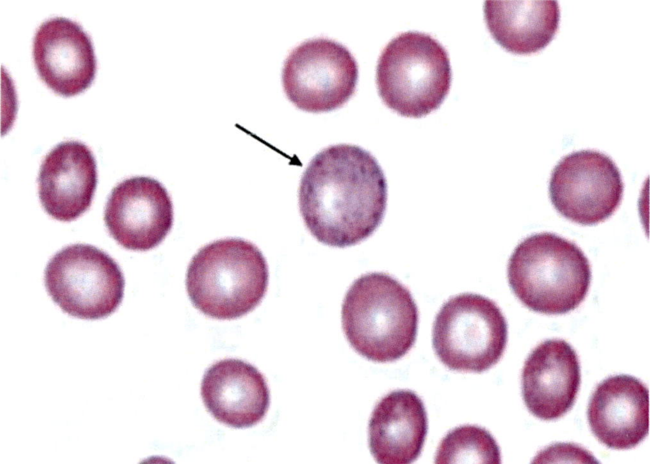

Fig. 1.8: Basophilic stippling

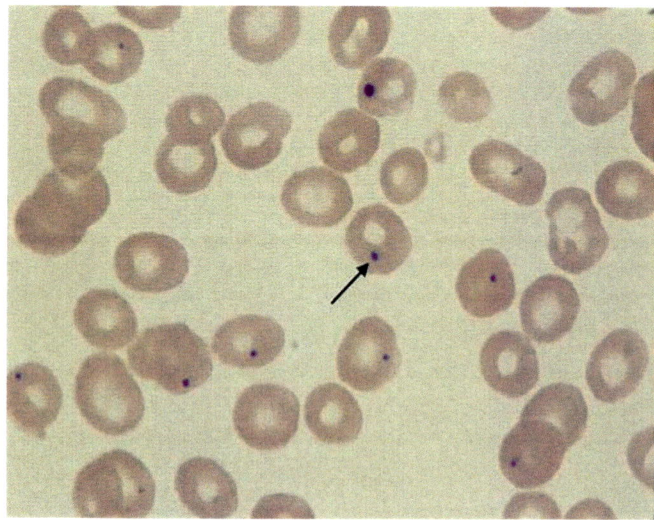

Fig. 1.9: Howell-Jolly bodies

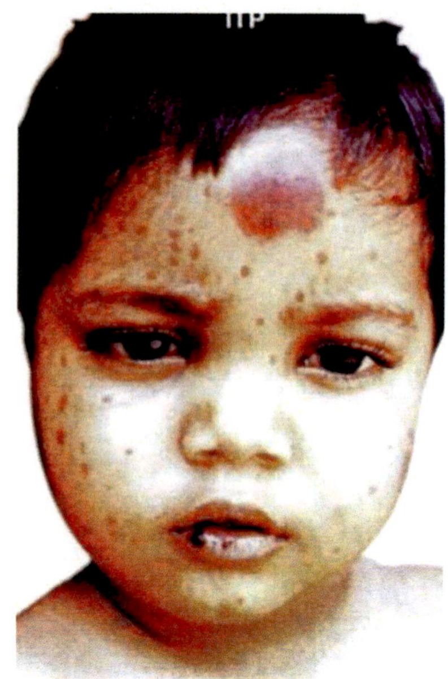

Fig. 17.1: Typical skin manifestations in a case of ITP (*Courtesy:* MR Lokeshwar)

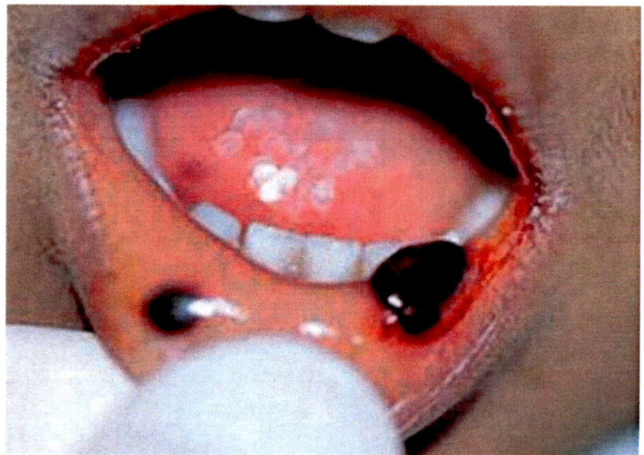

Fig. 17.2: Mucosal bleeds in the oral cavity in ITP (*Courtesy:* MR Lokeshwar)

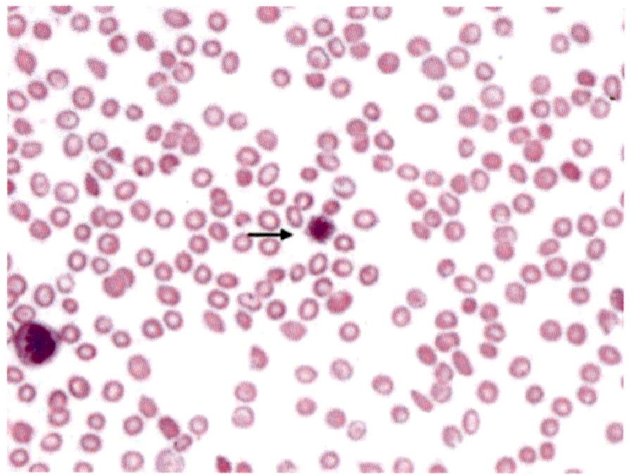

Fig. 17.3: Peripheral blood smear showing paucity of platelets and a giant platelet (arrow)

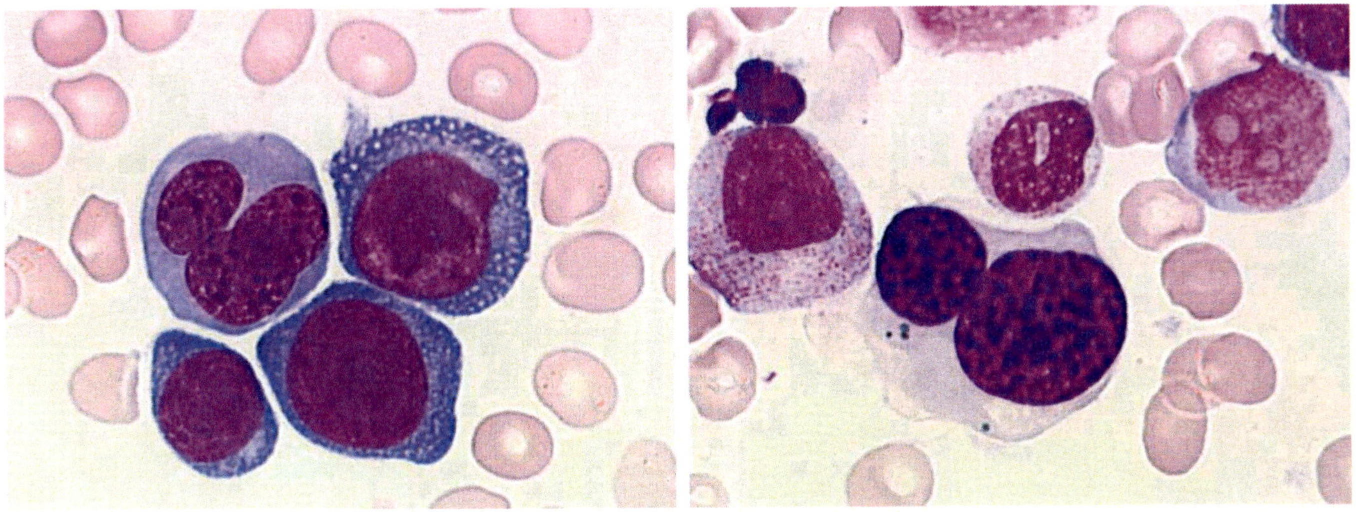

Fig. 32.1A: Dyserythropoiesis: BM

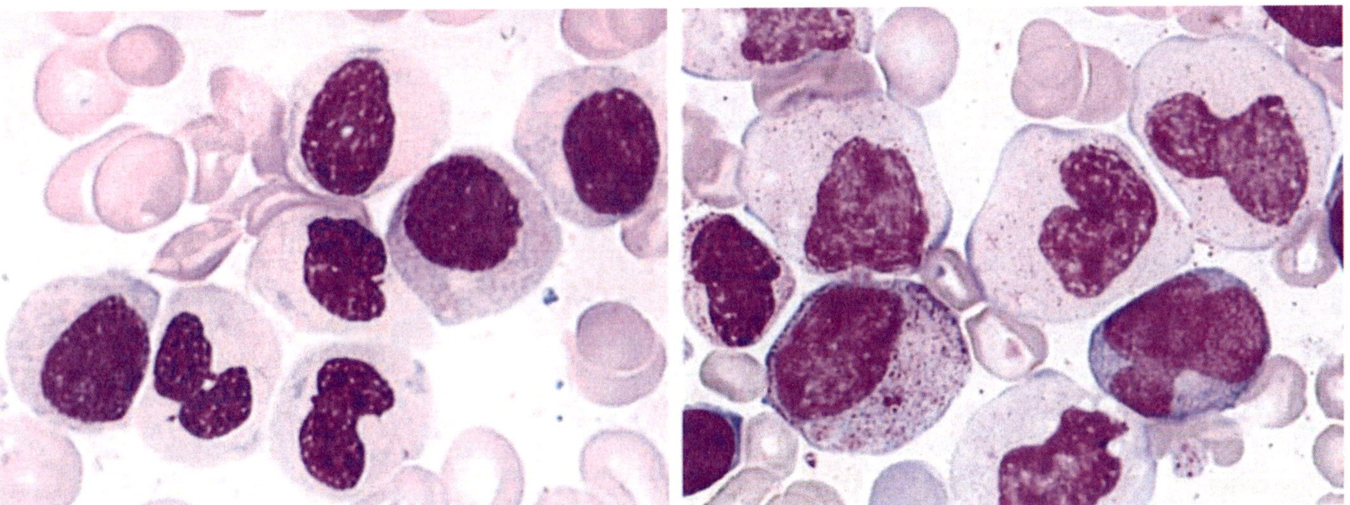

Fig. 32.1B: Dysgranulopoiesis: BM

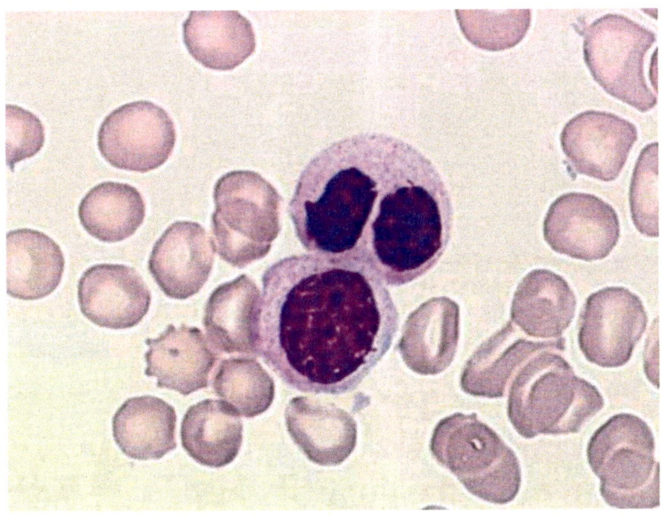

Fig. 32.1C: Dysgranulopoiesis: PB

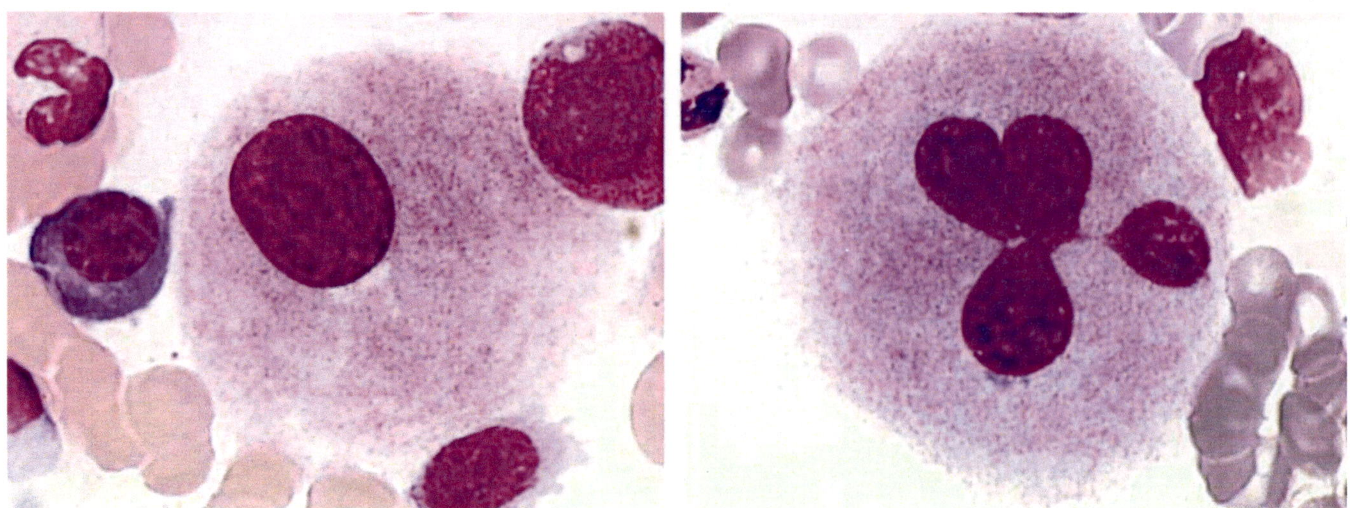

Fig. 32.1D: Dysmegakaryopoiesis BM

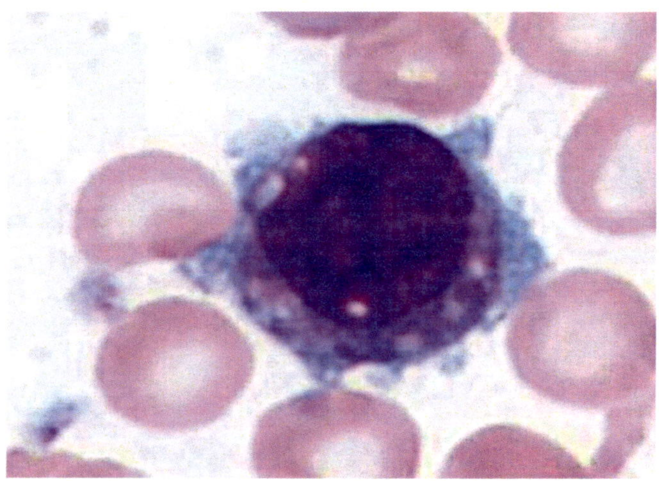

Fig. 32.1E: Micromegakaryocytes BM

1 Interpretation of the Complete Blood Count

Vikas Dua, Vinita Jain, SP Yadav, Anupam Sachdeva

The complete blood count (CBC) is a simple, inexpensive, test to order and interpret, but the results often are given only cursory appraisal. It tells us:
1. Whether the patient is anemic
2. Total leukocyte count (TLC) and differential leukocyte count (DLC) tell us about infection
3. Whether the platelet count is low or high enough to cause bleeding or thrombosis.

There are many nuances and clues from the CBC, which help us in many clinical situations to guide additional diagnostic evaluation. The CBC is a bargain; but its value is lost without appropriate analysis. The CBC consists of:
1. Hemoglobin concentration
2. Hematocrit (packed cell volume)
3. Mean corpuscular hemoglobin (MCH)
4. MCH concentration (MCHC)
5. Mean corpuscular volume (MCV)
6. Erythrocyte count
7. Leukocyte count
8. Platelet count.

When a child presents with anemia, it is important to establish whether the child has:
1. Single cell line (red blood cells) involvement or
2. Bi or trilineage problem (i.e. red cell, white cell, and platelets).

A two or three cell line problem usually indicates:
1. Bone marrow involvement as is seen in:
   a. Aplastic anemia
   b. Leukemia
2. Immunologic disorder leading to destruction of various components of blood:
   a. Connective tissue disease
   b. Acquired immunodeficiency syndrome (AIDS)
   c. Peripheral destruction of cells
      i. Immunoneutropenia
      ii. Idiopathic thrombocytopenic purpura (ITP)
      iii. Immune hemolytic anemia, singly or in combination
      iv. Sequestration of cells (e.g. hypersplenism).

The automatic instruments directly measure hemoglobin, MCV, and erythrocyte count, whereas MCH, mean corpuscular hemoglobin concentration (MCHC), and hematocrit are derived from the following formulas:

$$\text{MCH} = \text{Hb (g/L)/RBC} \quad (10^6/\text{dl})$$
$$\text{MCHC} = \text{Hb (g/dl)/HCT (\%)}$$
$$\text{HCT} = \text{MCV (fl)} \times \text{RBC} \quad (10^6/\text{dl})$$

Hemoglobin concentration is measured by absorbance spectrophotometry after complete lysis of erythrocytes.

RED CELL DISTRIBUTION WIDTH

The cells are made to pass singly through an electric field or through a light source, a small resistance is generated, from the pulse height, the size and number of times the resistance is generated erythrocyte number is determined. These data can be plotted as a histogram. In the histogram, the MCV as well as the distribution of cells that give rise to the MCV can be seen. This measure of dispersion of the erythrocyte size distribution is called the RBC distribution width (RDW), which is the coefficient in variation of the erythrocyte volume distribution expressed as a percentage. In other words it is a measure of the degree of anisocytosis in the blood.

HEMATOCRIT

The hematocrit is calculated rather than measured directly and this accounts for differences that occur when 'spun' and automated hematocrits are compared. In the manual hematocrit the degree of erythrocyte packing that occurs is optimal and not complete, because small pockets of plasma are trapped in the spaces between the incompletely packed erythrocytes. The amount of plasma that is trapped is estimated to be 3% under most conditions; however, this fraction is not constant over the spectrum of hematocrit values and becomes larger as the hematocrit increases. In addition, alteration in erythrocyte shape, density, and stiffness affects the fraction of trapped plasma; for example, certain erythrocyte shapes lead to more trapping of plasma as occurs in:[1]

- Spherocytes
- Sickle erythrocytes
- Hypochromic cells
- Reticulocytes.

RULE OF 3s

A simple rule of 3s for screening can be applied:

The measured Hb concentration is three times the RBC count, and the calculated hematocrit is three times the Hb level. A significant deviation means artifacts in the value estimated[2] or the RBCs are smaller or larger than normal . For example, failure of complete cell lysis causes interference with hemoglobin measurement. This occurs in conditions that create hyperosmolar plasma (e.g. uremia). In this situation, the hematocrit and MCV are artificially elevated. Agglutination of erythrocytes, which may occur in autoimmune hemolytic anemia because of cold-reacting IgM antibodies, also results in a markedly increased MCV unless precautions are taken to warm the blood thoroughly before analysis.[3] Elevated MCH and inaccurate hematocrit determination also may result. Another example is hyperleukocytosis (white blood cell count, >100,000/mm^3), which can cause elevation of the Hb, hematocrit, red blood cell count, and MCV.

BLOOD SMEAR

The examination of the blood smear can be useful particularly in evaluating a patient with anemia. Unfortunately, to become expert in recognizing alterations in blood cell morphology, blood smears must be examined with regularity and patience. The best place to search for properly spread erythrocytes is several millimeters inside the feathered edge of the smear.

Artifacts in the Blood Smear

Red Blood Cells

Erythrocyte shapes created by both artifact and disease includes target cells, spherocytes, and stomatocytes. Artifactual spherocytes are especially common and can be distinguished from the true spherocyte:

1. They are larger than normal erythrocytes.
2. The complete loss of central pallor in every cell, unlike in true spherocytes, in which central pallor still is present in many cells.
3. Finally, when erythrocyte morphology is truly abnormal, the alterations in erythrocyte shape are apparent in different areas of the same smear and on different blood smears.

Platelets and Leukocytes

Blood smear artifacts similarly can interfere with the evaluation of platelet and leukocyte morphology. Persistent-platelet-leukocyte satellitism (resulting in spurious thrombocytopenia).

Delay in making the blood smear can adversely affect platelet and leukocyte:

- Platelets become rounded and lose their granularity
- Granulocytes may loose toxic granulation
- Granulocytes may loose Dohle bodies
- Nuclei become pyknotic
- Cytoplasmic vacuolization also can increase.

Delay artifacts can obscure changes associated with infection.

Importance of the Blood Smear

The blood smear can provide important information about erythrocyte abnormalities.

In patients with severe hemolysis:

- Nucleated erythrocytes (sometimes accompanied by granulocytosis and thrombocytosis)
- Schistocytes in immune mediated hemolytic anemia and hereditary spherocytosis
- Spiculated erythrocytes
- Acanthocytes (spur cells) in pyruvate kinase deficiency
- Poikilocytosis 'bite' or 'blister' cells in glucose-6-phosphate dehydrogenase (G6PD) deficiency.

Some Specific Shapes and Characteristics

Target Cells

Altered erythrocyte surface area, which, in dried smears, results in the outward bulge of excess membrane into the region of central pallor, creating the characteristic target appearance.

Causes:

1. Iron deficiency
2. Liver disease
3. Hemoglobinopathies (hemoglobins C, D, and E)
4. Thalassemia
5. Postsplenectomy state
6. Hereditary xerocytosis
7. Lecithin cholesterol acyl transferase deficiency (LCAT deficiency).

Howell-Jolly Bodies

They are nuclear remnants that are not extruded from mature erythrocytes and indicate splenic hypofunction.

Basophilic Stippling

It is caused by aggregated ribosomes in the erythrocyte (for ribosomal DNA and mitochodrial fragments in lead poisonings) is seen with thalassemia and lead intoxication.

Rouleaux Formation

It occurs when plasma proteins block the negative charge on the erythrocyte surface, and red cells stack in long columns. Stacking occurs in several clinical conditions, especially when the erythrocyte sedimentation rate is elevated and is readily distinguishable from erythrocyte agglutination, in which erythrocyte aggregates are distorted and form clumps.

Leukocyte Abnormalities

Dohle bodies: They are bluish cytoplasmic inclusions that can be seen in the neutrophils from patients with:
- Bacterial infection
- Burns
- Myelodysplasia
- May-Hegglin anomaly
- Pregnancy.

Alder-Reilly bodies: They are coarse, dark granules found in the neutrophils from patients with mucopolysaccharidosis.

Chédiak-Higashi syndrome, giant azurophilic granules are present in lymphocytes, whereas granulocytes contain very large irregular granules.

Hemoglobin and Hematocrit Values

Hemoglobin and hematocrit values relate to the number and content of erythrocytes, and when the measured hemoglobin is depressed, that is, more than two standard deviations below the mean, anemia exists.

Polycythemia

Several conditions may result in elevation of the hemoglobin or polycythemia. These conditions include:
1. Primary (e.g. Polycythemia Vera)
2. Secondary
   a. Renal tumors
   b. Posterior fossa brain tumors
   c. Cyanotic heart disease
   d. Defects in synthesis of 2,3-diphosphoglycerate leading to left ward shifts in the oxygen and hemoglobin dissociation curve.[4,5]
   e. Alteration in the hemoglobin molecule that increase its affinity for oxygen.

Infants with hematocrit exceeding 65% are at risk for a hyperviscosity syndrome that can be accompanied by hypoglycemia and central nervous system injury.[6]

ROLE OF MCV, RDW AND RETICULOCYTE COUNT IN EVALUATING ANEMIA

CBC is a good way to organize one's thinking about anemia. The MCV and the RDW provide a classification of erythrocytes based on their size and size distribution[7] (Table 1.1). In children, the MCV is less than in adults and in children between the ages of 2 years and 10 years, the lower limit for MCV is approximately 70 fl + age (in years). The approximate upper limit for MCV is obtained by adding 0.6 fl per year to 84 fl beyond the first year of life until the upper limit of 96 fl in adults is reached. Erythrocytes in children with anemia can be

Table 1.1: Classification of anemia based on red cell MCV and RDW

MCV Low		*MCV Normal*		*MCV High*	
RDW–normal	*RDW–high*	*RDW–normal*	*RDW–high*	*RDW–normal*	*RDW–high*
Thalassemia trait	Iron deficiency	Normal	Mixed deficiency	Aplastic	Folate deficiency
Chronic disease	β-thalassemia	Chr ds.	Early Fe or folate	Preleuk. deficiency	B_{12} deficiency
Hb H	Sickle/HbC trait	Hemoglobinop.			Immune hemoglobin
	Fragmentation	Hereditary spherocytosis	Myelofibrosis		Cold agglutinins
		Transfusion	Sideroblastic anemia		CLL*
		Chemotherapy CLL, CML Hemorrhage			

*Caused by inclusion of leukocytes in the red cell volume distribution in CLL. Abbreviations: CLL: Chronic lymphocytic leukemia; CML: Chronic myelogenous leukemia; Hb: Hemoglobin; MCV: Mean corpuscular volume; RDW: Red cell distribution width

either small, large or normal in size, the RDW can be normal or increased.

Reticulocyte Count

Each day ~0.8% of the RBC pool needs to be replaced by young erythrocytes (reticulocytes) released from the marrow. Their number in the blood reflects the marrow's response to peripheral anemia. In anemia due to hemorrhage or hemolysis, erythropoietin (EPO) overdrive of the marrow results in reticulocytosis to compensate for the peripheral RBC deficit provided the marrow's capacity to produce RBC is intact. Reticulocytopenia in the presence of anemia indicates a disorder interfering with red cell production. Thus, reticulocyte count indicates whether the primary source of anemia is the bone marrow or the periphery.

Corrected Reticulocyte Count

Reticulocyte count needs to be corrected for anemia as it is a percentage of the total RBC count and is spuriously elevated when the number of RBC's falls in anemia. Reticulocyte percentage may be increased due to:

- More reticulocytes in circulation
- Fewer mature cells.

Hence, "correction" for the degree of anemia has to be done.

$$\text{Corrected reticulocyte (\%)} = \frac{\text{Patient PCV (L/L)}}{0.45} \times \text{Actual reticulocyte count}$$

Absolute Reticulocyte Count

$$\text{Retics/L} = \text{Retics (\%)} \times \text{RBC count}$$
$$[\text{Normal: } 50\text{–}100 \times 10^9/\text{L}]$$

An absolute reticulocyte count >100,000/dl indicates increased marrow activity.

Reticulocyte Production Index (RPI)

- The percentage of reticulocytes may be increased by premature release from the bone marrow (shift). The degree of "shift" is related to the intensity of stimulation by EPO.
- Thus, maturation time of the reticulocyte (in circulation) is:

1 day	if PCV = 0.45 L/L
1.5 days	if PCV = 0.35 L/L
2 days	if PCV = 0.25 L/L
2.5 days	if PCV = 0.15 L/L

$$\text{RPI} = \frac{\text{Reticulocyte (\%)}}{\text{Reticulocyte maturation time}} \times \frac{\text{Patient PCV (L/L)}}{0.45}$$

e.g. if PCV = 0.25 L/L and retics are 20%,

$$\text{RPI} = \frac{20}{2} \times \frac{0.25}{0.45} = 5.5$$

i.e. reticulocyte production has increased to 5.5 times the normal rate.

Increased MCV

Patients with increased erythrocyte volume may be classified according to their corresponding reticulocyte count.

Macrocytosis and Elevated Reticulocyte Count

- Acute blood loss
- Hemolysis.

Ancillary measures of erythrocyte destruction include:

- Serum bilirubin
- Lactate dehydrogenase (LDH).

Macrocytosis is caused by an increased number of reticulocytes, which have a large cellular volume (140-150 fl) (Fig. 1.1).

Anemia with Diminished Reticulocyte Count

Bone marrow failure: The macrocytosis is caused by the production of 'stress' erythrocyte, which display fetal characteristics, including increased fetal hemoglobin content and expression of *i* antigen.[8] For changes caused by stress erythropoiesis to occur, at least some

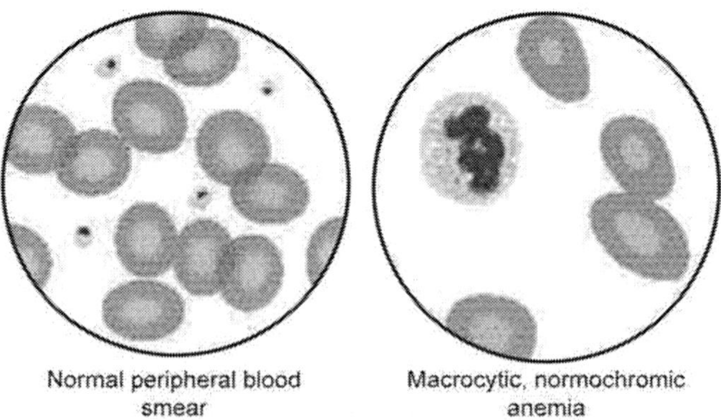

Fig. 1.1: Peripheral smear macrocytic anemia
(For color version, see Plate 1)

erythrocyte production is required, albeit at an insufficient rate. For this reason, in patients with severe aplastic anemia and pure red cell aplasia when erythropoiesis is absent, the resultant anemia may be normochromic and normocytic; however, stress erythropoiesis can be present in patients with these disorders with concomitant macrocytosis, making them difficult to distinguish from bone marrow failure syndromes like Fanconi's anemia and Diamond-Blackfan anemia (DBA).

Drugs are a common cause of macrocytosis:

- Valproate
- Zidovudine
- Immunosuppressive agents.[9]

Diamond-Blackfan anemia: A congenital hypoplastic anemia that most commonly presents in infancy, with 80% of cases occurring in the first 6 months of life.[10] This disorder is usually characterized by macrocytic anemia with reticulocytopenia, although many patients do not have an elevated MCV initially because of complete cessation of erythropoiesis. These patients become macrocytic, however, if some recovery of erythropoiesis occurs. White blood cells and platelet counts are generally normal, although the platelet count can be elevated.[11] Although most cases of DBA present before 1 year of age, as many as 5% of cases are identified later in life, for this reason, transient erythroblastopenia of childhood (TEC), which in 90% of cases, occurs in children more than 1 year of age, can be confused with DBA, TEC is a form of acquired anemia in which an immune reaction seems to occur against erythroid progenitor cells.[12] Some patients with TEC also may experience neutropenia.[13]

Because TEC is accompanied by cessation of erythropoiesis, the MCV is not increased initially; however, in the recovery phase of TEC, which is heralded by a marked reticulocytosis, the MCV is elevated. This recovery occurs within 1 to 2 months from the outset. Accordingly, expression of the *i* antigen and hemoglobin F production are low initially, increased during recovery from TEC (or following recovery from any marrow insult), and then return to normal following recovery. In addition, the erythrocyte adenosine deaminase level is increased in DBA (and other states of stress erythropoiesis) but is generally normal in patients with TEC.[14]

Other causes of macrocytic anemias are less common in childhood. These are associated with hypersegmentation of polymorphonuclear leukocytes and macro-ovalocytes. Examination of the bone marrow demonstrates megaloblastic changes that are diagnostic.

The megaloblastic disorders are:

1. Folate deficiency
2. Vitamin B_{12} deficiency
3. Inherited disorders of DNA metabolism (e.g. inborn errors of folate metabolism)
4. Alcohol causes a mild macrocytic anemia due to direct toxicity[15]
5. Folic acid antimetabolites like methotrexate produce pancytopenia more often than megaloblastic changes.
6. Other antimetabolites like trimethoprim can cause acute folate deficiency.
7. Hypothyroidism usually causes a normochromic normocytic anemia, but macrocytosis may develop.

Decreased MCV

Microcytic anemias (Fig. 1.2) are caused by insufficient hemoglobin synthesis, resulting in hypochromia (cells with an enlarged region of central pallor), target shapes, and in more severe cases, markedly deformed forms. In general, microcytosis is caused by:

1. Iron deficiency
2. The inability to utilize iron, as occurs in anemia of chronic disease
3. Thalassemia
4. Lead poisoning
5. Sideroblastic anemia.

Iron deficiency, is a common cause of microcytic anemia in children between 1 and 3 years of age. Iron deficiency may potentiate the toxic effects of lead poisoning; in most cases, the anemia seen with lead poisoning is caused by iron deficiency and not lead toxicity so that testing for lead poisoning in endemic regions may be warranted in the child with documented iron deficiency.[16,17]

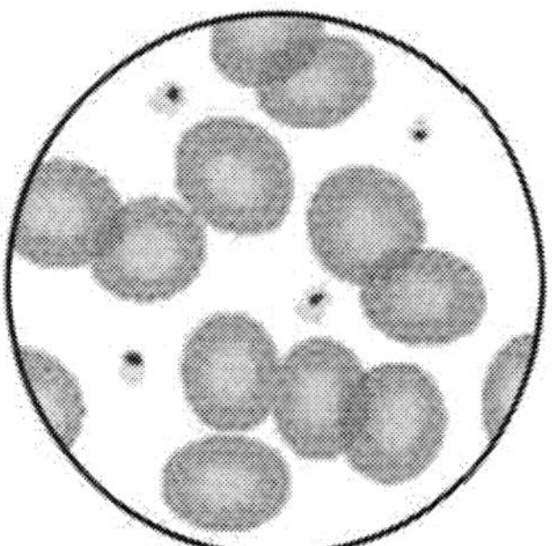

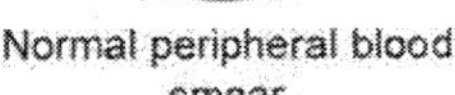

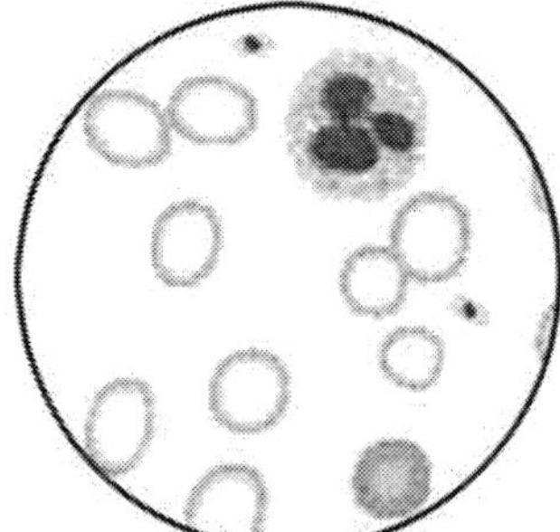

Fig. 1.2: Peripheral smear of microcytic hypochromic anemia *(For color version, see Plate 1)*

Inherited disorders of hemoglobin synthesis also cause microcytic anemia. Children with β-thalassemia major present during the first 6 to 24 months of life with profound anemia hepatosplenomegaly, jaundice, and growth retardation, β-thalassemia trait, the much more common heterozygous state, may be confused with iron deficiency. To differentiate between the two:

- Erythrocyte count is generally higher in the child with β-thalassemia trait.
- MCV is disproportionately low as compared to the Hb level in thalassemia trait.
- Free erythrocyte protoporphyrin (FEP) is elevated in iron deficiency.

DISCRIMINANT FUNCTION

Calculation	Iron deficiency	β-thalassemia trait	
MCV – (5 × Hb) – RBC – 3.4	>0	<0	(England and Fraser)
$\frac{MCV}{RBC}$	>13	<13	(Mentzer)
$\frac{MCH}{RBC}$	>3.8	<3.8	(Srivastava)
RBC count	<5.0	>5.0	(Klee et al)
$MCH \times \frac{(MCV)^2}{100}$	>1530	<1530	(Shine and Lal)

It is important to document that individuals suspected to have β-thalassemia trait must be iron replete prior to performing a diagnostic hemoglobin electrophoresis, because iron deficiency, which inhibits globin chain synthesis, obscures the elevation of Hb A_2 in these individuals.

Alpha-Thalassemia trait (with two of the four α-globin genes) results in microcytosis with a moderately severe hemolytic anemia. In these patients erythrocyte inclusions are seen following supravital staining with brilliant cresyl blue.

Sideroblastic anemias are rare in childhood, and caused by failure to incorporate iron into heme, resulting in a microcytic anemia.

1. Inherited form (X-linked)
2. Acquired forms
   - Myelodysplastic syndromes (microcytes and normal or macrocytic erythrocytes)
   - Drugs
     - Isoniazid
     - Ethanol
     - Others

The diagnosis of sideroblastic anemia is confirmed by demonstrating ringed sideroblasts on iron staining of the bone marrow. The presence of Pappenheimer bodies, (iron-laden mitochondria) in RBCs on smear support this diagnosis, but can be demonstrated in the postsplenectomy state.

Anemia with a Normal MCV

Normocytic anemia with an elevated reticulocyte count:

- Hemolysis
- Blood loss
- Balanced causes of macrocytic and microcytic anemia, such as iron deficiency combined with folate or B_{12} deficiency, i.e. dimorphic anemia.

However, patients with hemolysis may not be anemic if increased erythropoiesis is adequate to compensate for the shortened erythrocyte lifespan.

It is important to distinguish between erythrocytes of normal size versus a mixture of small and large erythrocytes creating a normal MCV or in other words dimorphic anemia.

In the latter case, the RDW is increased greatly, reflective of erythrocyte populations of different sizes.

Other causes of normocytic anemia:

- Acquired pure red cell aplasia
- TEC
- Aplastic anemia
- Hypothyroidism

These conditions also are often accompanied by macrocytic erythrocytes.

- Replacement of the marrow space by malignant cells in myelophthisis:
  - Leukemia
  - Lymphoma
  - Histiocytoses
  - Neuroblastoma
  - Ewing's sarcoma
  - Medulloblastoma
- Storage diseases in an advanced stage similarly can replace the marrow space.

Normocytic and normochronic anemias with a normal or low reticulocyte count:

Normal RDW

- Chronic infection
- Chronic inflammatory process
- Anemia of renal disease
- Liver disease.

Anemia of renal disease is due to:

- Erythropoietin insufficiency[18]
- Serum inhibitors of erythropoiesis may accumulate in the uremic patients

- Hyperparathyroidism may inhibit erythropoiesis by promoting myelofibrosis.[19,20]

With high BUN, acanthocytosis may develop, and RBC lifespan is shortened.

The anemia of liver disease is multifactorial and includes:
- Hypersplenism
- Concomitant vitamin-nutritional deficiency
- Blood loss.

The characteristic spur cell in liver disease, which is caused by an alteration in lipid composition of the membrane, is often a late and ominous development.

Mean Corpuscular Hemoglobin Concentration

The MCHC is a method for detecting erythrocyte cellular dehydration.
- Hereditary spherocytosis.
- Patients with sickle cell anemia.

These populations of cells are not readily detected by the Coulter electric impedence instrument but can be seen with instruments that rely on light scatter methodology to measure erythrocyte indices.

NEWBORN INFANTS

CBC determinations are done in the newborn period for:
- Infection
- Jaundice
- Pallor.

Method of collection becomes an important consideration. Blood samples can be obtained from a central site, via venepuncture, or central indwelling catheter (e.g. umbilical artery/vein), or pricking the skin of an extremity for collection of capillary blood. Blood samples collected from central sites are generally more reliable for hemoglobin determination; alternatively, capillary blood samples are much less reliable, with a tendency for capillary blood to overestimate the actual central hemoglobin. This occurs despite higher plasma content in smaller blood vessels (i.e. capillaries) and a somewhat larger erythrocyte volume among oxygen-carrying red cells in capillary blood. In fact, the ratio of hemoglobin values from capillary and central sites can be as high as 1.2:1, with the greatest disparity occurring in infants who are most ill (e.g. premature infants and neonates with hypotension, acidosis, or marked anemia).[21]

Although premature infants tend to have lower hemoglobin values because of the shorter period for hemoglobin synthesis *in utero*, the differences largely disappear after 32 to 33 weeks.[22] The erythrocyte size is increased in premature infants because of the relative abundance of larger fetal erythrocytes. The MCV at birth declines continuously with gestational age, which coincides with the switch from γ to β-globin chain synthesis, as does the reticulocyte count.

Anemia in the Newborn

- Blood loss
  - Placental transfusion, in which an infant may lose 10 to 20% of his or her blood
  - Fetal-maternal hemorrhage
  - Umbilical cord hemorrhage
  - Twin-twin hemorrhage
  - Internal hemorrhage
- Disorders of erythrocyte production and maturation (e.g. Diamond-Blackfan anemia)
- Hemolysis
  - Isoimmune
  - Infectious processes
- Hereditary disorders of hemoglobin and its production
- Disorders of the erythrocyte membrane (e.g. hereditary spherocytosis)
- Metabolism (e.g. G6PD deficiency).

Once anemia caused by blood loss has been diagnosed in neonates, differentiation between chronic and acute blood loss is likely to have an impact on management (Table 1.2).

Acute Blood Loss

- Normal MCV and MCH for age
- May have a normal hemoglobin initially then declines precipitiously[23]
- Clinically, present with distress, pallor, tachycardia, hypotension and no hepatosplenomegaly.

They require resuscitation with volume-expanding intravenous solutions and whole blood. After that, they need iron-replacement therapy in excess of that provided to normal neonates.

Neonates with Chronic Anemia

Caused by blood loss:
- Lowered Hb concentration
- Depressed MCV
- A peripheral blood smear shows hypochromic, microcytic picture.

Clinically, these infants are:
- Without distress
- Hepatosplenomegaly
- Signs of congestive heart failure

Table 1.2: Characteristics of acute and chronic blood loss in newborns

Characteristics	*Acute blood loss*	*Chronic blood loss*
Clinical features	Acute distress; pallor; shallow, rapid, and often irregular resp; tachycardia; weak or absent peripheral pulses; low or absent blood pressure; no hepatosplenomegaly	Marked pallor disproportionate to evidence of distress; on occasion signs of congestive heart failure including heart failure including hepatomegaly
Venous pressure	Low	Normal or elevated
Laboratory values		
Hemoglobin	May be normal initially; then drops quickly during first 24 hours of life	Low at birth
Red cell morphology	Normochromic and macrocytic	Hypochr. and microcytic; aniso. and poikilocytosis
Serum iron	Normal at birth	Low at birth
Course	Prompt treatment of anemia and shock necessary to prevent death	Generally uneventful
Treatment	Intravenous fluids and Whole blood; iron therapy later	Fe; packed red cells may be necessary on occasion

- Do not require acute intervention
- Transfusion of red cells is rarely necessary
- Iron replacement therapy is indicated for these infants.

At birth, the increased oxygen tension following conversion from maternal to environmental oxygenation results in a rapid decline in erythropoiesis, as shown by reduction in reticulocyte count, hemoglobin, and erythroid progenitors in the bone marrow. Eventually, as the hemoglobin-oxygen dissociation curve becomes progressively right-shifted, resulting from conversion of fetal to adult hemoglobin and as the hemoglobin level falls, a threshold of diminishing venous oxygen saturation is reached. A signal in the form of increased erythrocytes creates a physiologic hemoglobin nadir at 7 to 10 weeks of age in normal newborns.

Agents that either impair erythrocyte production or decrease red cell survival (e.g. infection, medications, or hemolysis) can lead to an earlier or lower nadir. This is commonly encountered in premature infants. Because of their smaller red cell mass, premature infants reach their nadir earlier than term infants and require a longer period of time to recover, in part because of an impaired erythropoietin response to tissue hypoxemia. Hemoglobin levels begin to fall by the end of the first week of life and may take as many as 4 months to recover. Because of this blunted response, premature infants will more likely develop symptoms related to inadequate tissue oxygen delivery and require transfusion of red cells or recombinant erythropoietin therapy.

Screening Hemoglobin at 4 to 6 Months of Age

Iron Deficiency

Collecting a hemoglobin and hematocrit value at 4 to 6 months of age to screen for anemia is a prudent practice among pediatricians. The most common causes of anemia in this age group are iron deficiency and intercurrent infection.[24]

Anemia caused by iron deficiency is a late step in the pathophysiology of iron deficiency. First, as iron stores become depleted, the serum ferritin concentration declines and the RDW increases. Next, serum iron concentration becomes depressed. Finally, iron deficiency begins to affect erythropoiesis, causing a decrease in the MCV and an increase in the free erythrocyte protoporphyrin with accompanying anemia.

The first hematologic manifestation of iron deficiency is increase in the RDW (normal range in children, 11.5 to 14.5%).

This alteration may be more sensitive in screening for iron deficiency than serum ferritin, transferrin saturation, or even serum iron level, some of which can be altered by inflammation or even variation in iron intake.[25]

Moreover, the increased RDW may be useful in discriminating microcytosis secondary to iron deficiency from thalassemia trait, in which the RDW is normal.[26]

Although rigorous testing may be required to be sure about the cause of anemia in the 4 month to 6 month hemoglobin screen a reasonable approach in this cost-conscious era has been a trial of oral, iron replacement for children whose hemoglobin levels fall below the 10th percentile. Thus, in patients with anemia accompanied by an increased RDW and a supportive history who respond to a trial of iron (defined as an increase of 1.5-2.0 g/dl in the hemoglobin after 1 months of therapy), a presumptive diagnosis of iron deficiency anemia usually can be made.

Although iron deficiency is common in children 9 months to 3 years of age and in teenage girls, iron deficiency anemia in children more than 3 years of age generally should prompt consideration of dietary history and occult blood loss.

PLATELETS

Alterations in platelet numbers and platelet size can provide important clues to disease processes. Platelet size is often determined from review of the peripheral smear, but mean platelet volume also can be derived by the coulter counter. Mean platelet volume (MPV) as determined by automated electronic counters; is normally between 8.9±1.5 fl.

In general, platelets tend to be larger when there is peripheral destruction, e.g. immune mediated or on a mechanical basis, and normal to small in size when production defects are present. In Wiskott-Aldrich syndrome, platelets are about half of normal size and look like dust particles. Large platelets are generally thought to be young which in part may be true, but increased mean platelet volume and large platelets also may be a reflection of stimulated thrombopoiesis.

Macrothrombocytes (MPV Raised)

- ITP or any condition with increased platelet turnover (e.g. DIC)
- Bernard-Soulier syndrome
- May Hegglin anomaly and other MYH-9–related diseases
- Swiss cheese platelet syndrome
- Montreal platelet syndrome
- Gray platelet syndrome
- Various mucopolysaccharidosis.

Normal Size (MPV Normal)

Conditions in which marrow is hypocellular or infiltrated with malignant diseases.

Microthrombocytes (MPV Decreased)

- Wiskott-Aldrich syndrome
- TAR syndrome
- Some storage pool diseases
- Iron-deficiency anemia.

The normal lifespan of platelets is 7 to 10 days. Approximately one-third of the body platelets are located in the spleen and two-thirds in the circulation. Practitioners most often are interested in qualitative aspects of platelets as well as quantitative. The CBC cannot answer functional questions, but the significance of thrombocytopenia and thrombocytosis can be clarified. There is a wide range of normal platelet counts, but thrombocytopenia generally is defined as a platelet count of less than 1.5 lac/mm^3 and thrombocytosis as values between 600,000/mm^3 and 1,000,000/mm^3 or more.

Thrombocytosis

Thrombocytosis in childhood rarely causes complications, although it is frequently a cause for concern.

Causes

- Primary
  - Polycythemia vera
  - Essential thrombocythemia, are unusual but have better outcome in children[27]
- Reactive
  - Iron deficiency anemia
  - Hemolytic anemia
  - Vitamin E deficiency
  - Hemorrhage
  - Collagen vascular disorder
  - Kawasaki syndrome (usually 2-3 weeks into the illness)
  - Nephrotic syndrome
  - Inflammatory bowel disease
  - Postsplenectomy
  - Postoperative state
  - Trauma
  - Various tumors
  - Myeloproliferative syndromes
  - Histiocytoses
  - Various drugs
    - Epinephrine
    - Corticosteroids
    - Vinca alkaloids[28]

Because no apparent sequelae exist to reactive thrombocytosis, antiplatelet therapy is rarely indicated (Kawasaki syndrome is a notable exception). Platelet morphology is usually normal, as is the bleeding time. Splenomegaly is absent unless caused by the underlying disorder, and the duration is transitory, usually measured in days to weeks.

Thrombocytopenia

When thrombocytopenia is reported, the most common cause is immune platelet destruction, but falsely low platelet counts may occur when inadequate anticoagulation of the blood-sample results in platelet clumping. The precision of platelet counting by automated instruments is reduced in the severe thrombocytopenia range (platelets fewer than 20,000/mm^3) because loss of measurement linearity occurs. Thrombocytopenia is associated with a wide range of infections and other conditions. The major issues confronting practitioners are the risk of life-threatening bleeding and the possibility of a serious underlying condition. Isolated thrombocytopenia without other hematologic abnormalities in an otherwise healthy appearing child without lymphadenopathy or hepatosplenomegaly almost never is associated with childhood acute leukemia. In such cases, idiopathic thrombocytopenia purpura (ITP) is usually the correct diagnosis. Intracranial hemorrhage occurs only rarely in children with ITP.[29]

WHITE BLOOD CELLS

The total and differential white blood cell count is often requested without much thought, but it can be a clue to underlying disorders. Its usefulness as a screening test is not great because both sensitivity and specificity are low; however, the reliability and low cost justifies these tests as part of the complete blood count although abnormalities and definitive characterizations still require examination of the peripheral smear. Practitioners generally are interested in the total and differential white blood cell count as clues to underlying infection. Interpretation of white count numbers is aided by the clinical context:

- The age of the patient
- The temperature
- General appearance
- Underlying conditions.

The white blood cell response to infection can be highly variable, the younger the patient and the higher the temperature, the more one becomes suspicious if the white blood cell count is either above or below the normal range.

Leukopenia is associated with a wide variety of viral and bacterial infections:

- Viral illness
- Epstein-Barr virus
- Hepatitis A and B
- Respiratory syncytial virus
- Rubella.

Changes usually are noted within 1 to 2 days of infection and often can persist for several weeks. If the clinical situation warrants, consideration should be given to:

- *Salmonella*
- Staphylococcal
- Mycobacterial infections.

Neutropenia (neutrophil count <1000/mm^3)

500–1000/mm^3: indicates a moderate risk for infection

<500/mm^3: indicates a severe risk of life-threatening infection. Causes include.

- Chemotherapy
- Immunosuppression (Steroid therapy)
- Chronic benign neutropenia of childhood
- Syndromes affecting the immune system.

Leukocytosis is part of the body's acute phase response to many conditions, including infections:

- Bacteria
- Virus
- Fungi
- Protozoa
- Spirochetes.

We are often left with the perplexing situation of determining which febrile child with leukocytosis requires additional diagnostic studies or treatment. As noted earlier, the practitioners skill and experience are critical in making a determination. In children 3 to 36 months of age with fever 39.5°C or more, bacteremia is highly correlated with white blood cell count.

TLC	Incidence of bacteremia
>15,000	16%
>20,000	25%
>30,000	40%[30]

Attention should also be paid to the band count when appreciable numbers of bands and more immature forms are present in the peripheral blood it is generally referred to as a left shift. Instead of using this term, considering the absolute number of band forms may be more useful.

Beyond the neonatal period >500 bands/mm^3 is an indication of infection regardless of the absolute white blood cell count. Although an increase in band forms classically has been thought to be associated with bacterial infections, a recent study of children with proven viral infections (e.g. influenza, enterovirus, respiratory syncytial virus, and rotavirus) showed significant elevations in absolute numbers of band forms. Further, if toxic granules (larger than normal granules that stain intensely), vacuolization, or Dohle bodies are reported on the peripheral smear, possible bacterial infection also should be suspected. In the end, no substitute exists for astute clinical judgment coupled with judicious interpretation of laboratory tests, especially when trying to differentiate a viral from bacterial process.

Monocytes are the second line of defense against infection. Monocytosis often is associated with monocytic leukemia, ulcerative colitis, viral diseases such as mononucleosis and herpes zoster, parasitic diseases such as rocky mountain spotted fever. Monopenia is seen in some forms of leukemia, bone marrow failure or suppression.

Eosinophilia often is associated with rashes, wheezes, and unusual diseases. Common examples of diseases are parasitic infections. Eosinophilia also is associated with drug hypersensitivity, asthma, cow's milk allergy, hay fever, urticaria, eczema, other skin disorders, job syndrome, and malignancy. Eosinopenia is associated with corticosteroid therapy, adrenocortical hyperfunction, stress, shock.

Lymphocytosis most often is associated with viral infections, including infectious mononucleosis, cytomegalovirus, rubella, mumps, and hepatitis. White blood cell counts of more than 30,000/mm^3 with 60 to 70% lymphocytes, especially if they are described as clefted or baby bottom may be caused by pertusis. Lymphopenia is associated with corticosteroid therapy, adrenocortical hyperfunction, stress, shock.

Basophilia most often is associated with chronic inflammatory and hypersensitivity reaction. Basopenia is seen with corticosteroid therapy, adrenocortical hyperfunction, stress and shock.

Distinguishing leukemoid from leukoerythroblastic reactions is important. In leukoerythroblastic reactions, nucleated red blood cells and immature white blood cells are found in a setting of underlying leukemia, myelophthisis, severe bleeding, or hemolysis. Leukemoid reactions, on the other hand, are elevations in the white blood cell count, in excess of 50,000/mm^3, sometimes leading to confusion with leukemia. There are many causes of leukemoid reactions, which can be either myeloid or lymphoid.

Heinz Bodies (denatured/aggregated hemoglobin)

- Normal newborn
- Thalassemia syndromes
- Unstable hemoglobins
- HMP shunt abnormalities (G6PD deficiency)
- Asplenia.

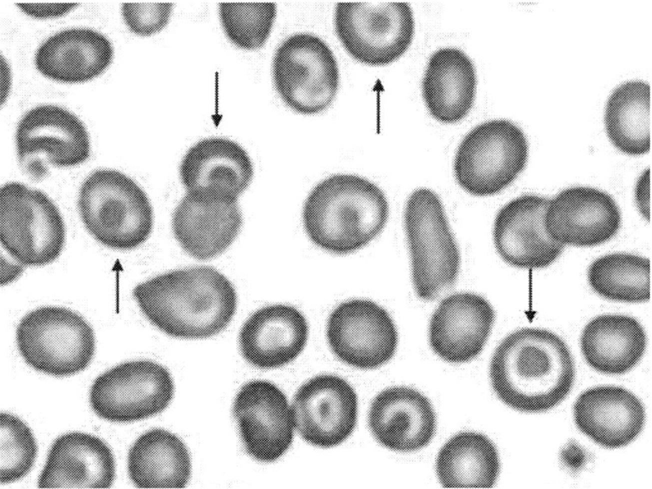

Fig. 1.3: Target cells *(For color version, see Plate 1)*

TARGET CELLS (FIG. 1.3)

Increased surface/volume ratio:

- Thalassemia
- Hemoglobinopathies
  - Hb AC or CC
  - Hb SS, SC, S-Thalassemia
- Obstructive liver disease
- Postsplenectomy or hyposplenic states
- Severe iron deficiency
- Hb E (heterozygote and homozygote)
- LCAT deficiency
- Abetalipoproteinemia.

SPHEROCYTES (FIG. 1.4)

Decreased surface/volume ratio, hyperdense (>MCHC)

- Hereditary spherocytosis
- ABO incompatibility
- Autoimmune hemolytic anemia
- Microangiopathic hemolytic anemia
- SS disease
- Hypersplenism
- Burns
- Severe hypophasphatemia
- Post-transfusion
- Pyruvate kinase deficiency
- Water dilution hemolysis.

ACANTHOCYTES (FIG. 1.5)

- Liver disease
- Disseminated intravascular coagulation
- Postsplenectomy or hyposplenic disorder
- Vitamin E deficiency

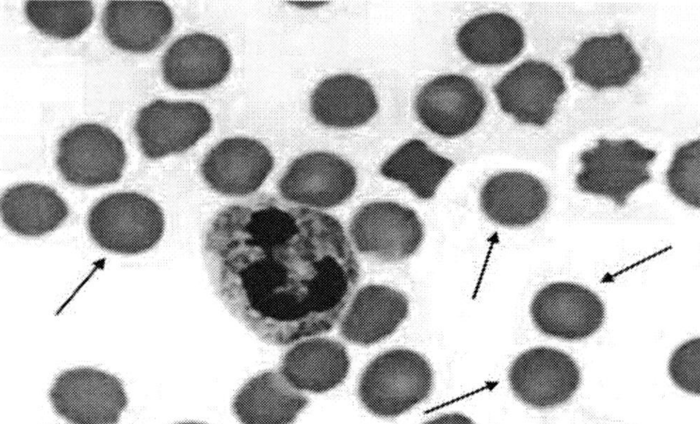

Fig. 1.4: Spherocytes *(For color version, see Plate 1)*

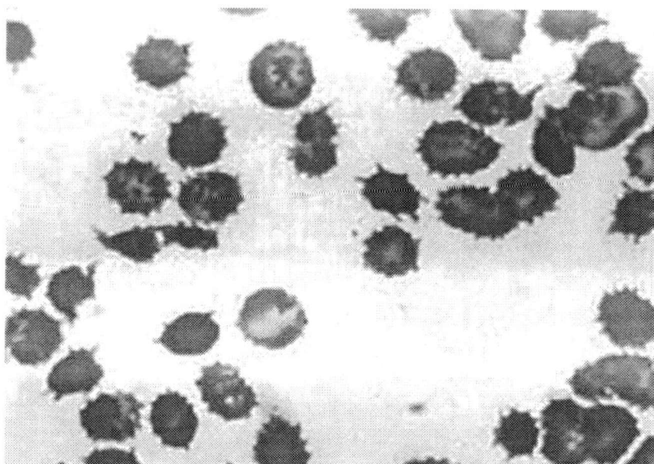

Fig. 1.5: Acanthocytes *(For color version, see Plate 1)*

- Hypothyroidism
- Abetalipoproteinemia
- Malabsorption states.

ECHINOCYTES (FIG. 1.6)

- Artifact
- Uremia
- Dehydration
- Liver disease
- Pyruvate kinase deficiency
- Peptic ulcer disease or gastric carcinoma
- After blood transfusion.

SCHISTOCYTES (FIG. 1.7)

- DIC
- Severe hemolytic anemia
- Microangiopathic hemolytic anemia
- HUS

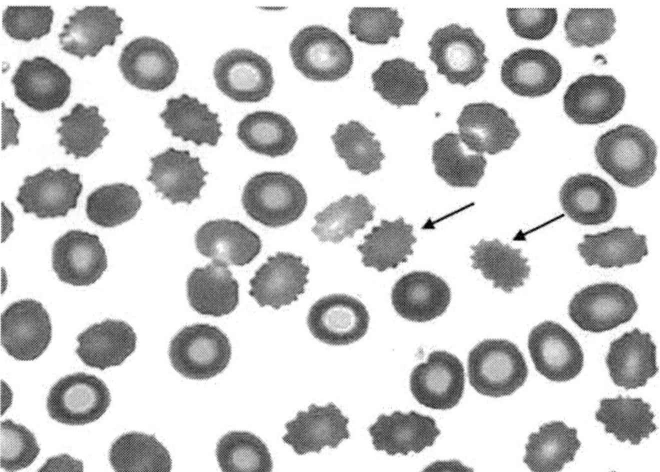

Fig. 1.6: Echinocytes *(For color version, see Plate 1)*

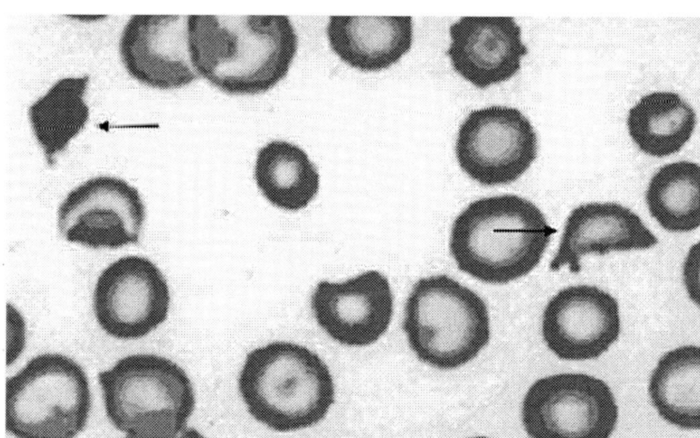

Fig. 1.7: Schistocytes *(For color version, see Plate 2)*

- Prosthetic cardiac valves
- Connective tissue disorders
- Kasabach-Merritt syndrome
- Purpura fulminans
- Renal vein thrombosis
- Burns
- Thrombotic thrombocytopenic purpura
- Uremia
- Malignant hypertension
- Systemic amyloidosis
- Liver cirrhosis
- Disseminated carcinomatosis.

BASOPHILIC STIPPLING (AGGREGATED RIBOSOMES) (FIG. 1.8)

- Hemolytic anemia, thalassemias, unstable hemoglobins
- Ineffective erythropoiesis

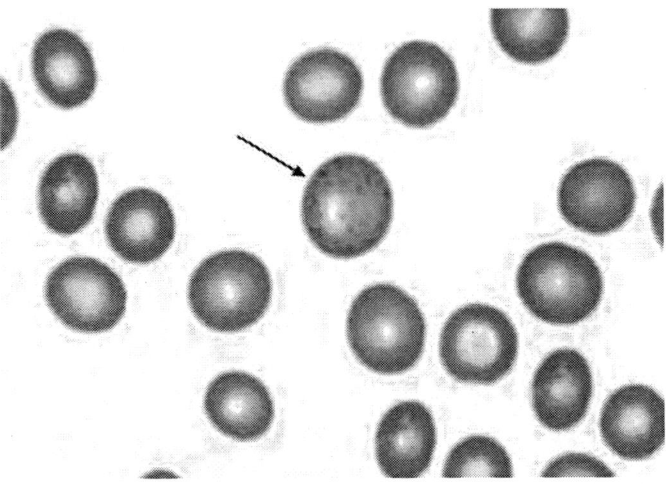

Fig. 1.8: Basophilic stippling *(For color version, see Plate 2)*

- Lead poisoning
- Pyrimidine 5′-nucleotidase deficiency
- Iron deficiency anemia.

HOWELL-JOLLY BODIES (FIG. 1.9)

- Postsplenectomy
- Newborn
- Megaloblastic anemia
- Dyserythropoietic.

SIDEROCYTES (NONHEMOGLOBIN IRON)

- Postsplenectomy
- Chronic infection
- Aplastic anemia
- Hemolytic anemias.

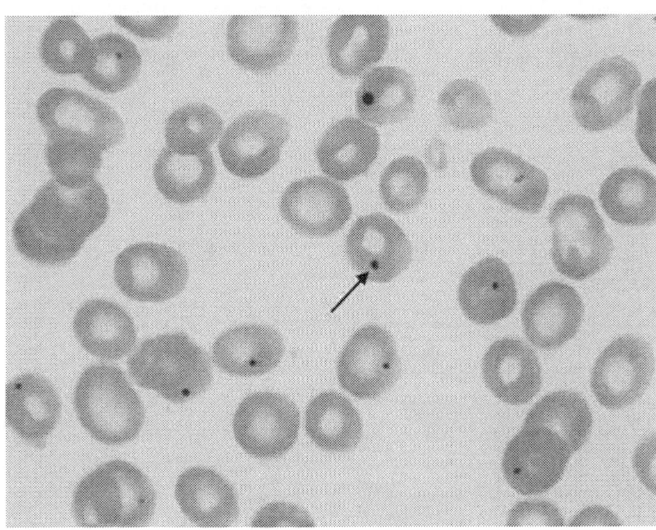

Fig. 1.9: Howell-Jolly bodies *(For color version, see Plate 2)*

CABOT'S RINGS (NUCLEAR REMNANTS)

- Hemolytic anemias
- Pernicious anemia
- Lead poisoning.

POLYCHROMASIA

- Reticulocytosis
- Hemolytic anemia
- Acute hemorrhage
- Response to 'hematinics' in nutritional anemia.

NUCLEATED RBCs

- Normal in neonates (first few days)
- Hemolytic anemia
- Acute hemorrhage.

ELLIPTOCYTES

- Hereditary elliptocytosis
- Hypochromic microcytic anemias
- Thalassemias.

SPICULATED/CRENATED CELLS

- Acute hepatic necrosis
- Uremia
- Abetalipoproteinemia
- Transiently after massive transfusion of stored blood.

BIZARRE POIKILOCYTES

- Red cell fragmentation syndromes (Microangiopathic hemolytic anemias)
- Acute oxidant injury
- Hereditary elliptocytosis in neonates.

Differentiation of Beta-Thalassemia Trait from Iron Deficiency

	Beta-thalassemia trait	IDA
Hb concentration	D/N	D/N
Hematocrit	D/N	D/N
RBC	I	D
MCV	D	D/N
MCH	D	D
MCHC	N	D
S. Iron	N	D
TIBC	N	I
% TS	N	D
Serum ferritin	N	D
Free erythrocyte proporphyrin	N	I
HbA_2	I	N/D

Abbreviations: D: Decreased; N: Normal; I: Increased

REFERENCES

1. Economou-Mavrou C, Tsengli C. Plasma trapping in the centrifuged red cells of children with severe thalassemia. J Clin Path. 1965;18:203.
2. Cornbleet J. Spurious results from automated hematology counters. Lab Med. 1983;14:509-14.
3. Bessman JD, Banks D. Spurious macrocytosis, a common clue to erythrocyte cold agglutinins. Am J Clin Pathol. 1980; 74:797.
4. Davidson M, Miranda AF, Bender AN, et al. Muscle phosphofructokinase deficiency: Biochemical and immunological studies of phosphofructokinase isozymes in muscle culture. J Clin Invest. 1983;72:545-50.
5. Tyndall MK, Tertel DF, et al. Serum erythropoietin levels in patients with congenital heart disease. J Pediatr. 1987; 110:538.
6. Black DB, Lubchenco LO, et al. Developmental and neurologic sequelae of neonatal hyperviscosity syndrome. Pediatr. 1982;69:426.
7. Bessman JD, Gilmer PR Jr, Gardner FH. Improved classification of anemias by MCV and RDW. Am J Clin Pathol. 1983;80:322-6.
8. Alter BP. Fetal erythropoiesis in stress hematopoiesis. Exp Hematol. 1979;7:200.
9. Pappo AS, Fields BW, Buchanan GR. Etiology of red blood cell macrocytosis during childhood: Impact of new diseases and therapies. Pediatrics. 1992;89:1063-7.
10. Alter BP. Childhood red cell aplasia. Am J Pediatr Hematol Oncol. 1980;2:121.
11. Buchanan GR, Alter BP, Holtkamp CA, et al. Platelet number and function in Diamond-Blackfan anemia. Pediatr. 1981;68:238.
12. Freedman MH, Saunders EF. Transient erythroblastopenia of childhood: Varied pathogenesis. Am J Hematol. 1983; 14:247.
13. Rogers ZR, Bergstrom SK, Amylon MD, et al. Reduced neutrophil counts in children with transient erythroblastopenia of childhood. J Pediatr. 1989;115:746.
14. Glader BE, Backen K. Elevated red cell adenosine deaminase activity, A marker of disordered erythropoiesis in Diamond-Blackfan anaemia and other haematologic diseases. Br J Haematol. 1988;68:165.
15. McCurdy P, Rath C. Vacuolated nucleated bone marrow cells in alcoholism. Semin Hematol. 1980;17:100.
16. Cohen AR, Trotzky MS, Pincus D. Reassessment of the microcytic anemia of lead poisoning. Pediatrics. 1981; 67:904-6.
17. Piomelli S, Young P, et al. Field screening of children for lead poisoning with the FEP test. Pediatr Res. 1973;7:350.
18. Blumberg A. Pathogenesis of anemia due to kidney disease. Nephron. 1989;51(suppl):15.
19. Caro J, Erslev AJ. Uremic inhibitors of erythropoiesis. Semin Nephrol. 1985;5:128.
20. Klahr S, Slatopolsky E. Toxicity of parathyroid hormone in uremia. Ann Rev Med. 1986;37:71.
21. Linderkamp O, Vesmold HT, et al. Capillary-venous hematocrit differences in newborn infants. I. Relationship to blood volume, peripheral blood flow, and acid-base parameters. Eur J Pediatr. 1977;127:9.
22. Forrestier F, Daffos F, et al. Hematological values of normal fetuses between 18 and 30 weeks of gestation. Pediatr Res. 1986;20:342.
23. Oski FA. The erythrocyte and its disorders. In Nathan DG, Oski FA (Eds). Hematology of Infancy and Childhood, 4th edn. Philadelphia, WB Saunders; 1993. pp. 18-43.
24. Oski FA. Iron deficiency in infancy and childhood. N Engl J Med. 1993;329:190-3.
25. Patton WW, Cave RJ, Harris RI. A study of changes in red cell volume and hemoglobin concentration during phlebtomy induced iron deficiency and iron repletion using the Technicon H_1. Clin Lab Haematol. 1991;13:153-61.
26. Bessman JD, Feinstein DI. Quantitative anisocytosis as a discriminant between iron deficiency and thalassemia minor. Blood. 1979;53:288-93.
27. Hoagland HC, Silverstein MN. Primary thrombocythemia in the young patient. Mayo Clinic Proc. 1978;53:578.
28. Chan KW, Kaikov Y, Wadsworth LD. Thrombocytosis in childhood: A survey of 94 patients. Pediatr. 1989;84:1064-7.
29. Woerner SJ, Abildgaard CF, French BN. Intracranial hemorrhage in children with idiopathic thrombocytopenic purpura. Pediatr. 1981;63:453.
30. Bass JW, Steele RW, Wittler RR, et al. Antimicrobial treatment of occult bacteremia: A multicenter cooperative study. Pediatr Infect Dis J. 1993;12:466-73.

2 Clinical Approach to a Child with Anemia

Nitin K Shah, Himani Manchanda, MR Lokeshwar

INTRODUCTION

Anemia is a global problem of immense health significance affecting persons of all ages and economic groups. It is ranked as the most common chronic malady mankind has ever suffered. Approximately 1500 million people, i.e. 30% of the world population suffers from iron deficiency state. It is more common in developing countries like ours. 30-50% of pregnant ladies and 60-80% of school going children are reported in some studies to be iron deficient.

APPROACH TO A CHILD WITH ANEMIA

When confronted with a case of anemia, one should try to answer following questions:

a. Is the patient anemic?
b. How severely is he/she affected?
c. What is the cause and type of anemia?
d. What treatment should he/she be offered?

IS THE PATIENT ANEMIC?

There are two points to be noted. One is the cut off values of Hb and blood indices appropriate for age. The other point is reliability of signs and symptoms, especially presence or absence of pallor as a marker of anemia.

DEFINITION

Anemia is generally defined as a reduction in the O_2 carrying capacity leading to tissue hypoxia. Ideally it is the 'functional anemia' at the tissue level which is more important, as is very well demonstrated in case of congenital cyanotic heart disease. However, there is no good marker of 'functional anemia' and hence one has to rely on values of red cell mass or hemoglobin levels to define anemia. Age appropriate cut off levels of Hb and blood indices are shown in Chapter on Laboratory Evaluation of Anemia (Chapter 3). It is clearly seen that a child with Hb of 10 g% will be labeled as severely anemic if he is a neonate, mildly anemic if he is an infant and mild to moderately anemic if he is an adolescent. Hence, age appropriate cut off levels are very important to interpret the CBC report.

CLINICAL JUDGMENT OF ANEMIA

The common symptoms and signs of anemia are pallor, tiredness, lassitude, easy fatiguability, weakness, lack of concentration, breathlessness, puffiness, edema feet, etc. However, these symptoms are also seen in other systemic illnesses like respiratory illness, cardiovascular diseases, congestive cardiac failure, renal disease, myxedema, etc.

Pallor is a common sign of anemia. However, all cases of anemia do not have pallor, especially mild cases of anemia. Icterus, cyanosis or dilatation of peripheral blood vessels, like in inflammation, may mask pallor. Similarly, pallor can also be seen in non-anemic conditions as color of the skin not only depends on the Hb content, but on the state of blood vessels of the skin, presence of edema, skin pigmentation and skin thickness. Hence, pallor can be seen in nephrotic syndrome or myxedema even in absence of anemia and, it is always prudent to rely on Hb or HCT estimation to detect anemia.

HOW SEVERE IS THE ANEMIA?

It is important to quickly assess the patient's clinical condition. If the patient is severely pale and sick looking, breathless, has tachycardia, raised JVP and tender hepatomegaly, it is suggestive of congestive cardiac failure (CCF). Such a patient needs immediate attention and prompt treatment including diuretics, restricted fluids, oxygen support and packed cell transfusion. One should not waste time in lengthy diagnostic tests and do as minimum tests as required. Even removing too much blood for various tests can be hazardous as it can precipitate cardiac failure. Instead one can arrange for packed cell transfusion and remove blood for various tests just before starting transfusion.

If the patient is pale but comfortable and not sick, there is neither need to give packed cell transfusion nor start 'gunshot' therapy without proper investigations and establishing the diagnosis. Remember, the clinical condition of the patient depends not only on the severity of anemia but also on the rate of drop of Hb. A child with 5 g% Hb, when it develops slowly like in iron deficiency, may be comfortable and come walking to your clinic whereas, if it deveops acutely due to G6PD deficiency, the child may be brought in a collapsed state.

WHAT IS THE TYPE AND CAUSE OF ANEMIA?

Anemia can be classified in two ways. One is the etiological classification, based on the disturbance of erythropoiesis, which makes it easy to understand why anemia develops in a case. Other is the morphological classification based on the objective and the subjective findings of red cell size and indices, which helps us to arrive at a diagnosis. Both these are not mutually exclusive and are often used together to come to a conclusion as to the cause of anemia.

In normal subjects the average lifespan of red cell is 120 days. These cells are destroyed everyday as they grow old. The aged cells are removed from the circulation by the reticuloendothelial cells, principally in the walls of sinusoids of RE system like liver and spleen where the flow of blood is slow. The cells destroyed everyday are replaced by new cells released from bone marrow with the result that red cell population will consist of cells which are 1 day old to 120 days old. Approximately, 1% or so of red cells are turned over everyday. Any disruption of this balance will lead to anemia which can occur due to decreased production, increased destruction or due to blood loss. The etiological classification is given in Table 2.1 and morphological classification is given in Table 2.2.

Table 2.1: Etiological classification of anemia

A. Decreased effective production
- Nutritional deficiency, e.g. deficiency of iron, folate, vitamin B_{12}, protien, zinc, copper.
- Bone marrow failure, e.g. aplastic anemia, constitutional hypoplastic anemia, pure red cell aplasia.
- Bone marrow infiltration, e.g. malignancies like leukemia, lymphoma, osteopetrosis, myelofibrosis.
- Impaired erythropoietin production, e.g. renal disease, prematurity, hypothyroidism, hypopituitarism, chronic inflammation, protein malnutrition, hemoglobin mutants with decreased affinity for oxygen.
- Ineffective erythropoiesis, e.g. Thalassemia, sideroblastic anemia, lead poisoning, primary dyserythropoietic anemia, erythropoietic protoporphyria, megaloblastic anemia.

B. Increased destruction (Hemolytic anemia)
- Extracorpuscular causes (usually acquired except PNH)
  1. Mechanical, e.g. prosthetic valve, DIC, HUS, cardiac bypass.
  2. Immune, e.g. acquired immune hemolytic anemia, ABO or Rh sensitization, mismatched transfusion.
  3. Infection, e.g. malaria
  4. Sequestration, e.g. hypersplenism
  5. Complement induced, e.g. paroxysmal nocturnal hemoglobinuria
- Intracorpuscular causes (usually congenital)
  1. Membrane defect—spherocytosis, stomatocytosis, elliptocytosis
  2. Enzyme defect—G6PD deficiency, PK deficiency
  3. Hemoglobin defect—Sickle cell anemia, thalassemia, HbC, HbD, HbE disease.
- Blood loss (Hemorrhage): Acute or chronic, internal or external
  1. Internal
     - Acute—Massive cephalhematoma, hemothorax
     - Chronic—Pulmonary hemosiderosis
  2. External
     - Acute—massive GI hemorrhage, trauma, hemoptysis
     - Chronic-peptic ulcer, rectal polyp, hookworm infestation

NB: In many diseases there is more than one cause or mechanism of anemia

Approach to Establishing Diagnosis

Approach to an anemic patient includes:

a. Detailed history
b. Thorough physical examination
c. Screening laboratory tests
d. Confirmatory laboratory tests.

History taking: Following factors are important in history while evaluating a case of anemia. At times, it may give clinching clue to establish diagnosis.

a. *Age of onset:* Nutritional anemia is not seen at birth. The commonest causes of anemia in a newborn include hemolysis and hemorrhage. Hemolysis may be due to ABO, Rh incompatibility. Rarely G6PD deficiency or spherocytosis can present at birth. Hemolysis is usually associated with icterus besides anemia. Hemorrhage can be internal like huge cephalhematoma, pulmonary hemorrhage, intraventricular hemorrhage or external like umbilical bleeding, fetoplacental or fetomaternal hemorrhage, GI hemorrhage like in vitamin K deficiency, etc.

   At around 4 months of age erythroblastopenia of infancy can occur. Rarely nutritional anemia can start very early, especially in preterms. Between 6 months to 2 years nutritional anemia and hemo-

Table 2.2: Morphological classification of anemia

A. Microcytic, hypochromic anemia
MCV < 70 u^3, MCH < 28 pg.
- Iron deficiency anemia
- Anemia of chronic infection or inflammation
- Thalassemia syndromes
- Sideroblastic anemia
- Lead poisoning
- Severe protein deficiency

B. Macrocytic anemia
MCV > 85 u^3
- Megaloblastic anemia
  1. Folate deficiency
  2. Vitamin B_{12} deficiency
  3. DNA metabolism defects like orotic aciduria
- Non-megaloblastic anemia
  1. Normal newborn
  2. Reticulocytosis
  3. Aplastic anemia
  4. Liver disorders
  5. Hypothyroidism
  6. Alcoholism
  7. Down's syndrome

C. Normocytic anemia
- High reticulocyte count—Early hemorrhage, hemolysis, nutritional anemia on treatment.
- Low reticulocyte count—Bone marrow failure, bone marrow infiltration, decreased erythropoietin production, infections, drugs.
- Normal reticulocyte count—Late phase of hemorrhage or hemolysis, sickle cell anemia, unstable hemoglobin disease, other hemoglobinopathies, osteopetrosis, dyserythropoiesis, myelofibrosis, enzyme deficiency, spherocytosis.

globinopathies can present as anemia. Fanconi's anemia usually presents around 4 to 6 years of age. In adolescents, especially females, folate deficiency is a common cause of anemia due to food fads.

b. *Sex:* X-linked diseases will be seen in males and this includes G6PD deficiency and PK deficiency. Only males are affected. Hence, there will be similar history in male siblings, maternal male cousins, maternal uncles and maternal grandfather.

   In adolescent age, anemia is more common in females due to nutritional deficiency as a result of food fads and menstrual loss of iron.

c. *Community:* G6PD deficiency is more commonly seen in *Parsis, Bhanushalis* and *Sindhis*. Certain communities are at high risk for certain hemoglobinopathies inherited in autosomal recessive manner. Beta-thalassemia is more common in *Kutchis, Lohanas, Punjabis, Sindhis, Gujarati Banias, Kolis, Mahars* and other Neo-Buddhists, Lingayat and Gaud communities. Sickle cell disease is more common in tribals and hilly areas of Nagpur, Vidarbha, Andhra Pradesh, Bilaspur and in Neo-buddhists. HbD disease is more common in Punjabis and HbE disease is seen in Eastern India including Bengalis.

d. *Inheritance:* A detailed pedigree chart should be drawn including 2-3 generations on both parents' side to see for anyone else being affected which will give clue to the type of inheritance. All hemoglobinopathies and thalassemia syndromes are inherited in autosomal recessive manner. There will be similar cases in siblings, cousins and distant relatives affecting both sexes equally. There may be history of consanguineous marriage. The parents are trait but clinically normal. This is also called as horizontal transmission.

   Spherocytosis is inherited as autosomal dominant condition. The parents can be affected. Siblings are affected and children can be affected. This is called as vertical transmission. Both sexes are equally affected. There may be skipped generations and variable penetrance with different severity amongst the affected in same family. Hence, a child with spherocytosis may be needing repeated transfusions, the father may have needed occasional transfusion whereas grandfather may just have mild anemia with splenomegaly without any transfusion needed in life time!

   X-linked inheritance is already discussed before.

e. *Diet:* A detailed diet history is very important especially in infant with anemia. Exclusive breastfeeding for 4 to 6 months, introduction of good home made weaning food thereafter, continuation of breast milk till 18 months, avoidance of animal milk in first year and balanced diet with occasional non-vegetarian food consumption makes nutritional anemia an unlikely diagnosis. Iron deficiency develops where there is poor breastfeeding and improper time and quality of weaning food, both of which are exaggerated by bottle-feeding. Prolonged breastfeeding especially with improper weaning food is also a cause of nutritional anemia in poor.

   Perverted appetite or pica is both an effect and a cause of iron deficiency besides being seen in lead poisoning. Eating clay or mud (geophagia), ice (phagophagia), starch (amylophagia), paper, cloth, raw cereals, paint flakes, etc. is commonly seen in iron deficiency. Clay or mud can bind whatever little iron is present in food which further precipitates iron deficiency.

Megaloblastic anemia due to folate deficiency is common in those villagers who consume a lot of goat milk. Similarly, folate deficiency is commonly seen in adolescents due to food fads.

f. *Drugs:* Drugs can induce anemia by many ways. Certain drugs can lead to aplastic anemia like chloramphenicol, sulpha drugs or analgesics. Drugs like penicillin, alpha methyldopa or stibophen can lead to immune hemolytic anemia. In a patient with G6PD deficiency certain drugs like aspirin, sulpha drugs, primaquine, etc. can precipitate hemolysis. Lastly certain drugs can precipitate iron deficiency like, chronic GI bleeding following NSAID abuse; or produce megaloblastic anemia as seen with sulpha drugs, phenytoin or folate antagonists.

g. *Infections and infestations:* History suggestive of intrauterine infection should be elicited when dealing with neonatal anemia especially when it is associated with hepatosplenomegaly, IUGR, icterus and thrombocytopenia. Hypoplastic anemia can be precipitated by hepatitis virus. G6PD deficiency induced hemolysis can be precipitated by many infections and drugs used to treat such infections. Hemolysis could also be induced by malaria. Bone marrow suppression can occur following many viral infections, falciparum malaria, kala-azar, fulminant sepsis or drugs used in such cases. Chronic infections and inflammations like tuberculosis, repeated respiratory or GI infections can lead to mild to moderate anemia of chronic inflammation. Nutritional anemia can be precipitated by worms due to malabsorption, nutrient deficiency and micro bleeding especially with hook worm infestations. Any acute infection can lead to drop in hemoglobin by 1-1.5 g% over next one week.

h. *Family history:* History of any other family member being affected by anemia by drawing a detailed pedigree chart. History to be elicited in family members includes history of blood transfusion, unexplained recurrent jaundice, gall stone removal, splenectomy, which suggest some hemolytic process in them. Similarly, history of anemia following drugs in other members will suggest G6PD deficiency.

Physical examination: A detailed head to toe examination is required to be done to decide the severity of affection and to achieve a diagnosis. Some physical signs help clinch the diagnosis (Table 2.3).

Table 2.3: Physical findings as clues to the etiology of anemia

Skin	Hyperpigmentation	Fanconi aplastic anemia
	Petechia, purpura thrombocytopenia,	Autoimmune hemolytic anemia with hemolytic-uremic syndrome, bone marrow aplasia, bone marrow infiltration
	Carotenemia	Suspect iron deficiency in infants
	Jaundice	Hemolytic anemia, hepatitis, and aplastic anemia
	Cavernous hemangioma	Microangiopathic hemolytic anemia
	Ulcers on lower extremities	S and C hemoglobinopathies, thalassemia
Facies	Frontal bossing, prominence of the maxillary bones	Congenital hemolytic anemias, thalassemia major, severe iron deficiency
Eyes	Microcornea	Fanconi's aplastic anemia
	Tortuosity of the conjunctival and retinal vessels	S and C hemoglobinopathies
	Microaneurysms of retinal vessels	S and C hemoglobinopathies
	Cataracts	Glucose-6-phosphate dehydrogenase deficiency, galactosemia with hemolytic anemia in newborn period
	Vitreous hemorrhages	S hemoglobinopathy
	Retinal hemorrhages	Chronic, severe anemia
	Edema of the eyelids	Infectious mononucleosis, exudative enteropathy with iron deficiency, renal failure
	Blindness	Osteopetrosis
Mouth	Glossitis	Vitamin B_{12} deficiency, iron deficiency
	Angular stomatitis	Iron deficiency
Chest	Unilateral absence of the pectoral muscles	Poland syndrome (increased incidence of leukemia)
	Shield chest	Diamond-Blackfan syndrome
Hands	Triphalangeal thumbs	Red cell aplasia
	Hypoplasia of the thenar eminence	Fanconi aplastic anemia
	Spoon nails	Iron deficiency
Spleen	Enlargement	Congenital hemolytic anemia, leukemia, lymphoma, acute infection, portal hypertension

a. *Ascertain severity:* Pulse, blood pressure and respiratory rate should be recorded. Look for puffiness, edema feet, sacral edema, jugulovenous pulse, heptic tenderness, hepatojugular reflux and basal crepitations. All these will help to diagnose congestive cardiac failure as such patients need urgent treatment. Hypertension may be seen in anemia due to renal diseases.
b. *Facies:* Hemolytic facies will have frontal and parietal bossing, large head, depressed bridge of nose, malar prominance, sallow complexion, irregular maxillary teeth with anterior overbite. Diamond-Blackfan syndrome will have box like face with patients resembling one another rather than their family members. Hypothyroidism will have typical cretin facies and may be missed unless one looks for it carefully. Look for periorbital puffiness which can suggest edema due to anemia, CCF or myxedema.
c. *Eyes: Mongols* will have mongoloid slant. Fanconi's anemia will have microcornea. Conjunctival vessels tortuosity is seen in sickle cell anemia and so is the presence of retinal hemorrhage or microaneurysms. Icterus in absence of high colored urine will suggest hemolytic anemia with indirect hyperbilirubinemia. Osteopetrosis patients will develop blindness as time passes by.
d. *Oral cavity:* Look for glossitis, angular stomatitis, bald tongue which will suggest nutritional anemia. Look for teeth abnormality for hemolytic anemia.
e. *Nail changes:* Platynychia, koilonychia, brittle nails are suggestive of iron deficiency. They are less common in children than in adults, but when present are pathognomonic of IDA. Dyskeratotic nails will be seen in dyskeratosis congenita.
f. *Lymphadenopathy:* Significant lymphadenopathy will suggest tuberculosis, HIV, infectious mononucleosis, leukemia, lymphoma as the cause of anemia.
g. *Hepatosplenomegaly:* Palpable tender liver with positive hepatojugular reflux is suggestive of CCF. Significant hepatosplenomegaly will suggest tuberculosis, other viral fever, HIV, leukemia, thalassemia, other hemoglobinopathies, lymphoma, myelodysplastic syndrome, JCML, malaria, kala azar, storage disorders as a cause of anemia.

   Isolated splenomegaly will go in favor of enteric fever, malaria, portal hypertension, lymphoma, CML, tropical splenomegaly or hypersplenism, immune hemolytic anemia, congenital spherocytosis as a cause of anemia.
h. *Bleeding manifestation:* Presence of bleeding tendencies with petechiae, purpura will suggest thrombocytopenia which can be seen in benign diseases like ITP or in serious diseases like aplastic anemia, malignancies or marrow infiltration. Patient

Table 2.4: Laboratory studies often helpful in the investigation of a patient with anemia

Usual initial studies
- Hemoglobin and hematocrit determination
- Erythrocyte count and red cell indices, including MCV and RDW
- Reticulocyte count
- Study of stained blood smear
- Leukocyte count and differential count
- Platelet count

Suspected iron deficiency
- Free erythrocyte protoporphyrin
- Serum ferritin levels
- Stool for occult blood
- ^{99m}Tc pertechnetate scan for Meckel's diverticulum
- Endoscopy (upper and lower bowel)

Suspected vitamin B_{12} or folic acid deficiency
- Bone marrow
- Serum vitamin B_{12} level
- Serum folate level
- Gastric analysis after histamine injection
- Vitamin B_{12} absorption test (radioactive cobalt) (Schilling test)

Suspected hemolytic anemia
- Evidence of red cell breakdown
  a. Blood smear
  b. Serum bilirubin level
  c. Urinary urobilinogen excretion
  d. Serum haptoglobin
- Evidence of red cell regeneration
  a. Reticulocyte count
  b. Blood smear
  c. Skeleton radiography
- Evidence of type of hemolytic anemia: Corpuscular
  a. Membrane
     — Blood smear
     — Osmotic fragility test
     — Autohemolysis test
  b. Hemoglobin
     — Sickle test
     — Hemoglobin electrophoresis
     — Hemoglobin F determination
     — Kleihauer-Betke smear
     — Heat-stability test
  c. Enzymes
     — Heinz-body preparation
     — Enzyme assay
- Evidence of type of hemolytic anemia: Extracorpuscular
  a. Immune
     — Antiglobulin test
     — Acid serum lysis test
     — Sucrose lysis test
     — Donath-Landsteiner antibody
     — ANA

with ITP is usually a well child without fever, hepatosplenomegaly, lymphadenopathy, weight loss or bony tenderness as compared to a patient with bone marrow failure or leukemia who will be a sick child with fever, weight loss, bony tenderness, lymphadenopathy and hepatosplenomegaly.

i. *Skeletal changes:* Patients with Fanconi's anemia, TAR syndrome, etc. have skeletal malformations like absent radius, absent or bifid thumb, triphalangeal thumb, polydactyly, syndactyly, short stature, microcephaly. Look for associated anomalies like mental retardation, skin hyperpigmentation, hypogonadism, renal anomalies in such cases.

j. *Skin changes:* Hyperpigmentation is seen in Fanconi's anemia. Icterus is seen in liver diseases as well as hemolytic anemia. Iron deficiency can be seen in patients with carotenemia. Non-healing ulcers over lower limbs are seen in any chronic hemolytic anemia especially in HbS and C disease. Lastly localized DIC like picture with anemia and thrombocytopenia are present in patients with giant cavernous hemangioma as seen in Kasabach-Merrit syndrome.

CONCLUSION

Detailed history and physical examination give many vital clues as to the severity, type and cause of anemia which can be further established by doing laboratory tests as discussed in Table 2.4. Clinical examination, a forgotten art, is very important in a case of anemia.

BIBLIOGRAPHY

1. Frank A Oski. Differential diagnosis of anemia. In: Nathan DG, Oski FA (Eds). Hematology of infancy and childhood. WB Saunders Company; 1997. pp. 346-53.
2. Nitin Shah, Lokeshwar MR, Bavdekar SB. Iron deficiency in India. In Suraj Gupte (Ed): Recent Advances in Pediatrics—special volume 7, Hematology. Published by Jaypee Brothers Medical Publishers, New Delhi, Edition 2000.

3 Laboratory Evaluation of a Patient with Anemia

Ushma Singh, Shirish Kumar, SP Yadav, Anupam Sachdeva

DEFINITION

A reduction in the blood hemoglobin concentration 2 standard deviations below the mean for the normal population with respect to age, gender and altitude of residence is known as anemia. This will result in 2.5% of the normal population classified as anemic. Some individuals with hemoglobin value apparently in the normal range may be deficient as can be shown by an increase in Hb following iron intake.

Locally prevalent values, i.e. mean value of a population MUST NOT be equated with normal values, as different lower standards do not apply to a particular subpopulation or geographic regions, e.g. hemoglobin, hematocrit, mean corpuscular volume are significantly lower in African-American than in whites (approximately 0.5 g/dl).

INTRODUCTION

Anemia is the reduction below normal in the red cell mass of the body that is assessed by measuring:
- Concentration of hemoglobin (Hb) or
- Hematocrit (Hct)/Packed cell volume (PCV) or
- Erythrocyte count in the blood.

The preferred measurement is Hb concentration as it is not only accurate and reproducible but its value is most indicative of the pathophysiologic consequences of anemia.

Anemia is not a diagnosis in itself but a sign of the presence of disease. Correct diagnostic terminology requires inclusion of the pathogenesis of anemia because proper treatment requires its understanding. Investigating anemia depends on the relative frequency of the causes of anemia at various ages and the normal values based on the age, sex and altitude of residence of the patient (Table 3.1).

MECHANISMS AND PATHOPHYSIOLOGY OF ANEMIA (TABLE 3.2)

Anemia occurs due to imbalance between RBC production and destruction. It can have many origins, and often may be multifactorial. It may arise due to a primary hematologic disorder within the bone marrow or due to accelerated loss/destruction in the periphery.

Anemia depends on:
- *Red cells mass,* i.e. total number or volume of RBCs in the circulation.
- *Blood volume,* i.e. total quantity of blood (RBCs + plasma) in circulation
- *Hematocrit,* i.e. ratio of red cell mass to blood volume which is a measure of concentration.

When the RBC mass decreases, the total blood volume remains nearly normal because of compensatory increase in plasma volume. Therefore, as a rule, reduction in RBCs and/or reduction in Hb concentration very nearly reflects reduction in the total quantity of red cells in circulation. This factor eliminates the need to measure blood volume to measure reduction in red cell mass. Even with acute hemorrhage or increase/decrease in plasma volume, there is no need to measure blood volume.

Alterations in plasma volume cause a problem in interpretation as Hb concentration, RBC count and PCV are all ratios. Their numerators are a RBC property while the denominator is the volume of circulating blood, which contains both erythrocytes and plasma. Thus, an elevated PCV may not always indicate raised RBC production but is often due to reduced circulating plasma volume as seen in conditions causing hypovolemia as happens in Dengue shock syndrome.

Similarly, steadily decreasing RBC values may indicate that the worsening 'anemia' is due to volume

Table 3.1: Red blood cell values at various ages

Age	Hb (g/dl)		PCV (%)		RBC count (× 10³/fl)		MCV (fl)		MCH (pg)		MCHC (g/dl)	
	Mean	–2SD*	Mean	–2SD*	Mean	–2SD	Mean	–2SD	Mean	–2SD	Mean	–2SD
Birth	16.5	13.5	51	42	4.7	3.9	108	98	34	31	33	30
1-3 days	18.5	14.5	56	45	5.2	4.0	108	95	34	31	33	29
1 week	17.5	13.5	54	42	3.1	3.9	107	88	34	28	33	28
2 week	16.5	12.5	51	39	4.9	3.6	105	86	34	28	33	28
1 months	14.0	10.0	43	31	4.2	3.0	104	85	34	28	33	29
2 months	11.5	9.0	35	28	3.8	2.7	96	77	30	26	33	29
3-6 months	11.5	9.5	35	29	3.8	3.1	91	74	30	25	33	30
0.5-2 years	12.0	11.0	36	33	4.5	3.7	78	70	27	23	33	30
2-6 years	12.5	11.5	37	34	4.6	3.9	81	75	27	24	34	31
6-12 years	13.5	11.5	40	35	4.6	4.0	86	77	29	25	34	31
12-18 years												
M	14.5	13.0	43	37	4.9	4.5	88	78	30	25	34	31
F	14.0	12.0	41	36	4.6	4.1	90	78	30	25	34	31

* Values less than 2SD denote anemia

Table 3.2: Dynamics of RBC

Erythrocytes	
Erythroid progenitors in the BM:	5 × 10^9
Number of RBCs produced	
3 × 10^9/kg/day (1/100th of total red cell mass)	
or	
10^{10} retics per hour	
Lifespan of erythrocytes	
Preterms	~20-30 days
Term neonates	~60-80 days
Adults:	90-150 days
Erythrocyte circulation	
300 miles in 120 days	
1,70,000 recirculations through the heart	

expansion. *Spurious anemia* reduced RBC concentration due to hemodilution.

Classification of Anemia

The classification of anemia can be kinetic, morphologic or etiologic. Usually, several broad categories can be considered (Table 3.3):

1. Decreased or increased production of RBCs.
2. Size of the red cells—Normal (*Normocytic*), large (*Macrocytic*) or small (*Microcytic*).
3. Impaired production, increased destruction or blood loss.

In practice, characteristic change in the size of the RBC and the Hb content along with the reticulocyte count are combined so as to enable a rational laboratory approach to diagnosis.

Approach to a Child with Anemia

It differs from that for an adult due to:

1. *Age differences in normal values for Hb/PCV (Table 3.4):* Children between the age of 6 months to 12 years appear anemic compared with adults. Their RBCs, however, have a higher concentration of 2,3-diphosphoglycerate and ATP with a consequent *right-shift of the oxygen dissociation curve*. The lower hemoglobin concentration is compensated by increased tissue oxygenation and the apparent anemia is thus, a physiologically appropriate adaptation of the red cell mass to increased efficiency of oxygen delivery.
2. *Iron deficiency anemia:* A frequent cause of anemia in children; is nearly always due to nutritional factors and requires less intensive follow-up evaluation.
3. *Sampling difficulty in neonates/young children:* Frequent use of capillary blood that should be obtained from a freely flowing stab wound made on a warmed tissue (heel or toe or finger). The initial blood drop should be discarded as it may be diluted with tissue fluid. Frequent sampling may lead to iatrogenic anemia.
4. *Absence of gender difference:* The male/female difference in Hb, RBC count and PCV is not present prior to puberty.

Table 3.3: Physiologic classification

A. Disorders of red cell production (with reticulocytopenia)
- *Marrow failure*
  a. Aplastic anemia (congenital or acquired)
  b. Pure red cell aplasia
     Congenital (Diamond-Blackfan syndrome)
     Acquired (Transient erythroblastopenia of childhood)
  c. Marrow replacement
     Malignancies
     Osteopetrosis
     Myelofibrosis (chronic renal disease and vitamin D deficiency)
  d. Pancreatic insufficiency marrow hypoplasia syndrome
- *Impaired erythropoietin production*
  a. Chronic renal disease
  b. Hypothyroidism; hypopituitarism
  c. Chronic inflammation
  d. Protein malnutrition
  e. Abnormal hemoglobins with reduced oxygen affinity

B. Disorders of erythroid maturation and ineffective erythropoiesis
- *Abnormalities of cytoplasmic maturation*
  a. Iron deficiency
  b. Thalassemia syndromes
  c. Sideroblastic anemias
  d. Lead poisoning
- *Abnormalities of nuclear maturation*
  a. Vitamin B_{12} deficiency
  b. Folic acid deficiency
  c. Thiamine-responsive megaloblastic anemias
  d. Hereditary abnormalities of folate metabolism
  e. Orotic aciduria
- *Primary dyserythropoietic anemias (CDA types I-IV)*
- *Erythropoietic protoporphyria*

C. Hemolytic anemias
- *Defects of hemoglobin*
  a. Structural mutants
  b. Synthetic mutants (Thalassemia syndromes)
- *Defects of red cell membrane*
- *Defects of red cell metabolism*
- *Antibody mediated*
- *Mechanical injury to red cell*
- *Thermal injury to red cell*
- *Oxidant-induced red cell injury*
- *Infectious agent-induced red cell injury*
- *Paroxysmal nocturnal hemoglobinuria*

D. Hemorrhage
- Acute
- Chronic

Classification of anemias based on red cell size (MCV)

A. Microcytic
- Iron deficiency (Nutritional and chronic blood loss)
- Thalassemia syndromes
- Chronic inflammation/disease
- Sideroblastic anemias
- Chronic lead poisoning

B. Macrocytic
- Megaloblastic bone marrow
  a. Vitamin B_{12} deficiency
  b. Folate deficiency
  c. Hereditary orotic aciduria
  d. Thiamine responsive anemia
  e. Myelodysplastic syndromes
  f. Drug-induced
- Non-megaloblastic
  a. Aplastic anemia
  b. Diamond-Blackfan syndrome
  c. Hypothyroidism
  d. Liver disease
  e. Bone marrow infiltration
  f. Dyserythropoietic anemias

C. Normocytic
- Congenital hemolytic anemias
  a. Hemoglobin mutants
  b. Red cell enzyme defects
  c. Red cell membrane disorders
- Acquired hemolytic anemias
  a. Antibody mediated
  b. Microangiopathic hemolytic anemias
  c. Secondary to acute infections
- Acute blood loss
- Splenic pooling
- Chronic renal disease

5. *Lower incidence of malignancy, cardiovascular disease or drug use:* There is a much lower incidence of these conditions in the pediatric age group as a direct or indirect cause of anemia.

Clinically significant anemia in childhood (other than nutritional), is frequently due to a primary hematologic abnormality (*hypoplastic or hemolytic anemia*) while in adults it is usually secondary to an underlying illness, i.e. a primary cause in the hemopoietic system is more frequent in children.

Evaluation of the Anemic Patient

Diagnostic approach should begin with a detailed history and physical examination followed by appropriate laboratory tests which are as follows (Fig. 3.1).

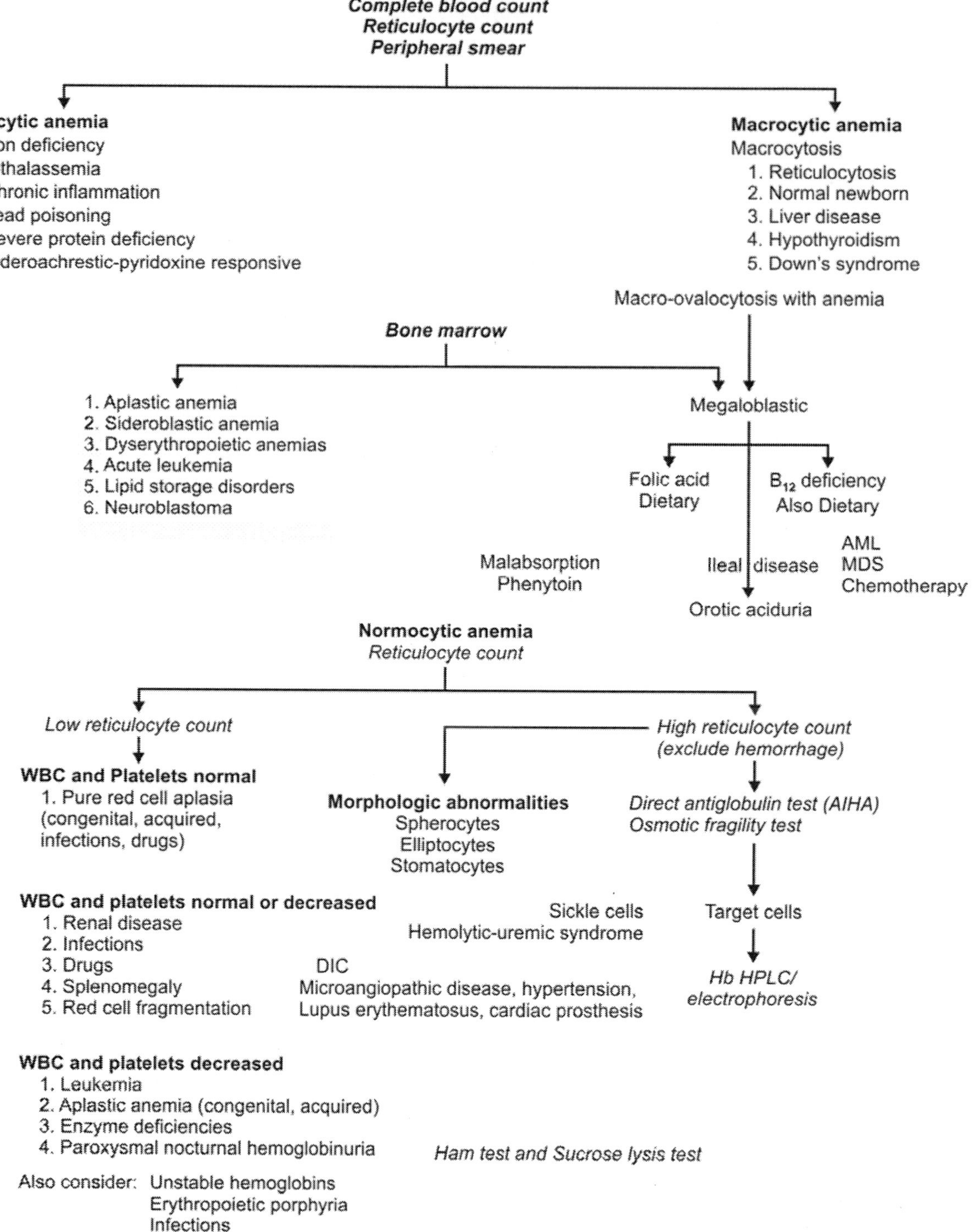

Fig. 3.1: Diagnostic approach to childhood anemia

Table 3.4: Causes of anemia at various age groups

Common causes of anemia at different ages	
Neonate	Blood loss Hemolysis
Neonate and early infancy	Physiologic anemia Pure red cell aplasia
6 months–2 years	Nutritional anemias Secondary to acute inflammation
Older children	Marrow infiltration (including leukemias)
Adolescence	Nutritional anemias

- Detection of the *presence* of anemia
  - Accurate measurement of pertinent values
  - Comparison with reference values
- Investigation of *pathogenesis* of anemia.

Initial investigations include:

1. Complete blood count (including differential count)
2. Reticulocyte count
3. Peripheral blood film examination
4. Other specific laboratory test, when indicated, include:
   a. Measurement of free erythrocyte porphyrins.
   b. Serum ferritin level estimation.
   c. Hemoglobin electrophoresis.
   d. Screening of presence of unstable hemoglobin.
   e. Direct and indirect Coombs' test (DAT).
   f. Glucose-6 phosphate dehydrogenase estimation.
   g. Supravital staining of erythrocytes.
   h. Vitamin B_{12} and folate level estimation.
   i. Examination of bone marrow.

Complete Blood Count

It is determined using hematology analyzers that employ electronic counting. They have the advantage of greater precision, reproducibility and speed. The red cell data generated by them (indices) include—Hb, RBC count, PCV, Mean cell volume (MCV, Mean cell hemoglobin (MCH), Mean cell hemoglobin concentration (MCHC), Red cell distribution width (RDW) and Hemoglobin distribution width (HDW). The MCV is the "average" volume of the red cells and helps in categorizing the types and causes of anemia (Table 3.5).

The RDW is derived from the RBC histogram and is an index of variation of the red cell size, i.e. *anisocytosis*. It is calculated as the coefficient of variation of the red cell volume distribution and reflects the ratio of the standard deviation (SD) and MCV. The RDW is calculated as follows:

$$RDW = SD/MCV \times 100$$

Normal value in infants and children: 11.5–15.0% (Adults: 11.5–14.5%)

The HDW is similarly calculated from the histogram for MCHC.

Histograms for MCHC are useful as they permit easy identification of dehydrated hyperchromic cells in hereditary spherocytosis, immune hemolytic anemia (IHA) and Sickle cell disease. A careful study of histogram may differentiate iron deficiency/beta thalessemia and hemoglobin H/hemoglobin CS disease.

The MCV and hemoglobin concentration histograms permit differentiation between iron deficiency and β-thalassemia trait and Hb H and Hb H/CS disease.

Reticulocyte Count

Each day ~0.8% of the RBC pool needs to be replaced by young erythrocytes (reticulocytes) released from the marrow. Their number in the blood reflects the marrow's response to peripheral anemia secondary to chronic hemorrhage or hemolysis resulting in erythropoietin (EPO) overdrive of the marrow and reticulocytosis to compensate for the peripheral RBC deficit

Table 3.5: Anemia classification based on MCV, RDW, MCHC and HDW

		MCV	
RDW	*Low*	*Normal*	*High*
Normal	Heterozygous α- and β-thalassemia	Normal Early iron deficiency Mixed nutritional deficiency	Aplastic anemia
High	Iron deficiency Hemoglobin H disease δ/β-thalassemia	Lead poisoning Liver disease	Neonates Prematurity B_{12}/folate deficiency
		High MCHC/RDW	*High MCHC/RDW*
		Immune hemolytic anemia Hereditary spherocytosis SS and SC disease	Immune hemolytic anemia

provided the marrow's capacity to produce RBC is intact. Reticulocytopenia in the presence of anemia indicates a disorder interfering with red cell production. Thus, reticulocyte count indicates whether the primary source of anemia is the *bone marrow* or the *periphery*.

Corrected Reticulocyte Count

Reticulocyte count must be corrected for anemia as it is a percentage of the total RBC count and is spuriously elevated when the number of RBCs falls in anemia. Reticulocyte percentage may be increased due to (i) more reticuclocytes in circulation or (ii) fewer mature cells, and hence, "correction" for anemia has to be done.

$$\text{Reticulocyte (\%)} = \frac{\text{Patient PCV (L/L)}}{0.45}$$

Absolute Reticulocyte Count

Retics/L = Retics (%) × RBC count

[Normal: 90×10^9/L]

An absolute reticulocyte count > 100,000/dl indicates *hemolytic anemia.*

Reticulocyte Index

The reticulocyte count is a total number of reticulocyte per volume of blood or as a percentage of the red cells. When a percentage is used, it should be corrected for the severity of anemia by multiplying it by the patient's hemoglobin (or hematocrit) divided by the normal hemoglobin (hematocrit).

When the anemia is severe (Hct ≤25) and polychromatophilia is prominent on the smear, a second correction is necessary. For the reticulocyte percentage to reflect erythrocyte production in these circumstances, it should be divided by 2. The reticulocyte percentage that emerges from these corrections is called the reticulocyte index.

Reticulocyte enumeration is especially important in the classification of anemia by physiologic mechanisms or red cell kinetics. It has three categories:

1. Hypoproliferative anemia, in which the bone marrow cannot increase its erythrocyte production;
2. Maturation defects, in which bone marrow hyperplasia occurs, but many cells die in the marrow, a situation called ineffective erythropoiesis;
3. Acute hemorrhage or hemolysis, in which the red cell production increases and erythrocytes leave the marrow intact but die prematurely in the peripheral circulation.

Assigning an anemia to one of these categories utilizes the reticulocyte index.

In the absence of anemia, the reticulocyte index is 1. With a moderately severe anemia (Hct<30) and a normal bone marrow, the reticulocyte index should exceed 3. This response typically occurs with hemolysis or acute hemorrhage. The reticulocyte index is less than 2 in hypoproliferative and maturation defect disorders The reticulocyte index, the bone marrow findings, and serum studies of LDH, Indirect bilirubin allow an accurate designation of the category of anemia:

In hypoproliferative anemias, the erythrocytes are usually normocytic, the reticulocyte index is <2, the E:M ratio is <1:2, and the indirect bilirubin and LDH are normal.

In maturation defects, the reticulocyte index is <2, the E:M ratio is >1:1 with severe anemias, the serum LDH and indirect bilirubin are elevated (except in iron deficiency), and polychromasia is present. Examples of nuclear maturation defects, which cause macrocytosis, are vitamin B_{12} and folate deficiencies. Cytoplasmic maturation defects produce microcytic erythrocytes, include thalassemias, certain hemoglobinopathies, some sideroblastic anemias.

In hemolysis, the reticulocyte index is >3, the E:M ratio is >1:1, serum LDH and indirect bilirubin are elevated, and polychromatophilia is prominent.

Peripheral Blood Film

Examination of the PBF is the single most valuable procedure in the evaluation of anemia. Characteristic morphologic changes in RBCs have diagnostic utility.

Approach to Anemia with Low MCV and Low Reticulocytes

Differential Diagnosis

a. Iron deficiency
b. Thalassemia trait (*defect in globin synthesis*)
c. Anemia of chronic inflammation (*failure of iron mobilization*)
d. Sideroblastic anemia (*defect in heme synthesis*).

Investigations

1. CBC
2. *Peripheral smear:* target cells, stippling
3. Serum iron, TIBC and ferritin (Table 3.6)
4. Hemoglobin HPLC/electrophoresis for evidence of thalassemia
5. *Bone marrow examination:* Iron stores, sideroblasts

Table 3.6: Levels of iron in the body

Normal iron status		
Marrow iron stores	: 2-3 +	(only direct measure of iron status)
Transferrin IBC (μg/dl)	: 330 ± 30	(estimate of body iron store)
Ferritin (μg/L)	: 100 ± 60	(estimate of body iron store)
Transferrin (Tf) receptor	: 5.5 ± 1.5	(reflects erythroid marrow activity)
Iron (μg/dl)	: 115 ± 50	(measures current iron supply to tissues)
Tf saturation (%)	: 35 ± 15	
Sideroblasts (%)	: 40–60	(correlate well with Tf saturation)
RBC protoporphyrin (μg/dl RBC)	: 30	(indicates iron supply to erythroid precursors)

Table 3.7: Causes of hypo- and hyperferritinemia ferritin

Low (<12 μg/L)	*Raised*
1. Practically diagnostic of iron deficiency • Hypothyroidism • Ascorbate deficiency (the only 2 conditions that lower it independently of decrease in iron stores)	1. Increased iron stores 2. Acute phase reactant fever, acute infections, RA, chronic inflammation 3. Acute and chronic damage to liver or ferritin rich parenchymal cells

Table 3.8: Causes of hypo- and hypertransferritinemia—transferrin concentration (TIBC)

Raised	*Decreased*
1. Depletion of storage iron	1. Iron overload
2. Pregnancy	2. Inflammation
3. Oral contraceptives	3. Infection
4. Malignancy	
5. Liver disease	
6. Nephrotic syndrome	
7. Malnutrition	

Iron Deficiency

- Absent marrow Fe; and sideroblasts absent or <10% of normoblasts
- Ferritin <12 μg/dl (may be normal if infection, inflammation, malignancy) (Table 3.7)
- Plasma Tf receptor levels elevated (ELISA)
- Low serum Fe and Tf saturation (<10%) with raised TIBC (Table 3.8)
- Elevated erythrocyte zinc protoporphyrin.

Anemia of Chronic Inflammation

- Normal to increased BM iron with decreased sideroblasts
- Elevated ferritin
- Normal plasma Tf receptor concentration
- Low serum Fe, low IBC, Tf saturation >10%

Thalassemia Trait

- Normal to raised serum iron, Tf saturation, ferritin and BM iron
- Normal free erythrocyte protoporphyrin
- Use of red cell indices for discriminant function (Table 3.9).

Approach to Anemia with Elevated MCV and Low Reticulocytes

Differential Diagnosis

1. Megaloblastic anemia
   a. Vitamin B_{12} deficiency
   b. Folate deficiency
   c. Myelodysplastic syndrome
   d. Drug-induced anemia
2. Non-megaloblastic anemia
   a. Liver disease
   b. Hypothyroidism
   c. Reticulocytosis.

Investigations

1. Serum vitamin B_{12} and red cell folate (Table 3.10)
2. *Peripheral smear examination:* hypersegmented neutrophils, giant platelets, megaloblasts
3. *Bone marrow examination:* Myelodysplastic features
4. Thyroid and liver function tests.

Table 3.9: Discriminant functions to differentiate iron deficiency from thalassemia trait

Calculation	Iron deficiency	β-thalassemia trait	
MCV – (5 × Hb) – RBC – 3.4	>0	<0	(England and Fraser)
$\frac{MCV}{RBC}$	>13	<13	(Mentzer)
$\frac{MCH}{RBC}$	>3.8	<3.8	(Srivastava)
RBC count	<5.0	>5.0	(Klee et al)
$MCH \times \frac{(MCV)^2}{100}$	>1530	<1530	(Shine and Lal)

Table 3.10: Normal levels of various nutrients in the body

	Normal level
Serum vitamin B_{12}	180-914 picogm/ml
Serum folate (ngm/ml)	3-17 ngm/ml
Red cell folate (ng/ml)	400-800 ngm/ml

Approach to Anemia with Normal MCV and Low Reticulocytes

Differential Diagnosis

a. Early or mild iron deficiency
b. Primary bone marrow failure
   i. Aplastic anemia
   ii. Pure red cell aplasia (Diamond-Blackfan syndrome)
   iii. Acquired red cell aplasia
   iv. Myelophthisis
   v. PNH
c. Secondary bone marrow failure
   i. Uremia
   ii. Endocrine disorders
   iii. HIV infection
   iv. Anemia of chronic inflammation.

Investigations

1. Serum iron, TIBC and ferritin
2. *Peripheral smear examination:* dacryocytes, helmet cells, etc.
3. Erythropoietin level
4. *Bone marrow aspiration and biopsy:* Assess cellularity, red cell production, iron stores
5. Hemosiderinuria, LAP score, sucrose lysis test and Ham's test
6. Renal and liver function tests, hormone levels, etc.

Table 3.11: Salient features of the causes of anemia with reticulocytosis

Hemolytic anemia
- Unconjugated hyperbilirubinemia
- Decreasing PCV

Hemorrhage
- PCV increases on subsequent determination
- In occult hemorrhage - reticulocytosis
  - unconjugated hyperbilirubinemia
  - decreased PCV

(But serial determinations: reticulocytes decrease, PCV increases and bilirubin decreases)

Approach to Anemia with Elevated Reticulocyte Count

Differential Diagnosis (Anemia with Signs of Accelerated Erythropoiesis) (Table 3.11)

a. Acute hemorrhage
b. Hemolytic anemia
c. Intentional or inadvertent treatment of nutritional anemia
d. Ineffective erythropoiesis (intramedullary hemolysis)
e. Recovery from bone marrow failure (e.g. drug/alcohol)
f. Splenic sequestration.

SIGNS OF ACCELERATED ERYTHROPOIESIS

Blood

- Reticulocytosis (polychromatophilia, basophilic stippling)
- Macrocytosis
- Erythroblastosis (usually <1% of all nucleated cells)
- Leukocytosis and thrombocytosis.

Bone Marrow

Erythroid hyperplasia.

Ferrokinetic

- Increased plasma iron turnover (PIT)
- Increased erythrocyte iron turnover (EIT).

Biochemical

Chemical markers of cell age (RBC creatine and some enzymes).

Hemorrhage

a. Phase of hypovolemia (2-3 days)
b. Phase of a (regenerative anemia), i.e. active erythrocyte regeneration
   - Decrease in plasma volume and red cell mass in proportion and thus PCV is normal (nadir of PCV at 3rd day)
   - Restoration of blood volume
   - Reticulocytosis within 3-5 days; maximal 6-11 days. Related to magnitude of hemorrhage but rarely >15%.
     RPI may reach 5.0 at 10 days
   - Polychromasia and macrocytosis
   - Neutrophilia, maximum at 2-5 hours ($10\text{-}20 \times 10^9$/L) up to 35,000/ml due to
     – Adrenalin mediated release from marginal pool
     – Release from marrow granulocyte reserve
- RBC reach normal level (4.5×10^9/L) in $\simeq$ 33 days Hb lags but restored in 6-8 weeks
- Morphologic evidence of red cell regeneration disappears in 10-14 days if no recurrence of hemorrhage TLC normal in 3-4 days
- Sustained reticulocytosis and persistent leukocytosis suggests continued bleeding.

Hemolytic Anemia

Hemolytic anemia is suspected by the:
- Presence of red cell abnormalities
- A reticulocytosis, and
- Unconjugated hyperbilirubinemia.

The clinical and laboratory phenomena of increased hemolysis reflect the:
- *Nature* of the hemolytic mechanism
- *Where* the hemolysis is taking place
- *Response* of the bone marrow to the anemia, namely,
  – erythroid hyperplasia
  – reticulocytosis

SIGNS OF ACCELERATED RBC DESTRUCTION

- Decreased RBC lifespan (^{51}Cr)
- Increased catabolism of heme
  – Unconjugated hyperbilirubinemia
  – Increased endogenous CO production
  – Increased rate of bilirubin production
  – Increased rate of urobilinogen excretion
- Increased serum LDH [LDH-2] Av: 580 U/ml (N: 240 U/ml)
- Absence of serum haptoglobin
- Reduced glycosylated Hb
- Signs of intravascular hemolysis
  – Hemoglobinemia
  – Hemoglobinuria
  – Hemosiderinuria
  – Methemalbuminemia
  – Reduced serum hemopexin
  – Fall in blood Hb @ >1 g/dl/week

INVESTIGATIONS FOR HEMOLYTIC ANEMIA

Evidence of Increased Hemolysis

a. Hb estimation
   Reticulocyte count
   PBF—spherocytes, schistocytes, irregularly-contracted cells or autoagglutination
b. Osmotic fragility test or glycerol lysis test
   Serum bilirubin estimation
c. Measurement RBC lifespan (^{51}Cr method)
   Demonstration of haptoglobins
   Test for increased urinary urobilinogen excretion.

Type of Hemolytic Mechanism

a. Direct antiglobulin test (DAT) with broad spectrum serum
b. Test for hemosiderinuria and hemoglobinuria
   Estimation of plasma Hb
   Schumm's test
   Flowcytometry for CD 55 and CD 59 in PNH.

Precise Diagnosis

1. If hereditary hemolytic anemia is suspected:
   - Osmotic-fragility determination after 24 hour incubation at 37°C
   - Autohemolysis test $\pm$ the addition of glucose
   - Red-cell instability at 45°C
   - Screening test for red cell G6PD deficiency, red cell pyruvate kinase assay; assay of other red cell enzymes involved in glycolysis
   - Estimation of red cell glutathione

- Electrophoresis for abnormal hemoglobins
- Estimation of HbA_2 and HbF
- Tests for sickling
- Tests for heat-labile Hb (Hb Koln, etc.).

2. If an autoimmune acquired hemolytic anemia is suspected:
   - Direct antiglobulin test using anti-Ig and anti-complement (C) sera
   - Tests for autoantibodies in the patient's serum
   - Titration of cold agglutinins
   - Donath-Landsteiner test
   - Electrophoresis of serum proteins
   - Demonstration of thermal range of autoantibodies
   - Assays of surface bound IgG by ELISA or Flow-cytometry.
3. If drug-induced hemolytic anemia is suspected:
   - Screening test for red cell G6PD
   - Glutathione stability test
   - Staining for Heinz bodies
   - Identification of methemoglobin (Hi) and sulphemoglobin (SHb)
   - Tests for drug-dependent antibodies.
4. In obscure hemolytic anemia
   - Acidified serum (Ham's) test for PNH
   - Sucrose lysis test
   - Warm reactive/cold reactive Erythrocyte Autoantibodies (in Infections).

Another approach to hemolytic anemias is based on history, peripheral smear examination and direct antiglobulin test. This can differentiate patients into five groups, which include:

a. Hemolytic anemia with obvious history suggesting malaria or exposure to drugs/chemicals
b. DAT-positive immune hemolytic anemia
   1. Detection of antibody and its measurement
   2. Thermal amplitude of antibody
c. DAT-negative spherocytic hemolytic anemia
   1. Osmotic fragility and incubation osmotic fragility (family studies)
   2. Membrane protein studies
d. Specific morphologic abnormalities of RBCs
   1. *Spherocytes*: HS, IHA, burns, chemical injury to RBC
   2. *Target cells*: Thalassemia, HbC, liver disease, postsplenectomy
   3. *Schistocytes*: Microangiopathic anemias (HUS, TTP), uremia
   4. *Acanthocytes*: Spur-cell anemia with liver disease, abetalipoproteinemia
   5. *Elliptocytes*: Hereditary ovalocytosis, megaloblastosis
   6. *Echinocytes*: Pyruvate kinase deficiency, uremia
   7. *Sickle cells*: Sickle cell disease
   8. *Autoagglutination*: Cold agglutinin disease
e. DAT-negative with no specific abnormality on peripheral smear
   1. Hemoglobin HPLC/electrophoresis
   2. Tests for unstable hemoglobins
   3. Screening tests for enzyme deficiency (G-6-PD and PK)
   4. Screening for PNH.

BIBLIOGRAPHY

1. Beutler E Waalen J. The definition of anemia: what is the lower limit of normal of the blood hemoglobin concentration? Blood. 2006;107:1747-50.
2. Dallman PR, Barr GD, Allen CM Shinefield HR. Hemoglobin concentration in white, black and oriental children: is there a need for separate criteria in screening for anemia? Am J Clin Nutr. 1978;31:377-80.
3. Dallman PR, Sijmans MA. Percentile curves for hemoglobin and red cell volume in infancy and childhood. J Pediatr. 1979;94:26-31.
4. Hillman RS, Finch CA. Erythropoiesis: Normal and abnormal. Semin Hematol. 1967;4(4):327-36.
5. Itano M. CAP comprehensive chemistry. Serum iron survey. Am J Clin Pathol. 1978;70(3 suppl):516-22.
6. Killman SA. on the size of normal human reticulocytes. Acta Med Scand. 1964;176:529-33.
7. Owren P. Congenital hemolytic jaundice. The pathogenesis of the 'hemolytic crisis'. Blood. 1948;3:231-48.
8. Ullrich C, Wu A, Armsby C, et al. Screening healthy infants for iron deficiency using reticulocyte hemoglobin content. JAMA. 2005;294:924-30.
9. Varat MA, Adolph RJ Fowler NO. Cardiovascular effects of anemia. Am Heart J. 1972;83(3)415-26.
10. Wintrobe's Clinical Hematology, 12th edn. Lippincott Williams and Wilkins, 2009.

4 Anemia of Prematurity

Himani Manchanda, Sachin Thakur, Dhiren Gupta, Anupam Sachdeva

Anemia is frequently observed in preterm babies admitted in the neonatal intensive care unit (NICU). Both term and preterm babies have a fall in the erythropoietin levels after birth when improved oxygenation decreases the stimulus for erythropoietin production. In full term babies, the hemoglobin falls for the first 2-3 months as erythropoiesis declines and then rises in the fourth to sixth month as erythropoietin (EPO) production increases. In preterm babies, the fall is much earlier and the nadir of hemoglobin is much lower as compared to the full-term infants. The hemoglobin falls to 7-8 g/dl or even lower in preterm babies who have not had much phlebotomy losses.[1] Anemia of prematurity (AOP) is seen more commonly in babies' with lower gestational age, lower birth weight and who are more sick and present by 3 to 12 weeks of age. The incidence is about 80% in very low birth weight babies (VLBW) and 95% in extremely low birth weight babies (ELBW). Babies >32 weeks of gestational age usually do not have significant AOP.

PATHOPHYSIOLOGY

The anemia of prematurity is due to a combination of decreased red blood cell (RBC) production, phlebotomy losses and shortened lifespan of the RBC. In the fetus the RBCs are first produced in the yolk sac followed by liver, which contributes to 50% of the RBC production at 32 weeks of gestation. Later, the bone marrow becomes the primary organ of erythropoiesis. Erythropoietin is initially produced in the yolk sac, followed by the liver and then by the peritubular cells of the kidney. The liver erythropoietin production responds to much lower levels of hypoxia and anemia and thus the preterm baby experiences limited erythopoietin production in spite of lower hemoglobin levels, as liver is still the major source of erythropoietin in them.[2,3]

Secondly, the lifespan of RBCs in preterm infants is 40-60 days (instead of 120 days as in adults) and this also contributes to lower hemoglobin levels. The shortened lifespan may be due to decreased enzyme levels in the RBCs and increased susceptibility to cell membrane peroxidation and fragmentation. Hemolysis may be seen more often in sick preterm babies and also in infections.

Finally, the phlebotomy losses, which are significant in a sick preterm baby, are one of the major causes of anemia. Due to the need to closely monitor a tiny infant, frequent samples of blood are removed for various tests. Because the smallest patients may be born with as little as 40 ml of blood in their circulation, withdrawing a significant amount of blood in a short period is relatively easy. Phlebotomy losses have been shown to strongly correlate with the number of transfusions a preterm baby requires.[4]

Concomitant nutritional deficiencies of vitamin E, vitamin B_{12} and folate may exaggerate the degree of anemia.

SIGNS AND SYMPTOMS

Though there are no specific symptoms of AOP, low hemoglobin has been associated with the following—apnea and bradycardia, increased oxygen requirements, tachypnea, tachycardia, pallor, lactic acidosis, flow murmurs and poor weight gain. Other than resolution of tachycardia and lactic acidosis with blood transfusion most of the other symptoms of anemia have not consistently responded to improvement of anemia in various trials.

EVALUATION

Laboratory evaluation should include a complete blood count (CBC), reticulocyte count, RBC indices (e.g. normocytic normochromic) for age, mother's blood group and Coombs' test (for immune mediated hemolytic anemia). Complete blood count shows low hemoglobin with normal white blood cell and platelet counts and no abnormal forms on peripheral smear. A normocytic normochromic anemia with a low reticulocyte count is consistent with the diagnosis of AOP in a premature baby. High reticulocyte counts or rising indirect bilirubin should prompt evaluation for a hemolytic process.

DIFFERENTIAL DIAGNOSIS

This includes other causes of neonatal anemia like hemolytic disease of the newborn, birth trauma, congenital bone marrow failure syndromes parvovirus B_{19} infection and others. A meticulous clinical history with special attention to timing of onset of anemia, blood losses, jaundice, maternal dietary, drug and medical history should be taken along with a detailed clinical examination.

TREATMENT

Low EPO levels in response to hypoxia or anemia is the hallmark of AOP.

Replacement of EPO is the definitive therapy though its routine use in the NICU is still not universally accepted.[5,6] The first trial of EPO in the preterm infants was conducted by Halperin et al[7] Various trials have been conducted since then to evaluate different doses, frequency of dosing, iron supplementation, and duration of EPO therapy, cost effectiveness, etc. Maier et al evaluated the effect of EPO on PRBC transfusions in $\leq$ 34 weeks gestational age babies (Birth weight 750-1499 g) given EPO 250 u/kg SC × 3/week along with iron supplementation (2 mg/kg/d). The EPO group received fewer transfusions (0.87 vs 1.25) and had greater success in maintaining hematocrit >35% without need for transfusion (44% in EPO group vs 28% in placebo group).[8]

Al-Kharphy et al in their study (EPO 200 u/kg SC × 3/week) reported less PRBC transfusions in the EPO group (3.48 $\pm$ 1.58 vs 5.68 $\pm$ 2.3 in placebo) without any increase in morbidity.[9]

Ohls et al evaluated EPO in $\leq$750 g birth weight. babies and demonstrated the efficacy of EPO in the first weeks of life (4.7$\pm$ 0.7 transfusions and 70 $\pm$ 11 ml/kg vs 7.5 $\pm$ 1.1 transfusions and 112 $\pm$ 17 ml/kg blood transfusion).[10] Iron supplements have been used from 2 mg/kg/d to 12 mg/kg/d and many studies have shown low ferritin levels when babies are put on EPO (suggesting rapid utilization of Fe). Adequate iron supplementation is absolutely essential for getting a good response to EPO and many studies have used levels of ferritin to adjust the iron supplementation (>65 μg/dl).[11]

Low dose EPO (750 u/kg/week) vs high dose EPO (1500 u/kg/week) courses were used in a European trail in babies from day 3 of life to 37 weeks of postconception (Birth weight <1000 g). There was no difference in the transfusion requirements in the two groups and nor was there any difference in the hematocrit achieved. Thus in <1 kg birth weight babies there was no improvement in outcomes using a higher dose of EPO.[12]

In a NICHD trial (multicenter, randomized, double-masked and placebo controlled), 290 babies were randomized to receive EPO (400 u/kg × 3/week) or a placebo. In this study, the EPO administration did not reduce the transfusion requirements compared to the placebo group, though the reticulocyte count and the hematocrit levels were higher in the EPO group. The placebo group also required fewer transfusions, when compared to the rest of the babies who were not in the study (thus underlining the importance of phlebotomy losses and strict blood transfusion guidelines). There were no adverse effects noted with EPO use or Fe supplementation in the study.[13]

Drug dosing schedule was compared by Brown and Keith in preemies reporting that a frequent dosing schedule (100 u/kg/d × 5/week vs 250 u/kg/d × 2/week) was more effective in stimulating erythropoiesis.[14] Another study has shown that a slow 24-hour intravenous infusion of the EPO dose to be as effective as the subcutaneous dose.[15] Lower efficacy of rapid IV infusions and fewer subcutaneous administrations of a higher dose may be due to rapid EPO excretion and decreased bioavailability of EPO.

No agreement regarding the timing, dosing, route or duration of therapy exists. The cost-benefit ratio for EPO has yet to be evaluated, and this medication is not universally accepted as standard therapy for AOP. When the family has religious objections to transfusions, the use of EPO is advisable.[15]

Reducing phlebotomy losses by planning various investigations in advance to prevent frequent sampling, rational investigative work-up, using new technology analyzers, which require small quantities of blood and transcutaneous monitors for hemoglobin oxygen saturation and partial pressure of carbon dioxide, etc. help in decreasing the blood loss and thus the transfusions required. This has been well documented in various studies.[16-18]

PRBC transfusions still remain the mainstay of therapy for AOP though there is disagreement regarding the timing, level of hematocrit and their efficacy. Over the last 2 decades the guidelines for transfusion have become more stringent though there is some hospital to hospital variation in the transfusion protocols. A combination of classic symptoms of anemia, cardiorespiratory status and hematocrit levels are taken into account for deciding the transfusion protocols. The guidelines for administering transfusions to newborns are given in the chapter on anemia in the newborn.

Reducing the donor exposure can decrease complications of PRBC transfusions. Using PRBCs stored in preservatives (e.g. Citrate-phosphate-dextrose-adenine, CPDA-1), allows the blood to be stored safely for up to 35-42 days. Assigning a unit of CPDA-1 blood for a baby may be adequate for all the transfusions during his/her hospital stay thus limiting donor exposure. Using leukocyte filters for decreasing the cytomegalovirus (CMV) exposure, irradiating the blood before transfusion or administering blood from CMV sero-negative donors also helps in decreasing the exposure to CMV infections.

AOP still remains a common problem in preemies under 32 weeks of gestational age. With stricter transfusion guidelines and less phlebotomy losses the transfusion requirements have decreased significantly over the last 2 decades. Addition of EPO likely decreases the need for transfusions, though issues regarding its efficacy and cost effectiveness remain, when compared to preventive measures and transfusions. Erythropoietin is usually discontinued before discharge at about 35-42 weeks of gestation. To prevent any exacerbation of AOP, which resolves naturally by 3-6 months of age we must provide adequate doses of vitamin E, vitamin B_{12}, folate and Fe (when using EPO). After discharge from hospital, regular hematocrit levels to determine a steady increase, are to be frequently documented on regular visits.

REFERENCES

1. Kling PJ, Schmidt RL, Roberts RA, et al. Serum erythropoietin levels during infancy: Associations with erythropoiesis. J Pediatr. 1996;128:791.
2. Erslev AJ, Caro J, Kansu E, et al. Renal and extrarenal erythropoietin production in anemic rats. Br J Haematol. 1980;45:65.
3. Zanjani ED, Poster J, Burlington H, et al. Liver as primary site of erythropoietin formation in the fetus. J Lab Clin Med. 1997;89:640.
4. Kling PJ, Sullivan TM, Leftwich ME, et al. Score for neonatal acute physiology and phlebotomy blood loss predict erythrocyte transfusions in premature infants. Arch Pediatr Adolesc Med. 1997;151:27.
5. Brown MS, Garcia JF, Phibbs RH, et al. Decreased response of plasma immunoreactive erythropoietin to "available oxygen" in anemia of prematurity. J Pediatr. 1992;120:292.
6. Stockman JA, Graeber JE, Clark DA, et al. Anemia of prematurity: Determinants of the erythropoietin response. J Pediatr. 1984;105:786.
7. Halperin DS, Wacker P, Lacourt G, et al. Effects of recombinant human erythropoietin in infants with the anemia of prematurity: A pilot study. J Pediatr. 1990;116:779.
8. Maier RF, Obladen M, Scigalla P, et al. The effect of epoetin beta (recombinant human erythropoietin) on the need for transfusion in very low birth weight infants. N Engl J Med. 1994;330:1173.
9. Al-Kharfy T, Smyth JA, Wadsworth L, et al. Erythropoietin therapy in neonates at risk of having bronchopulmonary dysplasia and requiring multiple transfusions. J Pediatr. 1996;129:89.
10. Ohls RK, Harcum J, Schibler KR, et al. The effect of erythropoietin on the transfusion requirements of preterm infants ≤750 g: A randomized, double blind, placebo-controlled study. J Pediatr. 1997;131:66.
11. Meyer MP, Meyer JH, Commerford A, et al. Recombinant human erythropoietin in the treatment of anemia of prematurity; Results of a double-blind, placebo controlled study. Pediatrics. 1994;93:918.
12. Maier RF, Obladen M, Kattner E, et al. High versus low dose erythropoietin in extremely low birth weight infants. J Pediatr. 1998;132:866.
13. Ohls RK, Ehrenkranz RA, Lemons JA, et al. A multi-centered, randomized, double-blind, placebo-controlled trial of erythropoietin administration to premature infants ≤1250 g birth weight. Pediatr Res. 1999;45:216.
14. Brown MS, Keith JF III. Comparison between two and five doses a week of recombinant human erythropoietin for anemia of prematurity: A randomized trial. Pediatrics. 1999; 104:210.
15. David P, Herbert M, Davies DP, et al. Erythropoietin for anaemia in a preterm Jehovah's baby. Early Hum Dev. 1991; 1:279-83.
16. Ohls RK, Veerman MW, Christensen RD. Pharmacokinetics of recombinant erythropoietin administered to preterm infants by continuous infusion in parenteral nutrition solution. J Pediatr. 1996;128:518.
17. Asch J, Wedgwood JF. Optimizing the approach to anemia in the preterm infant: Is there a role for erythropoietin therapy? J Perinatol. 1997;17:276.
18. Widness JA, Seward VJ, Kromer IJ, et al. Changing patterns of red blood cell transfusion in very low birth weight infants. J Pediatr. 1996;129:680.

5 Anemia in the Newborn

Neha Rastogi, Anupam Sachdeva, SP Yadav, Arun Soni

Neonatal anemia is defined as hemoglobin or hematocrit concentration of >2 standard deviation below the mean for postnatal age.[1] Rapid changes in normal hematological parameters take place throughout the neonatal period. Therefore, the diagnosis of anemia in the newborn is made in relation to gestation and postnatal age. Anemia during 1st week of life is defined as hemoglobin level less than 14 g/dl. Any significant fall in hemoglobin in a neonate, although, within normal range is suggestive of hemorrhage or hemolysis. For example, in a term newborn whose hemoglobin was 18.5 g/dl at birth, hemoglobin of 14.5 g/dl on D 7 of life is abnormal. Similarly, failure of hemoglobin to rise during first few hours of life may be the first clue to a hemorrhage or hemolysis in a newborn. Severe anemia present at birth (i.e. Hemoglobin < 8.0 g/dl) is usually due to immune hemolysis or hemorrhage.

FETAL ERYTHROPOIESIS

Fetal erythropoiesis occurs in yolk sac, liver and bone marrow. Initially between 10 and 14 days of gestation erythropoiesis occurs in yolk sac. By 6-8 weeks of gestation the liver replaces the yolk sac as primary site of production of red blood cells (RBCs). Hepatic erythropoiesis begins to diminish during second trimester. Myeloid (bone marrow production) of RBCs begins at around week 18 and, by the end of 30th week it is the major erythropoietic organ.[2]

The erythroid blood cell indices change with increasing gestation and continue to change throughout the first year of life. There is a gradual increase in circulating erythrocyte concentration during the second and third trimesters. Along with this increased erythrocyte concentrations, hematocrit also rises in second and third trimester. Mean cell volumes (MCVs) are inversely proportional to gestation and to life span of the cell. The mean cell volume (MCV) of erythrocytes is >180 fl in the embryo, decreases to about 130 fl by mid-gestation, then decreases to 110 fl by 40 weeks of gestation.[3] The red cell values on the first postnatal day during the last 16 weeks of gestation is shown in Table 5.1.

NORMAL HEMATOLOGICAL VALUES IN THE NEONATAL PERIOD

During neonatal period, RBC values are more variable than any other time of life and understanding of normal values of hemoglobin and other red cell indices is essential for diagnosing anemia in newborn (Tables 5.2 and 5.3).

Hemoglobin Concentration

The mean cord blood hemoglobin of healthy term infant ranges from 15.7 to 17.9 g/dl with a mean of 16.8 g/dl. Shortly after birth hemoglobin concentration rises. This rise is absolute as well as relative—absolute owing to placental RBC transfusion and relative owing to the reduction of plasma volume. This rise is around 17-20% of the initial value during the first 2 hours. At 16 weeks of gestation, hemoglobin concentration is around 10 g/dl and it rises to 15 g/dl at 32-34 weeks of gestation. Cord blood hemoglobin can be calculated in preterm infant as 7+ gestation age in lunar month g/dl. Normal hematocrit value ranges from 51.3 to 56% and it also rises during 1st few hours of life and reaches to original value of cord blood by one week.

Reticulocyte Count

The average reticulocyte count in a term newborn at birth ranges from 3 to 7%. It decreases to 1 to 3% by 4th day of life and reaches to less than 1% on 7th day of life. Persistent high reticulocyte count in a newborn is suggestive of blood loss, hemolytic anemia or hypoxia. In premature infants reticulocyte count is higher (6 to 10%) and may remain higher for a longer period of time.

Table 5.1: Red blood cell values on the first postnatal day

	Gestational age (weeks)							
	24-25 (7)	*26-27 (11)*	*28-29 (7)*	*30-31 (25)*	*32-33 (23)*	*34-35 (23)*	*36-37 (20)*	*Term (19)*
RBC count (× 10^6/mm^3)	4.65 ± 0.43	4.73 ± 0.45	4.62 ± 0.75	4.79 ± 0.74	5.0 ± 0.76	5.09 ± 0.5	5.27 ± 0.68	5.14 ± 0.7
Hb (g/dl)	19.4 ± 1.5	19.0 ± 2.5	19.3 ± 1.8	19.1 ± 2.2	18.5 ± 2.0	19.6 ± 2.1	19.2 ± 1.7	19.3 ± 2.2
Hct (%)	63 ± 4	62 ± 8	60 ± 7	60 ± 8	60 ± 8	61 ± 7	64 ± 7	61 ± 7.4
MCV (fl)	135 ± 0.2	132 ± 14.4	131 ± 13.5	127 ± 12.7	123 ± 15.7	122 ± 10.0	121 ± 12.5	119 ± 9.4
Reticulocytes (%)	6.0 ± 0.5	9.6 ± 3.2	7.5 ± 2.5	5.8 ± 2.0	5.0 ± 1.9	3.9 ± 1.6	4.2 ± 1.8	3.2 ± 1.4
Weight (g)	725 ± 185	993 ± 194	1174 ± 128	1450 ± 232	1816 ± 192	1957 ± 291	2245 ± 213	—

Abbreviations: Hb: Hemoglobin; Hct: Hematocrit; MCV: Mean corpuscular volume; RBC: Red blood cell

Table 5.2: Normal hematological values during the neonatal period of the term infant hemoglobin, hematocrit and RBC count

	Hb (g %)	*Hematocrit (%)*	*RBC (million/mm^3)*
Cord blood	16.2 ± 3.6	46.66 ± 5.1	4.9 ± 1.2
12-18 hours	18.79 ± 2.8	49 ± 4.8	5.3 ± 0.8
72 hours	17.38 ± 3.0	46.9 ± 5.3	5.2 ± 0.6
7 days	17.0 ± 2.4	45.0 ± 4.0	5.0 ± 1.1
15 days	16.36 ± 2.2	43.4 ± 4.1	5.01 ± 0.9
20 days	14.17 ± 2.4	42.1 ± 3.8	4.7 ± 1.0

Table 5.3: MCV, MCH, MCHC and normoblast count

	MCV (fl)	*MCH (pg)*	*MCHC (%)*	*Normoblasts (cells/mm^3)*
Cord blood	113.04 ± 5.3	34.33 ± 1.4	33.9 ± 0.8	600 ± 186
12-18 hours	108.96 ± 5	35.1 ± 1.9	34.4 ± 0.6	283 ± 122
72 hours	98.54 ± 2.9	35.82 ± 0.8	34.9 ± 0.5	36 ± 48
7 days	96.0 ± 3.4	34.0 ± 1.0	34.6 ± 0.8	
15 days	95.5 ± 4.0	33.2 ± 9.0	34.54 ± 0.5	
28 days	96.1 ± 3.2	31.6 ± 0.93	34.2 ± 0.7	

Nucleated Red Blood Cells

Term infant has 0-24 nucleated RBCs per 100 leukocytes at birth and preterm infant has higher number of nucleated RBCs. Nucleated RBCs generally disappear by 3-4 days of life in term infants and 7-10 days in preterm infant. The persistence of nucleated RBCs beyond this period suggests the possibility of hemorrhage or hemolysis.

Red Blood Cell Count

Normal red cell count varies from 4.6 to 5.2 million/cumm. It also rises rapidly during first few hours and returns to normal value of 5 to 5.2 million/cumm by the end of 1st week.

Red Cell Indices

Normal newborn RBCs are large and MCV ranges from 105 to 125 fl. By 10 weeks of life RBC approaches the size of older children (75-90 fl). In neonates microcytosis is defined as an MCV of less than 95 fl at birth. The RBC hemoglobin content of neonatal red cell, maternal and child health (MCH) ranges from 35 to 38 pg which is greater than that seen in older children (30-33 pg) and any value of MCH less than 34 pg is defined as neonatal hypochromia. Hypochromia and microcytosis generally occur together and are seen in thalassemic disorders and iron deficiency due to chronic blood loss.

ETIOLOGY

Anemia in neonatal period is due to three distinct causes:

1. *Hemorrhage:* Acute/chronic, prenatal/postnatal
2. *Hemolysis:* Immune/nonimmune
3. Failure of red cell production.

Hemorrhage

About 5 to 10% of the cases of severe neonatal anemia are due to hemorrhage and this may occur during prenatal, intranatal or postnatal period. In an anemic newborn not having jaundice and a negative Coombs' test, hemorrhage is the most probable cause.[4]

Prenatal Blood Loss

Transplacental fetomaternal blood loss: Spontaneous leakage of small amount of fetal Hb into maternal circulation occurs in 50% of all pregnancies, but in about 1% it is of sufficient magnitude to produce anemia in the infant. The frequency and magnitude of fetomaternal hemorrhage is increased by invasive procedures like amniocentesis and external cephalic version. Many maternal conditions like chorioangioma, choriocarcinoma, abdominal trauma, antepartum hemorrhage and pregnancy induced hypertension also cause transplacental fetomaternal bleed. Fetomaternal bleed is diagnosed by demonstrating fetal red cells in the maternal circulation by Kleihauer-Betke technique (Acid elution method of staining for fetal hemoglobin). But in presence of thalassemia minor, sickle cell anemia, hereditary persistence of fetal hemoglobin Kleihauer-Betke test is not useful. In such cases differential hemagglutination should be employed. Similarly in ABO blood group incompatibility, diagnosis may be missed as infant's A or B-cells are rapidly cleared from maternal circulation. The amount of blood lost in fetomaternal hemorrhage can be calculated by following formula:

$$\text{ml of fetal blood} = \frac{\text{Fetal RBC} \times 2400}{\text{Maternal RBC}}$$

Presence of 1 fetal RBC per 1000 maternal RBCs indicates 2 ml of fetomaternal hemorrhage.

Transplacental bleed may be acute or chronic. The characteristics of acute and chronic blood loss in a newborn are listed in Table 5.4.

Table 5.4: Characteristics of acute and chronic blood loss in the neonate

Acute blood loss	*Chronic blood loss*
Pallor	Pallor
Shallow tachypnea	Signs of cardiac failure
Poor peripheral perfusion	Cardiac enlargement
Hypotension	Tachypnea
No organomegaly	Hepatomegaly
Normochromic microcytic anemia	Ascites
	Hypochromic, microcytic anemia
	Reticulocytosis

Retroplacental Bleed

Abnormally implanted placenta and placental malformation can cause retroplacental bleed. This can be diagnosed by examination of placenta in an anemic newborn. Accidental incision of the placenta during cesarean section can also cause massive fetal hemorrhage.

Twin-to-Twin Transfusion

In 15-20% of monochorionic twins, significant twin to twin transfusion occurs. This condition should be suspected if there is difference of hemoglobin of over 5 g/dl between the twins. Typically the donor twin is smaller, pale and may show evidence of shock. The recipient twin is larger and polycythemic.

Postnatal Blood Loss

Postnatal blood loss may occur from a number of sites and may be internal or external. One of the most common causes of obvious bleeding in the newborn is slipped ligature of the cord. Traumatic delivery, especially forceps and breech delivery, results in subgaleal (scalp) intracranial or intra-abdominal hemorrhage. An infant with internal bleed may appear well for first 24 hours, but may then suddenly go into shock. Hemophilia, vitamin K deficiency and disseminated intravascular coagulation are also important causes of postnatal bleed.

Iatrogenic Anemia

Frequent sampling in neonatal care unit is a very common cause of anemia in newborn, especially in the preterm babies. One milliliter of blood represents about 1% of total blood volume in preterm babies. Removal of 8–10 ml of blood in a 1500 g baby constitutes 8% of the blood volume. Thus, excessive sampling should be avoided.

Hemolytic Anemia

Premature destruction of RBC leads to hemolytic anemia. Hemolysis as a cause of anemia should be suspected in presence of rapid fall of hemoglobin concentration with reticulocytosis, unconjugated hyperbilirubinemia and hemoglobinuria without any evidence of hemorrhage. Abnormal erythrocyte morphology also points towards hemolytic process. Hemolysis can be due to immune mediated or non-immune mediated mechanism. Nonimmune hemolytic anemia involves defects in either red cell membranes or hemoglogin or enzyme defects.[4]

Nonimmune Mediated Hemolytic Anemia

a. *Red cell membrane defects* such as hereditary spherocytosis, elliptocytosis stomatocytosis can cause significant anemia in newborn.[5] A family history of chronic anemia, cholelithiasis, unhealed leg ulcers, splenomegaly may be present in case of hereditary spherocytosis. Examination of peripheral blood smear and osmotic fragility test is diagnostic in hereditary spherocytosis.
b. *Hemoglobinopathies:* Defect or deficiency of production of globin chains result in hemolytic anemia. In the newborn period, α-globin defect tends to be the most common and most severe, because γ-chain defects are exceedingly rare and β-chain production does not usually peak until about 3 months of age. Homozygous alpha thalassemia is due to absence of all four alpha globin chains and is associated with severe intrauterine hemolytic anemia, hydrops fetalis with massive hepatosplenomegaly. Most affected children are stillborn, although some may live for few hours after birth. The RBC in alpha thalassemia is hypochromic, fragmented and bizarre in shape and erythroblastosis is also seen.

Gamma thalassemia: Large deletion within the beta globin gene cluster sometimes removes both gamma globin chains as well as delta and beta globin chain. The resulting gamma-delta-beta thalassemia is lethal in the homozygous state. In heterozygous state it produces a transient but moderate to severe anemia but this anemia improves spontaneously within first six months of life and afterwards the hematological picture is like thalassemia trait.[6]

RBC enzyme abnormalities: Most commonly encountered enzymopathy in newborn is sex-linked Glucose-6-phosphate dehydrogenase (G6PD) deficiency and others are pyruvate kinase deficiency, 5′ nucleotidase deficiency and glucose phosphate isomerase deficiency. In India G6PD deficiency is common in Parsi, Bhanushali, Sindhi and Punjabi communities. It can cause significant neonatal hemolysis resulting in anemia and hyperbilirubinemia due to exposure to known hemolytic agent and cases have been seen without any exposure to oxidant or infection. Normal value of G6PD level during acute hemolysis may not rule out G6PD deficiency as younger RBCs contain high level of enzyme. Hence, G6PD level should be repeated after 6 weeks of an episode of hemolysis.[7]

Infection: Both prenatal and postnatal infection causes anemia and other hematological abnormalities in the neonatal period. Intrauterine infections of *Toxoplasma*, cytomegalovirus, syphilis, rubella, malaria and parvovirus (TORCH) can cause hemolysis. The hemolytic process is due to direct injury to the red cell membrane. Congenital infection is suspected due to clinical findings of chorioretinitis, pneumonitis, central nervous system abnormalities, hepatosplenomegaly, growth retardation and skin changes. If the spleen is enlarged, hypersplenism can increase the rate of red cell destruction. Laboratory features include thrombocytopenia, leukocytosis with immature form and reticulocytosis. Postnataly acquired infection produce marrow suppression and hemolysis of RBC thereby causing anemia in newborn. Vertical transmission of malaria is rare. Features of malaria in a newborn are fever, irritability, hepatosplenomegaly with severe anemia and reticulocytosis.

Immune Mediated Hemolytic Anemia

The immune causes are mainly due to blood group incompatibility between fetus and the mother. This incompatibility may be Rh (D), ABO or minor blood groups such as anti-C, Duffy, anti-C, anti-E, Kell, etc.

a. *Rh isoimmunization:* Placental transfer of maternal antibodies directed against fetal RBC is the cause of hemolysis of neonatal RBC. Clinical features of Rh isoimmunization are anemia, which may be mild to severe, jaundice, hepatosplenomegaly. Laboratory investigations reveal blood group incompatibility, reticulocytosis and increased number of nucleated RBC's in peripheral blood smear and positive direct Coombs' test.
b. *ABO incompatibility:* In ABO incompatibility, maternal Anti-A or Anti-B antibodies enter fetal circulation and react with A or B antigen on the erythrocyte surface. ABO incompatibility frequently occurs during first pregnancy without prior sensitization. Hemolysis due to ABO incompatibility is clinically milder than Rh incompatibility but

occasionally severe hemolysis may occur. In most cases pallor and jaundice are minimal and hepatosplenomegaly is uncommon. Direct Coombs' test is frequently negative but indirect Coombs' test is positive. On peripheral smear, spherocytes are found so it is sometimes confused with hereditary spherocytosis.

Failure of Red Cell Production

Congenital

Pure red cell aplasia (Diamond-Blackfan anemia), Aase syndrome and Fanconi's anemia are congenital anemia in newborn. Diamond-Blackfan syndrome is characterized by the absence of recognizable erythroid precursor cells in bone marrow. Physical abnormalities associated with Diamond-Blackfan syndrome are triphalangeal or duplicated thumb, cleft palate, ocular defect, short or webbed neck, hypertelorism, ptosis. Diagnosis is confirmed by demonstrating virtual absence of erythroid precursors in bone marrow. Fanconi's anemia usually does not manifest in the newborn period.[8]

Anemia of Prematurity

In term infant the hemoglobin level reaches its nadir of 9-11 g/dl at approximately 8-12 weeks of life. This anemia is viewed as physiological adaptation of extrauterine life and is due to low erythropoietin level, shortened survival of fetal RBC's and rapid expansion of blood volume. In preterm babies the fall of hemoglobin is both more rapid and more profound and in baby weighing less 1500 g hemoglobin level can fall as low as 7-8 g/dl by 4-8 weeks of life. Clinically these infants have tachycardia, tachypnea, feeding problem, decreased activity and apneic attacks. The factors operating in physiological anemia of term baby is also present in preterm baby, but are exaggerated. The response to anemia or hypoxia to hepatic erythropoietin synthesis in preterm baby is poor as compared to that in term baby. Frequent sampling, low level of hematopoietic growth factors such as insulin like growth factor-1 and 2 and deficiency of folate, vitamin B_{12}. Vitamin E is also an important factor, which contributes to pathophysiology and severity of anemia of prematurity.[9]

DIAGNOSTIC APPROACH TO ANEMIA IN A NEWBORN

Medical history and physical examination can give a lead to the cause of anemia in a newborn. Family history of anemia, cholelithiasis, unexplained jaundice and splenomegaly points towards some hereditary hemolytic anemia. Obstetric history of difficult labor, instrumentation, bleeding or placental abnormalities correlate with hemorrhagic anemia. The age at which anemia becomes manifest also is of diagnostic importance. Significant anemia at birth is due to blood loss or alloimmunization. After 24 hours, internal hemorrhage and other causes of hemolysis manifest. Anemia of prematurity, hypoplastic anemia and abnormalities of synthesis of hemoglobin chain generally appear several weeks after birth.

Coombs test, reticulocyte count, mean corpuscular volume, MCH and blood smear are the key investigative tools for diagnosing the cause of anemia in newborn. Figure 5.1 shows a flow diagram of investigation of anemia in newborn.

TREATMENT OF ANEMIA IN NEWBORN

Treatment of anemia in a neonate depends on the clinical condition.[10] If the infant is in hypovolemic shock due to acute blood loss, 10-20 ml/kg of whole blood cross matched with mother should be transfused immediately through umbilical vein. In case of unavailability of cross-matched blood, O negative blood can be used. Asymptomatic anemic neonate with moderate hemorrhage or chronic blood loss does not require blood transfusion as such. The only therapy required for such a neonate is iron in the dose of 2 mg/kg three times a day for 3 months. Vitamin B_{12} and folate should also be supplemented on discharge to breastfed preterm infants. In severe anemia with congestive cardiac failure due to chronic blood loss partial exchange transfusion or packed cell transfusion is the treatment of choice.[11] RBC transfusion is indicated for asymptomatic infant with venous hematocrit $\leq$ 20% and absolute reticulocyte count less than 3%. In hemolytic anemia main concern is hyperbilirubinemia, which may require phototherapy or exchange transfusion. Infants with ABO incompatibility not requiring an exchange transfusion for hyperbilirubinemia may have protracted hemolysis and may require RBC transfusion several weeks after birth.

In a hemodynamically unstable infant, hyaline membrane disease or severe bronchopulmonary dysplasia, hemoglobin level is maintained at the level of 12-14 g/dl to improve oxygen delivery.[12]

Diamond-Blackfan syndrome is managed with corticosteroids and blood transfusion. Anemia of prematurity is treated with recombinant human erythropoietin. The dose of erythropoietin is 75-300 units/kg/week subcutaneously for 4 weeks starting at 3-4 weeks of age. To prevent iron deficiency, oral iron supplementation in a dose of 2 mg/kg/day is also given.

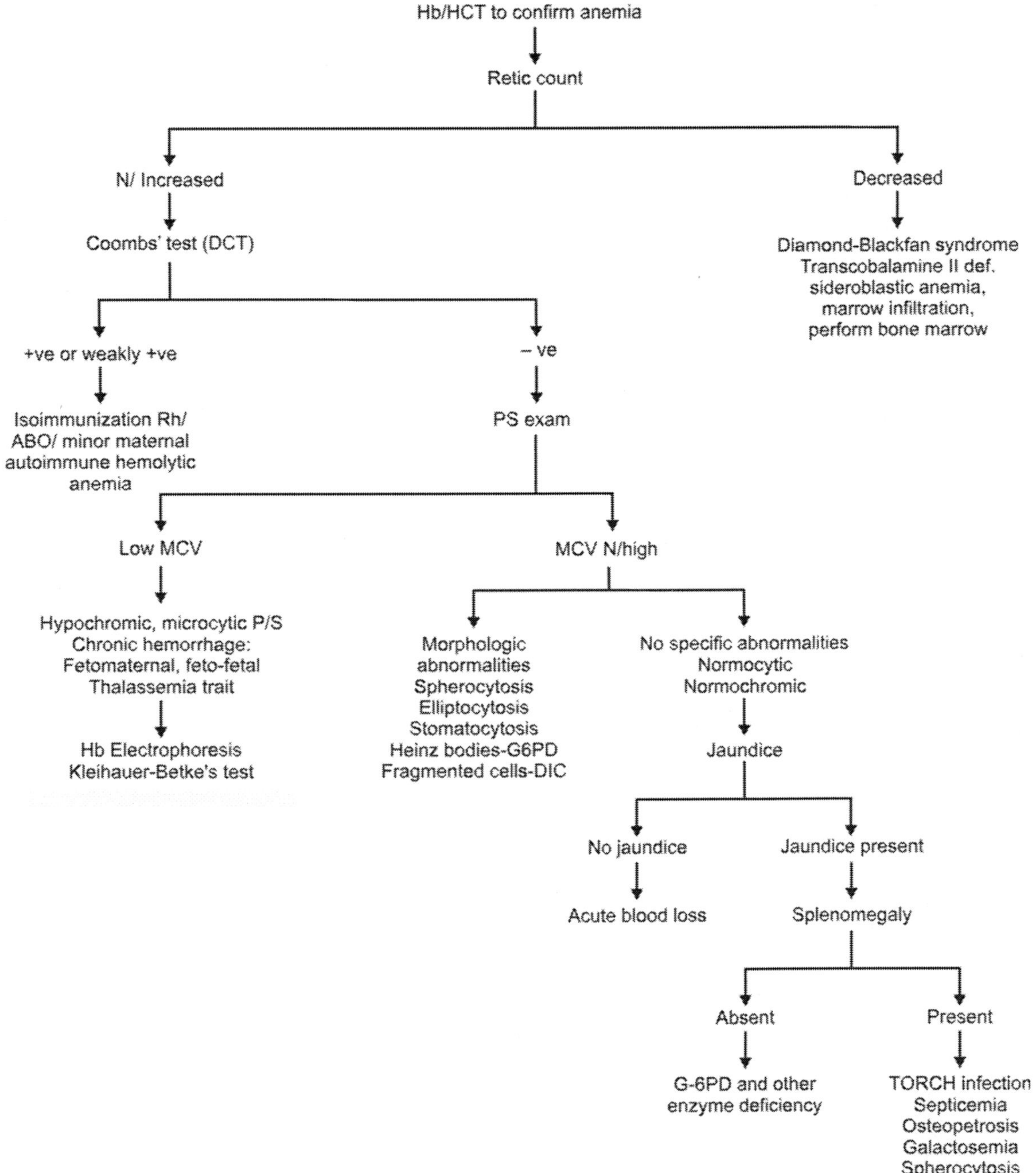

Fig. 5.1: Approach to neonatal anemia

Erythropoietin takes about 2 weeks to raise the hemoglobin to a biological significant degree. Erythropoietin therapy is safe and effective in reducing the number of transfusions but its cost is of concern. The criteria for transfusion of preterm infants are given in Table 5.5.

Table 5.5: Indications for small-volume RBC transfusions in preterm infants

Transfuse infants at hematocrit <30%
- a. If receiving <35% supplemental hood oxygen
- b. If on continuous positive airway pressure (CPAP) or mechanical ventilation with mean airway pressure <6 cm H_2O
- c. If significant apnea and bradycardia are noted (>9 episodes in 12 hours or two episodes in 24 hours requiring bag and mask ventilation) while receiving therapeutic doses of methylxanthines.
- d. If heart rate >180 beats/min or respiratory rate >80 breaths/min persists for 24 hours.
- e. If weight gain <10 g/day is observed over 4 days while receiving ≥100 kcal/kg/day in the absence of sepsis.
- f. If undergoing surgery.

Transfuse for hematocrit ≤ 35%
- a. If receiving >35% supplemental hood oxygen
- b. If intubated, on CPAP or mechanical ventilation with mean airway pressure <6-8 cm H_2O.

Do not transfuse
- a. To replace blood removal for laboratory tests alone
- b. For low hematocrit alone.

REFERENCES

1. Luchtman-Jones L, Schwartz AL, Wilson DB. The blood and hematopoietic system. In: Fanaroff AA, Martin RJ (Eds). Neonatal-perinatal medicine. Disorders of fetus and infant. 7th edn. St.Louis, MO: Mosby; 2002. pp. 1182-1254.
2. Finne PH, Halvorsen S. Regulation of erythropoiesis in the fetus and newborn. Arch Dis Child. 1972;47(255):683-7.
3. Robin K Ohls, Robert D Christensen. The Hematopoietic system. In: Robert M Kliegman, Richard E Behrman, Hal B Jenson, Bonita F Stanton (Eds). Nelson Textbook of pediatrics. 18th edn. Elsevier;2008.pp.1997-2003.
4. Aher S, Malwatkar K, Kadam S. Neonatal anemia. Semin Fetal Neonatal Med. 2008;13(4):239-47.
5. Tse WT, Lux SE. Red blood cell membrane disorders. Br J Haematol. 1999;104:2-13.
6. Kan YW, Forget BG, Nathan DG. Gamma-beta thalassemia: a cause of hemolytic disease of the newborn. N Engl J Med. 1972;286:129-34.
7. Brenda ES Gibson, Christina Halsey. Nonimmune neonatal anemias. In: Robert J Arceci, Ian M Hann, Owen P Smith, (Eds). Pediatric Hematology. 3rd edn. Blackwell Publishing Ltd; 2006. pp. 130-50.
8. Anemia during neonatal period. In: Philip Lanzkowsky (Ed). Manual of Pediatric Hematology and Oncology. 5th edn, Elsevier; 2011. pp. 14-37.
9. Widness JA. Pathophysiology of Anemia During the Neonatal Period, Including anemia of Prematurity. Neoreviews. 2008;9(11):e520.
10. Widness JA. Treatment and Prevention of Neonatal Anemia. Neoreviews. 2008;9(11):526-33.
11. Christou HA, Shannon K, Rowitch DH. Anemia. In: John P Cloherty, Eric C Eichenwald, Ann R Stark, (Eds). Manual of neonatal care. 6th edn. Lippincott Williams and Wilkins; 2008. pp. 436-44.
12. Luban NL. Management of anemia in the newborn. Early Hum Dev. 2008;84(8):493-8.

6 Nutritional Anemia

Neha Rastogi, Anupam Sachdeva, SP Yadav, Panna Choudhury

Anemia is the most prevalent problem in the world particularly in the developing countries.[1] The World Health Organization (WHO) has outlined the criteria for the diagnosis of anemia for various age and sex group by low hemoglobin (Hb) or hematocrit (Hct) (Table 6.1). Anemia is considered mild, when Hb concentrations are above 10 g/dl but below the cut-off value, moderate when the concentration is between 7 and 10 g/dl and severe when it is below 7 g/dl.[2] Epidemiological criteria for assessing the severity and magnitude of anemia in population have been defined by FAO/WHO[3] (Table 6.2).

Table 6.1: Hemoglobin and hematocrit cut-offs to define anemia

Age or sex group	*Hb below g/dl*	*Hct below (%)*
Children 6 months to 5 years	11.0	33
Children 6 to 14 years	12.0	36
Nonpregnant women	12.0	36
Pregnant women	11.0	33
Men	13.0	39

Table 6.2: Parameters for defining the magnitude of prevalence of anemia as a public health problem

Parameters	*Magnitude*		
	High	*Moderate*	*Low*
Percentage of population with less than defined cut-off	>40	10-39	1-9
Percentage of population with Hb <7 g/dl, especially women and children	>10	1-9	<1

PREVALENCE

National Family Health Survey (NFHS)-3 data shows that 7 out of every 10 children in the age-group of 6-59 months in India are anemic. Three percent of children (age 6-59 months) are severely anemic (less than 7.0 g/dl), 40 percent are moderately anemic (7.0-9.9 g/dl), and 26 percent are mildly anemic (10.0-10.9 g/dl).[4] Anemia among children is widespread throughout India. The prevalence of anemia varies from 38 percent in Goa to 78 percent in Bihar. More than half of young children in 24 states have anemia, including 11 states where more than two-thirds of children are anemic. A prevalence rate of over 65% in preschool children has been reported in various studies undertaken in rural and urban India.[5] In the adolescent period (10-19 years), in a multicentric study, it was found that the incidence of anemia is about 50% and increases from 10 years onwards and continues to remain high till 18 years of age.[6] By all accounts, India falls in the category of high magnitude prevalence for anemia.

Prevalence survey and surveillance data usually do not distinguish between different causative factors of anemia. As nutritional deficiencies account for most of the anemic cases, it is often referred to as nutritional anemia from public health view point. Iron deficiency (ID) is usually the most common cause of anemia. If in a population anemia prevalence exceeds 40%, all children <5 years of age and all women of childbearing age will be iron deficient.[7] Iron deficiency affects nearly 2170 million persons worldwide, and 1200 million of them are anemic, of which 90% are in the developing countries.[8] Besides iron deficiency anemia (IDA), the importance of other micronutrients in causation of anemia is being increasingly realized. In a recent study in an urban slum of Delhi, nearly half of the anemic young children had other nutritional deficiencies notably vitamin B_{12} and folic acid as the direct or associated cause.[9] The nutrients which cause anemia and their normal daily requirements are shown in Table 6.3.[10]

IRON DEFICIENCY ANEMIA

Etiology

A thorough understanding of iron requirement, intake and bioavailability is essential to explain why some individuals—infants, young children, women in

Table 6.3: Normal requirement of some vitamins that may cause anemia

Nutrients	*Infants*		*Preschool*	*School*	*Adolescents*
	0-6	*6-12 months*	*1-5 years*	*7-12 years*	*13-18 years*
Vitamin A (µg/L)	350		400	600	600
Vitamin B_6 (mg)	0.3	0.4	0.9	1.6	2.0
Thiamine (mg/1000 cal)			——0.5——		
Riboflavin (mg/1000 cal)			——0.6——		
Vitamin C (mg)			25	40	
Vitamin E	——0.8 mg/g essential FFA——				
Folate (µ)	25		40-50	60-70	100
Vitamin B_{12} (µ)	0.2			0.2-1.0	

Adapted from ICMR report[10]

Table 6.4: Recommended dietary (iron) allowances for Indians

Group	*Particulars*	*Body weight (kg)*	*Iron (mg/day)*
Children	1-3 years	12.2	12
	4-6 years	19.0	18
	7-9 years	26.9	26
Boys	10-12 years	35.4	34
	13-15 years	47.8	41
	16-18 years	57.1	50
Girls	10-12 years	31.5	19
	13-15 years	46.7	28
	16-18 years	49.9	30
Men		60	28
Women		50	30
Pregnant women		50	38
Lactation (0-6 months)		50	30

reproductive age group (particularly pregnant women)—are at a greater risk of developing IDA than others. The iron requirements for various age/sex groups are given in Table 6.4.[10] The balance between requirements and the amount of iron absorbed can be disturbed by several factors working in concert or individually.

a. *Inadequate iron supply:* Low overall dietary intake is one of the most important factors responsible for low iron intake. Low intake of iron rich foods further aggravates the situation.
b. *Bioavailability of dietary iron:* Factors enhancing or inhibiting iron absorption play a significant role in determining the bioavailability of dietary iron. During first 6 months of life, breastfed infants are usually not iron deficient, as bioavailability of iron from breast milk is very high. Infants receiving predominantly cereal based weaning foods thereafter are however prone to anemia as iron absorption from this cereal based diet is very low. It is estimated that in the wheat millet based diet, iron absorption is around 2% and in rice-based diet, iron absorption is around 5-8%.
c. *Decreased absorption of the iron:* High infection rates, Giardiasis and gastrointestinal problems interfere with food intake and the absorption. This may result in the development of anemia, particularly in young children when iron balance is precarious.
d. *Chronic blood loss:* Hookworm infestations and various gastrointestinal pathologies may cause iron losses. However, chronic blood losses leading to IDA generally do not constitute a public health problem.

Pathogenesis

Iron deficiency anemia is the end stage of a relatively long drawn process of deterioration in the iron status of an individual. It is only seen in the severe iron deficiency state, which may be divided into three functionally distinct stages of severity.

Stage I: Iron depletion with decrease in iron stores, reduction in ferritin levels and stainable iron in the bone marrow. Hemoglobin, serum iron, transferrin concentration and saturation are within normal limits.

Stage II: Iron deficient erythropoiesis leading to low serum ferritin, serum iron, and raised TIBC and free erythrocyte protoporphyrin. Hemoglobin may still be normal.

Stage III: Iron deficiency anemia (IDA) with significantly reduced hemoglobin production resulting in microcytosis and hypochromia.[6]

IRON METABOLISM

There are two major sources of food iron: heme and non-heme iron. Heme iron is highly bioavailable, since it is absorbed intact within the porphyrin ring and is not influenced by most inhibitory factors in the diet. It is present in meat, fish and poultry as well as in blood products. In the developing countries especially India, heme iron intake is lower or even negligible. The second type of dietary iron, non-heme iron, is a more important source and is found to varying degrees in all foods of plant origin. This non-heme iron enters an exchangeable pool, which is markedly affected by promotive and inhibitory iron binding ligands. Some forms of non-heme iron, notably ferritin and hemosiderin only partially enter the exchangeable pool and are poorly absorbed. Besides this, the diet may also contain exogenous iron originating from the soil, water, and dust or cooking vessels. This is more frequently the case in developing countries where the amount of such contamination iron in a meal may be several times greater than the amount of food iron. The cooking of foods in iron pots may increase the iron content of a meal several fold.

Iron is not absorbed from the stomach. Maximum absorption of iron occurs from the duodenum and it decreases as the food passes down the small intestine. The exact mechanism of iron absorption and its regulation are not clear. Two steps are involved in the absorption of iron: entry of iron from the intestinal lumen into the mucosal cell and its passage from the mucosal cell into the plasma. Only a fraction of the iron that enters the mucosal cell finds its way into the plasma the remainder being held in the cell as ferritin, which is lost from the body as the mucosal cell is desquamated into the lumen at the end of its life of 3-4 days. Iron status of the body at the time of the formation of the mucosal lining cells determines the amount of iron that is absorbed through these cells. With increased iron stores there is increased transferrin saturation and increased 'messenger' iron in the mucosal cell. This 'messenger' iron stimulates the production of apoferritin. Thus, whenever there is increased transferrin saturation, a larger fraction of the iron entering the mucosal cell is held back as ferritin and discarded, as the cell is desquamated. Excessive accumulation of iron by absorption is thus prevented. Iron absorption is increased with decreased iron stores, increased erythropoietic activity and during pregnancy.

Iron metabolism is also affected by hepcidin. Hepcidin is small peptide with a central position in the regulation of iron recycling and balance. Hepcidin is primarily expressed by the liver in response to acute-phase reactions, any further expression depends on the degree of hepatic iron storage, and hypoxia and/or anemia strongly down-regulate hepatic hepcidin release.[11] Movement of iron from the enterocyte into the bloodstream is mediated by the iron exporter ferroportin (FPN) (iron-regulated transporter-1). Ferroportin is located along the entire basolateral membrane of enterocytes, in tissue macrophages, in the liver (Kupffer's cells), spleen and bone marrow, predominantly in the intracellular vesicular compartment. This protein also serves as an iron exporter in circulating phagocytic cells that recycle iron from senescent erythrocytes. Greater than 60% of total iron is present in erythrocytes. Thus, efficient heme iron recycling is critical in iron homeostasis. Hepcidin inhibits cellular iron export through binding directly to the iron exporter ferroportin and inducing its internalization and degradation in HEK-293 cells. The direct hepcidin–FPN interaction allows an adaptative response from the body in situations that alter normal iron homeostasis (hypoxia, anemia, iron deficiency, iron overload, and inflammation). Hepcidin (i) inhibits intestinal iron absorption, (ii) blocks iron transport across the placenta, and (iii) induces iron sequestration in macrophages. When body iron requirements are high (decreased iron stores or increased rate of erythropoiesis), the expression of hepcidin is decreased; a decline in the iron requirements leads to a reverse process.[12]

CLINICAL FEATURES OF IDA

Clinical features of iron deficiency anemia are similar to those due to anemia of any type. As the fall of hemoglobin is very gradual the onset of symptoms is very insidious. Symptoms depend on the rate of fall of hemoglobin and homeostatic adjustment of various systems in the body. Initially, pallor, anorexia and irritability may be noticed. Hyperdynamic circulation may lead to palpitation, fatigue, and shortness of breath, decreased exercise intolerance and congestive heart failure. Koilonychia, platynychia, glossitis, stomatitis, angular cheilosis are the other common features. Formation of mucosal webs at the pharyngoesophageal junction causes dysphagia, which is much more for solids than liquids. The triad of dysphasia due to esophageal webs, koilonychia and splenomegaly in a patient with IDA is known as the Plummer-Vinson or Patterson Kelly syndrome. Gastritis is common in IDA but usually is asymptomatic. Mild degree of hepatosplenomegaly is also not uncommon. Pica is a well-documented feature of anemia in children. Craving to eat unusual substances such as dirt, clay, ice, laundry starch, salt, cardboard, etc. are seen in almost 70-80% of patients and usually are cured by prompt iron therapy. Pedal edema in IDA may be due to congestive heart failure, impaired renal function or associated protein deficiency. Rarely increased intracranial tension with papilledema may occur. Skull changes similar to those seen in congenital hemolytic anemia may be seen in children with iron deficiency since early life. These skeletal changes do not reverse with iron therapy.

There is increasing evidence that iron deficiency *per se* even in the absence of obvious anemia leads to many deleterious effects on various systems. Several morphological and biochemical changes at the tissue level have been shown to be the result of iron deficiency *per se*, independent of the hemoglobin level. Functional impairment of various tissues such as the myocardium, peripheral nerves, jejunum, cerebral cortex, kidney and liver have been demonstrated in patients of iron deficiency, which have been corrected by iron therapy before a significant rise in the hemoglobin level.

CONSEQUENCES OF IRON DEFICIENCY

There are studies to suggest that children with iron deficiency are at high-risk of long-term impairment in mental and motor development. They also suffer from lower scores in IQ test, lack of concentration, short attention span and easy distractibility. Such deficits in cognitive functions may eventually result in school dropouts. What is worrying is that developmental deficits that occur due to iron deficiency in infancy have been shown to be irreversible.[13] Thus prevention of IDA in infants and growing children is an urgent need as it may lead to a permanent deficit in IQ. Iron deficiency also adversely affects immune system thus increasing the susceptibility to infection. Another area of special significance is poor endurance and physical fitness even with mild anemia, which may be an obstacle to children for self-fulfillment and overall development[14] (Table 6.5).

Table 6.5: Benefits of effective IDA control program

Population group	*Benefits*
Children	Improved behavioral and cognitive development Where severe anemia is common, improved child survival
Adolescence	Improve cognitive development In girls, better iron stores for later pregnancy
Pregnant women and their infants	Decreased low birth weight and perinatal mortality Where severe anemia is common, decreased maternal mortality and obstetrical complications
All individuals	Improved fitness and work capacity Improved recognition

ASSESSMENT OF IRON STATUS AND SCREENING FOR ANEMIA

When negative iron balance ensues in a setting of normal body iron stores, the ultimate development of iron deficiency anemia is preceded by a number of different phases. The individuals begin to suffer from the adverse effects of iron deficiency well before they become frankly anemic. Initially iron is drawn from the stores to meet the needs of erythropoiesis. Exhaustion of body iron reserves is associated with decrease in stainable iron in the bone marrow, fall in serum ferritin to levels below normal and increase in iron absorption and iron binding capacity. These measurements are useful in evaluation of iron stores. Changes in hemoglobin concentration (Hb), serum iron, transferrin saturation (TS), free erythrocyte protoporphyrin (FEP) and marrow sideroblasts occur after the iron reserves are depleted. These tests are useful measures of functional iron (Table 6.6).[2]

Table 6.6: Laboratory screening for iron deficiency

- Single measures
  - Hemoglobin
  - Serum ferritin
  - Erythrocyte protoporphyrin
  - Serum transferrin receptor
- Dual measures
  - Serum ferritin + hemoglobin
  - Erythrocyte protopophyrin + hemoglobin
  - Serum transferrin receptor + hemoglobin
  - Serum ferritin + serum transferrin receptor

Laboratory Evaluation of Iron Status

Hemoglobin Concentration (Hb)

Both hemoglobin and hematocrit (Hct) are equally useful tests and are interpreted similarly. On average hematocrit values are roughly equivalent to three times the hemoglobin concentration. A fall in Hb or Hct represents anemia without any indication to its etiology. Hemoglobin (Hb) estimation, by cyanmethemoglobin method is considered sensitive, rapid and inexpensive investigation for routine practice and field level. Hb estimation by hemocue hemoglobin photometer has also been found simple and reliable, though it may be costly. The major limitation of Hb measurement is its low specificity. The Hb concentration alone does not distinguish between iron deficiency anemia and anemia due to other causes.

Erythrocyte Morphology and Red Cell Indices

In a mild iron deficiency, red cell morphology and other red cell indices, e.g. MCV, MCH and MCHC are not altered. However, in iron deficiency anemia, RBCs become microcytic hypochromic and red cell indices are low, i.e. MCV <80 fl, MCH <27 pg and MCHC <33%. MCV is more sensitive than MCH, but up to 30% cases of IDA could be misdiagnosed if only these indices are relied upon.

Red Cell Size Distribution

Electronic counters can provide red cell size distribution. The variability in red cell sizes is reported as red cell distribution width (RDW). An elevated red cells distribution width (RDW) more than 14.5% is strongly suggestive of iron deficiency. In thalassemia trait and anemia of chronic disease the RDW is normal.

Serum Ferritin

The serum ferritin is a sensitive laboratory index of iron status. It is estimated that each ng/ml of serum ferritin is equivalent to 8-10 mg of storage iron. A serum ferritin value of <12 ng/ml is highly specific for iron deficiency but gives no information about its magnitude. Another major limitation of serum ferritin is that its level is increased in chronic disorders, e.g. chronic infection and thus coexisting iron deficiency anemia can be missed.

Serum Iron, Total Iron Binding Capacity (TIBC) and Transferrin Saturation (TS)

A normal serum iron level varies considerably, as it has a diurnal variation and peaks in the morning and decreases in the evening. Serum iron concentration may also be affected by chronic infection, malignancy and chemotherapy. Serum iron value of <40 μg/dl (<12 mcg/dl in young children) is considered diagnostic of iron deficiency uncomplicated by infection or other disorders which affect iron metabolism.

TIBC is the measure of transferrin circulating in the blood. Usually, there is enough transferrin present in 100 ml of serum to bind about 250-450 μg of iron. Since normal serum iron concentration is 100 μg/dl, transferrin may be found to be one-third saturated with iron. In iron deficiency states, TIBC is increased and transferrin saturation level is less than 16% (<14% for children). TIBC <200 μg/dl is characteristic of inflammatory disease.

Transferrin saturation = Serum iron/TIBC × 100

Free Erythrocyte Protoporphyrin (FEP) and Protoporphyrin:Heme (P:H) Ratio

Erythrocyte protoporphyrin, the precursor of heme accumulates in red blood cells when it has insufficient iron to combine with to form heme. The FEP can be measured by a simple fluorescence assay performed directly on the thin film of blood. Therefore, both FEP and P:H ratio is elevated in iron deficiency. Normal values of FEP are 30-40 μg/dl RBC and P:H ratio 16 (±5.3). FEP values above 70 μg/dl RBC and of P:H ratio above 32 is thought to represent iron deficiency.

Serum Transferrin Receptor (sTFR)

The serum transferrin receptor increases with enhanced red cell production but iron deficiency is the only disorder in which there is increased serum receptor combined with a low level of red cell production. Unlike the serum ferritin, which only identifies iron deficiency, the serum transferrin receptor measures its severity. Values above 9 mg/L are considered abnormal, mean levels in healthy male and female subjects are 5.6 mg/L. Unlike many other iron measurements, the level remains normal in patients with anemia of chronic inflammation or infection and therefore assists in identifying iron deficiency in population where chronic infection is common. The serum receptor is measured by the same ELISA system as the ferritin and requires only a few microliter of plasma or serum.

Stainable Iron in the Bone Marrow

Bone marrow aspirates can be stained for hemosiderin by Perl's reaction and iron content is graded from 0 to 4. Although it is the most accurate technique to evaluate iron status, it is an invasive procedure and therefore impractical.

Response to Therapy

In uncomplicated IDA, administration of iron shows a predictable reticulocytosis and a rise in Hb. Hb concentration remains the most dominant predictor of response to therapy in uncomplicated iron deficiency. A positive response to therapy can be defined as a daily increase in Hb concentration of 0.1 g/dl (0.3 or 1% rise in Hct) from the 4th day onwards.

Multiple Indices

Hemoglobin remains a key screening measurement, but it has a low sensitivity and specificity. Its utility can be enhanced combining it with a more specific index of iron status. A very useful combination of measurements is the hemoglobin and serum ferritin. If both measurements are normal, iron deficiency is excluded; if both are low, iron deficiency anemia is unequivocally identified. If the serum ferritin is low but the hemoglobin is normal, the individual is at risk of iron deficiency, while if the hemoglobin is low but the serum ferritin is normal further hematological assessment is required to identify the cause of anemia.[15,16]

TREATMENT

Treatment of anemia depends upon the severity and associated complications. Cases with Hb level <5 g/dl may require hospitalization, as some of the patients may already be in congestive cardiac failure. Blood transfusion is required only in most severe cases with Hb concentration <3 g/dl. Young children may have to be transfused at Hb level less than 4-5 g/dl due to higher risk of congestive cardiac failure or when superimposed infection may interfere with the response. Rapid correction of anemia by transfusion may be dangerous due to the risk of hypervolemia and cardiac dilatation. Packed or sedimented red cells should be slowly administered, preferably 2-3 ml/kg at one time.[17]

Medicinal Iron Therapy

For infants and children, the recommended therapeutic dose is 3 mg of iron per kg per day.[1] For women (15 years +) with severe anemia (Hb <7 g/dl) National Nutritional Anemia Control Program (NNACP) recommends three tablets of iron-folate per day (each tablet containing 100 mg of elemental iron and 500 µg of folic acid) for a minimum of 100 days.[18] Although the desired Hb level is usually reached in 2 months, iron therapy should continue for another 2 months to build up iron stores to 250-300 mg or the serum ferritin level to 30 µg/L.

Preparations of Iron Tablets

Practically all medicinal preparations now contain ferrous compounds, which are better absorbed than ferric iron. Ferrous sulfate, gluconate and fumarate are the compounds mostly used. Other ferrous compounds previously or still in use include ferrous succinate, lactate, glycine sulfate, glutamate, citrate, tartrate and pyrophosphate. Although ferrous succinate is probably more completely absorbed, these compounds, in addition to being more expensive, offer no advantages over ferrous fumarate, gluconate or sulfate. Iron absorption is comparatively poor from carbonate, citrate, choline citrate, calcium citrate and pyrophosphate salts and combinations. Table 6.7 shows the iron content of some preparations.

Table 6.7: Elemental iron content of various iron tablets

Preparation	*Approximate iron content (%)*
Ferrous sulfate, exsiccated	30
Ferrous sulfate ($7H_2O$)	20
Ferrous sulfate, anhydrous	37
Ferrous fumarate	33
Ferrous gluconate	12
Ferrous carbonate	16
Ferrous glycine sulfate	23
Ferrous succinate	35
Iron choline citrate	12
Ferric chloride	44
Ferric sulfate	27
Ferric hydroxide	50
Ferric ammonium citrate	18
Ferric saccharate	10
Ferric pyrophosphate	25
Ferric orthophosphate	28
NaFeEDTA	14
Hemoglobin	0.34
Elemental iron powders	
Hydrogen-reduced iron	97
Electrolytically reduced iron	98
Carbonyl-reduced iron	98

Combination with Other Nutrients

Folic acid can be combined with iron at negligible extra cost. Tablets with combination of folate and ferrous sulfate, are usually available and particularly useful for pregnant women. Addition of vitamin C (200 mg) increases the absorption of iron by about 30%, but addition of vitamin C may add to the cost significantly. Vitamin B_{12} may need to be given in non-responders or those with evidence of megaloblastic anemia.

Side Effects

Side effects are seen in about 14% cases and not related to any particular iron compounds. Intolerance to oral iron is basically related to the dose of iron. Usual side effects are nausea, vomiting, constipation, diarrhea, and abdominal discomfort.[17] Non-compliance is stated to be more often due to poor counseling and lack of motivation. Patients discontinue therapy as soon as they feel better and/or experience discomfort with the medications. Difficulty of sustaining motivation for two to three months in subjects who do not perceive themselves to be ill has posed a great challenge to health educators. It is essential to continue the therapy, if necessary, at a lower dose or the tablets may be given with meals if that improves compliance. Iron taken with a meal is better tolerated, though absorption is reduced. The required amount may also be given in two divided doses, which will reduce side effects.

Parenteral Iron Therapy

Parenteral route should usually be avoided and is indicated in cases having severe side effects on oral therapy, noncompliance or gastrointestinal bleeding, which is aggravated by oral iron therapy. Complete iron requirement can be given in a single dose, known as total dose infusion. However, infusions can be given only in a hospital as anaphylactic reactions may occur. Iron dextran complex is the most commonly used preparation. The desired level of Hb to be increased can be precisely calculated. Keeping in account 50% or more iron for replenishing body store, the iron requirement can be determined from the equation:

Iron (mg) = Weight (kg) × Hb deficit (g/dl) × 80/100 × 3.4 × 1.5 or Weight (kg) × Hb deficit (g/dl) × 4.

Adverse reactions of parenteral iron therapy include anaphylaxis, skin rash, myalgia, arthralgia, etc.

Response to Therapy

Rapid hematologic response can be confidently predicted in iron deficiency. There is no evidence that the rate of Hb response is different in oral or parenteral therapy. Whether iron is given orally or parenterally the response to therapy should be carefully followed. Iron absorption, is maximum during the initial phase of therapy and declines from 14% in the 1st week to 7% in the 4th week to 2% after 4 months. A positive response to therapy can be defined as a daily increase in hemoglobin concentration of 0.1 g/dl (0.3 or 1% rise in hematocrit) from the 4th day onwards. Approximately 2 months are required to achieve a normal Hb level. Reticulocytes increase within 3-5 days and reach a maximum at 5-10 days, reticulocyte counts being 8-10 % in severe anemia. The maximum rate of recovery from severe anemia in a child may be 0.25–0.4 g/dl per day increase in Hb or a 1% per day rise in hematocrit, which is more rapid than is anticipated in the adult. The expected clinical and hematological response to iron therapy are described in Table 6.8.

Table 6.8: Response to iron therapy in iron deficiency anemia

12-24 hours	Replacement of iron enzymes; subjective improvement; decreased irritability; increased appetite
36-48 hours	Initial bone marrow response; erythroid hyperplasia
48-72 hours	Reticulocytosis, peaking at 5-7 days
4-30 days	Increase in Hb level
1-3 months	Repletion of stores

Nonresponders to Iron Therapy

This is evidenced by absence of rise in Hb or reticulocyte response, after 2 weeks of adequate therapy and needs to be investigated. Associated chronic infection may interfere with proper utilization of iron. Nutritional megaloblastic anemia is often associated and is seen in 2% preschool children in countries where malnutrition is common. Addition of folic acid as low as 100-200 µg per day will show fast response to treatment and reticulocytosis in 2-4 days in majority of cases. However, excess folate has no deleterious effect and hence recommended dose is 1-5 mg per day. Vitamin B_{12} deficiency may be present in children, particularly infants and needs to be added if there is no response to iron-folate therapy. Nonresponse to therapy should also arouse suspicion for possibilities like thalassemia, pure red cell aplasia, renal failure and chronic blood loss, e.g. hereditary hemorrhagic telangiectasia (Table 6.9).

PREVENTION OF NUTRITIONAL ANEMIA

The three basic approaches to the prevention of IDA are:
1. Supplementation with medicinal iron
2. Dietary modification
3. Fortification of food with iron.

Table 6.9: Poor response to oral iron

- Noncompliance
- Ongoing blood loss
- Insufficient duration of therapy
- High gastric pH
  - Antacids
- Histamine-2 blockers
- Gastric acid pump inhibitors
- Inhibitors of iron absorption/utilization
  - Lead
  - Aluminum intoxication (hemodialysis patients)
  - Chronic inflammation
  - Neoplasia
- Incorrect diagnosis
  - Thalassemia
- Sideroblastic anemia

For the control of nutritional anemia the effective convergence of all the three approaches is recommended.[19]

Supplementation with Medicinal Iron

Iron store present at birth and the highly bioavailable iron in breast milk protects an infant from IDA up to 6 months. Supplementation with medicinal iron has been recommended by WHO for all children beyond 6 months of age till 12 months of age and low birth weight babies from 2 months onwards till 24 months of age.[20] According to ESPGHAN guidelines, prophylactic entral iron supplementation in newborn less than 1800 g, should be started at 2-6 weeks of age (2-4 weeks in extremely low birth weight infants) at the dose of 2-3 mg/kg/day. Iron supplementation should be continued at least until 6-12 months of age.[21]

Daily Versus Weekly Supplementation

In humans, intestinal mucosal turnover time is five to six days and is used as the basis for the weekly preventive supplemental regimen. This could be a community based long-term and targeted regimen aiming at prevention of iron deficiency and at increasing iron reserves among adolescents and women. Recent results from a one-month supplementation study show that iron deficient and anemic women can absorb as much as 30-40 mg of iron per week from a single 60 or 120 mg dose of iron ingested on an empty stomach, demonstrating that if there is a high demand for iron as much as the equivalent of 4.3-5.7 mg of iron daily (30-40 mg/week divided by 7) can be absorbed from the supplement provided. This, plus the dietary iron absorption could supply increased iron demands. Indeed, weekly dosing preserves the absorption of 3 mg of iron ascorbate at higher levels than daily dosing suggesting that food iron absorption is better maintained, adding to the total amount of iron absorbed.[22] (supplemental plus food iron).[23] A recent meta-analysis on utility of weekly iron supplementation concludes that this modality provides therapeutic and prophylactic benefits. The effect on hemoglobin is only marginally lower than daily supplementation.[24] In the public health scenario, weekly supplementation has the advantage of being offered under supervised conditions. On the basis of a recent multicentric study in India National consultation has now recommended that adolescent girls on attaining menarche should consume weekly dosage of one IFA tablet containing 100 mg elemental iron and 500 µg folic acid once a week accompanied by appropriate dietary consultation. Thus, a pack of 25 tablets would provide requirement for 6 months. Weekly dose is considered as cost-effective, with fewer side effects and better compliance.[25] Amongst 1-5-year-old children, daily versus weekly supplementation in a dosing of 3-4 mg/kg showed similar results at the end of a 60-day trial.[26]

Table 6.10: Iron content of food articles

Class of food	*Iron content mg/100 g*	*Articles rich in iron >10 mg/100 g*
Cereals	2.5-14.0	*Bajra*, barley, *kangri*, *ragi*, rice flakes, whole wheat flour
Pulses and legumes	2.7-11.0	Bengal gram, soyabean
Leafy vegetables	0.9-40.0	Amaranth, beet greens, bengal gram leaves, coriander, potato leaves, *pudina*, *neem*, radish top, turnip greens, spinach, *methi*, lettuce.
Roots and tubers	0.4-13.9	
Nuts and oil seeds	2.5-100	Gingelly, mustard, pistachio
Fruits	0.1-10.0	Dates, raisins
Seafood	1.0-115	Fish, crab
Meat	2.0-18.8	
Milk	0.2-0.8	
Miscellaneous		Jaggery, yeast

Dietary Modification

Food based approach, though not suitable for treatment purposes, constitutes the most desirable and sustainable methods of preventing iron deficiency. Once the child has been weaned, dietary modification can help increase iron intake through iron rich foods. On the basis of currently recommended dietary allowances, it seems that the overall intake of iron is adequate (Table 6.10). However, the major limiting factor has been the poor bioavailability of iron due to presence of inhibitors like phytates in cereal-based diet. Phenolic compounds, including tannin present in tea and coffee are also strong absorption inhibitors. Absorption promoter of iron like vitamin C plays a crucial role to prevent iron deficiency. Indian diet has been shown to be deficient in vitamin C as well. Just inclusion of guava fruits with lunch and dinner meals for one month have shown to raise Hb level by 2.2 g/dl.[5] Absorption promoters and inhibitors (Table 6.11) can make a significant difference in the availability of iron from the food in an individual. Fermentation and germination can enhance iron absorption by increasing vitamin C content and lowering phytic acid content. Heme iron

Table 6.11: Factors influencing dietary iron absorption

Heme iron absorption
- Amount of heme iron especially as meat
- Content of calcium in meal
- Food preparation (time, temperature)

Nonheme iron absorption
- Iron status of subjects
- Amount of potentially available non-heme iron (adjustments for fortification iron and contamination iron)
- Balance between positive and negative factors

Positive factors	*Negative factors*
Ascorbic acid	Phytate
Meat, poultry, fish	Iron binding polyphenols including tannin
Germination	Calcium
Fermentation	Soy protein

present in meat is not only better absorbed, but increases absorption of non-heme iron of vegetable foods. In India vegetarianism is practiced widely and as such iron and vitamin C rich food items like green leafy vegetables and fruits probably hold the key for successful prevention of iron deficiency.

Fortification of Foods

Fortification of foods with iron is a cost-effective, long-term measure for improving the iron status of the entire population. India does not have any iron fortification program currently. A formula for double fortified salt, i.e. salt fortified with iodine and iron has been developed and is being field-tested. It could be a very cost-effective measure if found effective.

MACROCYTIC-MEGALOBLASTIC ANEMIA

After iron, vitamin B_{12} and folate deficiency are the most important causes of nutritional anemia and lead to megaloblastic anemia. Newborns and infants are prone to deficiency, if their mother is deficient in these micronutrients.[27]

Vitamin B_{12} (cobalamin) is found in animal tissues but not in vegetable matter. Microorganisms like bacteria and fungi synthesize it. The daily requirement of vitamin B_{12} is 1.0 μg. Milk, vegetables, cereals, pulses, etc. are poor sources of B_{12} so that a vegetarian diet is deficient in it. Liver, kidney, meat, fish, salmon, crabs, oysters, egg-yolk, etc. are rich sources. The steps of cobalamin absorption in the gastrointestinal tract are discussed below. Cobalamin is released by enzymatic digestion from protein complexes in food in the acid pH of the stomach, where it binds to R binder present in saliva and gastric juice. This binder is closely related to transcobalamin (TC) I present in plasma, and is similar to a binder in milk and other fluids. After release from R binder in the duodenum by pancreatic proteases, cobalamin binds to intrinsic factor (IF), which is synthesized by gastric parietal cells. Cobalamin in bile is also attached to R binder and complexes with IF in the duodenum. The IF–cobalamin complex attaches to its receptor cubulin on the ileal brush border. Within the enterocyte, the IF–cobalamin complex is digested, probably within lysosomes, and the cobalamin appears in portal blood attached to TCII. In the plasma, cobalamin can bind to either TCI or TCII. The cobalamin bound to TCII is transported into various tissues where it is available for its metabolic function. Cobalamin is stored by hepatocytes and is lost from the body with a half-life of about 400 days. Depletion thus requires a prolonged period of poor intake or absorption.[28]

The daily requirement of folic acid in humans as per WHO recommendations is 3 μg/kg/day of food folate for adults[29] with supplements for pregnant and lactating women and infants. Folate is widely distributed in foods and is selectively concentrated in a few tissues like liver, kidney and spinach. Egg, milk and meat are poor sources. Folic acid is absorbed from the whole length of small intestine. In the body, folate is stored in the liver but the major route of utilization of hepatic folate appears to be by secretion into the bile and reabsorption from the gut. The normal total body folate stores are 5-10 mg and one-third of this is in the liver. With the deficient intake, folate stores get exhausted within a few weeks.

Vitamin B_{12} deficiency usually manifests in children over 2 years as body store is 3-5 mg and the daily loss is just 2-4 μg per day. In contrast folate deficiency manifest as early as 4 months despite store of 5-20 mg as the daily loss is 100 μg per day.

As far as blood tests are concerned, it is not possible to differentiate B_{12} and folate deficiencies. Effects of deficiency of either of the two are conditioned by the status for the other.

Nutritional deficiency occurs:
- In newborns and infants, born to deficient mothers.
- In older children and adolescents having poor intake of diet causing malnutrition or practicing vegetarianism diet which leads to B_{12} deficiency. Folate being heat labile is also lost up to 80% in cooked food.

- Impaired absorption due to absence of intrinsic factor or diseases involving ileum or bypassing it also leads to malabsorption like tropical sprue, celiac disease, regional ileitis, idiopathic steatorrhea.
- Defective utilization in liver diseases due to reduction in the enzymes involved in folate metabolism. Anticonvulsants like hydantoin, phenobarbitone, antimalarials like pyrimethamine and antimetabolites like aminopterine block folic acid metabolism.
- Increased requirements particularly infants like preterm babies due to rapid growth. The requirement also increases during increased bone marrow activity in conditions like hemolytic anemias, bleeding, leukemias and other myeloproliferative disorders.

Clinical Features

Megaloblastic anemia has a gradual onset but varied clinical presentation and at times may even mimic a hematological malignancy.[27,30] Hyperpigmentation of dorsum of hands and fingers is a characteristic feature. Vitamin B_{12} deficiency may cause impaired maturation of cells of the mucosa of the mouth, tongue, and esophagus leading to gastrointestinal features like glossitis, nausea, constipation, diarrhea, loss of appetite and weight loss. Failure to thrive, growth retardation, poor cerebral development, infantile tremor syndrome, convulsions may be seen. Neurological features as seen in subacute combined degeneration of spinal cord are however, seen basically in pernicious anemia and not generally seen in nutritional B_{12} deficiency. Folate deficiency may be associated with neurological features like depression, psychosis, peripheral neuropathy; cardiovascular disease associated with atherosclerosis and thrombosis. There is also evidence to suggest that mothers deficient in folate may give birth to baby with neural tube defects.

Diagnosis

1. *Peripheral blood smear:* Demonstrating multilobed neutrophils can make the diagnosis. The red cells show macro-ovalocytes. There may be leukopenia and thrombocytopenia. The reticulocyte count is normal or low in an untreated case. Occasionally, megaloblasts may be seen in the peripheral smear.
2. *Bone marrow examination:* Bone marrow examination will show presence of megaloblasts, which are larger than the normoblasts of a corresponding developmental stage. The nucleus shows an open chromatin network with a normal cytoplasm and normal hemoglobinization. The cells of myeloid series are often called giant myelocytes and giant metamyelocytes.
3. *Estimation of serum B_{12} and folic acid:* A serum B_{12} level of <100 pg/ml and a serum folate level of <3 ng/ml are diagnostic of their respective deficiencies. However, deficiency of one produces changes in the serum level of the other. In patients with severe deficiency of folate, the concentration of cobalamin in plasma may be subnormal. This will become normal over a period of days after folate treatment is begun. Reduced erythrocyte folate levels (<150 ng/ml) are diagnostic of folate deficiency. Red blood cell assays are less affected by recent changes in diet or medications.
4. *FIGLU test:* In folate deficiency the conversion of formiminoglutamic acid (FIGLU) to glutamic acid is impaired. Thus when a loading dose of histidine which gets converted to FIGLU is given to a person with folate deficiency, he is not able to convert this FIGLU to glutamic acid resulting in excessive excretion of FIGLU in the urine which can be estimated.
5. *Schilling test:* Absorption of B_{12} can be tested by this test. 1000 μg of B_{12} is given parenterally to saturate the stores. Now, Co-58 labeled B_{12} is given orally and the amount of radioactivity in the urine is measured by a scintillation counter. Reduced excretion of Co-58 labeled B_{12} in the urine is diagnostic of impaired B_{12} absorption.
6. Serum methylmalonic acid is elevated in cobalamin but not folate deficiency. It is also elevated in renal failure, thyroid disease, hemoconcentration, small bowel bacterial overgrowth and pregnancy. Serum homocysteine is elevated in both folate and cobalamin deficiency. Homocysteine levels are less specific and are elevated in renal dysfunction, hypothyroidism, vitamin B_6 deficiency and with certain medications such as cholestyramine, carbamazepine and valproic acid. Hence, patients with suspected cobalamin or folate deficiency and normal serum levels should be investigated with plasma or serum methylmalonic acid and homocysteine levels.

However, the most practical, cheap and easily available test is a *therapeutic trial*. Here, 100-1000 μg of B_{12}, i.e. cyanocobalamin or hydroxycobalamin is given intramuscularly. *Diagnosis of B_{12} deficiency* is made if: (1) The megaloblastic changes in the erythroid series in bone marrow normalize in 48 hours. (2) At least two of the following occur: (i) serum iron decreases by 50% in 24 hours; (ii) reticulocyte count increases in 5-10 days; (iii) correction of thrombocytopenia in 2 weeks; (iv) correction of neutropenia in 2 weeks; (v) decrease in MCV by 5 fl in 2 weeks after reticulocytosis has subsided; (vi) decrease in plasma methylmalonic acid (MMA) and total homocysteine levels in two weeks; (vii) correction of anemia in 2-4 weeks; (viii) decrease in neutrophil lobe count in 4 weeks. To detect *folate deficiency* 0.5 mg/day of oral folate is given for 2-3 days. Within 2 weeks reticulocytosis and metabolic normalization is seen.

Correction of Vitamin B_{12} and Folate Deficiency

The deficiency of both vitamin B_{12} and folic acid can be corrected by either oral or parentral supplementation of the respective vitamin. Injection of vitamin B_{12} should be given by parentral route if there is any doubt about the absorptive function. Vitamin B_{12} injection of 100 µg may be given every 3-4 days for 3-4 weeks followed by oral route. Alternatively, 1000 µg of vitamin B_{12} is given weekly for 5 weeks. Oral dose of folic acid is 1.0 mg daily for 2-3 weeks. By parenteral route 5.0 mg. of folic acid every week should be an adequate dose. In cases of megaloblastic anemia, the response can be judged by the reticulocyte response seen between 5 and 10 days after starting the treatment. This is followed by a rise in hemoglobin.

In cases of combined deficiency vitamin B_{12} should be supplemented before the folic acid for the fear of precipitation of neurological complications. Megaloblastic anemia associated with antimetabolite (antifolic acid) therapy does not respond to folic acid but to folinic acid. Similarly, folate deficiency in liver disease, which is due to reduction in the enzymes concerned with folate metabolism, will also respond to folinic acid. Treatment of the cause leading to deficiency like tape worm infestation, malabsorption states, etc. should be treated simultaneously. Reduction of nutritional anemia should receive top priority for national health and wealth. This will require a multipronged approach with better utilization of health infrastructure through proper planning and full participation of communities.

REFERENCES

1. DeMaeyer EM, Dallmen P, Gurney JM, Hallberg L, Sood SK, Srikantia SG. Prevention of iron deficiency anemia. In: Preventing and Controlling Iron Deficiency Anemia through Primary Health Care. Geneva, World Health Organization; 1989. pp. 34-42.
2. Dubey AP. Iron deficiency anemia: epidemiology, diagnosis and clinical profile. In: Sachdev HPS, Choudhury P (Eds): Nutrition in Children: Developing Country Concerns. New Delhi, Cambridge Press; 1994. pp. 492-524.
3. FAO/WHO. Inter sectoral Conference on Nutrition-Major issues of Nutrition Strategies. FAO/WHO 1992; Theme Paper no. 6, Page 12.
4. Report. National Family Health Survey-3 2005-06. International Institute of Population Sciences, Mumbai, 2009.
5. Seshadri S. Nutritional anemia in south Asia. In: Malnutrition in South Asia: A Regional Profile. ROSA Publication No.5. UNICEF. November, 1997.
6. Vir S. Iron deficiency anemia control-A public health program priority. Proc Nutr Soc Ind. 1999;47:45-73.
7. Dallmen PR, Vip R. Prevalence and causes of anemia in United States 1976. Am J Clin Nutr. 1984;39:437-55.
8. ACC/SCN, 1991. Statement on Iron Deficiency Control. State of the Art Series, Nutrition Policy Discussion 1990; Paper 9.
9. Gomber S, Kumar S, Rusia U, Gupta P, Agarwal KN, Sharma S. Prevalence and etiology of nutritional anemias in early childhood in an urban slum. Indian J Med Res. 1998;107:269-73.
10. Nutrient requirements and recommended dietary allowances for Indians. A report of the expert group of the Indian Council of Medical Research. New Delhi: Indian Council of Medical Research; 1990.
11. Deicher R, Hörl WP. New insights into the regulation of iron homeostasis. Eur J Clin Inv. 2006;36:301-9.
12. Atanasiu V, Manolescu B, Stoian I. Hepcidin–central regulator of iron metabolism. Eur J Haematol. 2007;78:1-10.
13. Lozoff B, Jimenez E, Wolf AW. Long term developmental outcome of infants with iron deficiency. New Eng J Med 1991;325:687-94.
14. Viteri FE. Iron deficiency. In: Proceedings of Ending Hidden Hunger. Montreal, Quebec, Canada, October 10-12, 1991.
15. Seshadri S. Prevalence and implication of nutritional anemia in children. Proceeding of National Symposium cum workshop on Child Nutrition. The Indian Scene; 1990. pp.223-68.
16. Satyanarayana K, Pradhan DR, Ramnath T, Prahlad Rao N. Anemia and physical fitness of school children of rural Hyderabad. Indian Pediatr. 1990;27:715-21.
17. Choudhury P. Management of iron deficiency anemia in clinical practice. In: Sachdev HPS, Choudhury P (Eds). Nutrition in Children: Developing Country Concerns. New Delhi, Cambridge Press; 1994. pp. 237-44.
18. National Nutritional Anemia Control Programme. Policy on Control of Nutritional Anemia. Ministry of Health and Family Welfare, Government of India; 1991. pp. 1-8.
19. Choudhury P, Vir S. Prevention and strategies for control of iron deficiency anemia. In Sachdev HPS, Choudhury P (Eds). Nutrition in Children: Developing Country Concerns. New Delhi, Cambridge Press; 1994. pp. 492-524.
20. Rebecca J Stoltzfus, Michele L Dreyfuss. Who guidelines for the use of iron supplements to prevent and treat iron deficiency anemia. International Nutritional Anemia Consultative Group. ILSI PRESS.
21. Agostoni C, et al. Enteral Nutrient Supply for Preterm Infants: Commentary From the European Society for Paediatric Gastroenterology, Hepatology, and Nutrition Committee on Nutrition. J Pediatr Gastroentrol Nutr. 2010; 50;85-91
22. Report of the USAID/ UNICEF Consultation on Iron/ Micronutrient Supplements for Young Children. Copenhagen, Denmark, UNICEF, August, 1996.

23. Viteri FE. Control of iron deficiency anemia-New approaches. NFI Bulletin. 1999;20:5-7.
24. Sharma A, Prasad K, Rao KV. Identification of an appropriate strategy to control anemia in adolescent girls of poor communities. Indian Pediatr. 2000;37:261-7.
25. Report. National Consultation on Control of Nutritional Anemia in India. Ministry of Health and Family Welfare. Government of India, 1998.
26. Dubey AP, Rana M, Sachdev HPS, Choudhury P. Daily vs. weekly supplementation in anemic children (Abstract). Paper presented at 5th International Congress of Tropical Pediatrics, Jaipur Feb 10-15, 1999.
27. Dubey AP. Megaloblastic anemia. P.H.O. Review. Bulletin of IAP Subspecialty Chapter on pediatric Hemato-Oncology. 1995;8:5-7.
28. Cooper BA. Nutritional macrocytic anemia. In: Fomon, S Zoltkin (Eds): Nutritional Anemias. Nestle Nutrition Workshop Series. 1992;30:39-51.
29. Beaton G. Requirements of vitamim A, iron, folate and vitamin B_{12}: Report of a Joint FAO/WHO Expert Consultation. Rome: FAO, 1988.
30. Gomber S, Kela K, Dhingra N. Clinico-hematological profile of megaloblastic anemia. Indian Pediatr. 1998;35: 55-8.

7 National Nutritional Anemia Control Program

Neha Rastogi, Panna Choudhury, Anupam Sachdeva

Iron deficiency anemia (IDA) affects nearly two billion persons, of which 90% are in the developing countries.[1,2] In India, anemia is a major public health problem and especially affects women in the reproductive age group and young children. In a large scale study conducted by the Indian Council of Medical Research (ICMR), about 53% of children were found to be anemic.[3] Estimates suggest that about 25-50% girls become anemic by the time they reach menarche.[4] The prevalence of anemia in pregnancy ranges from 34.6% to as high as 98.3% with severe anemia accounting for 5.8-48.7% cases.[5,6] Anemia is an important cause of maternal mortality and accounts for 19% of the maternal deaths.[7,8]

NATIONAL NUTRITIONAL ANEMIA PROPHYLAXIS PROGRAM

The National Nutritional Anemia Prophylaxis Program (NNAPP) was launched in 1970 with the main intervention of distribution of iron and folate preparations amongst the vulnerable population, i.e. expectant mothers and children between 1 and 11 years of age. For control of anemia during pregnancy, the standard intervention undertaken by health agencies consisted of administration of 60 mg of iron and 500 µg of folate in the last 100 days of pregnancy as a part and parcel of antenatal care. Children were provided with a small tablet or 2 ml of syrupy liquid containing 20 mg elemental iron and 100 µg folate.

EVALUATION OF IRON SUPPLEMENTATION PROGRAM

It has been shown that NNAPP did not have the desired impact on anemia prevalence. A multicentric study by ICMR revealed that 17% of pregnant women had hemoglobin (Hb) levels less than 9 g/dl before iron supplementation was started and compliance rate was unsatisfactory in a considerable proportion of cases.[9] Non-reduction of prevalence of nutritional anemia has been attributed to non-delivery of the tablets to the women, poor quality of tablets, non-consumption due to women's lack of awareness about the importance of iron, particularly during pregnancy, for their health and the health of their unborn child. Side effects of oral iron therapy have also been mentioned as a reason for non-compliance but these are probably more highlighted than real.[10,11] Another revealing fact was that as high as 38% of women who had consumed the tablets regularly for more than 90 days during the last trimester had hemoglobin level less than 10 g/dl and in nearly 20% less than 9 g/dl at the end of pregnancy.[12] It is felt that a dose of 60 mg per day may be inadequate and there is need to build up hemoglobin levels in pregnant women at a much earlier stage.[13]

The above observations led to the suggestion that the focus of anemia program should be on control of anemia and not only on prophylactic measures.[9] Following this suggestion, since 1991 the program has been renamed as the National Nutritional Anemia Control Program.[14]

NATIONAL NUTRITIONAL ANEMIA CONTROL PROGRAM

The National Nutritional Anemia Control Program (NNACP) aims at significantly decreasing the prevalence and incidence of anemia in women in reproductive age group, especially pregnant and lactating women, and in preschool children.

Objectives

The specific objectives of the program are:

1. To assess the baseline prevalence of nutritional anemia in mothers and young children through estimation of Hb levels (The Government says that in young children estimation of Hb need not be undertaken in view of its limitations and risk of spread of diseases. Severe anemia should be identified clinically).

2. To put the mothers and children with low Hb levels (less than 11 g/dl and less than 8 g/dl, respectively) on anti-anemia treatment.
3. To put the mothers with Hb level more than 11 g/dl and children with Hb more than 8 g/dl on the prophylaxis program.
4. To monitor continuously the quality, distribution and consumption of the IFA tablets.
5. To assess periodically the Hb levels of the beneficiaries.
6. To motivate the mothers to consume the tablets through relevant nutrition education (and to pass on the information to their children).

Beneficiaries

The beneficiaries are children 1-5 years of age, pregnant and nursing mothers, and female acceptors of terminal methods of family planning and intrauterine devices (IUDs).

The target beneficiaries of the scheme are 50% of total pregnant and nursing mothers, and 25% of total women acceptors of terminal methods and IUDs. The target child population is 50% of total population in the age group of 1-5 years. Presently, 27 million adult and 30 million child beneficiaries are being covered under the program. Coverage of all pregnant mothers with IFA tablets has also been made an integral part of services under CSSM Program.

Organization

The program is implemented through the Primary Health Centers (PHCs) and subcenters. The multipurpose workers (F) and other paramedical personnel working in the PHCs are responsible for the distribution of iron tablets (adult and pediatric doses) to pregnant and lactating women, IUD users and children aged 1-5 years. Opinion had been expressed that linking of nutrition interventions with UIP Plus and ICDS program could possibly strengthen the implementation of NNACP. The functionaries of Integrated Child Development Services (ICDS) Program, under the Women and Child Development, assist in the distribution of iron tablets to children and mothers in the ICDS Blocks and for imparting education to mothers on prevention of nutritional anemia.

Activities and Services

The program focuses on the following strategies:

1. Promotion of regular consumption of foods rich in iron.
2. Provision of iron and folate supplements in the form of tablets (folifer tabets) to the high risk groups.
3. Identification and treatment of severely anemic cases.
4. Treatment of hookworm infection in areas where hookworm prevalence rates are high or when infection is suspected.
5. Birth-spacing among women by at least 3 years.

Promotion of Regular Consumption of Iron Rich Foods

Food based approach (i.e. dietary modification for control of anemia), though not suitable for treatment purposes, consists of the most desirable and sustainable method for preventing iron deficiency. Approaches should include dietary diversity and improving the year round availability, access to and utilization of foods, which promote the increased intake and absorption of dietary iron. It is also desirable to encourage the addition of an absorption enhancer to the meal and discourage consumption of inhibitors. Vitamin C appears to have greater potential of success as enhancers for the absorption of non-heme iron from the same meal.

Tannin and phytates are the important inhibitors. The drinking of tea or coffee with or shortly after the meal has a marked inhibitory effect on iron absorption, because of tannins. Common household processing methods like germination, malting, and fermentation enhance the iron absorption by increasing the vitamin C content, by lowering the tannin and phytic acid content or both.[15,16]

Taking the above facts into consideration, NNACP promotes consumption of iron rich food and emphasizes on:

1. Regular dietary intake of iron and folic acid rich foods by pregnant and lactating mothers, adolescent girls and children under 5 years of age should be promoted.
2. The mothers attending antenatal clinics, immunization sessions as well as women beneficiaries in the ICDS program should be made aware of the importance of preventing nutritional anemia.
3. Regular consumption of iron rich foods, such as green leafy vegetables, cereals such as wheat, *ragi*, *jowar* and *bajra*, pulses (especially sprouted pulses) and gur (jaggery) must be promoted widely. In addition, wherever culturally and economically feasible, consumption of animal flesh foods such as meat, liver, etc. must be encouraged.
4. Ensure incorporation of iron rich liver, etc.
5. Ensure incorporation of iron rich foods such as green leafy vegetables in the weaning food of infants.

6. Vitamin C (ascorbic acid) promotes absorption of iron. Regular consumption of vitamin C rich food such as lemon, orange, guava, amla, green mango along with iron rich food must be promoted.
7. For increasing availability of iron rich foods, growing of iron rich foods in home gardens and consumption of these must be promoted.
8. Tea inhibits absorption of iron in the stomach. Advise a reduced consumption of tea, especially during pregnancy, for improving the absorption of iron and prevention of anemia.

Promoting Consumption of Iron and Folic Acid Supplements

1. As a priority, all pregnant women, irrespective of hemoglobin levels, must be provided with the recommended dose of iron and folic acid (folifer) supplements.
2. In addition, if supplies are readily available, iron and folic acid supplements must be provided to lactating women and IUD users.
3. Preschool children, especially those in tribal areas and ICDS blocks, should be given the recommended dosage of iron and folic acid supplements on priority.
4. The contact during administration of tetanus toxoid should be utilized for distribution of Folifer tablets to pregnant women. Ensure every mother is provided with complete recommended dosage of Folifer tablets during pregnancy.
5. For monitoring distribution as well as consumption of Folifer tablets by pregnant and lactating women and children 12-24 months, the mother-infant immunization card should be used. The growth monitoring cards/registers used for monitoring the growth of preschool children under the ICDS program should be used for monitoring the distribution of folifer tablets to children 1-5 years.
6. In addition, records of under fives and antenatal care maintained under the MCH services and ICDS Program should be used for identifying beneficiaries (pregnant and lactating women, preschool children) as well as for recording and monitoring the distribution of iron and folic acid supplements.

Recommendations of Dosage by the National Nutritional Anemia Control Program

Pregnant women: One big (adult) tablet per day for 100 days (each tablet containing 100 mg of elemental iron and 500 mcg of folic acid). These tablets should be provided to women after the first trimester of pregnancy. Lactating women and IUD acceptors, one big (adult) tablet per day for 100 days. Preschool children (1-<5 years) One small (pediatric) tablet containing 20 mg iron and 100 mcg folic acid daily for 100 days every year. It needs to be stressed that tea inhibits absorption of iron in stomach. Therefore, drinking tea should be avoided within a few hours of taking folifer tablets.

Identification and Treatment of Severe Anemia

Women with hemoglobin levels below 7 g/dl are considered to be severely anemic. Testing of blood for hemoglobin concentration at field levels is neither considered safe nor practical. Therefore, as far as possible, severely anemic cases should be identified on the basis of clinical signs. All health workers should be able to identify such anemic cases.

The recommended therapeutic dose for anemic women in the reproductive age group is one tablet (big) of iron three times daily for a minimum of 100 days.[17] Further, cases of severe anemia should be referred to the PHC medical officers for diagnosis of the causative factors and treatment.

REFERENCES

1. WHO Report. The Prevalence of Anemia in Women: A Tabulation of Available Information, 2nd edn. Geneva, WHO/MCH/MSM/92.2,1992.
2. DeMaeyer EM, Dallmen P, Gurney JM, Hallberg L, Sood SK, Srikantia SG. Prevention of iron deficiency anemia. In: Preventing and Controlling Iron Deficiency Anemia Through Primary Health Care. Geneva, World Health Organization; 1989. pp. 34-42.
3. Indian Council of Medical Research. Studies on preschool children. Technical Report Series No. 26, New Delhi, ICMR, 1977.
4. Vasanthi G, Pawashi AB, Susie H, Sujatha T, Raman. Iron nutritional status of adolescent girls from rural area and urban slum. Indian Pediatr. 1994;31:127-32.
5. Collaborative Study on High Risk Pregnancies and Maternal Mortality. An ICMR Task Force Study, New Delhi, ICMR, 1990.
6. Field Supplementation Trial in Pregnant women. An ICMR Task Force Study, New Delhi, ICMR, 1992.
7. Anemia in pregnancy. Leading cause of maternal and perinatal mortality. CSSM Review. 1993;6:1-8.
8. Government of India Report. Child Survival and safe Motherhood Program - India. New Delhi, Ministry of Health and Family Welfare, Government of India, 1991.
9. Indian Council of Medical Research. Field Supplementation Trial in Pregnant Woman with 60 mg, 120 mg, and 180 mg of iron with 500 mcg of Folic Acid: ICMR Task Force Study. New Delhi, Indian Council of Medical Research; 1992.

10. Indian Council of Medical Research Report. Evaluation of the National Nutritional Anemia Prophylaxis Programme. New Delhi, An ICMR Task Force Study; 1989.
11. Government of India/ UNICEF Report. Study of Existing System of Procurement, Distribution and Management of Drugs Under the National Nutritional Anemia Prophylaxis Programme and the National Programme for Prevention of Nutritional Blindness Due to Vitamin A Deficiency in Selected States of India. Ministry of Health and Family Welfare, Government of India/UNICEF, January, 1991. pp. 1-54.
12. Gopalan C. Micronutrient deficiencies - Public health implications. Bul NFI. 1994;15:1-6.
13. Narasinga Rao BS. Prevention and control of anemia in India. In Gopalan C, Kaur H (Eds): Towards Better Nutrition. Problems and Policies New Delhi, Nutrition Foundation of India. Special Publication Series 9; 1993. pp. 315-23.
14. National Nutritional Anemia Control Program, Policy on Control of Nutritional Anemia. Ministry of Health and Family Welfare, Government of India; 1991.pp. 1-8.
15. Hallberg L, Brune M, Rossander L. Effect of ascorbic acid on iron absorption from different types of meals. Studies with ascorbic acid rich foods and synthetic ascorbic acid given in different amounts with different meals. Hum Butr Appl Nutr. 1986;40:97-113.
16. Oski FA. Iron deficiency in infancy and childhood. N Eng J Med. 1993;329(3):190-3.
17. Kumar A. National Nutritional Anemia Control Programme in India. Indian J Public health. 1999;43(1):3-5.

8 Aplastic Anemia: Current Issues in Diagnosis and Management

Bharat R Agarwal, Nivedita Dhingra

Aplastic anemia (AA) is a disease characterized by pancytopenia and hypocellular (or fatty) bone marrow. It can be classified into congenital bone marrow failure syndromes and acquired AA. The predictable marrow aplasia that occurs after chemotherapy and/or radiotherapy is excluded from the diagnosis of acquired AA. The incidence of acquired aplastic anemia in Europe and North America is around 2-6/million population/year[1,2] and is even higher in India and Japan, resulting from differences in population immunogenetics and environmental factors. The age distribution is biphasic, with peaks occurring between 10 and 25 years and above 60 years. There is no significant difference in incidence between males and females.[3]

Congenital aplastic anemia is very rare, the commonest type being Fanconi anemia, which is inherited as an autosomal recessive disorder in most cases. In majority of the cases of acquired AA, the etiology remains unknown (idiopathic AA). In other cases it may be related to drug and chemical use, viral infections, post-hepatitis notably seronegative hepatitis and rarely paroxysmal nocturnal hemoglobinuria (PNH).

PANCYTOPENIA IN CHILDREN

Many conditions present in childhood with pancytopenia, some of which may also feature a hypocellular marrow. Conditions that may cause pancytopenia in children are detailed in Table 8.1. Some children will have reversible infectious, metabolic or nutritional causes. Infections may account for 10-20% of children presenting with pancytopenia. Others will have acute lymphoblastic or myeloid leukemia (ALL, AML) or myelodysplastic syndrome (MDS). ALL is the most common hematological malignancy to present with pancytopenia and BM hypoplasia. About 1-2% of cases of childhood ALL are preceded by a period of pancytopenia, often with a hypocellular marrow. Subsequent recovery of blood counts may occur, followed by development of overt leukemia, usually within a few months.

IMMUNE PHYSIOLOGY OF AA

Most cases of acquired aplastic anemia can be pathophysiologically characterized as T-cell–mediated, organ specific destruction of bone marrow hematopoietic cells.[4] In an individual patient, the aberrant immune response can sometimes be linked to a viral infection or to drug or chemical exposure. There is much less evidence for other mechanisms, such as direct toxicity for stem cells or a deficiency of stromal-cell or hematopoietic growth factor function. Furthermore, the variability in clinical course and response to treatment can be explained by the quantitative degree of stem-cell destruction and qualitative variations in immune response.

DIAGNOSIS OF AA

The following investigations are required to: (i) confirm the diagnosis; (ii) exclude other possible causes of pancytopenia with a hypocellular bone marrow; (iii) exclude inherited aplastic anemia; (iv) screen for an underlying cause of aplastic anemia; and (v) document or exclude a coexisting abnormal cytogenetic clone or a PNH clone. Table 8.2 for a summary of investigations required for the diagnosis of aplastic anemia.

Full Blood Count, Reticulocyte Count, Blood Film and % HbF

The full blood count (FBC) typically shows pancytopenia although usually the lymphocyte count is preserved. Anemia is usually severe (hemoglobin of about 3 g/dl). In most cases the hemoglobin level, neutrophil and platelet counts are all uniformly depressed, but in the early stages isolated cytopenia, particularly thrombocytopenia, may occur. In about 40% of cases erythrocytes are macrocytic. Reticulocytes

Table 8.1: Differential diagnosis of childhood pancytopenia

Category	*Condition*	*Bone marrow appearance*
Aplastic anemia	Idiopathic	Hypocellular
	Inherited bone marrow failure syndrome	Hypocellular
	Drug/toxin associated	Hypocellular
Megaloblastic anemia	Acquired	Hypercellular
	Congenital deficiency	Hypercellular
Malignant infiltration	ALL/AML	Hyper- or hypocellular
	MDS	Hyper- or hypocellular
	Hodgkin's disease	Infiltrated
	Solid tumors	Infiltrated
	Histiocytic syndromes	Hypocellular with hemophagocytosis
Non-malignant infiltration	Storage disorders	Infiltrated
	Osteopetrosis	Increased bony trabeculae
Infection	CMV, EBV, Parvovirus, HHV-6, Hepatitis (non-A, non-B), HIV	Hypocellular (Pro-erythroblasts in Parvovirus)
Immune disorders	SLE	Hypercellular
	Evans' syndrome	Hypercellular
	Autoimmune lymphoproliferative syndrome	Hypercellular
	Thymoma	Hypocellular
Acquired clonal bone marrow failure disorder	Paroxysmal nocturnal hemoglobinuria	Variable
Metabolic	Hypothermia	Variable
	Anorexia nervosa	Hypocellular with fat necrosis
Others	Hypersplenism	Hypercellular

Table 8.2: Summary of investigations required for the diagnosis of aplastic anemia

1. FBC and reticulocyte count
2. Blood film examination
3. HbF% in children
4. Bone marrow aspirate and trephine biopsy, including cytogenetics
5. Peripheral blood chromosomal breakage analysis to exclude Fanconi's anemia
6. Flow cytometry for GPI-anchored proteins
7. Urine hemosiderin if Ham test positive or GPI-anchored protein deficiency
8. Vitamin B_{12} and folate
9. Liver function tests
10. Viral studies: Hepatitis A, B and C, EBV, HIV (CMV)
11. Anti-nuclear antibody and anti-dsDNA
12. Chest X-ray
13. Abdominal ultrasound scan and echocardiogram
14. Peripheral blood gene mutation analysis for dyskeratosis congenital DKC1, TERC, ?TERT) if clinical features or lack of response to immunosuppressive therapy

are usually decreased, but occasionally are inexplicably excessive for the anemia. Careful examination of the blood film is essential to exclude the presence of dysplastic neutrophils, abnormal platelets, blasts and other abnormal cells. Platelet size is usually decreased (cf immune thrombocytopenias). HbF may be increased, especially in genetic types and those with macrocytosis. As a result of diminution in the erythron, serum iron and transferrin saturation are increased; B_{12} and folate may be increased. The first sign of recovery is a rise in reticulocyte count, followed by increase in hemoglobin, then neutrophils, with platelets slowest to recover; if at all.

Marrow

Both a bone marrow aspirate and trephine biopsy are required. Bone marrow aspiration and biopsy may be performed in patients with severe thrombocytopenia without platelet support, provided that adequate surface pressure is applied.[5] Erythropoiesis is reduced or absent, dyserythropoiesis is very common and often marked, so this alone should not be used to make a diagnosis of MDS. Megakaryocytes and granulocytic cells are reduced or absent; dysplastic megakaryocytes and granulocytic cells are not seen in aplastic anemia Lymphocytes, macrophages, plasma cells and mast cells appear prominent. Hypoplasia may be patchy, especially early in the disease. Thus, a good quality trephine of at least 2 cm is essential to assess overall cellularity, to assess the morphology of residual hemopoietic cells and to exclude an abnormal infiltrate. Increased blasts are not seen in aplastic anemia, and their presence either indicates a hypocellular MDS or evolution to leukemia.[6-8]

Cytogenetic analysis of the bone marrow should be attempted although this may be difficult in a very hypocellular bone marrow and often insufficient metaphases are obtained. In this situation, one should consider fluorescence *in situ* hybridization (FISH) analysis for chromosomes 5 and 7 in particular. It was previously assumed that the presence of an abnormal cytogenetic clone indicated a diagnosis of MDS and not aplastic anemia, but it is now evident that abnormal cytogenetic clones may be present in up to 12% of patients with otherwise typical aplastic anemia at diagnosis.

Once the diagnosis of AA has been established, the severity of the disease needs to be defined. The severity of the disease is graded according to the blood count parameters and bone marrow findings as summarized in Table 8.3.

Other tests include vitamin B_{12} and folate levels to exclude megaloblastic anemia which, when severe, can present with pancytopenia, an autoantibody screen as rarely SLE may occur with a hypocellular marrow. Liver function tests should be performed to detect antecedent hepatitis, but in post-hepatitic aplastic anemia the serology is most often negative for all the known hepatitis viruses. Blood should be tested for hepatitis A antibody, hepatitis B surface antigen, hepatitis C antibody and Epstein-Barr virus (EBV). Cytomegalovirus (CMV) and other viral serology should be assessed if BMT is being considered. Human immunodeficiency virus (HIV) is not a recognised cause of aplastic anemia, but it can cause isolated cytopenias. Paroxysmal nocturnal hemoglobinuria should be excluded by performing flow cytometry.[12] The Ham test and sucrose lysis test have been abandoned by most centres as diagnostic tests for PNH. Analysis of glycosylphosphatidylinositol (GPI)-anchored proteins, such as CD55 and CD59 by flow cytometry, is a sensitive and quantitative test for PNH enabling the detection of small PNH clones which occur in up to 50% of patients with aplastic anemia, the proportion depending on the sensitivity of the flow cytometric analysis used.[13-15]

Table 8.3: Definition of severity of aplastic anemia

Severe AA (SAA)[9]	BM cellularity <25%, or 25-50% with <30% residual hemopoietic cells* 2/3 of the following: Neutrophil count <0.5 × 10^9/L Platelet count <20 ×10^9/L Reticulocyte count < 20×10^9/L
Very severe AA (vSAA)[10]	As for severe AA but neutrophils < 0.2×10^9/L
Non-severe AA	Patients not fulfilling the criteria for severe or very severe aplastic anemia

*Cellularity should be determined by comparison with normal controls[11]

ETIOLOGY OF APLASTIC ANEMIA: RECOGNIZED CAUSES

Drugs

Drugs may cause: (a) predictable, dose-related reversible marrow suppression, and (b) unpredictable dose-unrelated, idiosyncratic, usually irreversible damage.

Drugs, which can seriously damage marrow, usually do so in an unpredictable and devastating fashion and in only in a minuscule proportion of those exposed. Susceptibility is presumably genetic. This effect usually does not occur until after cessation of the drug—with chloramphenicol at least 6-10 weeks, and up to 12 months later. In a study conducted by Kauffman et al[16] data from several large-scale series studying the relationship of drugs in the etiology of AA was incorporated. Comparisons were made between 454 patients with AA and 6458 controls. The strongest associations between AA and drugs were for penicillamine, gold, and carbamazepine. The other associated drugs include butazones, indomethacin, diclofenac, sulfonamides, and furosemide. Chloramphenicol exposures were too few to provide an estimated risk (Table 8.4).

Some drugs, e.g. chloramphenicol, have both dose-related and idiosyncratic effect, rarely one following the other. Pediatric drug and toxins with, or with suspected capacity to cause marrow aplasia are listed in Table 8.5. Some (e.g. benzol) have a potential for causing leukemia, which usually does not occur until many years after exposure.

Viral Infection

As with idiosyncratic reaction to drugs, hypoplasia occurs in only a minuscule proportion of those exposed.

Table 8.4: Dose-related effects of chloramphenicol

	Timing
Reticulocytopenia, increase in serum Fe	2-5 days
Marrow	
Erythroblast depletion	3-7 days
Vacuolation of precursor cells	
Anemia	5-10 days
Thrombocytopenia (mild)	10-14 days
Neutropenia	10-21 days

Table 8.5: Pediatric drugs and chemicals which may cause marrow aplasia

Cytotoxics	
Antibacterial	Chloramphenicol (more often oral than intravenous)
	Sulphonamides (some)
Antimalarial	Mepacrine
	Quinacrine
	Chloroquine
	Trimethoprim
	Pyrimethamine
Antihistamine	Cimetidine
	Ranitidine
	Chlorpheniramine
Anticonvulsant	Phenytoin, other hydantoins
Tranquilizer	Promazine Chlorpromazine
	Carbamazepine
Anti-inflammatory	Indomethacin
	Diclophenac
	Gold
Antipurines	Azathioprine
Antidiabetic	Chlorpropamide
	Tolbutamide
Antithyroid	Propylthiouracil
	Methimazole
Other drugs	Allopurinol
	Quinidine
	Acetazolamine
	Penicillamine
Solvents	Benzol
	White spirit (benzene, naphtha and other synonyms)
	Carbon tetrachloride
	Kerosene
	Glue (sniffing)
	Model aeroplane 'dope' Hair dyes
Insecticides	DDT
	Lindane
	Chlordane
	Organophosphates

However, viral infection is probably an under-diagnosed cause: EBV for instance may be demonstrable in patients without the typical clinical features of infective mononucleosis and acyclovir may produce hematologic improvement when a virus etiology cannot be proven. The destructive effect of virus may be due to direct action or an immune effect such as T-lymphocyte mediated suppression.

The best known association is with viral hepatitis-usually non-A,-B,-C. Hypoplasia is usually severe, though the preceding hepatitis may not be, and manifests at a mean of 9-10 weeks after onset of hepatitis.[17] Hypoplasia occurs in isolated instances of infection with EBV,[18] HIV,[19] varicella, dengue-type viruses,[20] CMV[21] measles, mumps[22] and parvovirus.[23,24] Although the effect of parvovirus is ordinarily restricted to the erythron, panhypoplasia occasionally occurs in apparently normal persons. Transient hypoplasia may also occur in rickettsial infections, e.g. Q fever and Ehrlichiosis.

Fanconi's Syndrome

This classical marrow failure disorder is typically inherited in an autosomal recessive manner with a heterozygote frequency of about 1 in 300, and occurs in all racial and ethnic groups. At presentation patients may have either a classic phenotype comprising physical anomalies and abnormal hematology, or typical physical anomalies but normal hematology, or normal physical features but abnormal hematology. Data from the International FA Registry showed that out of 202 patients tested, 39% had aplastic anemia and anomalies, 30% had aplastic anemia without anomalies and 24% had physical anomalies only.[25] It is a chromosomal instability disorder which is diagnosed most reliably by quantitation of chromosomal breaks on cultured blood lymphocytes or fibroblasts, induced by the DNA cross-linking agent, dieopoxybutane (DEB) or mitomycin C. Abnormal fragility appears to be specific for Fanconi's anemia and is detectable from birth and before onset of cytopenias. A scoring system for diagnosis, using other characteristics, has been devised (Table 8.6).

Fifteen FA linked genes (FANC genes) also known as complementation groups have been discovered so far which account for more than 95% of the cases. The cells in these patients accumulate DNA damage at an increased rate. Unrepaired DNA damage can activate pro-apoptotic pathways, leading, for example, to depletion of hematopoietic stem cells, causing pancytopenia. Alternatively, defective DNA repair in FA cells can lead to mutations and translocations that cause inactivation of cell cycle barriers and result in AML and other blood and solid tumors.

Blood abnormalities are rare before 18 months and may not manifest till about 20 years. Average age at onset of pancytopenia is about 7 years (range: birth to

Table 8.6: Assessment of likelihood of Fanconi's syndrome

Characteristic	*Score*
Growth retardation	+ 1
Skin	
Pigmentation (cafe-au-lait spots) + Hypopigmented areas	+ 1
Thumb and radius	
Absent or triphalangeal thumb, Hypoplasia of 1st metacarpal, Absent radius one or both sides with Absence of corresponding thumb.	+ 1
Microphthalmia	+ 1
Kidney, urinary tract	
Absence of one kidney Horse-shoe kidney, Double ureters	+ 1
Thrombocytopenia	+ 1
Other skeletal defects	− 1
Learning difficulties	− 1
Total score-1 Probability of Fanconi's	0.00
0	0.20
1	0.31
2	0.75
3	0.92
4	0.98

31 years).[26] Thrombocytopenia is usually the first sign, and may be misdiagnosed as idiopathic if the association with somatic anomalies is not recognized; granulocytopenia and then anemia follow, evolving over months to years. Fetal features, e.g. macrocytosis and increased HbF are frequent. Dyserythropoiesis is common on bone marrow examination, with megaloblastosis, internuclear bridges, karyorrhexis and defective hemoglobinization. In the presymptomatic period the marrow may appear normal or show hyperplasia. There is a risk (about 20%) of malignancy, especially AML - M4 and squamous cell carcinoma especially of head and neck. Occasionally it may be the presenting feature.

Table 8.7 summarizes the inherited marrow failure syndromes.

Dyskeratosis Congenita

This rare disorder is characterized by ectodermal dysplasia,[27,28] bone marrow failure,[29] cancer predisposition[29] and extreme telomere shortening.[30] In most cases it is inherited in an X-linked or autosomal recessive manner and usually presents in adolescence with aplastic anemia. The initial hematologic change is usually thrombocytopenia, anemia, or both, followed by pancytopenia. The red cells are often macrocytic and the hemoglobin F can be elevated. Oddly, early bone marrow aspirations and biopsies may be hypercellular;

Table 8.7: Genetic syndromes and marrow panhypoplasia

Syndrome	*Age/gender*	*Hematological presentation*	*Associated clinical features*	*Gene mutation*	*Inheritance pattern*	*Specific diagnostic test*
Fanconi's anemia	Usually first decade Equal gender distribution	Typically thrombocytopenia followed by progressive pancytopenia with marrow hypoplasia	Skin pigmentation, abnormal thumbs/ radii, renal/urinary tract malformations	>13 *FANC* genes identified	AR X-linked	Increased chromosomal breakage by DNA cross-linkers in hematopoietic cells (90%) or fibroblasts (100%)
Dyskeratosis congenita	Second decade Male > female	Macrocytosis Thrombocytopenia Pancytopenia with marrow hypoplasia	Dyskeratotic nails, reticular rash, oral lesions	*DKC1* *TERC?*	X-linked AD AR	None (shortened telomeres seen in some cases)
Shwachman-Diamond syndrome	0-5 years Equal gender distribution	Neutropenia, pancytopenia with marrow hypoplasia	Short stature Pancreatic exocrine insufficiency	*SBDS*	AR	Decreased serum trypsinogen/isoamylase levels
Amegakaryocytic thrombocytopenia	0-5 years Equal gender distribution	Thrombocytopenia with absent megakaryocytes, Pancytopenia with marrow hypoplasia	Bleeding	*C-MPL*	AR	None

however, with time all cellular elements decline. The non-hematological manifestations include skin pigmentation and nail changes which appear in the first 10 years of life, mucosal leukoplakia and excessive ocular tearing appear later.

Cancer develops in at least 10-15% of patients, usually in the third or fourth decades of life. The types of malignancies are similar to Fanconi's anemia, although in DC solid tumors are more common than hematologic malignancies.

Shwachman's Syndrome

Shwachman-Diamond syndrome (SDS) is an autosomal recessive multisystem disorder first described in the early 1960s by several groups.[31,32] This syndrome comprises a triad of bone marrow failure, pancreatic insufficiency and skeletal abnormalities.[33] In addition, the liver, kidneys, teeth, and immune system may also be affected.[34,35] SDS is also associated with a propensity for MDS and leukemia. Exocrine pancreatic insufficiency (fatty replacement) is associated with neutropenia, metaphyseal dyschondroplasia and growth retardation. Neutropenia is intermittent rather than constant and may be cyclic, although not as predictably as in true cyclic neutropenia. The neutrophil count may rise with infection, and is responsive to administration of G-CSF. Monocytes are usually not increased.

About 50% of patients have anemia; however this is persistent in only a minority. Increase in HbF is common even without anemia, but substantial increase (to 30%) is unusual. About 70% have thrombocytopenia, which varies independent of the neutrophil count and may be severe ($<60 \times 10^9/L$). About 10% have pancytopenia.

Marrow hypoplasia of varying degree is common, even without pancytopenia. Maturation arrest in myeloid cells or sparsity of myeloid precursors may be noted. The erythron is normal (patchy disease). Rarely Gaucher-like cells may be noted.

The relation of pancreatic insufficiency to the cytopenias is not clear. Inheritance is thought to be autosomal recessive; defective neutrophil mobility may be demonstrable in parents. There is a risk (about 5%) of leukemia (ALL, AML, Juvenile CML).

Differential diagnosis is from other pancreas-marrow syndromes: Pearson's and atypical cystic fibrosis.

Congenital Amegakaryocytic Thrombocytopenia

Congenital amegakaryocytic thrombocytopenia (CAMT) is a rare autosomal recessive disorder which usually presents in infancy with isolated thrombocytopenia due to reduced or absent marrow megakaryocytes, and frequently evolves into pancytopenia of varying degrees. In untreated cases, MDS with monosomy 7 and AML can develop at a later stage.[36] Non-hematologic manifestations occur in about a quarter of the patients. Mutations in the *MPL* (thrombopoietic receptor) gene are the cause of the disorder in most patients with CAMT, particularly,[37] but not exclusively,[38] in those without physical anomalies. Both alleles were mutated, confirming an autosomal recessive mode of inheritance.[37,38]

Immune Destruction of Marrow

Graft vs Host Disease

Marrow destruction is severe, with high mortality. Transfused, un-irradiated lymphocytes are a high risk if an immunocompetent (or incompetent) recipient shares an HLA haplotype with an HLA-homozygous donor (facilitates engraftment of viable donor lymphocytes).

PNH (Exceptionally Rare in Childhood)

A variety of cells are abnormally sensitive to lysis by complement, due to a defect in the glycosylphosphatidyl-inositol anchor, which binds proteins to the cell membrane (including those which protect against complement).

Diagnosis might be considered in cases with hemolysis of obscure origin. Chronic hemolysis is more common than sleep-induced hemoglobinuria, and hemosiderinuria is constant. The DAT is negative. Reticulocytes may be inappropriately low (marrow hypoplasia, ineffective erythropoiesis, iron deficiency from hemosiderinuria). The MCV is often high for the reticulocyte count, but microcytosis may result from the iron deficiency. Hemolysis may be exacerbated by exercise, infection, vaccination and blood transfusion (increase in blood temperature or acidity, infusion of complement).

About 25% of patients with PNH proceed over a period of years to marrow aplasia (5-10% of patients with various aplasias, e.g. drug-induced, Fanconi, evolve to PNH). Marrow storage iron may be subnormal from hemosiderinuria, in contrast to the excess usual in aplasia. Dyserythropoiesis is not conspicuous.

SLE and Marrow Hypoplasia

Marrow depletion is rare in SLE and may be global or affect only the erythron. Maternal SLE is a cause of marrow depletion in the neonate.

Flow chart 8.1: Algorithm for non-severe AA

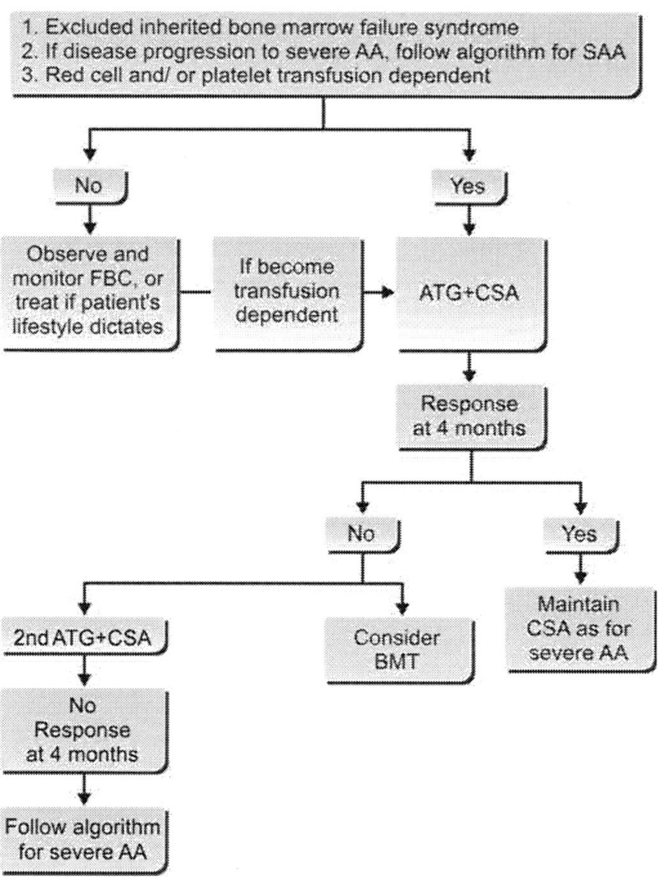

Flow chart 8.2: Algorithm for management of severe AA

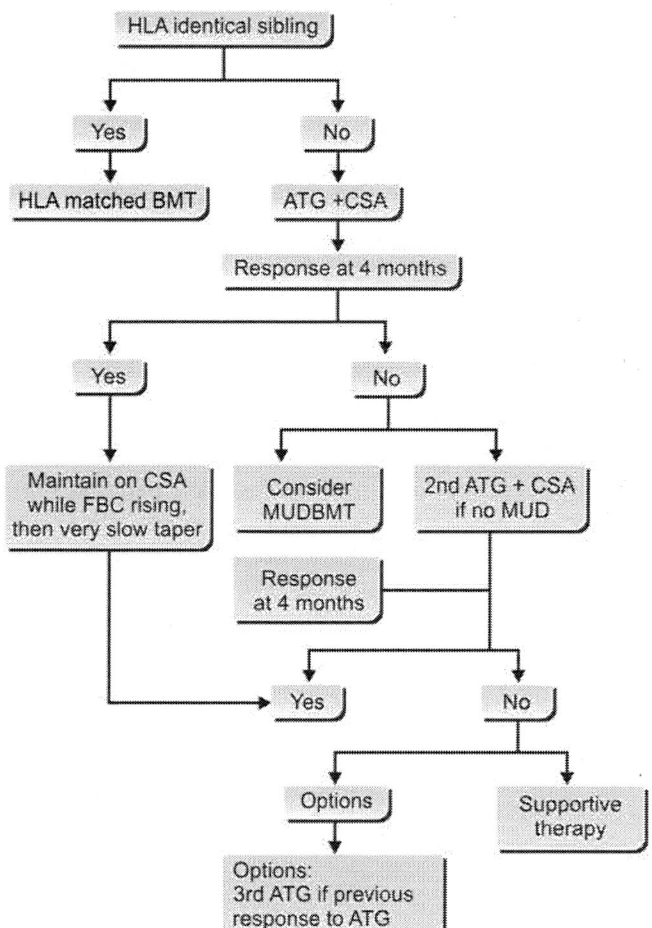

Chronic Mucocutaneous Candiadiasis

Aplasia occurs in some patients. Aplasia, T-cell dysfunction in handling of candida and endocrinopathy (parathyroid) are attributed to autoimmune effect.

Thymoma

Association with hypoplasia (erythroblastopenia or panhypoplasia) is very rare in childhood.

MANAGEMENT OF APLASTIC ANEMIA

Most of the patients with marrow failure can be cured. Besides various forms of 'definitive therapy' availability and access to long-term adequate 'supportive care' decides the outcomes. The treatment strategy of AA is based on consideration of the severity of the disease (Flow chart 8.1), data on the response rate to different kinds of treatment options, and the natural history of disease. Patients with severe AA should be treated immediately (Flow chart 8.2). The preferred treatment for severe and very severe aplastic anemia is allogeneic hematopoietic stem cell transplantation (allo-HSCT). However, this treatment is not always applicable, due to unavailability of matched HLA donors and age restriction of the recipients. The alternative to allo-HSCT is immunosuppressive therapy (IST) consisting of antithymocyte globulin (ATG)/antilymphocyte globulin (ALG) and/or cyclosporine A (CsA) with or without the addition of hematopoietic growth factors (HGF). Of those patients who die, the majority will die during the first 4 months and/or during the first two years (approximately 60%).

The natural history of the disease is characterized by the development of late hematologic complications, such as acute leukemia, paroxysmal nocturnal hemoglobinuria (PNH), etc. Interestingly, this incidence has risen from 5-15% to more than 57% in those patients treated with immunosuppressive therapy; these factors should be taken into account when treatment is planned.

Supportive Care

Transfusional Support

Support with red cell and platelet transfusions is essential for patients with aplastic anemia to maintain a safe blood count. The most feared complication is spontaneous intracranial hemorrhage, which can be fatal. Steroid therapy, stress and infections can lead to GI, GU and pulmonary hemorrhage. Aspirin must be avoided. Coagulation defects due to antibiotics and vitamin K deficiency must be corrected.

It is recommended to give prophylactic platelet transfusions when the platelet count is $<10 \times 10^9/L$ (or $<20 \times 10^9/L$ in the presence of fever) (Grade C recommendation; level IV evidence), rather than giving platelets only in response to bleeding manifestation.[39] A common problem in multi-transfused patients with aplastic anemia, compared with leukemia patients, is that they may develop alloimmunization to leukocytes present in red cell and platelet transfusions by generating HLA or non-HLA (minor histocompatibility) antibodies. This can result in platelet refractoriness, as well as an increased risk of graft rejection after allogeneic BMT.[40] Routine pre-storage leukocyte depletion of all units of red cells and platelets is likely to reduce the risk of alloimmunization.[41] Red cell transfusions should be given to maintain a hemoglobin level > 8 g/dl. Directed blood donations from family members should be strongly discouraged due to risk of alloimmunization and graft rejection in case BMT is planned in the future. Apart from platelet transfusional support, other important practical measures to help prevent bleeding include good dental hygiene, the use of oral tranexamic acid and control of menorrhagia with norethisterone.

Granulocyte transfusions can also be used as supportive therapy in patients with life-threatening neutropenia. Adverse events, such as febrile reactions, HLA alloimmunization and transfusion-related acute lung injury (TRALI) are well-recognized complications following granulocyte transfusions. The use of irradiated granulocyte transfusions should therefore be limited to patients in whom the possible benefits outweigh the hazards.

Hemopoietic Growth Factors

The routine use of rHuEpo (recombinant Erythropoietin) in aplastic anemia is not recommended as there may be severe and/or sudden worsening of anemia due to red cell aplasia from anti-rHuEpo antibodies.[42] A short course of G-CSF may be considered for severe systemic infection that is not responding to intravenous antibiotics and anti-fungal drugs, but should be discontinued after 1 week if there is no increase in the neutrophil count.

Prevention of Infection

The risk of infection is determined by the patient's neutrophil and monocyte counts.[43,44] Patients with aplastic anemia are at risk of bacterial and fungal infections. *Aspergillus* infections have a very high mortality in patients with severe aplastic anemia because of the frequent prolonged periods of severe neutropenia. Prophylactic antibiotic and antifungal drugs should be given to all patients with neutrophil counts $<0.2 \times 10^9/L$. Broadspectrum full dose parenteral antibiotic therapy is needed to control sepsis which is a major cause of mortality in aplasia anemia. "Ceftazidime with Aminoglycoside" is the usual regimen. Systemic antifungal therapy should be introduced into the febrile neutropenia regimen early if fevers persist.

Iron Chelation Therapy

Iron overload can cause significant problems in heavily transfused patients. Subcutaneous desferrioxamine should commence when the serum ferritin is >1000 ug/L, although the evidence base for this is lacking.

DEFINITIVE THERAPY

The following options are available:

A. Bone marrow transplantation (BMT)
B. Immunomodulation
   Anti-lymphocyte globulin (ALG)
   Anti-thymocyte globulin (ATG)
   Cyclosporine-A (CA)
   Methylprednisolone (MP)
C. Androgens

Bone Marrow Transplantation

It is an effective modality of treatment for SAA. However, problem areas include:

Donor availability as a full house HLA matched family member, almost always a sibling, is needed as a donor. Success rate from HLA identical but unrelated donor or transplant across HLA barriers from blood relatives is very low. Unfortunately HLA-matched sibling donors are not available for large number of patients.

Age

Elderly patients have high incidence of graft versus host disease. Hence BMT is often deferred after the age of 40-45 years.

Transfusion History

Heavily pretransfused patients especially where blood products are used without leukocyte filters, suffer from high incidence of graft rejection.

Infection at Time of Transplant

This always increases the problem. Thus, a good candidate for BMT should satisfy following criteria: untransfused, infected, young patient with HLA-matched sibling being available as a donor such patients have 60-70% chance of long-term survival following BMT. Rest may succumb following BMT due to acute graft vs host disease (GVHD), interstitial pneumonitis, other infections or veno-occlusive disease (VOD). In addition, chronic GVHD is a serious multisystem disease with high morbidity. Other long-term problems secondary to BMT are those due to chemotherapy and radiation. These include poor pulmonary function, endocrine dysfunction including infertility, cognitive disorders, leukoencephalopathy and occurrence of second malignancy. In AA, there is a higher incidence of graft rejection due to the same pathophysiological mechanisms that had resulted in failure of patient's own marrow. Lastly, in India, funds and facilities also matter.

Immunomodulation

The second line of treatment for patients with AA is immunosuppressive therapy (IST) with antithymocyte globulin (ATG). The response rates reported using the combination of ATG and cyclosporin are between 60 and 80% with current 5-year survival rates of around 75-85%. However, the true response rate to ATG seems to be between 40 and 60%.[45,46] One should be aware that complete normalization of the blood count with any form of therapy is not usual. Long-term follow-up indicates that after 10 years 85% of patients had a normal blood count, 80% of patients had normal neutrophils, and 66% a normal platelet count. Late spontaneous improvements are also possible. Infection or uncontrolled bleeding should be treated first before giving immunosuppressive therapy.

ATG

There are two preparations of ATG—equine and rabbit. Equine ATG is used in higher dose, i.e. 40 mg/kg/day for 5 days, while the dose for rabbit ATG is 3.75 mg/kg/day for 5 days. Its efficacy is believed to be similar to the equine preparation. Equine ATG has been withdrawn from most European countries since 2007 due to manufacturing problems related to quality control. Duration of treatment varies from 5 to 10 days. The briefer treatment regimen is more rational as body produces IgG antibodies against the products within about one week.

Anaphylaxis could be lethal, but fortunately it is rare. A skin test is useful and may indicate the need for desensitization. Other allergic reactions like fever, chills and urticaria are common. Serum sickness after about 10 days of therapy is also common. Administration of methylprednisolone prior to ATG infusion is helpful in avoiding allergic reactions as well as serum sickness. There is increase in requirement of platelet and blood during and immediately after ATG therapy. Antibiotic requirement may also increase. Antithymocyte globulin must not be given as an out-patient. The patient should remain hospitalized from the start of ATG through the period when serum sickness occurs.

It takes a few months for overt improvement to occur. A second course of ATG may be considered if there is no response at 3 months. Overall long-term survival after immunosuppressive therapy is comparable to BMT. However, late clonal hematological diseases like PNH, MDS, etc. can occur after apparent recovery from aplasia.

Cyclosporin-A

This drug in doses up to 12-15 mg/kg/day for 6-12 months, when combined with ATG, produces remission rates of about 70%. Nephrotoxicity can be dose limiting. All patients on Cyclosporin must receive *Pneumocystis jiroveci* prophylaxis.

High Dose Corticosteroids

Popular in Europe and probably effective in patients treated within few weeks of diagnosis, this therapy is reserved for occasional patients due to tremendous toxicity. The dose of methylprednisolone is 100 mg/kg for a week tapered over a month. We use it only for the patients, who cannot afford ATG.

Other Immunosuppressive Agents

High dose cyclophosphamide and Mycophenolate mofetil are other agents which have been evaluated in the management of AA but have not been found to be useful. High dose cyclophosphamide without stem cell support was associated with prolonged neutropenia

Table 8.8: Criteria for response to immunosuppressive therapy in AA

Response criteria for severe aplastic anemia	
None	Still severe
Partial	Transfusion independent No longer meeting criteria for severe disease
Complete	Hemoglobin normal for age Neutrophil count $>1.5 \times 10^9/L$ Platelet count $>150 \times 10^9/L$
Response criteria for non-severe aplastic anemia	
None	Worse or not meeting criteria below
Partial	Transfusion independence (if previously dependent) or doubling or normalization of at least one cell line or increase of baseline hemoglobin of >30 g/L (if initially <6) or increase of baseline neutrophils of $>0.5 \times 10^9/L$ (if initially <0.5) or increase of baseline platelets of $>20 \times 10^9/L$ (if initially <20)
Complete	Same criteria as for severe disease

and high mortality. Alemtuzumab (Campath-1H) is currently under evaluation for the treatment of refractory aplastic anemia in prospective trials at NIH in USA, and retrospectively by the EBMT, following reports of its efficacy in patients with autoimmune cytopenias, particularly autoimmune neutropenia.[47]

Androgens

Androgens have a mixed reputation. Probably dose makes the difference. We use Nandrolone Decanoate at 5 mg/kg/week IM for at least 3 months. The advantage of this preparation is freedom from hepatotoxicity.

Response to Therapy

Response to therapy should be confirmed by two or more blood counts at least 4 weeks apart, and should ideally be measured in patients who are not receiving hemopoietic growth factors. The criteria for response to immunosuppressive therapy are summarized in Table 8.8.

APPENDIX 1: PRACTICAL ISSUES WITH IMMUNOSUPPRESSIVE THERAPY IN APLASTIC ANEMIA

Shorter intervals of treatment with antithymocyte globulin (ATG) (5-10 days) are probably as efficacious as longer therapy (28 days). Although ATG does not seem to influence death-outcome in moderate AA, as compared with androgen therapy, about 30% of patients are transfusion independent in a 3 months period, as compared with virtually 0 in an androgen treated group. ATG can cause severe anaphylactic and allergic reactions. Serum sickness is described in about 47% of patients. Because of this skin testing with 0.1 ml of 1:1,000 dilution of ATG in saline should be done before treatment with ATG. A severe local reaction (>0.5 cm induration or erythema) or an immediate systemic reaction warrants exclusion from treatment. The usual way of administering ATG is to give methylprednisolone (MP) (40 mg) with the daily dose (40 mg/kg) of ATG, diluted in 500 ml of physiologic saline.

ATG is then given as an infusion over 4-5 hours through a microaggregate filter. The rest of the total daily dose of prednisolone (1 mg/kg) is given orally. Antihistamines and Meperidine are usually given for allergic symptoms.

Cyclosporine is usually given orally twice a day in a dose of 12 mg/kg/day (adults). Doses are usually adjusted to achieve trough blood levels between 100-150 µg/L. Cyclosporine levels are usually determined at 2 weeks intervals. Interestingly, there is no significant correlation between cyclosporine blood levels and toxicity. Toxicity typically develops between 3 weeks and 3 months. Major adverse effects are reflected in liver toxicity. When transaminases are up, the clinician should stop therapy for 1-4 days and resolve treatment with a lower dose. If this does not help, therapy should be stopped.

REFERENCES

1. Issaragrisil S, Kaufman D, Anderson T, et al .The Aplastic Anaemia Study Group. The epidemiology of aplastic anaemia in Thailand. Blood. 2006;107:1299-1307.
2. Montane´ E, Ibanez, L, Vidal X, et al. The Catalan Group for the Study of Agranulocytosis and Aplastic Anemia, Epidemiology of aplastic anemia: a Prospective multicenter study. Haematologica. 2008;93:518-23.
3. Heimpel H. Epidemiology and aetiology of aplastic anaemia. In: Schrezenmeier H, Bacigalupo A (Eds). Aplastic Anaemia: Pathophysiology and Treatment. Cambridge University Press, Cambridge, UK. 2000. pp. 97-116.
4. Young NS, Maciejewski J. The pathophysiology of acquired aplastic anemia. N Engl J Med. 1997;336:1365-72.
5. Kelsey P, Murphy MF, Brown M, et al. Guidelines for the use of platelet transfusions. Br J Haematol. 2003;122:10-23.
6. Tichelli A, Gratwohl A, Nissen C, et al. Morphology in patients with severe aplastic anaemia treated with antilymphocyte globulin. Blood. 1993;80:337-45.
7. Marin P. Clinical presentation, natural course and prognostic factors. In: Schrezenmeier H, Bacigalupo A (Eds). Aplastic Anaemia: Pathophysiology and Treatment.

Cambridge University Press, Cambridge, UK; 2000. pp. 117-36.
8. Bennett JM, Orazi A. Diagnostic criteria to distinguish hypocellular acute myeloid leukemia from hypocellular myelodysplastic syndromes and aplastic anemia: recommendations for a standardized approach. Haematologica. 2009;94:264-8.
9. Camitta BM, Rappeport JM, Parkman R, et al. Selection of patients for bone marrow transplantation in severe aplastic anemia. Blood. 1975;45:355-63.
10. Bacigalupo A, Hows, JM, Gluckman E, et al. Bone marrow transplantation (BMT) versus immunosuppression for the treatment of severe aplastic anaemia (SAA): areport of the EBMT SAA Working Party. Br J Haematol. 1988;70:177-82.
11. Tuzuner N, Bennett JM. Reference standards for bone marrow cellularity. Leuk Res. 1994;18:645-7.
12. Parker C, Omine M, Richards S, et al. The International PNH Interest Group-Diagnosis and management of paroxysmal nocturnal haemoglobinuria. Blood. 2005;106: 3699-3709.
13. Dunn DE, Tanawattanacharoen P, Boccuni P, et al. Paroxysmal nocturnal hemoglobinuria cells in patients with bone marrow failure syndromes. Ann Intern Med. 1999; 131(6):401-8.
14. Socie G, Rosenfeld S, Frickhofen N, et al. Late clonal diseases of treated aplastic anemia. Semin Hematol. 2000; 37(1):91-101.
15. Sugimori C, Chuhjo T, Feng X, et al. Minor populations of CD55/ CD59 blood cells predicts response to immunosuppressive therapy and prognosis in patients with aplastic anaemia. Blood. 2005;107:1308-14.
16. Kaufman DW, Kelly JP, Jurgelon JM, et al. Drugs in the aetiology of agranulocytosis and aplastic anaemia. Eur J Haematol Suppl. 1996;60:23-30.
17. Linet MS, McCaffrey LD, Morgan WF, et al. Incidence of aplastic anemia in a three county area in South Carolina. Cancer Res. 1986;46:426-9.
18. Baranski B, Armstrong G, Truman JT, et al. Epstein–Barr virus in the bone marrow of patients with aplastic anemia. Ann Intern Med. 1988;109:695-704.
19. Shah I, Murthy AK. Aplastic anemia in an HIV infected child. Indian J Pediatr. 2005;72:359-61.
20. Nakao S, Lai CJ, Young NS. Dengue virus, a flavivirus, propagates in human bone marrow progenitors and hematopoietic cell lines. Blood. 1989;74:1235-40.
21. Sing GK, Ruscetti FW. The role of human cytomegalovirus in haematological diseases. Baillière's Clin Haematol. 1995; 8:149-63.
22. Kook H, Kim GM, Kim HJ, et al. Rubella-associated aplastic anemia treated by syngeneic stem cell transplantations. Am J Hematol. 2000;64:303-5.
23. Goto H, Ishida A, Fujii H, et al. Successful bone marrow transplantation for severe aplastic anemia in a patient with persistent human parvovirus B19 infection. Int J Hematol. 2004;79:384-6.
24. Qian XH, Zhang GC, Jiao XY, et al. Aplastic anaemia associated with parvovirus B19 infection. Arch Dis Child. 2002;87:436-7.
25. Kutler DI, Singh B, Satagopan J, et al. A 20-year perspective on the International Fanconi Anemia Registry (IFAR). Blood. 2003;101:1249-56.
26. Butturini A, Gale RP, Verlander PC, et al. Hematologic abnormalities in Fanconi anemia: An International Fanconi Anemia Registry Study. Blood. 1994;84:1650-5.
27. Zinnsser F. Atrophia cutis reticularis cum pigmentatione, Dystrophia unguium et leukoplakiaoris. Ikonogr Dermatol (Hyoto). 1906;5:219-23.
28. Cole HN, Rauschkolb JC, Toomey J. Dyskeratosis congenital with pigmentation, dystrophia unguis and leukokeratosisoris. Arch Dermatol Syphili graph. 1920;21: 71-95.
29. Dokal I. Dyskeratosis congenita in all its forms. Br J Haematol. 2000;110:768-79.
30. Vulliamy TJ, Knight SW, Mason P, et al. Very short telomeres in the peripheral blood of patients with X-linked and autosomal dyskeratosis congenita. Blood Cells Mol Dis. 2001;27:353-7.
31. Shwachman H, Diamond LK, Oski FA, et al. The syndrome of pancreatic insufficiency and bone marrow dysfunction. J Pediatr. 1964;65:645-63.
32. Bodian M, Sheldon W, Lightwood R. Congenital hypoplasia of the exocrine pancreas. Acta Paediatr. 1964;53:282-93.
33. Aggett PJ, Cavanagh NP, Matthew DJ, et al. Shwachman's syndrome. A review of 21 cases. Arch Dis Child. 1980;55: 331-47.
34. Mack DR, Forstner GG, Wilschanski M, et al. Shwachman syndrome: exocrine pancreatic dysfunction and variable phenotypic expression. Gastroenterology. 1996;111:1593-1602.
35. Dror Y. Shwachman-Diamond syndrome. Pediatr Blood Can. 2005;45(7):892-901.
36. Shaw PH, Haut PR, Olszewski M, et al. Hematopoietic stem-cell transplantation using unrelated cord-blood versus matched sibling marrow in pediatric bone marrow failure syndrome: one center's experience. Pediatr Transplant. 1999;3:315-21.
37. van den Oudenrijn S, Bruin M, Folman CC, et al. Mutations in the thrombopoietin receptor, Mpl, in children with congenital amegakaryocytic thrombocytopenia. Br J Haematol. 2000;110:441-8.
38. van den Oudenrijn S, Bruin M, Folman CC, et al. Three parameters - plasma thrombopoietin levels, plasma glycocalicin levels and megakaryocyte culture, distinguish between different causes of congenital thrombocytopenia. Br J Haematol. 2002;117:390-8.
39. Kelsey P, Murphy MF, Brown M, et al. Guidelines for the use of platelet transfusions. Br J Haematol. 2003;122:10-23.
40. Kaminsky ER, Hows JM, Goldman JM, et al. Pretransfused patients with severe aplastic anaemia exhibit high numbers of cytotoxic T lymphocyte precursors probable directed atnon-HLA antigens. Br J Haematol. 1990;76:401-5.
41. Killick SB, Win N, Marsh JC, et al. Pilot study of HLA alloimmunisation after transfusion with pre-storage leucodepleted blood products in aplastic anaemia. Br J Haematol. 1997;97:677-84.

42. Casadevall N, Nataf J, Viron B, et al. Pure red cell aplasia and anti erythropoietin antibodies in patients treated with recombinant erythropoietin. N Eng J Medicine. 2002;346: 469-75.
43. Bodey, GP, Bolivar R, Fainstein, V. Infectious complications in leukaemic patients. Semin Hematol. 1982;19:193-226.
44. Keidan, AJ, Tsatalas C, Cohen J, et al. Infective complications of aplastic anaemia. Br J Haematol. 1986;63:503-8.
45. Bacigalupo A, Brand R, Oneto R, et al. Treatment of acquired severe aplastic anaemia: bone marrow transplantation compared with immunosuppressive therapy—The European Group for Blood and Marrow Transplantation experience. Semn Hematol. 2000;37(1):69-80.
46. Bacigalupo A, Bruno B, Saracco P, et al Antilymphocyte globulin, cyclosporine, prednisolone, and granulocyte colony-stimulating factor for severe aplastic anemia: an update of the GITMO/ EBMT study on 100 patients. European Group for Blood and Marrow Transplantation (EBMT) Working Party on Severe Aplastic Anemia and the Gruppo Italiano Trapianti di Midolio Osseo (GITMO). Blood. 2000;95:1931-4.
47. Willis F, Marsh J, Bevan D, et al. The effect of treatment with Campath-1H in patients with autoimmune cytopenias. Br J Haematol. 2001;114:891-8.

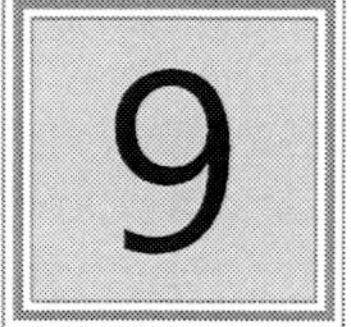

Approach to the Diagnosis of Hemolytic Disorders

Mohammed Ramzan, SP Yadav, Anupam Sachdeva

Hemolysis is the destruction or removal of red blood cells from the circulation before their normal lifespan of 120 days. While hemolysis can be a lifelong asymptomatic condition, it most often presents as anemia when erythrocytosis cannot match the pace of red blood cell destruction. Hemolysis also can manifest as jaundice, cholelithiasis, or isolated reticulocytosis.

Hemolytic disorders are conditions in which the rate of destruction of red blood cells is increased, and the bone marrow response to anemia is not compromised. Stated otherwise, the lifespan of the red blood cells is shortened and the red blood cell production is accelerated. The bone marrow has a capacity to increase red blood cell production by 6 to 8 folds. Thus, shortening of erythrocyte lifespan to a corresponding degree remains compensated and anemia does not manifest (Hemolytic disorder). When shortening of red blood cell lifespan is beyond the regenerative capacity of bone marrow hemolytic anemia manifests. In several diseases, the red blood cell lifespan is slightly reduced and there is an associated marrow failure. Accelerated hemolysis is thus, not the primary cause of anemia in these conditions and they are not categorized as hemolytic disorders. Anemia's due to vitamin B_{12} deficiency/ folate deficiency, iron deficiency, chronic disorders, chronic renal failure, dyshemopoietic disorders and many other conditions fall in this category. There are two mechanisms of hemolysis. Intravascular hemolysis is the destruction of red blood cells in the circulation with the release of cell contents into the plasma. Mechanical trauma from a damaged endothelium, complement fixation and activation on the cell surface and infectious agents may cause direct membrane degradation and cell destruction. The more common extravascular hemolysis is the removal and destruction of red blood cells with membrane alterations by the macrophages of the spleen and liver. Circulating blood is filtered continuously through thin walled splenic cords into the splenic sinusoids (with fenestrated basement membranes), a sponge like labyrinth of macrophages with long dendritic processes. A normal 8-micron red blood cell can deform itself and pass through the 3-micron openings in the splenic cords. Red blood cells with structural alterations of the membrane surface (including antibodies) are unable to traverse this network and are phagocytosed and destroyed by macrophages. Breakdown of red blood cells is associated with biochemically definable abnormalities. Specific alterations, in red blood cell morphology and biochemical changes occur in many hemolytic disorders. Further, some disorders have characteristic clinical features and these should be correlated with the laboratory evaluation.

HISTORY AND PHYSICAL EXAMINATION

Anemia most often is discovered through laboratory tests, but the history and physical examination can provide important clues about the presence of hemolysis and its underlying cause. The patient may complain of dyspnea or fatigue (caused by anemia). Dark urine and, occasionally, back pain may be reported by patients with intravascular hemolysis. The skin may appear jaundiced or pale. A resting tachycardia with a flow murmur may be present if the anemia is pronounced. Lymphadenopathy or hepatosplenomegaly suggest an underlying lymphoproliferative disorder or malignancy; alternatively, an enlarged spleen may reflect hypersplenism causing hemolysis. Leg ulcers occur in some chronic hemolytic states, such as sickle cell anemia. Different medical centers and physicians vary in their approach to diagnosis of hemolytic anemia. In general one has to first establish evidence of accelerated hemolysis based on reticulocyte count and level of unconjugated bilirubin. It is a common practice at many laboratories to establish whether the anemia is intravascular or extravascular. This approach limits the number of causative disorders. Hence, fewer confirmatory tests are required to reach a final diagnosis. Reticulocytosis must be correlated with hematinic therapy and recent blood transfusion. These markedly alter reticulocyte counts. When reticulocyte count and serum bilirubin value are inconclusive, two other tests are added (Flow chart 9.1). These are determination of serum haptoglobin and serum LDH. Serum haptoglobin is depleted not only in intravascular hemolytic anemias but also in hemolytic anemias, which are predominantly extravascular. Its depletion is a reliable index of accelerated hemolysis. Its limitation however is that being an acute phase reactant, haptoglobin levels are elevated in inflammatory and neoplastic conditions. Conversely, the levels may fall in diseases associated with a fall in synthetic function of the liver. Elevation of serum LDH, even though a non-specific finding, is common to all types of hemolytic anemias. Isoenzyme 2 is responsible for this rise. (In megaloblastic anemia, the rise in serum LDH is much greater and is due to a marked rise in isoenzyme 1). Theoretically, determination of red blood cell life span is an excellent test but is often not required. Secondly, it is cumbersome and does not give reliable results if the patient is receiving blood transfusions. Rise in urinary urobilinogen is considered by some to be a very reliable test of accelerated hemolysis. It is affected by many variables and hence, the test is often not carried out. Besides hemolytic anemias, urinary urobilinogen levels are elevated in dyshemopoietic anemias and liver dysfunction. In some conditions none of these tests provides conclusive evidence of hemolytic anemia. One of these is paroxysmal nocturnal hemoglobinuria (PNH). In this condition, however, hemosiderinuria is a consistent finding even if the patient is in a relatively quiescent phase. In patients who have been administered multiple blood transfusions, more specific tests such as acidified-serum test, sucrose lysis test and cold antibody lysis test may be of little value. In cases of severe intravascular hemolysis, the binding capacity of haptoglobin is exceeded rapidly, and free hemoglobin is filtered by the glomeruli. The renal tubule cells may absorb the

Flow chart 9.1: Evaluation of hemolytic anemia

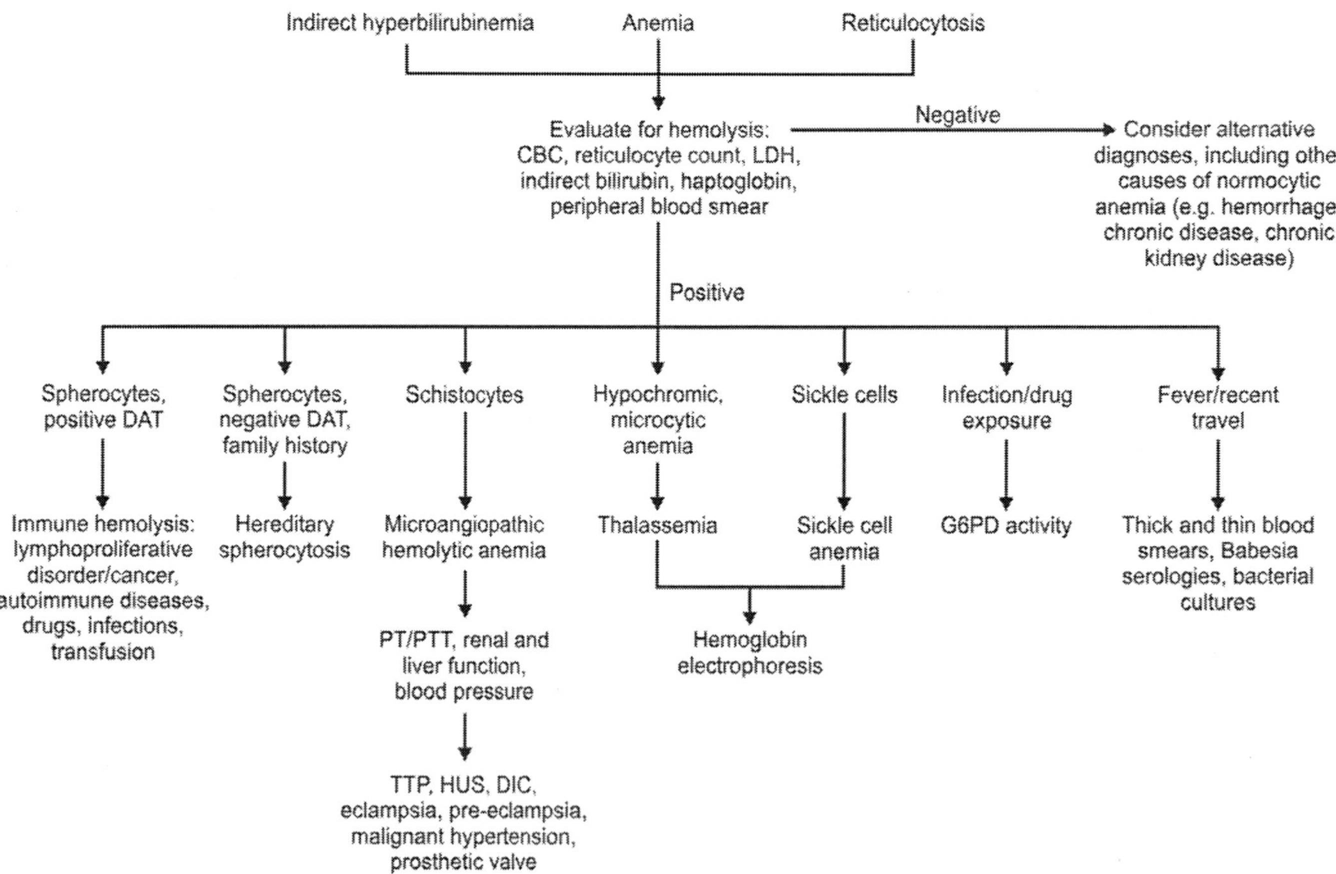

Abbreviations: CBC: Complete blood count; LDH: Lactate dehydrogenase; DAT: Direct antiglobulin test; G6PD: Glucose-6-phosphate dehydrogenase; PT/PTT: Prothrombin time/partial thromboplastin time; TTP: Thrombotic thrombocytopenic purpura; HUS: Hemolytic uremic syndrome; DIC: Disseminated intravascular coagulation)

hemoglobin and store the iron as hemosiderin; hemosiderinuria is detected by Prussian blue staining of sloughed tubular cells in the urinary sediment approximately one week after the onset of hemolysis. Hemoglobinuria, which causes red-brown urine, is indicated by a positive urine dipstick reaction for heme in the absence of red blood cells.

Investigations that establish accelerated hemolysis include demonstration of:

1. Shortened lifespan of red blood cells by ^{51}Cr labeling
2. Accelerated erythropoiesis.
   a. Erythroid hyperplasia in the bone marrow
   b. Reticulocytosis/polychromasia
3. Increase in catabolic products of hemoglobin in blood
   a. Unconjugated hyperbilirubinemia
   b. Hemoglobinemia (intravascular hemolysis)
   c. Hemoglobinuria (intravascular hemolysis)
   d. Hemosiderinuria (intravascular hemolysis)
   e. Increased urinary urobilinogen
   f. Increased CO excretion
4. Increased concentration of products released from the breakdown of red blood cells particularly LDH.
5. Effects due to release of hemoglobin
   a. Depletion of plasma/serum haptoglobin
   b. Depletion of plasma/serum hemopexin

Magnitude of anemia is estimated by determination of hemoglobin concentration. The CBC however, provides much valuable information and should be carried out in all patients suspected of having a hemolytic disorder. Acute hemolytic episode may be associated with neutrophilia, thrombocytosis and normoblastemia. On the other hand, many anemias may present with pancytopenia. PNH, autoimmune hemolytic anemia, hypersplenism and aplastic or megaloblastic crises in sickle cell anemia are few of the classical examples. Very often, the blood film helps in determining the type and etiology of hemolytic anemia.

SPECIFIC TESTS TO ESTABLISH THE CAUSE OF HEMOLYSIS

1. Microscopic examination of blood film for:
   a. Spherocytes, schistocytes, elliptocytes, sickle cells, target cells, acanthocytes, stomatocytes, pyropoikilocytes, polychromasia, basophilic stippling, agglutination, phagocytosis, parasites and normoblastemia
   b. Demonstration of Heinz bodies, hemoglobin H inclusions with special stains
2. Investigations for hereditary hemolytic anemias:
   a. Tests for red blood cell membrane abnormality:
      i. Osmotic fragility, incubation osmotic fragility, autohemolysis
      ii. Identification of specific membrane abnormality
3. Identification of abnormal hemoglobin:
   a. Electrophoresis, isoelectrofocussing (IEF), HPLC*
   b. Hb A_2 by microcolumn chromatography
   c. Hb F by alkali denaturation
   d. Intracellular Hb F distribution
   e. Quantitation of α- and β-chains by HPLC or electrophoresis
   f. Hb S by sickling test, solubility test
   g. Tests for unstable hemoglobins
   h. DNA analysis for detection of mutations.
4. Screening tests or quantitative analysis for enzymopathies
5. Investigations for acquired hemolytic anemias
   a. Immune hemolytic anemias
   b. PNH.

SALIENT LABORATORY FEATURES OF COMMON DISORDERS ASSOCIATED WITH HEMOLYTIC ANEMIA (TABLE 9.1)

Thalassemias

Trait: RBC indices (RBC $\geq$ 5 mill/dl, MCV < 70 fl, MCH >24 pg, normal RDW and various discriminant functions), microcytic hypochromic anemia, basophilic stippling.

β-*thal trait:* Hb A_2 > 3.5%; Hb F may be normal or mildly elevated

β-*thal major:* Hb A_2 reduced or normal, Hb F elevated

(Specific mutation may be defined by DNA analysis especially where prenatal diagnosis is planned).

Major: Mis-shapen RBC, microcytosis, hypochromia, basophilic stippling, normoblastemia, elevated Hb F Parents are obligate carriers

(Diagnosis difficult at <6 months of age and in multiply transfused).

*Electrophoretic mobility (on acid and alkaline pH) and HPLC elution pattern of several abnormal hemoglobins show considerable overlap. Diagnosis of abnormality is presumptive. Findings should be correlated with clinical features, family studies and other supportive or confirmatory tests. Confirmation of abnormal hemoglobin requires mass spectroscopy, peptide analysis or DNA analysis. IEF separates many more variants than gel electrophoresis. HPLC elution patterns should be interpreted with caution. In the frequently used Bio-Rad "Variant" system "Beta thal short programme", Hb A_2 value of more than 8% generally represents some other abnormal Hb commonly Hb E but it can also be Hb Lepore or even some others. When an abnormal Hb is about 10-20%, it is likely to be α-chain variant as only one of the 4 α-genes may be affected.

Table 9.1: Overview of the hemolytic anemias

Type	*Etiology*	*Associations*	*Diagnosis*	*Treatment*
Acquired*				
Immune-mediated	Antibodies to red blood cell surface antigens	Idiopathic, malignancy, drugs, autoimmune disorders, infections, transfusions	Spherocytes and positive DAT	Treatment of underlying disorder: removal of offending drug, steroids, splenectomy, IV gamma-globulin, plasmapheresis, cytotoxic agents, or danazol (Danocrine), avoidance of cold
Microangiopathic	Mechanical disruption of red blood cell in circulation	TTP, HUS, DIC, pre-eclampsia, eclampsia, malignant hypertension, prosthetic valves	Schistocytes	Treatment of underlying disorder
Infection	Malaria, babesiosis, *Clostridium* infections		Cultures, thick and thin blood smears, serologies	Antibiotics
Hereditary†				
Enzymopathies	G6PD deficiency	Infections, drugs, ingestion of fava beans	Low G6PD activity measurement	Withdrawal of offending drug, treatment of infection
Membranopathies	Hereditary spherocytosis		Spherocytes, family history, negative DAT	Splenectomy in some moderate and some severe cases
Hemoglobinopathies	Thalassemia and sickle cell disease		Hemoglobin electrophoresis, genetic studies	Folate, transfusions

Abbreviations: DAT: Direct antiglobulin test; IV: Intravenous; TTP: Thrombotic thrombocytopenic purpura; HUS: Hemolytic uremic syndrome; DIC: Disseminated intravascular coagulation; G6PD: Glucose 6-phosphate dehydrogenase

*Other select causes of acquire hemolysis (not discussed in this chapter) incude splenomegaly, end-stage liver disease/spur cell (acanthocyte) hemolytic anemia, paroxysmal cold hemoglobinuria, paroxysmal nocturnal hemoglobinuria, insect stings, and spider bites

†Other select causes of inherited hemolysis (not discussed in this chapter) include Wilson's disease and less common forms of membranopathy (hereditary elliptocytosis), enzymopathy (pyruvate kinase deficiency), and hemoglobinopathy (unstable hemoglobin variants)

Hb Bart's hydrops fetalis: Severe erythroblastemia, Hb electrophoresis.

Bart's: In many patients, especially those presenting with thalassemia intermedia like picture, β-thalassemia globin chain polymorphism for Xmn-1 mutation should be studied. Those with the mutation respond to therapy with hydroxyurea.

Sickle Cell Disorders

Sickle cell anemia is an inherited disorder caused by a point mutation leading to a substitution of valine for glutamic acid in the sixth position of the β-chain of hemoglobin.

Sickling test, solubility test, Hb electrophoresis on alkaline and acid pH, HPLC and DNA analysis are useful in identification of both sickle cell trait and sickle cell anemia. DNA analysis is rarely required.

Clinical severity of sickle cell anemia is reduced by elevated Hb F level, coinheritance of β-thalassemia and certain types of α-gene cluster haplotypes.

Other Hemoglobinopathies

Hb E disease is common in eastern part of India and in homozygous state, may produce thalassemia trait-like picture. Patients doubly heterozygous for β-thalassemia and Hb E disease produce a highly varied clinical picture ranging from thalassemia trait to thalassemia intermedia/major. The diagnosis depends upon hemoglobin electrophoresis.

Hb D is frequently seen in Northern India. At alkaline pH, mobility of Hb D and Hb S is same. Acid electrophoresis and HPLC allow easy differentiation. Its identification is important, as in heterozygous state it is asymptomatic. In homozygous state, it may cause mild anemia. In those doubly heterozygous for Hb D and β-thalassemia, it may cause significant anemia. Differentiation between these two is often difficult. Hb A_2 estimation and family studies provide useful information. Hb G and several other hemoglobins have same electrophoretic mobility as Hb D.

Unstable Hemoglobins

The following tests are useful in the diagnosis of unstable hemoglobins and are within the reach of most laboratories: Heat instability test, isopropanol/n-butanol stability test, test for methemoglobin, measurement of oxygen dissociation curve.

Membranopathies

Hereditary spherocytosis is an autosomal dominant disorder caused by mutations in the red blood cell membrane skeleton protein genes. With a weakened protein backbone anchoring its lipid bilayer, the membrane undergoes a progressive deterioration in structure, resulting in a spherocyte, the characteristic abnormality seen on peripheral smear. The diagnosis is based on the combination of spherocytosis noted on peripheral smear, a family history (in 75% of cases), and a negative DAT. The mean corpuscular hemoglobin concentration frequently is elevated.

The blood film shows spherocytosis and the osmotic fragility (especially after 24 hours incubation) is enhanced. Positive autohemolysis test is corrected by glucose, though cumbersome, is a very useful test. Special studies to define abnormalities of membrane proteins can be done using polyacrylamide gel electrophoresis (PAGE). Demonstration of abnormality in one of the parents is almost a conclusive evidence of hereditary spherocytosis.

Enzymopathies

Most patients have no clinical or laboratory evidence of ongoing hemolysis until an event—infection, drug reaction or ingestion of fava beans—causes oxidative damage to hemoglobin. The oxidized and denatured hemoglobin crosslinks and precipitates intracellularly, forming inclusions that are identified as Heinz bodies on the supravital stain of the peripheral smear. Heinz bodies are removed in the spleen, leaving erythrocytes with a missing section of cytoplasm; these "bite cells" can be seen on the routine blood smear. The altered erythrocytes undergo both intravascular and extravascular destruction. Older red blood cells are most susceptible, because they have an intrinsic G6PD deficiency coupled with the normal age-related decline in G6PD levels. Hemolysis occurs two to four days following exposure and varies from an asymptomatic decline in hemoglobin to a marked intravascular hemolysis. Even with ongoing exposure, the hemolysis usually is self-limited, as the older G6PD-deficient cells are destroyed. There is no specific therapy other than treatment of the underlying infection and avoidance of implicated medications. In cases of severe hemolysis, which can occur with the Mediterranean—variant enzyme, transfusion may be required. G6PD activity levels may be measured as normal during an acute episode, because only nonhemolyzed, younger cells are assayed. If G6PD deficiency is suspected after a normal activity-level measurement, the assay should be repeated in two to three months, when cells of all ages are again present. Several screening tests for enzyme deficiency are sensitive and reproducible. Methylene blue reduction test is inexpensive and sensitive and often detects even heterozygotes. Enzyme quantitation is now frequently available in many laboratories in India. Specific mutations can be defined by DNA analysis.

Pyruvate kinase deficiency: Diagnosis is made by the presence of spicules on irregularly contracted RBC and demonstration of enzyme deficiency by screening or quantitative assay.

Paroxysmal Nocturnal Hemoglobinuria

Peripheral blood film findings are variable—anemia may be normocytic normochromic or microcytic hypochromic. Reticulocyte count may be elevated or normal. Pancytopenia is common. Hemosiderinuria (an evidence of intravascular hemolysis) is almost a constant feature. Specific tests include those, which demonstrate sensitivity of red blood cells to complement. Abnormality of membrane proteins can be demonstrated by CD markers (especially CD55 and CD59) through flowcytometry. Neutrophil alkaline phosphate activity is reduced.

Autoimmune Hemolytic Anemia

Blood film shows spherocytosis, polychromasia, reticulocytosis and mild erythroblastemia. Direct antiglobulin test with potent broad-spectrum and monospecific sera is positive. A negative antiglobulin test is very rare. Further definition requires tests such as indirect antiglobulin test, determining thermal amplitude of antibody, test for Donath-Landsteiner antibody and tests for SLE. Expanded blood group antigen should be done in all cases of proven AIHA to further characterize the subclass of the antibodies.

Red Blood Cell Fragmentation Syndromes

Schistocytosis is a salient feature of red blood cell fragmentation syndromes (RFS) RFS whether arising from large vessel abnormality or from small vessel microangiopathy. Evidence of intravascular hemolysis such as hemosiderinuria, hemoglobinemia, hemoglobinuria, depletion of haptoglobin and elevated levels of serum LDH isoenzyme is often present. A variety of disorders can cause RFS and further investigations depend upon the clinical history and age of the patient. Early diagnosis and treatment of microangiopathic conditions such as hemolytic uremic syndrome and thrombotic thrombocytopenic purpura is often rewarding.

As already stated, many clinical entities and laboratory tests are not included in this discussion. The laboratory investigations should be planned according to the clinical features and CBC values. After evidence of accelerated hemolysis is established, further tests depend upon red blood cell morphology and, whether the hemolysis is intravascular or extravascular. Etiology of hemolytic anemias in many patients in India remains unestablished. Very few laboratories have facilities to screen for common enzymopathies and there is not a single reference laboratory, which carries out tests for unusual enzymopathies. There is no center where reference material for hemoglobinopathies is available.

BIBLIOGRAPHY

1. Bolton-Maggs PH. The diagnosis and management of hereditary spherocytosis. Baillieres Best Pract Res Clin Haematol. 2000;13:327-42.
2. Chadburn A. The spleen: anatomy and anatomical function. Semin Hematol. 2000;37(suppl 1):13-21.
3. Tabbara IA. Hemolytic anemias. Diagnosis and management. Med Clin North Am. 1992;76:649-68.
4. Walters MC, Abelson HT. Interpretation of the complete blood count. Pediatr Clin North Am. 1996;43:599-622.

10 Management of β-Thalassemia Major

Mohammed Ramzan, SP Yadav, Anupam Sachdeva

Thalassemia is an inherited disorder of hemoglobin that causes reduced or absent globin synthesis, results in an imbalanced accumulation of globin chains and ineffective erythropoiesis with hemolysis.[1] The hallmarks of treatment include regular red blood cell (RBC) transfusions with iron chelation therapy for transfusion-related iron overload and supportive care to treat the complications of iron overload.[2,3]

However, the only curative therapy is replacement of the defective gene by hematopoietic cell transplantation.[4-6] It is estimated that about 100,000 children with transfusion dependent thalassemia are born worldwide annually. Out of these, 8,000 to 10,000 are born in India alone. In the absence of treatment, most patients with β-thalassemia major die before the age of five years. The management of thalassemia has undergone metamorphosis over the last three decades. With the modern management, most of the patients with thalassemia major are free of complications of anemia and compensatory bone marrow expansions. They have near normal development throughout childhood with a better quality of life.

Management of thalassemia involves a multidisciplinary therapeutic team approach. The treating doctor should remain the same to ensure continuity of specialized care and to develop supportive relationship with each patient. It is equally important to have dedicated nurses and to have regular checkups by specialists such as a hematologist, cardiologist, endocrinologist, ophthalmologist, orthopedic surgeon, neurologist and a psychologist.

The mainstay of current recommended treatment for thalassemia is regular blood transfusion and chelation. Bone marrow transplantation, a curative form of treatment is available to a small proportion of patients. Other forms of therapies such as pharmacological stimulation of fetal hemoglobin are still experimental as far as thalassemia major is concerned. The definite treatment with gene therapy is still a long way off.

TRANSFUSION THERAPY

Blood transfusion remains the cornerstone of therapy in β-thalassemia major. The decision to initiate life long regular transfusions in patients with β-thalassemia should be based on the molecular defect, severity of symptoms, and clinical criteria such as failure of growth, development and bone changes. The goals of transfusion are:

- Prevention of chronic hypoxia.
- Suppression of erythropoiesis to reduce compensatory marrow hyperplasia and gastrointestinal absorption of iron.
- To prevent serious growth, neurological and skeletal complication of thalassemia major.
- To prevent hypervolemia (secondary to marrow hyperplasia).
- To prevent early splenomegaly and hypersplenism.

In the 1960s, Wolmans proposed a palliative transfusion therapy for thalassemia major. It was aimed at maintaining the hemoglobin level at 8.5 g%. This led to improved survival, but the chronic illness, bone disease and cardiomyopathy persisted. To overcome these problems, Piomelli and workers suggested maintaining the hemoglobin level above a minimum of 10 g%. These vigorous regimens were termed as hypertransfusion, although normotransfusion may be a more descriptive term. Hypertransfusion promotes normal growth and development, prevents the onset of severe hepatosplenomegaly and hemolytic facies, lowers the absorption of gastrointestinal iron and reduces the anemic cardiomyopathy changes.

In 1980s, Propper and colleagues introduced a further improvised regimen called supertransfusion, and maintained a pretransfusion hemoglobin of above 12 g%. However, this did not prove significantly superior to hypertransfusion and was given up. Hypertransfusion remains the most accepted regimen in most parts of the world. However, in Europe, a yet newer regimen termed the 'moderate transfusion regimen' has been adopted and recommended by the Thalassemia International Federation. In this regimen, pretransfusion hemoglobin is maintained between 9 and 10.5 g%.

The current recommendation is to maintain a mean hemoglobin (Hb) level of 12 g/dl and to transfuse at a level of 9-10.5 g/dl. Post-transfusion hemoglobin should not rise above 15 g/dl. This regime ensures adequate marrow suppression, and relatively lower rates of iron accumulation. Maintaining higher pre-transfusion hemoglobin increases the blood requirement and thus increases the iron overload.

Type of Blood to Give

A thalassemia child should receive red blood cells with the least possible amount of white blood cells or plasma as these can induce antibody formation and allergic reactions. To avoid allosensitization of clinically important blood group antigens, patient's ABO, Rhesus, Kell, Kidd and Duffy system should be typed before institution of transfusion therapy. Patient's blood should be matched with donor's blood ABO, Rhesus and Kell systems. To prevent non-hemolytic febrile transfusion reactions (NHFTR) it is recommended to use filters from the beginning. Bedside leukocyte-filters have 99.9% white cell removal efficiency and are easy to use. Those patients who develop NHFTR in spite of filtration should have their blood filtered at the source. Reduction of leukocyte to $<5 \times 10^6$ per unit is considered the critical threshold for eliminating adverse reactions attributed to contaminating white cells. Other advantages of leucodepletion are to avoid HLA alloimmunization, prevent CMV infection, improved storage of erythrocytes and their flow cytometric evaluation if required. Pre-storage filtration is a method of leukocyte depletion that offers a high efficiency filtration and prevents the leukotrienes from leaking into the plasma due to degeneration of the white cells.

Blood Products for Special Patient Population

- Washed red cells are beneficial for patients who have repeated severe allergic reactions.
- Frozen red cells are useful for patients who have rare blood group or unusual red cell antibodies.
- Neocyte transfusions reduce the blood requirement but expose the patients to a high number of donors and increase the cost, risk of transmission of infections and risk of alloantibodies.
- Erythrocytopheresis or automated red cells exchange also reduces the blood requirement. However, this procedure is expensive, exposes the patient to a number of donors, which increases the risk of infection and alloimmunization.

Table 10.1: Transfusion interval in relation to pre- and post-transfusion hemoglobin*

Weeks between transfusion	*Hb level g/dl*		
	Pre-transfusion	*Post-transfusion*	*Mean*
2	11.0	13.0	12.0
3	10.5	13.5	12.0
4	10.0	14.0	12.0
5	9.5	14.5	12.0
6	9.0	15.0	12.0

*Adapted from Management Protocol for the Treatment of Thalassaemia Patients. Thalassaemia International Federation. Nicosia, Cyprus, 1997[7]

Frequency of Transfusion

The volume and rate of blood transfusion depends on patient's age, their clinical status, solutions added to preserve red blood cells, hematocrit of donor's RBC's and target level of hemoglobin. Transfusion interval is usually influenced by many factors such as the distance from the patient's home to the transfusion center and social and psychological impact on the patient of each hospital visit. To avoid wastage, blood transfusion interval is adjusted to allow transfusions of a whole unit (except in small children). The average rate of fall in hemoglobin is approximately 1 g per week. This allows easy calculation of pre-transfusion hemoglobin necessary to maintain a mean Hb of 12 g/dl for a given transfusion interval (Table 10.1).

How much Blood to Transfuse

The amount of blood to be transfused varies with different anticoagulant, procoagulant solutions and the hematocrit. For CPD-A units with a hematocrit of 75%, the volume per transfusion is 10-15 ml/kg. Units with additive solutions may have hematocrit of 60-70% and thus larger volume may be required to deliver the same red cell mass as delivered by CPD-A unit with a high hematocrit.

Guidelines for Choosing Amount of Blood for Transfusion

The amount of packed cells to be transfused depends on the hematocrit of the donor packed cells and the target increase in hemoglobin level. This is depicted in the Table 10.2.

Table 10.2: Increase in hemoglobin level based on the hematocrit of the donor red cells*

Target increase in Hb Level	*Hematocrit of donor red cells* 50%	60%	75%	80%
1 g/dl	4.2 ml/kg	3.5 ml/kg	2.8 ml/kg	2.6 ml/kg
2 g/dl	8.4 ml/kg	7.0 ml/kg	5.6 ml/kg	5.2 ml/kg
3 g/dl	12.6 ml/kg	10.5 ml/kg	8.4 ml/kg	7.8 ml/kg
4 g/dl	16.8 ml/kg	14.0 ml/kg	11.2 ml/kg	10.4 ml/kg

*Adapted from technical manual 'Guidelines for the Clinical Management of Thalassaemia'. Thalassaemia International Federation, November 2008.[8]

Rate of Transfusion

Where there is no cardiac problem it is acceptable to give 5 ml/kg/hr of packed cells. When cardiac failure is present or the Hb level is less than 5 g/dl it is recommended to give 1-2 weekly transfusion of 5 ml/kg at the rate of 2 ml/kg/hr.

Evaluation of Transfusion Treatment

The most useful indicator of appropriate management is the annual pure red cell consumption. The average pure red cell consumption for splenectomized patients with a mean Hb of 12 g/dl is 130 ml of pure red cells/kg/ year (range 100-200 ml/kg/year). Non-splenectomized patients have higher blood requirement, which may be 30% more than splenectomized patients. The main causes of higher blood consumption are hypersplenism, red cell incompatibility and poor quality of transfused blood. One can calculate the annual pure red cell consumption and from that the transfusional iron overload (Table 10.3).

Complications of Blood Transfusion

This includes transfusion-transmitted infections. It is essential that the donor blood be tested for HIV, HCV, HBV and syphilis. Hepatitis B vaccine should be administered to all newly diagnosed thalassemia patients and to those older patients who lack demonstrable antibodies to hepatitis B.

Adverse Reactions

Adverse reactions because of blood transfusions can be reduced by leukodepletion, finding ways to reduce transfusion requirement and the number of donor exposures. Adverse reactions associated with transfusion include:

- Non-hemolytic febrile transfusion reactions can be minimized by use of leukocyte filters.
- Allergic reactions are mainly due to plasma proteins. They can be reduced by removal of plasma and patients prone to allergic reactions should be transfused with washed red cells.
- Acute hemolytic reactions most commonly result from errors in blood typing and cross matching.
- Autoimmune hemolytic reactions, a serious complication is mainly due to alloimmunization. This is more frequent in patients who begin transfusion therapy later in life. Steroids, immunosuppressive drugs and intravenous immunoglobulins are recommended to manage these complications. Delayed transfusion reactions develop as a result of alloantibodies and are all characterized by anemia, malaise and jaundice, and occur 5-10 days after transfusions.
- Transfusion related acute lung injury and graft versus host disease are rare but serious complications.

Table 10.3: Calculation of annual blood requirement and transfusional iron loading*

- Patient wt: 40 kg
- Transfusion amount and schedule: 600 ml every 4 weeks
- Average hematocrit of transfused red cells: 60%
- Annual blood requirement: 13 transfusions × 600 ml/40 kg = 195 ml/kg
- Annual pure red cells requirement: 195 ml/kg/yr × 60% (avg hematocrit) = 117 ml/kg/year
- Annual transfusional iron loading: 117 m/kg/yr of pure red cells × 1.08 mg iron per ml pure red cells = 126 mg iron
- Daily transfusional iron loading: 126 mg iron/yr/365 days = 0.34 mg/kg

*Adapted from technical manual. 'Guidelines for the Clinical Management of Thalassaemia'. Thalassaemia International Federation, November 2008.[8]

- Transmission of infectious agents such of viruses, bacteria, and parasites is a potential risk due to blood transfusions.
- Transfusion-induced graft versus host disease is caused by viable lymphocytes in units of transfused red cells. It is a rare but often fatal complication of transfusion. Immunosuppressed patients are at particular risk.

SPLENECTOMY

Currently recommended management of thalassemia may delay or even prevent hypersplenism thereby reducing the need for splenectomy. Splenectomy should be considered when:

- Annual blood requirement exceeds 1.5 times the basal requirement for a patient maintaining pre-transfusion Hb about 10 gm/dl. When transfusion requirement increases to more than 200-220 ml/kg/year of packed red cells (assuming hematocrit of transfused blood is 75%), splenectomy should be considered.
- Massive spleen enlargement posing a risk of splenic rupture or when splenic enlargement is associated with left upper quadrant pain or early satiety.
- Presence of leukopenia or thrombocytopenia due to hypersplenism.

Splenectomy should be delayed till the patient is five years of age as there is a risk of overwhelming sepsis below this age.

Risk of post-splenectomy serious infections can be reduced by:

- Immunization against pneumococcal, meningococcal, and *Haemophilus influenzae-B* and *Salmonella typhi* infection at least 3 weeks before splenectomy. Chemoprophylaxis with oral penicillin, 125 mg twice a day for children up to 2 years and 250 mg twice a day for children two years and above. Chemoprophylaxis is recommended for at least 2 years while some advocate this for whole life. In the presence of early signs of infection treatment should be started immediately with broad-spectrum antibiotics without waiting for the result of laboratory tests.
- Post-splenectomy, there may be transient or persistent thrombocytosis. Aspirin 50-100 mg/day is recommended for patients whose platelet count exceeds 8,00,000/mm^3.

FOLIC ACID

Folic acid should be given to untransfused or low transfused patients because they have increased folate consumption and may develop folic acid deficiency. Supplements (1 mg/day) may be given. Thalassemics on high transfusions rarely develop folic acid deficiency and usually have no need for supplements.

CHELATION THERAPY

Iron overload is an inevitable consequence of regular long-term transfusion therapy. In addition to transfusion, thalassemics have excessive intestinal absorption of iron because of increased and ineffective erythropoiesis, which further aggravates the already existing iron overload. When iron accumulation exceeds the storage capacity of ferritin, pathological quantities of metabolically active iron are released intracellularly in the form of hemosiderin and in the labile pool as free iron. The principal target organ systems vulnerable to iron toxicity are the heart, liver and endocrine glands. The heart is more vulnerable to damage than the liver, which produces more of protective ferritin. Endocrine complications, namely diabetes, hypothyroidism and hypoparathyroidism, are also seen. Liver disease with fibrosis and eventually cirrhosis, particularly if concomitant chronic hepatitis is present, is also a serious complication. In the absence of any mechanism of the human body to excrete excess iron, chelation therapy is essential and constitutes the second important arm, besides transfusion therapy, of the clinical management of these patients.

Initiation of Chelation Therapy

It is important to initiate chelation therapy at an appropriate time to prevent the manifestations of iron overload in various organs of the body. The optimal time to start chelation therapy has not been defined so far. It should be started when:

a. Serum ferritin approaches 1000 ng/dl.
b. Patient has received 15-20 transfusions.
c. Hepatic iron concentration exceeds 3.2 mg/g dry weight.

IRON CHELATORS

Desferrioxamine Therapy

Desferrioxamine has been in clinical use since the 1970's and widely used as subcutaneous infusions since 1980. DFO takes up iron from various iron containing proteins in the body including ferritin and hemosiderin. The plasma half life of DFO is 20 minutes. The iron desferrioxamine compound (ferrioxamine) is easily excreted in the urine (70-80%) and in the stools (20-30%). Excreted ferrioxamine imparts red color to the urine.

The factors that influence degree of iron excretion in response to DFO include:

- Body iron overload.
- Route of administration.
- Duration of infusion: Non-transfusion bound iron (NTBI) which is thought to be the most damaging to heart and other organs, falls significantly in patients given a continuous infusion of DFO either subcutaneously or intravenously.

If treatment is begun within 2-3 years of beginning transfusion therapy, administered regularly and administered in adequate doses, desferrioxamine has a well established impact on survival and on cardiac and other complications of iron overload.[9]

Dosage: The recommended dosage of DFO with different serum ferritin levels is given below:

Serum ferritin	*Dose of DFO*
<2000 μg/L	25 mg/kg/day
2000-3000 μg/L	35 mg/kg/day
>3000 μg/L	55 mg/kg/day*

*Not to exceed 100 mg/kg/day

Mode of Administration

Subcutaneous: DFO can be effectively administered by this route using a portable infusion pump that can be attached to the body (Fig. 10.1). It is infused over 8-12 hours as a 10% solution with the help of a fine gauge needle inserted subcutaneously in the abdomen, upper arm or thigh.

Recently a convenient infusion needle set called "Thala Set" has been introduced (Figs 10.2A and B). It consists of a vertical 8 mm needle with a polyethylene tubing to reduce allergic reactions and a transparent built-in adhesive strap to avoid extra dressing.

Recently it has been reported that twice-daily subcutaneous bolus injections of DFO are as effective as the same dose administered by subcutaneous infusion. It needs confirmation by further long-term trials.

Intravenous: Continuous intravenous transfusion is recommended for:

- Patients with severe cardiomyopathy.
- Patients having local drug reaction to DFO given subcutaneously.
- Non compliant patients.
- In preparation for a planned pregnancy with high serum ferritin.

DFO can be infused continuously through an intravenous access device 'port-a-cath' implanted subcutaneously. Treatment with continuous intravenous desferrioxamine has been shown to improve myocardial iron, even in the most overloaded hearts, with average myocardial T2* values of <6 ms.[10] The average rate of improvement at this level of iron loading of the heart

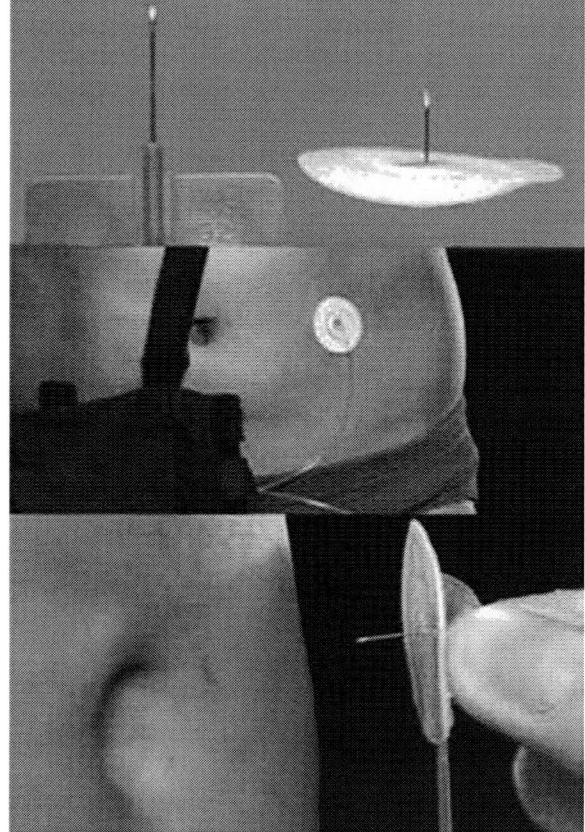

Fig. 10.1: Insertion of needles for desferrioxamine infusion

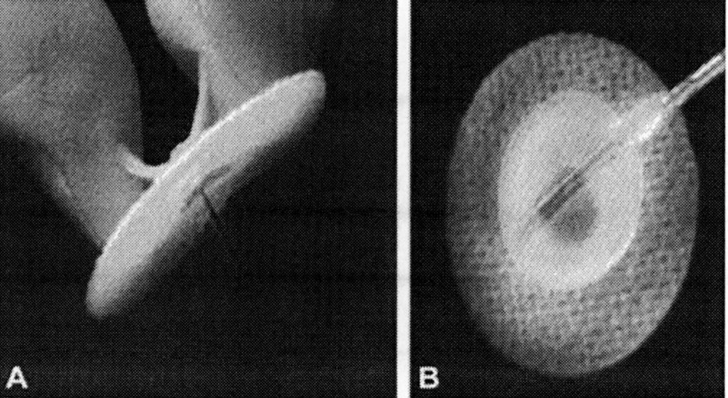

Figs 10.2A and B: Thala set

*If the only abnormalities are high ferritin or LIC, it would be usual to try to increase the dosing (e.g. to 50-60 mg/kg) or the duration or the frequency of subcutaneous infusions

is about 3 ms/year in severely overloaded hearts: if improvement is linear it would take several years to normalize the T2* to >20 ms.[11]

Intramuscular: This is less effective than intravenous or subcutaneous route because of rapid plasma clearance of DFO.

Consideration of Intensive Therapy

- Severe iron overload
  - Persistently very high ferritin value*
  - Liver iron >15 mg/g dry weight*
- Significant cardiac disease:
  - Significant cardiac dysrhythmias
  - Evidence of falling left ventricular function
  - Evidence of very severe heart iron loading (T2* <6 ms)
- Prior to pregnancy or bone marrow transplantation, when rapid reversal of iron loading may be desirable

Intensification of treatment through continuous, 24 hours infusion of deferrioxamine via an implanted intravenous delivery system (e.g. Port-a-cath)[12] or subcutaneously[13] has been shown to normalize heart function, reverse heart failure, improve myocardial T2* and lead to a better long term survival, provided treatment is maintained.

Supplementation with Vitamin C

Iron excretion with DFO can be enhanced by supplementing it with vitamin C. It should be given on the days when patient receives DFO and should be administered 30-60 minutes after starting the infusion. The recommended dose of vitamin C for children up to 10 years is 50 mg/dose, for older children it is 100 mg/dose while for adults it is 200 mg/dose.

Side Effects

DFO is a drug with low toxicity. Local reaction in the form of pain, itching, erythema and swelling may be observed. These may be decreased by restricting the concentration of the infusion to 10%, by changing the site of injection and by adding hydrocortisone in a dose of 1 mg/ml to the infusion solution. Systemic side effects are infrequent. Auditory and visual complications are dose related and have been observed in heavily chelated patients with low iron burden. These adverse effects are reversible on withdrawing the drug. Growth retardation and skeletal changes also occurred at high doses. Patients on DFO therapy have an increased susceptibility to some infection like Yersinia spp, hence DFO therapy should be temporarily discontinued in the presence of fever, pain abdomen, diarrhea and pharyngitis.

Regular estimation of iron overload and adjustment of the dose of DFO as to maintain Porter index value*[14] below 0.025 can avoid toxic effects of DFO.

$$\text{Porter's Index} = \frac{\text{Mean daily dose of DFO (mg/kg)}}{\text{Serum ferritin } (\mu g/L)}$$

*Mean daily dose = (actual dose received on each infusion x doses per day/7).

DEFERIPRONE (FERRIPOX, KELFER, L1) THERAPY

Deferiprone is an orally absorbed world's first oral iron chelator that began clinical trials in the UK in the 1980 and India was the first country to approve it for clinical use. It chelates iron from parenchymal tissue, reticuloendothelial stores and transferrin. It has a half-life of 135 minutes and is excreted mainly in urine. Vitamin C does not enhance urinary iron excretion when given to patients on L1 therapy. According to the official European Medicines Evaluation Agency (EMEA), deferiprone could be used as a second line drug, for removing iron in patients who are unable to use desferrioxamine or in whom DFO therapy has proven ineffective.

Dosage: The optimal dose is 75 mg/kg/day given in 2-4 divided doses. This may be increased to 100 mg/kg/day, but the incidence of side effects increases at higher dose. L1 is available as capsules of 250 mg and 500 mg strength.

Side effects: Most of the side effects are dose dependent.

- Vomiting and abdominal pain have been observed in 5% cases.
- Neutropenia, agranulocytosis and thrombocytopenia are the most serious side effects associated with L1 therapy. They are observed in 1-4% cases. Recently, 46 cases of agranulocytosis, were reported, in Europe with nine related deaths.[15] The mechanism of this toxicity remains unclear but is possibly an idiosyncratic reaction. Patients on L1 need monitoring in the form of total and differential counts at 2-4 weeks interval and the drug should be discontinued whenever:
  - total white cell count drops to less than 3000/mm^3
  - an absolute neutropenia count falls to less than 1000/mm^3
  - platelet count drops to less that 1,00,000/mm^3
- Arthropathy and musculoskeletal pains are seen in 10-30% of the cases. They are dose related, more common in heavily iron-loaded patients.

- Zinc deficiency may develop in patients during L1 therapy, especially in patients with diabetes mellitus.

L1 should be used as first line of treatment for patients not receiving DFO because of high cost, toxicity or poor compliance of the later.

Combined Therapy with Desferrioxamine and Deferiprone

The principle involve behind combination therapy is that if the drugs are given at the same time (simultaneously), they may interact in a process that involves the 'shuttling' (shuttle hypothesis) of iron, which may lead to additional chelation of iron from cells or plasma and so improved iron removal. However, there is also a possibility of chelation from metallo-enzymes, leading to increased drug-related toxicity. Chelators can be given at the same time as each other (simultaneously) or following one another (sequentially). There is considerable variation in the way in which sequential treatment can and has been administered. Some investigators have used the term 'alternating therapy' to describe the use of two drugs administered on alternate days, reserving the term 'sequential therapy' for when desferrioxamine is given at night and deferiprone during the day. In practice regimes may involve a component of 'sequential' and 'alternating' therapy, such as when desferrioxamine is given three times a week (alternate nights) and deferiprone every day. Most regimes have tended to give deferiprone daily, at standard doses, combined with varying frequency and dosing of desferrioxamine. In short, the simultaneous use of combination of these drugs has not been tested formally in large enough patient groups to allow firm, evidence-based recommendations about efficacy and safety.

Effects of Sequential Use on Serum Ferritin

Four randomized studies have compared levels of serum ferritin in patients using combined treatments with those under other treatment regimes. One study[16] found the decrease in serum ferritin achieved with five days of desferrioxamine monotherapy (n=11) to be similar to that achieved with two nights of desferrio-xamine plus seven days of deferiprone at 75 mg/kg (n=14). Another randomized study, involving 30 patients and three different treatments[17] found that the decrease in serum ferritin was greatest with five nights of desferrioxamine, albeit not significantly different from that achieved with a combined treatment of desferrioxamine two nights a week plus deferiprone seven days a week. A third randomized study, involving 60 patients[18,19] found no difference in the level of decrease in serum ferritin in patients randomized to combined treatment (two days desferrioxamine at 33 mg/kg + seven days deferiprone at 75 mg/kg) or to desferrioxamine five nights a week at 33 mg/kg. Taken together, these studies suggest that serum ferritin can be controlled with a relatively small dose of desferrioxamine given twice a week, when combined with deferiprone at standard doses (75 mg/kg/day). In a more recent randomized study of 65 patients,[18] serum ferritin was decreased more by combined treatment (desferrioxamine five days a week plus deferiprone seven days a week) than with standard desferrioxamine monotherapy (40 mg/kg five times a week).[20]

NEWER CHELATING AGENTS

Deferasirox (Exjade, Asunra)

Deferasirox was developed by Novartis as a once-daily, oral monotherapy for the treatment of transfusional iron overload. The drug has been licensed as first-line monotherapy for thalassemia major in over 70 countries worldwide, including the US (2005) and the EU (2006). This is an orally absorbed iron chelator, with two molecules binding each iron atom. The tablet is dissolved in water (or apple juice) using a non-metallic stirrer, and consumed as a drink once daily, preferably 30 minutes before a meal. The tablets must not be chewed or swallow. Due to the long plasma half-life (9–11 hours), once-daily administration provides 24-hour chelation from labile plasma iron.[21,22] A starting dose of 20 mg/kg is recommended for thalassemia major patients who have received 10-20 transfusion episodes and currently receive standard transfusion at rates of 0.3-0.5 mg of iron/kg/day. In those patients in whom there is a higher rate of iron intake from transfusion (>0.5 mg/kg/day or >14 ml/kg/month) or in patients with pre-existing high levels of iron loading, where a decrease in iron loading is clinically desirable, 30 mg/kg/day is recommended. For patients with a low rate of iron loading (< 0.3 mg/kg/day or less than 7 ml/kg/month), a dose of 10-15 mg/kg may be sufficient to control iron loading. For patients already well-managed on treatment with deferoxamine, a starting dose of deferisirox that is numerically half that of the deferoxamine dose could be considered. At this time, evidence of effectiveness is confined to serum ferritin and liver iron.

It is recommended that serum ferritin level should be monitored every month and that the dose of deferisirox should be adjusted if necessary every 3 to 6 months based on the trends in serum ferritin. Dose adjustment may be made in steps of 5 to 10 mg/kg and are to be tailored to the individual patient's response and therapeutic goals. Doses above 30 mg/kg are not recommended because there is only limited experience with doses above this level. However, recent data has shown that one can go up to 40 mg/kg.

Unwanted Effects with Deferasirox

Gastrointestinal disturbances—typically mild and transient - occurred in 15% of patients and included abdominal pain, nausea and vomiting, diarrhea and constipation, lasting a median of less than eight days. Skin rashes occurred in (11%) of patients and were typically pruritic, maculopapular and generalized, but occasionally confined to palms and soles of the feet. A rash typically developed within two weeks of starting treatment. A minority of patients may require permanent discontinuation of therapy, but mild rashes often resolved without dose modification. An increase in serum creatinine ≥30% on at least two consecutive readings was observed in 38% of patients receiving deferasirox, most frequently at doses of 20 mg/kg and 30 mg/kg.[23] No agranulocytosis, arthropathy or growth failure was associated with deferasirox administration. Deferasirox is contraindicated in patients with renal failure or significant renal dysfunction. For patients with evidence of significant heart dysfunction (e.g. LVEF below reference range) there is very limited clinical experience and treatment cannot be recommended at this time for patients with heart failure or poor LV function. The combined use of deferasirox with other iron chelators has also not been formally assessed and therefore cannot be recommended at this time. The drug should not be used in pregnant women.

BONE MARROW TRANSPLANTATION

Bone marrow transplantation (BMT) is an alternative to life long transfusion and chelation therapy. However since 1981, more than 1500 bone marrow transplants have been performed worldwide. The donor should be a histocompatible (HLA compatible) sibling or occasionally a parent. The procedure is associated with a significant risk of infection, drug related toxicity, graft versus host disease and relapse. However, the result of BMT has remarkably improved due to the use of cyclosporin, more effective treatment for cytomegalovirus infection, and improvement in aseptic techniques.[4]

The risk factors which significantly influence the outcome of BMT are:

- Inadequate iron chelation therapy
- Presence of liver fibrosis
- Hepatomegaly.

Patients in class 1 have none of these factors, patients in class 2 have one or two and patients in class 3 have all the three factors (Table 10.4).

Table 10.4: Results of bone marrow transplantation

	Survival	*Disease free survival*	*Risk of rejection*	*Mortality*
Class I	93%	91%	2%	8%
Class II	87%	83%	3%	15%
Class III	79%	58%	28%	19%

Bone marrow transplantation in thalassemics should be considered for patients at an early age before the complications due to iron overload appear.

HLA-matched Sibling Donors

The general applicability of bone marrow transplantation is limited by the availability of a related HLA-matched donor. There is a one in four chance that any given sibling will be HLA identical, with the likelihood of a thalassemic patient having an HLA identical sibling donor varying according to family size.

Matched Unrelated Donor Transplantation

Because most patients with thalassemia do not have a compatible sibling donor, there is interest in using unrelated but otherwise matched donors. Unfortunately, the complication rates of transplants using matched unrelated donors are generally much higher than with sibling matched transplants.

CORD BLOOD TRANSPLANTATION

The use of stem cells obtained from umbilical cord blood has recently received considerable interest. There are several possible advantages to this approach. First, stem cells can be obtained easily at birth, and often in sufficient quantity for a successful donation - thus avoiding the bone marrow harvest of a donor at a later age. Second, it has been suggested that graft versus host disease (GVHD) may be less severe when stem cells are obtained at this early point in life. Third, the routine collection of cord blood stem cells from all births would provide a wider pool of donors for BMT therapy. Some patients have been successfully treated with cord blood transplantation[24] but further studies are required to assess its overall value in treatment of this condition.

ALTERNATIVE THERAPIES IN THALASSEMIA

Activation/Modulation of Fetal Hemoglobin

The basic defect in thalassemia is the imbalance of α and non-α chains. Stimulation of HbF synthesis leads to correction/reduction of this imbalance, ameliorating the severity of the disease. Fetal hemoglobin is the predominant non-α globin produced in humans until immediately after birth, when it is typically suppressed and the production of β globin is increased. This pattern is the norm even when the genes are mutated, as in, β thalassemia. Patients with, β thalassemia who continue to produce high levels of fetal globin, such as those with hereditary persistence of fetal hemoglobin, have less globin imbalance and less severe anemia. The therapeutic stimulation of fetal globin could therefore benefit many patients, even rendering some transfusion independent. Following compounds have been tried for stimulation of HbF synthesis:

5-Azacytidine: It was the first compound to be tried to stimulate fetal hemoglobin synthesis, its administration leads to increased globin chain synthesis but has been found to be carcinogenic, and so was considered inappropriate for clinical use.

Short Chain Fatty Acid Derivatives

Short chain fatty acid derivatives induce activity from the fetal globin gene promoter, resulting in two-to-six-fold higher fetal globin mRNA in some patients, especially those who have at least one, β-thalassemia mutation and EPO levels >140 mU/ml.[25,26] Several preliminary trials with intravenous butyrate and oral phenylbutyrate compounds have shown increases in fetal and total hemoglobin levels in patients with thalassemia intermedia, while a few previously transfusion-dependent thalassemia major patients have been maintained transfusion-independent on home therapy for 5-7 years. Isobutyramide has induced fetal globin and reduced transfusion requirements in thalassemia intermedia and major.[27,28] Continuation of therapy with this compound causes "drug tolerance". Its combination with other agents like hydroxyurea or erythropoietin may be beneficial.

Erythropoietin: Erythropoietin has been found effective, mainly in thalassemia intermedia. It gives a significant dose related response with no major side effects. Its parentral mode of administration and cost are limiting factors. Combination with hydroxyurea has been found to give better result.

Hydroxyurea (HU): Hydroxyurea causes acute depletion of normal erythropoietic marrow and proliferation and differentiation of erythroid precursors which maintain gamma chain synthesis. Benefit of HU in sickle cells disease and thalassemia intermedia is well documented. Its response in β thalassemia major is less consistent. After prolonged daily administration of HU, there may be blunting of response. Its hematological toxicity is unpredictable and requires regular monitoring of blood counts. Further trials are required to look for long-term complications. Favorable response has also been noticed in some patients of β thalassemia major who have specific mutations or presence of XMN 1 polymorphism. HU shows a synergistic response with other agents like erythropoietin and butyrate.

With a proper balance between disease and treatment an individual with thalassemia major can enjoy a near normal life style and experience regular physical and emotional development from childhood to adulthood.

GENE THERAPY

A number of major discoveries and technical advances in gene therapy over the last 20 years, particularly since 2000, mean that, at long last, gene therapy for the hemoglobinopathies looks a serious possibility in the not too distant future. In 1987, a group led by Professor Frank Grosveld discovered the master regulator of the β-globin gene family, known as the 'locus control region' (LCR). It was found that linking the LCR to a β-globin gene unit enables the gene to be efficiently and reproducibly switched on, and to produce a sufficiently high level of, γ globin protein to be of therapeutic benefit, if reproduced in a gene therapy context.[29]

REFERENCES

1. Rund D, Rachmilewitz E. Beta-thalassemia. N Engl J Med. 2005;353(11):1135-46.
2. Borgna-Pignatti C, Rugolotto S, De Stefano P, et al. Survival and complications in patients with thalassemia major treated with transfusion and deferoxamine. Haematologica. 2004;89(10):1187-93.
3. Morris CR, Singer ST, Walters MC. Clinical hemoglobinopathies: iron, lungs and new blood. Curr Opin Hematol. 2006;13(6):407-18
4. Lucarelli G, Galimberti M, Polchi P, et al. Bone marrow transplantation in patients with thalassemia. N Engl J Med. 1990;322(7):417-21.
5. Angelucci E, Baronciani D. Allogeneic stem cell transplantation for thalassemia major. Haematologica. 2008;93(12): 1780-4.

6. Gaziev J, Sodani P, Lucarelli G. Hematopoietic stem cell transplantation in thalassemia. Bone Marrow Transplant. 2008;42(suppl 1):S41.
7. Cao A, Gabutti V, Galanello R, et al. Management protocol for the treatment of thalassemia patients. Nicosia, Cyprus: Thalassemia International Federation (TIF); 1997.
8. Cappellini MD, Cohen A, Eleftheriou A, et al. Guidelines for the Clinical Management of Thalassaemia. 2nd Edition revised. Nicosia, Cyprus: Thalassemia International Federation; 2008.
9. Borgna-Pignati C, Cappellini MD, De Stefano P, et al. Cardiac morbidity and mortality in Desferrioxamine or Deferiprone treated patients with thalassemia major. Blood. 2006;107(9):3733-7.
10. Anderson LJ, Westwood MA, Holden S, et al. Myocardial iron clearance during reversal of siderotic cardiomyopathy with intravenous desferrioxamine: a prospective study using T2* cardiovascular magnetic resonance. Br J Haematol. 2004;127(3):348-55.
11. Porter JB, Davis BA. Monitoring chelation therapy to achieve optimal outcome in the treatment of thalassaemia. Best Pract Res Clin Haematol. 2002;15:329-68.
12. Davis BA, Porter JB. Long-term outcome of continuous 24-hour deferoxamine infusion via indwelling intravenous catheters in high-risk betathalassemia. Blood. 2000;95:1229-36.
13. Davis BA, O'Sullivan C, Jarritt PH, Porter JB. Value of sequential monitoring of left ventricular ejection fraction in the management of thalassemia major. Blood. 2004;104: 263-9.
14. Porter JB, Jawson MS, Huehns ER, East CA, Hazell JW. Desferrioxamine ototoxicity: evaluation of risk factors in thalassemic patients and guidelines for safe dosages. Br J Haematol. 1989;73:403-9.
15. Swedish Orphan, safety alert, 2006. Clinical Guidelines Iron Overload; Electronic Infrastructure For Thalassaemia Research Network. http//portal.ethanet. eu page no.29 downloaded on 05/08/2011.
16. Mourad FH, Hoffbrand AV, Sheikh-Taha M, et al. Comparison between desferrioxamine and combined therapy with desferrioxamine and deferiprone in iron overloaded thalassaemia patients. Br J Haematol. 2003;121:187-9.
17. Gomber S, Saxena R, Madan N. Comparative efficacy of desferrioxamine, deferiprone and in combination on iron chelation in thalassemic children. Indian Pediatr. 2004;41: 21-7.
18. Galanello R, Kattamis A, Piga A, et al. A prospective randomized controlled trial on the safety and efficacy of alternating deferoxamine and deferiprone in the treatment of iron overload in patients with thalassemia. Haematologica. 2006a;91:1241-3.
19. Galanello R, Piga A, Forni GL, et al. Phase II clinical evaluation of deferasirox, a once-daily oral chelating agent, in pediatric patients with beta thalassemia major. Haematologica. 2006;91:1343-51.
20. Tanner MA, Galanello R, Dessi C, et al. A randomised, placebo-controlled, double-blind trial of the effect of combined therapy with deferoxamine and deferiprone on myocardial iron in thalassaemia major using cardiovascular magnetic resonance. Circulation. 2007;115(14):1876-84.
21. Nisbet-Brown E, Olivieri NF, Giardina PJ, et al. Effectiveness and safety of ICL670 in iron-loaded patients with thalassaemia: a randomised, double-blind, placebo-controlled, dose-escalation trial. Lancet. 2003;361:1597-602.
22. Galanello R, Piga A, Alberti D, Rouan MC, Bigler H, Sechaud R. Safety, tolerability, and pharmacokinetics of ICL670, a new orally active iron-chelating agent in patients with transfusion-dependent iron overload due to beta-thalassemia. J Clin Pharmacol. 2003;43:565-72.
23. Cappellini MD, Cohen A, Piga A, et al. A phase 3 study of deferasirox (ICL670), a once-daily oral iron chelator, in patients with beta-thalassemia. Blood. 2006;107:3455-62.
24. Miniero R, Rocha V, Saracco P, et al. Cord blood transplantation (CBT) in hemoglobinopathies. Eurocord. Bone Marrow Transplant. 1998;22(Suppl 1):S78-9.
25. Perrine SP. Foetal globin induction - Can it cure beta-thalassaemia? Hematology, Am Soc Hem Education Programme, December 2005.
26. Perrine SP, Castaneda SA, Boosalis MS, et al. Induction of foetal globin in beta-thalassaemia: Cellular obstacles and molecular progress. Ann N Y Acad Sci. 2005;1054:257-65.
27. Cappellini MD, Graziadei G, Ciceri L, et al. Oral isobutyramide therapy in patients with thalassemia intermedia: Results of a phase II open study. Blood Cells Mol Dis. 2000;26:105-11.
28. Reich S, Buhrer C, Henze G, et al. Oral isobutyramide reduces transfusion requirements in some patients with homozygous beta-thalassaemia. Blood. 2000;96:3357-63.
29. Stamatoyannopoulos G Prospects for developing a molecular cure for thalassemia. Hematology. 2005;10(Suppl 1):255-7.

11 Hemolytic Anemia (Other than Thalassemia) Management

MB Agarwal

Hemolytic anemias can be classified in various ways, e.g.

1. Intracorpuscular vs extracorpuscular
2. Intravascular vs extravascular
3. Inherited vs acquired
4. Acute vs chronic.

Table 11.1 gives a simplified etiological classification of hemolytic anemias. Hereditary hemolytic anemias are usually due to intracorpuscular or intrinsic red cell defects while acquired ones are a result of extracorpuscular or extrinsic defect. Exceptions do occur, e.g. in paroxysmal nocturnal hemoglobinuria (PNH), the red cell defect is an acquired one but hemolysis is due to intracorpuscular defect.

Following is an account of management of various individual hemolytic disorders (except thalassemia).

HEREDITARY HEMOLYTIC ANEMIAS (INTRACORPUSCULAR DEFECT)

Membrane Defect

Hereditary Spherocytosis

Hereditary spherocytosis (HS) is the most common of hemolytic anemias secondary to membrane defect. It is due to defective structural protein (spectrin) of the red cell membrane. The greater the deficiency of spectrin, the more severe is hemolysis. There are many genetic lesions resulting in variable degree of hemolysis due to the loss of membrane, which is also responsible for the spherical shape of the red cells. As the spherical cells are unable to pass through the splenic microcirculation, they die prematurely. Hereditary spherocytosis is inherited as an autosomal dominant disorder but the phenotypic expression is variable.

The treatment is splenectomy which almost always normalizes the hemoglobin, even though microspherocytes remain. Until splenectomy, folic acid should be given regularly. Pneumococcal vaccine is given prior to splenectomy and oral penicillin prophylaxis is given postsplenectomy to avoid sepsis due to encapsulated organisms. From the same angle, splenectomy is avoided in early childhood. Mild cases do not need splenectomy unless gallstones develop.

Hereditary Elliptocytosis (H. ovalocytosis)

Hereditary elliptocytosis (HE) has clinical and laboratory features similar to that of HS except for the characteristic red cell morphology and overall milder course. Majority of the patients can be left alone. Occasionally, splenectomy is required. Inheritance is autosomal dominant. Occasionally homozygous or doubly heterozygous cases of elliptocytosis may present with a more severe hemolytic anemia called hereditary pyropoikilocytosis.

Enzyme Defects

Glucose-6-phosphate Dehydrogenase Deficiency

Glucose-6-phosphate dehydrogenase (G6PD) functions to reduce nicotinamide ademine dinucleotide phosphate (NADP) while oxidizing glucose-6-phosphate. Various normal genetic variants of the enzyme G6PD are known. The most common being Type B and Type A in Africans. In all, over 400 variants of the enzyme have been characterized which show less activity than normal. It has been estimated that over 200 million people are deficient in G6PD enzyme. Usually, G6PD deficiency is an asymptomatic entity. The main clinical problems are due to an acute hemolytic crisis, which occurs in response to an oxidant stress (drugs, fava beans or infections). Rarely neonatal jaundice or even a congenital nonspherocytic-hemolytic anemia can occur.

The inheritance is sex linked, female being a carrier showing approximately half the normal red cell G6PD values. The female heterozygote has an advantage of resistance to falciparum malaria. Approximately 1% of Indian males are G6PD deficient. It is relatively more

Table 11.1: Etiological classification of hemolytic anemias

Congenital

A. Hemolytic anemias due to intracorpuscular (intrinsic) defect
   - *Membrane defects:*
     1. Hereditary spherocytosis
     2. Hereditary elliptocytosis
     3. Hereditary xerocytosis and hydrocytosis
   - *Enzyme defects (Nonspherocytic congenital hemolytic anemia):*
     1. Due to deficiency of glucose-6-phosphate dehydrogenase or other enzymes of the pentose phosphate pathway.
     2. Due to deficiency of pyruvate kinase or other enzymes of the Embden-Meyerhof pathway.
     3. Associated with abnormalities of nucleotide metabolism.
   - *Hemoglobin defects:*
     1. Thalassemia syndrome
        β-thalassemia major
        Hb-H disease
        Others
     2. Hemoglobinopathies
        Sickle cell anemia
        Other abnormal hemoglobins (Hb-C, Hb-E, Hb-D, etc.)
        Unstable hemoglobin disease

Acquired

A. Hemolytic anemias due to extracorpuscular (extrinsic) detect
   - *Immune mechanisms:*
     Autoimmune hemolytic anemia
     1. Warm antibodies
     2. Cold antibodies
        — Alloimmune hemolytic anemia
        — Hemolytic disease of the newborn
        — Incompatible blood transfusion
   - *Nonimmune mechanisms:*
     1. Mechanical hemolytic anemia
     2. Microangiopathic hemolytic anemia
     3. March hemoglobinuria
     4. Miscellaneous:
        — Hemolytic anemia due to chemicals including lead infestation
        — Hemolytic anemia due to infection
        — Hemolytic anemia due to burns
        — Paroxysmal nocturnal hemoglobinuria (an intrinsic but acquired detect)

common in Parsees (15%), Bhanushali (11%), Khatri (5%), Punjabi (3%), Kutchi (3%) and Muslims (2.5%). The world distribution shows highest prevalence in the tropical zone chiefly West Africa, the Mediterranean, Middle East and South East Asia. The deficiency is of variable degree. Most severely affected cases are seen in the Mediterranean countries and the orientals. Rarely, severe cases also occur in Caucasians.

The treatment includes stoppage of the offending drug, blood transfusion, maintaining high urine output and if required, hemodialysis. If neonatal jaundice is severe, newborns may need phototherapy or even exchange transfusion.

All other red cell enzyme deficiencies are rare.

Hemoglobin Disorders (Other than Thalassemia)

Sickle Cell Disease

Sickle cell disease is another group of hereditary hemoglobin disorders characterized by transformation of red cells into sickle shape on deoxygenation. This is a result of polymerization of sickle hemoglobin and is clinically characterized by two major problems, i.e. anemia and vaso-occlusive complications. Sickle cell disease includes sickle cell anemia (homozygous hemoglobin-S disease), sickle cell/beta-thalassemia, sickle cell/hemoglobin-C disease and others.

Management

This can be divided into three groups:
1. General care
2. Management of specific complications:
   a. Management of infections
   b. Blood transfusions
   c. Pain management
3. Newer therapeutic modalities.

General Care

This includes treatment to relieve pain, prevention of dehydration, treatment of fever and psychosocial support. Dietary advice includes adequate calorie intake, adequate folic acid, vitamin C, vitamin E and zinc support.

Specific Complications

a. *Management of infections:* These include:
   i. Prophylactic penicillin
   ii. Immunization to prevent infection: Pneumococcal vaccination at age of 10 months followed by boosters every 5 years are recommended. Immunization against *H. influenzae* is suggested by age of 18 months. Hepatitis B vaccination is also a must.
   iii. Evaluation and treatment of the febrile episodes.
b. *Transfusions:* Transfusions are associated with three important problems, i.e. transmission of viral diseases, iron overload and alloimmunization. Although, they can be used to treat each and every complications of sickle cell disease, their value has

been demonstrated for only a few of them. Chronic transfusion therapy has been used with a reasoning that suppression of Hemoglobin-S would lead to decreased vaso-occlusive episodes. Even exchange-transfusions have been carried out for immediate alteration in the blood.

c. *Pain management:* This is the most frequent requirement of a sickler.
   The guidelines include:
   i. Aggressive use of appropriate analgesics
   ii. Ensuring fluid supplement
   iii. Looking for the etiology especially an infectious cause.

Newer Therapeutic Modalities

Many chemical agents have been developed which may act as anti-sickling agents. None of them have been of any great therapeutic benefit. The most promising agent recently licensed by US FDA is Hydroxyurea, which has the ability to induce fetal hemoglobin synthesis. It decreases the number of vaso-occlusive episodes. Co-administration of other hematopoietic agents such as erythropoietin or butyric acid may also be useful.

Bone marrow transplantation has been carried out in over 100 patients with total cure. However, only 35% of patients would have immunologically compatible donors and one must also consider the risk-benefit issue. Very soon, gene therapy may become applicable to sickle cell disease.

Prenatal diagnosis by chorionic villous biopsy is possible. Unfortunately, deoxyribonucleic acid (DNA) analysis does not predict the clinical severity, and many parents do not consider sickle cell disease as a serious enough problem for pregnancy to be terminated.

ACQUIRED HEMOLYTIC ANEMIAS

Autoimmune Hemolytic Anemia (AIHA)

Hemolysis secondary to antibodies against red cell antigens is called immune-hemolysis. In autoimmune hemolysis, the antibodies are against own red cells. Fifty percent of cases of AIHA are primary or idiopathic, while the rest have an underlying cause like infections, drugs, systemic autoimmune diseases or malignancies. According to the temperature at which the antibody reacts with the red cell, one has warm or cold antibody.

Warm Antibody Autoimmune Hemolysis

This disease is common in adults after the age of 40 years. Females are more often involved. The onset is insidious. Occasional patient has associated immune thrombocytopenia and this combination is called Evan's syndrome. Acute events are associated with intravascular hemolysis. Underlying etiological cause must be investigated in all patients. The clinical course is exceedingly variable. Patients could have asymptomatic mild hemolysis for the whole life to a life-threatening acute hemolysis with renal failure. Spontaneous remissions occur. In secondary cases the prognosis is largely of the underlying disease.

Treatment includes corticosteroids, splenectomy, immunosuppressive drugs and blood transfusions. Any significant hemolysis is first treated with corticosteroids with prompt response in about 80%. Adults receive 60 mg of prednisolone daily. Parenteral methyl prednisolone is often used in acutely ill patients. After 3-4 weeks, steroids can be tapered. However, many would need a maintenance therapy. Most of the patients who do not respond to steroids and require large maintenance dosage, are candidates for splenectomy. Splenectomy results in good control over the disease in 60% of patients. If significant hemolysis continues despite splenectomy, immunosuppressive therapy like azathioprine or cyclophosphamide are used. Due to risk of malignancy, they are avoided in younger people.

All patients must receive oral folic acid supplements and treatment of underlying cause, if any. Intravenous gammaglobulin, Danazol, Cyclosporine, antithymocyte globulin, etc. are used in occasional refractory cases. Blood transfusions are reserved for patients where life is threatened due to severe anemia or there is significant morbidity because of hypoxia. The transfused red cells may be rapidly destroyed and both grouping and cross-matching are difficult due to presence of antibodies. Selection and slow administration of red cell units, which are least incompatible is the usual advice.

Cold Antibody Autoimmune Hemolysis

These are immune hemolysis where antibodies best react at temperature below 37°C. They are relatively less frequent. Two forms are recognized:

1. Cold hemagglutinin disease (CHAD)
2. Paroxysmal cold hemoglobinuria (PCH).

1. *Cold hemagglutinin disease:* It is a disorder where red cells are agglutinated at low temperature. It is a chronic insidious disease most common in adults aged over 50 years. It can occur in both primary and secondary forms.

   Most of the patients remain clinically well and protective clothing during cold weather, use of leather gloves and stocking or moving to a warmer climate is all that is needed. Steroids and splenec-

Table 11.2: Nonimmune acquired hemolytic anemia

S.No.	Causes	Examples	Mechanisms
1.	Infections and infestations	Malaria Meningococcal sepsis Pneumococcal sepsis Gram-negative sepsis Hemorrhagic fevers *Clostridium perfringens*	Intracellular organisms Enzymatic toxins
2.	Drugs, chemical and physical agents	Drugs Industrial/domestic substances Burns Drowning	Oxidative hemolysis Membrane damage Osmotic lysis
3.	Mechanical lysis	Diffuse intravascular coagulation Vasculitis Cardiac prostheses	Microangiopathic hemolytic anemic
4.	Acquired membrane disorder	Liver disease Paroxysmal nocturnal hemoglobinuria	Lipid abnormalities Somatic mutation

tomy are often ineffective, while Chlorambucil is more useful. Transfusions are rarely necessary. However, if needed, blood must be warmed to the room temperature, before and during administration. Plasmapheresis helps severe cases.

2. *Paroxysmal cold hemoglobinuria:* PCH is a rare disorder secondary to a cold reacting autoantibody having strong lytic activity. It is most commonly seen in children as an idiopathic disorder or secondary to viral illnesses. Occasionally, it occurs in adults where it has a chronic form with recurrent acute episodes precipitated with exposure to cold. During an acute attack, hemoglobinuria, pallor and jaundice develop and spleen becomes palpable. The antibody involved is demonstrable by Donath Landsteiner test. It is a complement binding IgG antibody having specificity against P blood group antigen. The antiglobulin test may be positive only during the episode of hemolysis.

Nonimmune Acquired Hemolytic Anemias

Table 11.2 enlists various miscellaneous conditions, which lead to nonimmune acquired hemolytic anemias. Management of some of these is discussed underneath:

Hemolysis Secondary to Infections and Infestations

Bacterial infections secondary to *Clostridium welchii* regularly cause hemolysis due to effects of toxins on the red cells. This occurs as a part of septic abortion or puerperal sepsis. Patients are acutely ill with septicemia, toxemia and acute severe hemolysis.

Malaria, commonly falciparum, can lead to severe hemolysis. Although, degree of anemia is variable, it often does not correlate with the parasitic index. Marrow suppression, hypersplenism and immunological destruction adds to the problem. Organisms may not be easily detectable. Black-water fever is a rare but serious complication of falciparum infection. It is often precipitated by antimalarial drugs, usually quinine. There may be underlying G6PD deficiency.

Treatment revolves around blood transfusion, management of primary infection and folic acid.

Hemolytic Anemias Due to Drugs, Chemicals and Physical Agents

Drugs causing hemolysis can be divided into three major groups:

1. Direct drug toxicity (dose related phenomenon).
2. Hemolysis secondary to hereditary metabolic defect in the red cell, e.g. enzyme deficiency or unstable hemoglobin.
3. Drugs causing immune-hemolysis.

Hemolysis due to direct drug toxicity: Usually these drugs (or chemicals) are powerful oxidants. The effect is dose-related but smaller doses could be dangerous if the person is G6PD deficient or he has unstable hemoglobin. Common examples are sulphones, sulphonamide and para-aminosalicylic acid. Young children swallowing mothballs containing naphthalene can suffer.

Such patients have irregularly contracted "blister" or "bite" cell, Heinz body formation and occasionally methemoglobinemia as well. Treatment consists of withdrawal of drug and if required, packed cells support.

Drugs causing hemolysis in G6PD deficiency: G6PD deficiency has been discussed earlier.

Drug induced immune hemolysis: Many drugs can lead to immune hemolytic anemia. Approximately 20% of immune-hemolytic anemias are secondary to drugs.

Drugs like penicillin and cephalosporine have a strong affinity for the red cell membrane. Hence, they bind to the membrane and the antibody is formed against the drug adsorbed on the cells. This is called adsorption mechanism.

Other drugs like Quinine, Rifampicin and Para-aminosalicylic acid lead to hemolysis by immune complex mechanism. Here, antibodies are formed against the drug and this complex deposits on the red cell membrane leading to complement activation.

Lastly, drugs like methyldopa, after chronic administration lead to formation of antibodies against the red cells, which in occasional person can lead to insidious onset of hemolysis. Treatment consists of withdrawal of incriminating drug.

CHEMICAL AGENTS

Regarding chemicals, lead is an important cause leading to basophilic stipplings of the red cells and moderate anemia. Often, there is reticulocytosis, at least mild and the bone marrow, besides erythroid hyperplasia shows ring sideroblasts. Treatment consists of avoiding further heavy metal exposure/ingestion, blood support (if needed) and metal chelators.

PHYSICAL AGENTS

March hemoglobinuria is a very rare disorder where prolonged march or running (in soldiers and athletes) results in passage of red urine lasting for many hours or even few days. This is secondary to traumatic intravascular hemolysis related to mechanical damage to the cells within the vessels of soles.

Hemolysis is also common in severely burnt patients.

Physical injury during circulation through narrowed vascular system leads to red blood cell (RBC) fragmentation. Such cells are prematurely destroyed and thus a hemolytic anemia results. This is called microangiopathic hemolytic anemia and its causes are listed in the Table 11.2.

Aortic and occasionally mitral valve replacement can also lead to hemolytic problems. In such cases, malfunction of the prosthesis is invariably present. This results in turbulent blood flow. Anemia, reticulocytosis, indirect hyperbilirubinemia and raised lactate dehydrogenase (LDH) are common. In severe cases, evidence of intravascular hemolysis is present. Surgery to replace the valve may be needed.

PAROXYSMAL NOCTURNAL HEMOGLOBINURIA

This is a rare disorder secondary to an acquired defect in the red cell membrane, which makes it unsually sensitive to lysis by the complement. It is characterized by chronic hemolysis with episodic hemoglobinuria. Hemolysis is secondary to activation of complement by the alternate rather than the classical pathway.

The disorder has a definite relationship to aplastic anemia with 25% of patients commencing as pancytopenia with hypocellular marrow. The evidence of paroxysmal nocturnal hemoglobinuria (PNH) may be restricted to laboratory tests. On the other side, patient may show a classical hemolytic PNH disease where marrow aplasia develops as a secondary event much later. Occasional patient goes on to develop myelodysplasia or even acute leukemia.

There is no specific treatment. Management is largely supportive. Transfusion with saline washed red cells given through leukocyte filters, folic acid supplement and iron replacement form the sheet anchor of therapy. Androgens, steroids and antithrombotic drugs are used occasionally. Bone marrow transplantation is curative.

BIBLIOGRAPHY

1. Dacie JV. The hemolytic anemias. In: the Autoimmune Hemolytic Anemias (3rd edn). New York; Churchill Livingstone, 1992.
2. Embury S. The clinical pathophysiology of sickle cell disease. Ann Rev Med. 1986;37:361.
3. Engelfried CP, Overbeeke MAM, von dem Borne AEGKr. Autoimmuno hemolytic anemia. Semin Hematol. 1992;29:3.
4. Garatty G (Ed.) Symposium on drug-induced immune cytopenia. Transfusion Med Rev. 1983;7:213.
5. Honig GR, Adams JG III. Human Hemoglobin Genetics. New York. Springer-Verlag; 1986.
6. Kazazian HH Jr. The thalassemia syndromes: Molecular basis and prenatal diagnosis in 1990. Semin Hematol. 1990;27:209.
7. Lubin B, Vichiasky E. Sickle cell disease. In: Hoffman R, et al (Ed). Hematology Basic Principles and Practices. New York: Churchill Livingstone; 1991. pp. 450-75.
8. Palek J. Anemias due to increased destruction of erythrocytes with abnormal shape and membrane defects. In: Williams WJ, et al. (Ed). Hematology. New York McGraw-Hill; 1989. p. 558.
9. Schwartz E, Benz Jr E. The thalassemia syndromes. In: Hoffman R, et al. (Eds). Hematology Basic Principles and Practices. New York : Churchill Livingstone; 1991.pp.392-421.
10. Valentine WN (moderator). Hemolytic anemias and erythrocyte enzymopathies. Ann Intern Med. 1985;103:245.

12 Thrombocytosis

Vikas Dua, SP Yadav, Vinita Jain, Anupam Sachdeva

Thrombocytosis in children is defined by an elevated platelet count, as in adults. It requires the knowledge of normal values and information about the method of platelet counting.

NORMAL UPPER THROMBOCYTE LEVELS IN CHILDHOOD

The platelet count will depend on the method of sampling (venous or capillary blood) and of counting. Thrombocytosis in children is defined by an elevated platelet count, as in adults. The definition of normal platelet counts in the range of 150000/mm^3 and 450000/mm^3 is generally accepted for healthy neonates, infants, children and adolescents. However, the definition of thrombocytosis varies between platelet counts of >400 × 10^9/L and >1001 × 10^9/L.[1] Generally, the following arbitrary classification of thrombocytosis has been chosen in current textbooks:

Mild	500-700 × 10^9/L
Moderate	701-900 × 10^9/L
Severe	901-1000 × 10^9/L
Extreme	>1001 × 10^9/L[1]

PHYSIOLOGY OF PLATELET PRODUCTION

Thrombopoietin (Tpo) promotes the proliferation of combined megakaryocyte progenitors, and their maturation. There are three stages of development.

Stage I: Extends from stem-cells to promegakaryocytes.

Stage II: It is the stage of endomiotic reduplication or polypolidization.

Stage III: It is the stage of cytoplasmic maturation of megakaryocytes.

At the end of their maturation process, megakaryocytes divide their cytoplasm into several 1000 fairly uniform platelets. Platelets are not only produced in the bone marrow but also in the lung, most probably in the pulmonary microvasculature, by physical fragmentation of megakaryocyte. Megakaryocytes or large cytoplasmic fragments leave the bone marrow and travel to the pulmonary circulation.

CLASSIFICATION

Thrombocytosis is common in infancy and childhood, occurring in 3 to 13% of children.[2] Extreme thrombocytosis (platelets >1000 × 10^9/L) is uncommon, occurring in less than 2% of children,[3] but may be more common in critically ill children.[4] The term thrombocythemia-corresponding to leukemia—is used for thrombocytosis due to an autonomous stem cell defect [e.g. in myeloproliferative disorders (MPD's)], where the term 'essential thrombocythemia' is applied.

More practical is the classification of thrombocytoses according to their origin into primary and secondary forms (Table 12.1). An increase in platelet count generally has one of three causes;

1. A primary disorder, such as a myeloproliferative or dysplastic syndrome classified as essential (or primary) thrombocytosis (ET).
2. Increased production due to stimuli.
3. A shift in platelets from the splenic pool into the peripheral circulation[2] and these two causes are referred to as reactive (or secondary) thrombocytosis (RT).

Essential thrombocytosis is extremely rare in children. In a recent large series of 1500 children with thrombocytosis there was not even one case of ET.

ESSENTIAL THROMBOCYTOSIS

Essential thrombocytosis is very rare in children. Approximately 50 pediatric cases have been published in literature.[5] In a single-center study of 220 children with thrombocythemia, 0.5% were diagnosed with ET.[6] In another study, the annual incidence of ET was estimated 0.09 per million between the ages of 0 and 14 years.[7] Patients most often are middle aged (average age, 50-60 years) at the time of diagnosis, and there is no gender predilection, although a higher prevalence in females of age 30 years has been noted.[8] Essential

Table 12.1: Differences between essential and reactive thrombocytosis

	Essential (primary)	*Reactive (secondary)*
Age (years)	Mostly >20 years Often >40 years	Mostly <20 years
Duration	Over 2 years	Days or weeks sometimes months.
Origin	Stem-cell defect	Reaction to hypoxia, infection, platelet loss; shift of platelet pool
Microvascular symptoms	Often	Extremely rare
Thrombosis	Often	Extremely rare
Bleeding	Often	Extremely rare
Splenomegaly	Often	Rare
Platelet count ($\times 10^9$/L)	Mostly >1000	Mostly <1000
Platelet morphology	Large, dysmorphic	Large, normal appearance
Platelet function	Disturbed	Normal
Platelet distribution	Elevated	Normal width
Iron stores	Normal	Low
Acute phase reagents such as IL-6, CRP fibrinogen	Normal	High, if thrombocytosis caused by infection

thrombocytosis results from a stem-cell defect and is associated with MPD's such as idiopathic thrombocythemia, polycythemia vera (PCV), chronic myeloid leukemia and idiopathic myelofibrosis. The platelet count usually persists at more than 1000×10^9/L in ET. In ET platelet function is usually disturbed and spontaneous aggregation as well as hypofunction can be observed. This may explain why the bleeding time in these patients is frequently prolonged despite thrombocytosis.

In ET as well as RT the number of megakaryocytes in the bone marrow is elevated. Morphological abnormalities of platelets in ET include bizarre forms, giant platelets, platelet conglomerates, circulating megakaryocytic fragments and hypogranularity. About 30% of children experience thromboembolic or hemorrhagic complications at the time of diagnosis or during the course of the illness and 15% will eventually die because of the underlying disease or from development of leukemia or myelofibrosis. Hence, ET like polycythemia vera is a premalignant condition. Several attempts have been made to formulate positive criteria for distinguishing patients with ET from those with RT. The diagnostic criteria for ET have changed substantially during the last 30 years. Table 12.2 outlines the current 2008 World Health Organization (WHO) classification.

CLINICAL MANIFESTATIONS

In patients of ET (aged 6-12 years) and persistent elevated platelet counts in excess of 1000×10^9/L; majority have splenomegaly, few have recurrent mucocutaneous bleeding and/or bleeding after minor surgery and some developed bleeding symptoms during long-term treatment with aspirin 500 mg/day or recurrent attacks of headache. They may present with microcirculatory disturbances, including acrocyanosis, myocardial infarction, focal transient cerebral ischemic attacks (TIA), atypical TIA's such as dysarthria and hemianopia and headache.

TREATMENT OPTIONS

Procedures to prevent obstruction of large vessels or disturbances of microvascular circulation include:

1. Platelet-lowering therapy (e.g. hydroxyurea, apheresis, busulfan, anagrelide, interferon, radioactive phosphorus)
2. Platelet aggregation inhibitors (e.g. aspirin and dipyridamole).

Indications for treatment are not well established in asymptomatic patients, but patients with thromboembolic or hemorrhagic complications and those with extreme thrombocytosis (>1000×10^9/L) and prolonged bleeding times may deserve treatment. Dror et al[9] from the Hospital for Sick Children in Toronto reviewed the clinical course of 36 children with ET, of whom only 15 had symptoms directly related to their hematological problem, including 9 who had severe thromboembolic and hemorrhagic complications. Symptomatic patients had significantly higher platelet counts (2,419,000/µL versus 904,000/µL P<0.001). However, 3 patients with platelets <800,000/µl had thrombotic events. Moreover, 3 patients who had thrombotic events and did not

Table 12.2: World Health Organization criteria (2008) for essential thrombocythemia

Proposed criteria for ET
Sustained platelet count ≥450 × 10^9/L*
Bone marrow biopsy specimen showing proliferation mainly of the megakaryocytic lineage with increased numbers of enlarged, mature megakaryocytes; no significant increase or left-shift of neutrophil granulopoiesis or erythropoiesis
Not meeting WHO criteria for PV•, PMF∆, CML◊, MDS§ or other myeloid neoplasm
Demonstration of JAK2 617V>F or other clonal marker, or in the absence of a clonal marker, no evidence for reactive thrombocytosis¥
Diagnosis requires meeting all 4 criteria.

*During the work-up period.
• Requires the failure of iron replacement therapy to increase hemoglobin level to the PV range in the presence of decreased serum ferritin. Exclusion of PV is based on hemoglobin and hematocrit levels, and red cell mass measurement is not required.
∆ Requires the absence of relevant reticulin fibrosis, collagen fibrosis, peripheral blood leukoerythroblastosis, or markedly hypercellular marrow for age accompanied by megakaryocyte morphology that is typical for PMF-small to large with an aberrant nuclear/cytoplasmic ratio and hyperchromatic, bulbous or irregularly folded nuclei and dense clustering.
◊ Requires the absence of BCR-ABL.
§ Requires absence of dyserythropoiesis and dysgranulopoiesis.
¥ Causes of reactive thrombocytosis include iron deficiency, splenectomy, surgery, infection, inflammation, connective tissue disease, metastatic cancer, and lymphoproliferative disorders. However, the presence of a condition associated with reactive thrombocytosis does not exclude the possibility of ET if the first three criteria are met.

receive therapy went on to have a benign clinical course.[9] From these data, it is evident that it is almost impossible to give evidence based guidelines for therapy in children with ET due to the rarity of this condition and its heterogeneous clinical course.

Platelet apharesis may be used in emergency situations, such as major bleeding at platelets counts more than 1000 × 10^9/L.

REACTIVE THROMBOCYTOSIS

Thrombocyte production increases after peripheral loss of platelets, e.g. after immunologic, septic, oncogenic or traumatic events, blood loss or hypoxia of respiratory or cardiac origin. Megakaryocytes are increased in the bone marrow of affected patients. Increased ploidy (more than 16 N) is seen in patients with RT. In immune thrombocytopenia (ITP), megakaryocytes in the bone marrow are markedly increased. Morphologic peculiarities have not been described; inert ingestion of other bone marrow cells by megakaryocytes (emperipoiesis) is physiologic and is increased in patients with ET and RT. Elevated levels of TPO have been found in patients with malignant liver tumors, hepatoblastoma and hepatocellular carcinoma, active lung tuberculosis and acute megakaryocytic leukemia. They also imply that the local marrow environment may contain a factor that increases megakaryocyte production. Such a putative growth factor might be elevated by activated T-cells or natural killer (NK) cells.

Another reactive cause of thrombocytosis is a shift of the splenic pool into the peripheral blood. This can be provoked by exercise or stress situations or by injection of epinephrine and isoprenaline, and can be found with functional or anatomical asplenia.

Thrombocytosis in childhood is seen in 6 and 13% in hospitalized children and 15% in pediatric outpatients.[10] The variation is due to different definitions of the degree of thrombocytosis. In general, there is no difference in frequency between boys and girls, but in children with thrombocytosis due to infections, a significantly high number of boys were observed. Infections, both viral and bacterial, are by far the most common cause of secondary thrombocytosis in childhood. Presently, infections of the respiratory tract account for 60-80% of cases of secondary thrombocytosis in children[11,12] followed by infections of the urinary and gastrointestinal tracts and of the bones. In most cases, thrombocyte numbers are only slightly elevated. The causes of RT are given in Table 12.3. Between 78 and 86% of children with thrombocytosis had a platelet count between 500 and 700 × 10^9/L. Some of them had moderately elevated counts but only a few had severe form with a platelet count exceeding 900 × 10^9/L; 3% had platelet counts more than 1000 × 10^9/L (platelet millionaires).

The frequency of thrombocytosis to be exceptionally high in neonates, infants and young children; 72% occurred in patients under 2 years of age, 56% in infants and 25% during the first 2 months of life, due to the

Table 12.3: Conditions associated with reactive thrombocytosis (predominantly in infants and young children)

- Infection (bacterial, viral)
  - Respiratory
  - Meningitis
  - Gastrointestinal
- Tissue damage (surgery, trauma)
- Splenectomy
- Hypoxia
  - Anemia
  - Iron-deficiency anemia
  - Hemolytic anemia
  - Anemia due to blood loss, chemotherapy
  - Anemia caused by nephrotic disease
- Respiratory disease
- Cardiac hypoxia
- Autoimmune disease
  - Juvenile rheumatoid arthritis
- Kawasaki syndrome
- Henoch-Schönlein disease
- Renal disease
- Malignancy
  - Hepatoblastoma
  - Hodgkin's disease
  - Histiocytosis
  - Sarcoma
  - Acute lymphoblastic leukemia and non-Hodgkin's lymphoma
- Prematurity
- Stress situation
- Medication
  - Epinephrine (adrenaline)
  - Corticosteroids
  - Vinca alkaloids
  - Miconazole
  - Penicillamine
  - Methadone (during pregnancy)
  - Hydantoin (during pregnancy)
- Miscellaneous
  - Gastroesophageal reflux
  - Caffey's disease

fact that the precursor cells in the bone marrow of young children have an intensified ability to react to stress. Another reason might be that infants normally have higher platelet values, and therefore develop mild thrombocytosis with the slightest platelet producing stimulus. This is particularly true for low-birth-weight infants.

Infection

Infection is by far the most common cause of thrombocytosis. Nearly 51 to 65% of the children under the age of 10 years with thrombocytosis had infection. The plasma level of CRP was inversely related to the thrombocyte aggregation. The rise in platelets in the course of an infection could be considered a compensatory, exaggerated platelet production following initial thrombocyte consumption by septic processes with intravascular coagulation, CRP induction and loss of platelets due to defence mechanisms. Fourty-nine percent of children with bacterial meningitis after the first week of treatment developed thrombocytosis.

Elevated platelets are seen in sepsis after the neonatal period. It has been seen that respiratory tract infections are the most common cause of thrombocytosis due to infection. It has been seen that thrombocytosis occurs in 92.5% of patients with pneumonia and empyema.[10,11] No correlation between thrombocytosis and prognosis was found. Inflammatory pulmonary disorders such as bronchitis and bronchopneumonia also induced elevation of pulmonary megakaryocytes. Rarely in ulcerative colitis and Crohn's disease one can see thrombocytosis, which can lead to lethal, thromboembolic complications.

TISSUE DAMAGE

Thrombocytosis occurs after trauma or surgical tissue damage. The highest elevation of platelet count is observed between the first and second postoperative weeks. The increased platelet numbers is due to bleeding or platelet consumption to restore hemostasis, which is especially pronounced after splenectomy. Thrombosis has been reported when additional risk factors, such as cyanotic heart disease and cardiac arrhythmia, are present or when splenectomy has been performed because of myeloproliferative syndrome.

Whether thrombocytosis, which develops after splenectomy, indicates a risk for thromboembolic complications is controversial. Thromboembolic complications are very rare in children; however, they have been observed after splenectomy for hematologic abnormalities such as autoimmune hemolytic anemia and portal hypertension although by and large there is no need for antiplatelet agents to be administered.

HYPOXIA

Anemia or respiratory distress syndrome leading to hypoxia can cause thrombocytosis. Premature infants with respiratory distress can have thrombocytosis. Iron deficiency and hemolytic anemia of different origin can also lead to thrombocytosis. Anemia due to chronic blood loss and anemia of renal disease with transient erythroblastosis can also present with thrombocytosis. Iron deficiency as a cause of thrombocytosis was described as early as 1904. Thirty-five percent of children with iron-deficiency anemia have thrombocytosis. Sickle cell anemia is a congenital hemolytic anemia associated with thrombocytosis due to increased bone marrow platelet production, but also due to functional asplenia from the repetitive splenic auto infarcts. Thrombocytosis has also been observed in infants with blood loss due to vitamin K deficiency bleeding and after extreme hemodilution in open heart surgery.

AUTOIMMUNE DISEASE

Autoimmune diseases, such as juvenile rheumatoid arthritis (JRA),[12] small and large vessel vasculitides including polyarteritis nodosa,[13] and Wegener's granulomatosis,[14] Kawasaki disease (KD), Henoch-Schönlein purpura,[15] and inflammatory bowel diseases[16] account for <10% of cases of reactive thrombocytosis in children. In patients with systemic-onset JRA, serum IL-6 levels correlate with platelet counts and with the extent and severity of joint involvement.[13] Regarding KD, thrombocytosis typically occurs in the second week of the illness, and it is therefore not helpful in making a timely diagnosis. Moreover, the absence of thrombocytosis during convalescence does not exclude the disease. Tpo in conjunction with IL-6 contributes to the thrombocytosis of patients with KD. Tpo serum levels are also increased in patients with inflammatory bowel diseases, irrespective of disease activity, platelet counts and clinical characteristics of the patients.[17]

GASTROINTESTINAL DISEASE WITHOUT INFECTION

In gastroesophageal reflux one can see thrombocytosis. The increased platelet production could reflect a reaction of the esophageal mucosa to constant irritation by acid gastric contents. Regurgitation and aspiration frequently result in recurrent bronchitis. Vomiting of hematin may in some cases lead to iron-deficiency anemia. Thrombocytosis has been reported in children with allergy to cow's milk, which in some cases leads to colitis. Of patients with Crohn's disease, 75% presented with thrombocytosis.

RENAL DISEASE

Thrombocytosis can occur in renal disease esp. with anemia due to macrohematuria or renal failure. Thrombocytosis in children with nephrotic syndrome is not rare especially in those in whom there is a propensity to infections due to decreased splenic function.

ONCOLOGIC DISEASE

Children with malignancies of the CNS, ALL, malignant liver disease, such as hepatoblastoma and hepatocellular carcinoma can all have thrombocytosis.[18,19]

MEDICATIONS

The following medications are known to cause thrombocytosis in children; epinephrine (adrenaline), corticosteroids, cyclosporine, vinca alkaloids, miconazole, penicillamine and citroforum. Epinephrine increases the platelet count by shifting the splenic pool into the peripheral blood.

In immune thrombocytopenias, advantage is taken of the fact that corticosteroids suppress platelet phagocytosis by macrophages. It is possible that the rise in platelets in patients who have been treated with corticosteroids is due to the same mechanism. Therefore, the inclusion of corticosteroid therapy in the differential diagnosis of thrombocytosis is recommended.

Transient thrombocytosis has been described in infants born to mothers taking methadone during pregnancy. Thrombocytosis as part of the fetal hydantoin syndrome has also been observed.

OTHER CAUSES

Prematurity

Elevated thrombocyte counts have been observed in otherwise healthy premature babies. These values may be physiologic as they are within the limits set for premature infants. The 95% range is between 160 and $675 \times 10^9/L$ with a median value of $375 \times 10^9/L$.

Exercise

The human spleen normally retains about one-third of the total platelets in an exchangeable pool, which can be released into the circulation on alpha-adrenergic stimulation. Redistribution of this pool into the peripheral blood stream immediately leads to marked thrombocytosis. It has not been possible to explain the association between thrombocytosis and various diseases, such as allergies, metabolic disease, myopathies, convulsive disorders (without steroid treatment), preoperative stages and deformities of the skeletal system in pediatric and adult patients.

COMPLICATIONS

Only two pediatric patients developed thrombosis in the course of iron-deficiency anemia with RT. One was a 22-month-old boy with iron-deficiency anemia who on admission had a hemoglobin of 4 g/dl and a thrombocyte count of $1000 \times 10^9/L$. On day 2 of his hospital stay he developed headache, confusion and convulsions. The CT showed infarction of the basal ganglia and thalamus and MRI indicated hemorrhagic infarction. Control of the blood count revealed hemoglobin of 6 g/dl, a mean corpuscular volume (MCV) of 57 fl and a thrombocyte cound of 540 × 10^9/L.

The second case was an 8-month-old Japanese girl who had developed left hemiparesis after a mild head injury. Her CT and MRI demonstrated a cerebral infarction. Laboratory findings revealed iron deficiency anemia and thrombocytosis (1075 × 10^9/L). Serum iron was only 18 μ/dl.

Interestingly, thrombotic complications in connection with thrombocytosis due to iron-deficiency anemia have been reported in rare adult cases. The rigidity of the iron-deficiency in patients with polycythemia because of cyanotic heart disease with constant hypoxia may act as continuous stimulation for erythro and thrombocytogenesis. Thus in polycythemia, increased rigidity of iron deficient erythrocytes and thrombocytosis combine to give a high-risk for thrombosis. The vicious circle is better interrupted by therapy with iron than with anticoagulants. The stimulant effect of erythropoietin on thrombocytogenesis is controversial. Three newborns in whom there was subcutaneous fat necrosis that appeared between the 4th and 21st day of life showed a marked increase in platelets before the onset of clinical manifestations. The question is raised whether thrombocytosis might lower blood perfusion with relative hypoxia and hypothermia and thus lead to necrosis of adipose tissue.

Thrombosis is the severest complication of thrombocytosis after splenectomy; however, it is not yet proven that the elevated number of platelets is a causative or concomitant factor.

INDICATIONS FOR PROPHYLAXIS

Reactive thrombocytosis in children does not justify general prophylaxis with anticoagulants or platelet aggregation inhibitors. Even an RT of 1000 × 10^9/L or more has no clinical importance in terms of morbidity. No prophylaxis with platelet aggregation inhibitors should be recommended. Individually tailored thrombosis prophylaxis should be considered if additional risk factors exist, such as immobilization in a cast, some cases of leukemia, alterations of other plasmatic thrombophilic factors, iron deficiency anemia, cyanotic heart disease and cardiac arrhythmias after Fontan surgery, splenectomy, disease such as autoimmune hemolytic anemia, or increased incidence of thrombosis in connection with postoperative thrombocytosis after pancreas transplantation.

PRIMARY FAMILIAL THROMBOCYTOSIS

Few familial, recessive, dominant, as well as X linked forms of primary thrombocytosis have been reported.[20,21] Spontaneous formation of megakaryopoietic progenitors and increased sensitivity to Tpo are thought to be the primary mechanisms. In several pedigrees, overproduction of Tpo has been shown to be responsible for the disease. In some adult patients mutations in the Tpo gene locus have been found. These mutations typically occur in the 5′ untranslated region of the Tpo gene and result in deletions of untranslated open reading frames and overproduction of Tpo. In children with familial thrombocytosis, platelet counts are lower than in ET, splenomegaly is usually absent, almost no thrombotic or hemorrhagic complications occur, and treatment is not typically required.

In conclusion, thrombocytosis even when marked is typically a benign, reactive phenomenon in children that does not require treatment. Although it is more common in hospitalized children who suffer from a variety of underlying conditions, it can also be seen in normal children during routine blood work, usually as a result of a recent self-limited infection. A repeat hemogram in a few weeks, provided that the child remains well, will show normalization or at least a substantial drop in the platelet count. In most cases, consultation with a pediatric hematologist is not required unless the primary physician and/or the parents are anxious and in cases that thrombocytosis is unexplained, prolonged, or symptomatic, i.e. it is associated with thrombotic and/or hemorrhagic complications. In these cases, ET cannot be excluded, and timely consultation is necessary.

REFERENCES

1. Sutor AH. Pediatric Hematology, 2nd edn. Churchill Livingstone; 1999. pp. 455-64.
2. Sutor AH. Thrombocytosis in childhood. Semin Thromb Hemost. 1995;21:330-9.
3. Yohannan MD, Higgy KE, Al-Mashhadani SA, Santhosh-Kumar CR. Thrombocytosis. Etiologic analysis of 663 patients. Clin Pediatr. 1994;33:340-3.
4. Denton A, Davis P. Extreme thrombocytosis in admissions to paediatric intensive care: no requirement for treatment. Arch Dis Child. 2007;92:515-6.
5. Dror Y, Blanchette VS. Essential thrombocythaemia in children. Br J Haematol. 1999;107:691-8.
6. Chen HL, Chiou SS, Sheen JM, et al. Thrombocytosis in children at one medical centre of southern Taiwan. Acta Paediatr Taiwan. 1999;40:309-13.

7. Hasle H. Incidence of essential thrombocythaemia in children. Br J Haematol. 2000;110:751.
8. Tsimberidou AM, Giles FJ. Essential thrombocythemia (ET): moving from palliation to cure. Hematology. 2002;7: 315-23.
9. Dror Y, Zipursky A, Blanchette VS. Essential thrombocythemia in children. J Pediatr Hematol Oncol. 1999;21:356-63.
10. Wolach B, Morag H, Drucker M, Sadan N. Thrombocytosis after pneumonia with empyema and other bacterial infections in children. Pediatr Infect Dis J. 1990;9:718-21.
11. Vlacha V, Feketea G. Thrombocytosis in pediatric patients is associated with severe lower respiratory tract inflammation. Arch Med Res. 2006;37:755-9.
12. de Benedetti F, Massa M, Robbioni P, Ravelli A, Burgio GR, Martini A. Correlation of serum interleukin-6 levels with joint involvement and thrombocytosis in systemic juvenile rheumatoid arthritis. Arthritis Rheum. 1991;34:1158-63.
13. Al Mazyad AS. Polyarteritis nodosa in Arab children in Saudi Arabia. Clin Rheumatol. 1999;18:196-200.
14. Le Thi Huong DU, Wechsler B, Cabane J, Piette JC, Herreman G, Guillevin L, et al. Wegener's granulomatosis. Clinical aspects, nosologic problems. Review of the literature apropos of 30 cases. Ann Med Interne (Paris). 1988; 139:169-82.
15. Lin CY, Yang YH, Lee CC, Huang CL, Wang LC, Chiang BL. Thrombopoietin and interleukin-6 levels in Henoch-Schoenlein purpura. J Microbiol Immunol Infect. 2006;39: 476-82.
16. Halfdanarson TR, Litzow MR, Murray JA. Hematologic manifestations of celiac disease. Blood. 2007;109:412-21.
17. Kapsoritakis AN, Potamianos SP, Sfiridaki AI, Koukourakis MI, Koutroubakis IE, Roussomoustakaki MI, et al. Elevated thrombopoietin serum levels in patients with inflammatory bowel disease. Am J Gastroenterol. 2000;95:3478-81.
18. Carrington PA, Carr TF, Stevens RF, Evans DI. Thrombocytosis associated with solid tumors in children. Pediatr Hematol Oncol. 1992;9:289-91.
19. Blatt J, Penchansky L, Horn M. Thrombocytosis as a presenting feature of acute lymphoblastic leukemia in childhood. Am J Hematol. 1989;31:46-50.
20. Fujiwara T, Harigae H, Kameoka J, Yokoyama H, Takahashi S, Tomiya Y, et al. A case of familial thrombocytosis: possible role of altered thrombopoietin production. Am J Hematol. 2004;76:395-7.
21. Cohen N, Almoznino-Sarafian D, Weissgarten J, Alon I, Zaidenstein R, Dishi V, et al. Benign familial microcytic thrombocytosis with autosomal dominant transmission. Clin Genet. 1997;52:47-50.

13 Hemostasis: Developmental Aspects and Rare Congenital Bleeding Disorders

Nivedita Dhingra, SP Yadav, Anupam Sachdeva

Bleeding problems are often seen in the neonatal period, particularly in the sick neonate. Although thrombocytopenia is the most common cause, coagulation problems also occur often and the two may coexist. Majority of the coagulation disorders in the neonatal period are acquired but a number of inherited conditions can also present at this time. A prompt diagnosis and management of these conditions depend on early recognition and initiation of appropriate investigations. Although acquired disorders most often present in sick term or preterm infants, many inherited disorders manifest in otherwise, healthy neonates. Recognition of the clinical setting in which bleeding occurs is, therefore, an important clue to the underlying diagnosis. In this chapter the causes, diagnosis and management of coagulation problems in the newborn infants are discussed.

NEONATAL HEMOSTASIS

Neonatal hemostasis is a highly complex process, which is dependent on a series of interactions occuring between endothelial cells, platelets and hemostatic proteins. The liver is the site of synthesis of most coagulation proteins; the surfaces of platelets and endothelial cells are the sites of most protein activation. Our understanding of this process has improved considerably in recent years, and it is now accepted that traditional models of hemostasis do not adequately reflect the events *in vivo*, and are an oversimplification of the processes involved. It is now recognized that the traditional extrinsic pathway, involving tissue factor and factor VIIa, is the major pathway by which coagulation is initiated.[1]

An understanding of the hemostatic system and the features unique to early weeks of life is important when it comes to the investigation of a neonate with a hemorrhagic problem. The hemostatic system is profoundly influenced by age, and the concentrations of many hemostatic proteins are dependent on both the gestational and postnatal age of the infant. Plasma levels and activities of most coagulation proteins are low at the time of term birth and reach adult levels in weeks to months postnatally. Maturation is accelerated after preterm birth. Despite the diminished capacity of neonatal plasma to generate thrombin, regulate clot formation, and subsequently lyse the formed clot, hemostasis is generally well balanced, and there is a low incidence of either inappropriate bleeding or clotting in the term infant. However, when stressed with extraordinary conditions, the neonatal hemostatic system is easily overwhelmed.

Evaluation of Neonatal Hemostasis

Evaluation of the neonatal hemostasis system, with the intention of identifying bleeding diathesis, should be performed similar to any other clinical problem in the neonatal period.

Maternal History

A history of previous pregnancies and their outcomes may be informative especially when there is a suspicion of neonatal alloimmune thrombocytopenia(NAIT).[2] A history of maternal drug intake or connective tissue disorders may also be linked to neonatal thrombocytopenia.

Family History

In diagnosing congenital bleeding disorders, parental ethnic background and whether there is consanguinity in the marriage are very important. Some bleeding disorders are more common within certain ethnic groups (e.g. incidence of factor XI deficiency is increased in Ashkenazy Jews).[3] Consanguineous marriages will increase the risk for birth of neonates with autosomal recessive bleeding disorders. The presence of family history for a bleeding disorder will also provide insight into the heritable basis for the hemorrhagic state. However, absence of family history for a bleeding disorder cannot exclude occurrence of severe bleeding disorders. For example, approximately a third of severe hemophilia A patients do not have a positive family history.

Neonatal History

A thorough evaluation of the neonate is essential for identification of the underlying pathology. Bleeding diathesis in a well baby is usually secondary to NAIT or transfer of maternal antibodies. Coagulopathies, however, tend to develop more often in sick neonates. Congenital infections, sepsis, metabolic disorders are some of the conditions which can lead to a derangement of the coagulation profile. It should also be ascertained whether vitamin K was administered at birth or not to rule out vitamin K deficiency bleeding. A history of abnormal bleeding in the newborn period should be sought with specific reference to delayed bleeding from the umbilical stump.

Lab Evaluation

The fetal and neonatal hemostatic system are totally different from the pediatric and adult system. Coagulation proteins do not cross the placenta but are synthesized in the fetus from around the tenth week of gestation. The concentrations of coagulation protein are dependent on gestational and postnatal age of the infant. Data is now available for both term and preterm infants on the normal levels of procoagulant proteins, inhibitors of coagulation, proteins involved in the fibrinolytic system, and screening tests of coagulation prothrombin time (PT) activated partial thromboplastin time (APTT) and thrombin clotting time (TCT) at sequential stages of postnatal development.

Mean levels of the vitamin K-dependent factors (II, VII, IX and X) in the term infants are around 50% of normal adult values and are reduced further in the premature infant. Factor VII levels reach the adult range by 5 days, while the other factors increase gradually over the first six months of life. Although within the normal adult range mean levels remain usually on the lower side of the adult range during infancy.

The contact factors (XI, XII, prekallikerin [PK] and high molecular weight kininogen [HMWK] are reduced to around 30-50% of normal at term. HMWK increases rapidly, whereas the other factors show a more gradual increase. Factors VIII (FVIII) levels on day one are the same as the adult values and remain so throughout the neonatal period. von Willebrand factor (vWF) levels are increased at birth and although they decline slightly, they remain high. In addition neonatal vWF is made up of multimers which are more active, as indicated by increased platelet aggregation in response to ristocetin. Thus, the diagnosis hemophilia A can be made safely whereas the diagnosis for more common forms of von Willebrand disease (vWD) cannot be made in the neonatal period (can be made at 6 months).

Mean levles of factors V (FV) are at the normal adult range at birth and show a minor drop by day five. Fibrinogen levels are normal in both term and preterm neonates. A transient increase in fibrinogen is observed at day five but thereafter levels are stable throughout the neonatal period. Fetal fibrinogen has increased content of sialic acid, similar to the situation seen in patients with chronic liver disease. The functional significance of fetal fibrinogen is unknown, however, the TCT is normal provided calcium is included in the buffering system. FXIII is 70% of normal at birth and increases to adult level by day five. Many of the coagulation factors increase gradually as the gestational age increases. There is, however, an accelerated maturation pattern in these preterm babies postnatally and levels of coagulation proteins are usually similar by 6 months of age.

Prothrombin time is only minimally prolonged in the normal term infant. APTT, can be markedly prolonged, particularly in the preterm infants due to the reduced levels of contact factors, which have a disproportionate effect on APTT compared with reduced levels of FVIII and FIX. The TCT, is normal if calcium is added to the buffering system; otherwise it is prolonged reflecting the effects of fetal fibrinogen.

Antithrombin III (ATIII), heparin cofactor II (HC II) and α_2 macroglobulin (α_2-M), are all inhibitors of thrombin and are increased at birth and continue to rise till 6 months, at which time they are twice normal adults values. Protein C and protein S, being vitamin K-dependent are <50% of normal at birth. They reach adult levels by early teenage years. Protein C, like fibrinogen circulates in a fetal form which does not affect the function of the moleule. In adults, 60% of protein S circulates as a complex with C4b-binding protein, in which form it contributes to complement regulation but not coagulation regulation. Neonatal plasma contains negligible levels of C4b-binding protein. Consequently, essentially all neonatal protein S is free to function as a cofactor to protein C. Tissue factor pathway inhibitor (TFPI) or extrinsic pathway inhibitor (EPI) levels are around 65% of adult values. Thrombin generation capacity is reduced to around 50% of adults values. The activity of clot-bound thrombin form is reduced and both of these effects have been shown to be related to reduced levels of prothrombin.

The fibrinolytic system in the neonate is immature. At birth plasminogen levels are around 50% of adult values in the term infants and slighty lower than this in preterm infants and reach normal adult level by 6 months. The levels of both tPA and PAI-1 appear to be transiently increased on day 1 of life in both term and preterm infants due to release form endothelial cells at the time of delivery. As well as being reduced at birth, plasminogen is present in a 'fetal' form. Akin to fetal fibrinogen with both reduced functional activity and decresed binding to cellular receptors. The reduced ability to generate plasmin, suggests that the neonate may have an impaired ability to lyze thrombi.

The platelet count is within the normal range in both the term and preterm infants. They have reduced reactivity to thrombin and ADP, adrenaline. The bleeding time in the neonate is shorter than in adults due to increased level of vWF antigen and activity together with the increased red cell size and hematocrit.[4,5]

The Coagulation Cascade and its Different Pathways

Bleeding is stopped by:

- Primary hemostatic plug formation with platelet adhesion and aggregation
- Secondary plug formation with coagulation and insoluble fibrin mesh.

Initially, circulating platelets adhere to the site of vessel injury. von Willebrand factor (vWF) forms a link between glycoprotein Ib (GpIb) receptors on the platelets and collagen of the subendothelium. This is followed by activation, shape change and aggregation of platelets. Then fibrinogen binds to GpIIb/IIIa receptors on the surface of adjacent activated platelets and crosslinks them resulting in the formation of the primary hemostatic plug. Activated platelets are a source of negatively charged phospholipids for amplification of the coagulation cascade which results in the formation of the fibrin clot.

After a vascular injury the coagulation process is initiated by exposure to tissue factor (TF), and membrane glycoprotein that is located in subendothelial tissues. Tissue factor binds tightly to factor VII (FVII); in the presence of calcium ions and phospholipid, FVII is converted to its active form, FVIIa. The TF-FVIIa complex then activates factor X (FX) to FXa and factor IX (FIX) to FIXa. These reactions occur on negatively charged cell membrane surfaces. The initial formation of FXa generates thrombin and triggers activation of platelets and a number of coagulation proteins, such as FXI, FIX, FVIII and FV. The initial stimulus for coagulation is quickly inhibited by the regulator tissue factor pathway inhibitor (TFPI) through the formation of an inactive quarternary FXa-FVIIa-TF complex. The secondary reactions stimulated by the initial generation of thrombin, especially the activation of FIX, are then essential for maintenance of the hemostatic response. Thus severe deficiencies of the contact factor (FXII), prekallikrein, high molecular weight kininogen (HMWK) are not asociated with a clinically significant bleeding disorder due to the key role of FVII in initiating coagulation. The role of FIX in maintaining the coagulation response explains why individuals with a severe deficiency of this factor have a clinically significant bleeding disorder.

In conditions where the initial quantity of FIXa generated is insufficient, or the processes opposing coagulation such as fibrinolysis, are particularly active, FXIa plays an important role in maintaining hemostasis. This supportive role is consistent with the clinical observation that spontaneous hemorrhage or hemorrhage following surgical procedures is rare in FXI-deficient patients unless the level of FXI is extremely low, whereas bleeding is common when trauma or surgery involves tissues with high fibrinolytic activity such as the oral cavity and urinary tract. The hemostatic system in the neonates is immature with reduced levels of many hemostatic proteins.

Homeostasis-general

Involves formation of blood clots to stop bleeding from damaged vessels, and activation of natural anticoagulation and fibrinolytic systems to limit clot formation to sites of injury. Bleeding disorders are due to defects in clot formation or overative fibrinolytic systems. Hypercoagulability disorders result from defects in the anticoagulant system or under active fibrinolytic systems.

INTRINSIC PATHWAY

Involves factors VIII, IX, XI, XII (Hageman factor), prekallikrein, high molecular weight kininogen and merges with extrinsic pathway into common pathway. This pathway is activated when factor XII binds to negatively charged "foreign" surface exposed to blood.

Then sequentially activates factors XI, IX, X then factor II (prothrombin to thrombin) which converts fibrinogen to fibrin (see common pathway). Once extrinsic pathway is inhibited by TFPI-Xa complex (see extrinsic pathway) factor VIIIa/IXa complex becomes the dominant generator of factor Xa, thrombin and fibrin.

EXTRINSIC PATHWAY

Involves tissue factor (TF, factor III), originally considered "extrinsic" to blood since it is present on cell surfaces not normally in contact with (i.e. extrinsic to) the circulatory system. This pathway is believed to be the primary mechanism of coagulation pathway *in vivo,* as tissue factor binds to factor VII or activated factor VII (FVIIa).

TF-FVIIa complex activates factors X and IX. Activated factor IX activates more factor X with cofactors activated factor VIII, anionic phospholipids (from activated platelets) and calcium. Activated factor X convers prothrombin to thrombin, with activated factor V, anionic phospholipids (from activated platelets) and calcium as cofactors. After initial activation, this pathway is inhibited by the binding of tissue factor pathway inhibitor (TFPI) to factor Xa which inhibits TF-FVIIa complex, and further coagulation is dependent on the intrinsic pathway.

COMMON PATHWAY

Involves fibrinogen (factor I), factors II (prothrombin), V, X. Thrombin acts on fibrinogen; releases fibrinopeptides A and B; and the remaining fibrin monomers polymerize to form insoluble fibrin. Thrombin also binds to antithrombin, which inhibits thrombin to prevent excessive clotting. Thrombin may also activate factor XI (part of intrinsic pathway), factors V, VIII, XIII, XI and platelets. Factor XIII cross links fibrin to increase stability of the fibrin clot.

PROTEIN C/PROTEIN S ANTICOAGULANT PATHWAY

This pathway is a physiologic anticoagulant system to limit blood clot formation (i.e. fibrinogen to fibrin conversion) at the site of vessel injury. The major anticoagulant systems are protein C and protein S, antithrombin and tissue factor pathway inhibitor (TFPI).

Protein C and S are vitamin K dependent anticoagulant proteins produced mainly in liver. The endothelial cell protein C receptor binds to thrombin- thrombomodulin complex, which activates protein C. Activated protein C binds to free protein S on the surface of endothelial cells or platelets and this protein C/protein S complex degrades factors Va and VIIIa which reduces fibrin formation. Resistance of FVa to degradation by activated protein C is known as Factor V Leiden mutation, which is the most common inherited procoagulant state in the west.

THROMBOMODULIN

Intrinsic membrane glycoprotein on luminal surface of endothelial cells that binds thrombomodulin and facilitates the activation of protein C. C/T dimorphism at nucleotide 1418 is associated with premature myocardial infarction, but no definite association with venous thromboembolism.

ANTITHROMBIN

Formerly called antithrombin III, functions as an anticoagulant by inhibiting activated factors II, IX, X, XI, XII, kallikrein, plasmin and probably factor VII. Activity is accelerated 1000x by interaction with heparin or heparin sulfate (located on endothelial cells).

FIBRINOLYSIS PATHWAY

It is a process of degrading the fibrin clot when it is no longer needed. Also prevents the extension of clot beyond site of injury. It is initiated by tPA (tissue plasminogen activator) or uPA (urokinase-like plasminogen activator) which converts plasminogen to plasmin in the presence of fibrin by cleaving the Arg561-Val562 peptide bond. Plasmin degrades the fibrin clot and intact fibrinogen to soluble fibrin/fibrinogen degradation products (FDP). Plasmin also inactivates factors Va and VIIIa (as does protein C and protein S). tPA is produced by endotheial cells; its activation of plasminogen is the major mechanism for lysis of fibrin clots. uPA is produced by urine and plasma; keeps renal tracts free of blood clots and is also important for initiating non-fibrinolytic activities of plasmin.

Excessive fibrinolysis is prevented by plasmin inhibitor (antiplasmin, formerly called alpha2-antiplasmin) and plasminogen activator inhibitor 1 (PAI-1, inhibits tPA and uPA). PAI -1 is synthesized by hepatocytes and endothelial cells, is present in platelets and plasma; can bind to fibrin and inhibit plasminogen activators tPA and uPA. Homozygous deficiency of plasminogen is associated with ligneous conjunctivitis (rare form of chronic pseudomembranous conjunctivitis); replacement therapy with plasminogen is therapeutic. Neither plasminogen deficiency (0.5 to 2.0% of patients with thrombosis) nor tPA is reported to be associated with an increased risk of thrombosis.

CAUSES OF NEONATAL BLEEDING (DERANGED HEMOSTASIS)

Platelet Disorders

A. **Thrombocytopenia** (platelet count <150 × 10^9/L) occurs in 1-4% of term newborns, 40-72% of sick preterms and 25% of ICU admissions; of these 75% present before 72 hours of life. Causes include:
   i. Decreased platelet production occurs in:
      - Congenital infections (e.g. CMV, Rubella, HIV)
      - Certain syndromes (e.g. Thrombocytopenia Absent Radius, Fanconi), sepsis and hemolytic disease of newborn.
   ii. Increased platelet consumption occurs in:
      - Maternal autoimmune disease (e.g. ITP, SLE)
      - Asphysia/Shock
      - Neonatal alloimmune thrombocytopenia
      - IUGR with toxemia of pregnancy
      - Necrotizing enterocolitis
      - Thrombosis (due to catheters, hemangiomas)
      - Hemolytic disease of the newborn
      - Exchange transfusion
      - Hepain induce thrombocytopenia
      - Polycythemia/Hyperviscosity

B. Impaired platelet function is rare in the newborn except for decreased platelet adhesiveness sassociated with indomethacin theraphy and von Willebrand's disease.

Coagulation Protein Disorders

A. Congenital factor deficiencies:
   - *X-linked recessive:* Hemophilia A (Factor VIII) and hemophilia B (Factor IX)
   - Autosomal recessive (rare): Factors V, VII, X, XI, XII, XIII and afibrinogenemia

B. *Acquired deficiencies:* Most common is vitamin K deficiency.

Combined Platelet and Coagulation Factor Disorders

A. Disseminated intravascular coagulation (DIC) occurs secondary to inappropriate systemic activation of normal clotting mechanisms after endothelial injury. Infants have low platelet counts and fibrinogen levels, prolonged PT, APTT, and elevated fibrin degradation products.

B. Hepatic dysfunction due to several causes (e.g. shock, infection, inherited conditions); most have prolonged PT and decreased factor and fibrinogen levels.

Disorders of Vascular Integrity

Such as hemangiomas or vascular malformations that may rupture and directly bleed, or sequester platelets and secondarily cause bleeding.

Platelet disorders are covered in the chapter on *Neonatal Thrombocytopenia.* In the following section bleeding disorders in the neonatal period secondary to defects in coagualtion proteins are reviewed. Table 13.1 summarizes the lab investigations required in neonatal coagulation disorders.

HEMOPHILIAS A AND B

Hemophilias A and B together with von Willebrand's disease account for more than 90% of all inherited bleeding disorders. Currently, it is estimated that 1 in 10,000 males are affected by severe hemophilia A and 1 in 50,000 males by severe hemophilia B.

Table 13.1: Lab investigation of neonatal coagulation disorder

Condition	*PT*	*APTT*	*Fibrinogen*	*Platelets*	*Useful diagnostic test*
Inherited disorders					
Hemophilia A	N	↑	N	N	FVIII assay
Hemophilia B	N	↑	N	N	FIX assay
vWD (type II)	N	↑	N	N/↓	FVIII, vWD assay
FVII	↑	N	N	N	FVII assay
FX	↑	↑	N	N	FX assay
Fibrinogen	N/↑	N/↑	↓	N	Fibrinogen assay
FXII	N	N	N	N	
Acquired disorders					
DIC	↑	↑	↓	↓	D-dimers
Vitamin K deficiency	↑	N/↑	N	N	FII, VII, IX and X assay
Liver disease	↑	↑	N/↓	N/↓	Factor assay

CLINICAL FEATURES

The hemophilias are the most common inherited bleeding disorder to present neonatally. It has been reported that 10-20% of severly affected neonates and 2 to 5% of those with mild or moderate disease had abnormal bleeding in the immediate neonatal period (i.e. within 7 days of birth).

The pattern of bleeding observed in neonates tends to differ from that typically seen in older children with hemophilia, where joint and muscle bleeds predominate. The majority of cases present with bleeding which is iatrogenic in origin. Bleeding after circumcision, continued oozing or excessive hematoma formation following venepunture, heel stab sampling and intramuscular vitamin K have all been observed. Umblical bleeding is relatively uncommon in hemophilia. Cephalhemtomas, subgaleal hematomas and intracranial hemorrhage (ICH) also occur.[6] Recent evidence suggest that the actual incidence of ICH is much higher if asymptomatic cases detected accidentally on cranial imaging are taken into account.[7,8] Less common sites of bleeding include gastrointestinal hemorrhage and intra-abdominal bleeding.

Inhibitors in Newborns with Hemophilia

Inhibitors, while rare, have been reported to occur in the newborn period. Risk factors included hemophilia severity, intron 22 inversions and intensity of factor exposure.[9,10] There is little data regarding inhibitor development and risk factors in newborns with hemophilia B.

Diagnosis

The diagnosis of hemophilia A is confirmed by finding a reduced level of FVIII activity. Diagnosing hemophilia B is complicated by the physiologic reduction in FIX during the neonatal period. While the diagnosis of severe (<1 u/dl) and moderate (1-5 u/dl) hemophilia B can be made, the diagnosis of mild (>5 u/dl) cases is problematic and repeat testing when the infant is older is necessary.

Management

Neonates requiring treatment should receive replacement therapy with FVIII or FIX concentrates as appropriate.

VON WILLEBRAND DISEASE

von Willebrand disease (vWD) is the most common inherited bleeding disorder with an estimated prevalence of 0.8-1.3%. It is caused by either a quantitative or qualitative deficiency of von Willebrand Factor (vWF). In most families vWD is inherited as an AD disorder and the bleeding tendency is usually mild. vWF is physiologically increased in the neonatal period and high molecular weight multimeric forms are also disproportionately increased at this time, thus making the diagnosis of this disease difficult in the neonatal period.[11]

Clinical Features

Bleeding in the neonatal period due to vWD is seen only in severe homozygous type 3 disorder in which there is a marked reduction in the levels of both FVIII and vWF. Type 3 disease is rare and accounts for <1% of all patients with vWD.

Diagnosis

Type 3 disease is confirmed by low levels of both FVIII activity and vWF antigen activity. Most other forms of vWD are marked by physiologically elevated levels of vWF and cannot be diagnosed neonatally other than by molecular analysis. The only other exception to this is type 2B vWD associated with thrombocytopenia, which has been recognized in infancy and should be included in the differential diagnosis of neonatal thrombocytopenia.

Management

Treatment of bleeding in type 3 vWD requires the use of a virucidally-treated factor concentrate which contains both FVIII and vWF. Recombinant vWF has been developed but is not widely available.

DEFICIENCIES OF THE INTRINSIC PATHWAY CONTACT ACTIVATING SYSTEM

Three proteins are involved in the contact activation pathway:

- Factor XII (Hageman factor);
- Prekallikrein (Fletcher factor);
- High molecular weight kininogen (HMWK; Williams-Fitzgerald-Flaujeac factor).

Hereditary deficiencies of these factors have been described.

Structure and Function

Coagulation Factor XII (Hageman factor, FXII) is produced and secreted by the liver. It is the product of a single gene that maps to chromosome 5.[12] FXII autoactivates upon exposure to negatively charged surfaces to become the enzyme Factor XIIa (α-FXIIa), which then activates FXI, prekallikrein (PK), and C1 esterase (a subunit of the complement cascade). The consequence of FXI activation by α-FXIIa is the initiation of a series of proteolytic reactions resulting in thrombin generation, which precedes clot formation. Activation of PK by α-FXIIa results in the formation of plasma kallikrein that can reciprocally activate more FXII and liberate bradykinin from high-molecular weight kininogen (HMWK). Bradykinin, is a potent vasodilator and also stimulates the formatin of prostacyclin (an inhibitor of platelet aggregation) and the release of tissue plasminogen activator.[13] α-FXIIa when cleaved by plasma kallikrein forms Factor β-XIIa (β-FXIIa), which then activates the macromolecular complex of the first component of complement, resulting in classic complement system activation; plasma kallikrein also directly activates complement components C3 and C5.[14,15] Thus, the activation of FXII results in coagulation and complement activation with bradykinin liberation.

Although deficiencies of the contact factors are characterized by a marked prolongation of the activated partial thromboplastin time (APTT), affected individuals do not have a clinically significant bleeding disorder and recent evidence suggests that the contact system has little to do with the initiation of hemostasis. Recently, Spronk et al demonstrated that tissue factor (TF) is the physiologic initiator of blood coagulation leading to hemostasis.[16]

In the revised view of the contact system, these proteins have been found to have antithrombotic and profibrinolytic actions that occur on negatively charged cell surfaces. Two pathways have been identified. The kininogens selectively inhibit α-thrombin-induced platelet activation. Secondly, activation of prekallikrein bound to HMWK on endothelial cells and platelets results in the activation of pro-urokinase and an increase in plasminogen activation. A number of individuals with congenital deficiencies of FXII, PK and the kininogens, including the index cases, John Hageman and Mayme Williams, experienced significant thrombotic events.

Inheritance

FXII, prekallikrein, HMWK and LMWK deficiencies are inherited in an AR fashion. The defects maybe quantitative or qualitative defects. Individuals with quantitative defects lack both functional and antigenic material and are designated cross-reacting material negative (CRM–), whereas those with qualitative defects have cross-reacting material and are designated (CRM+).

Clinical Features

The individuals with deficiencies of FXII, prekallikrein, HMWK and LMWK do not manifest clinically significant bleeding disorders.

Laboratory Features

The laboratory abnormality characteristic of the inherited contact factor deficiencies is a marked prolongation of the APTT. The diagnosis is established by a reduced level of functional FXII, prekallikrein or HMWK and LMWK in the absence of an alternative cause of the deficiency state.

Treatment

No requirement for replacement therapy as a measure either to prevent or treat bleeding.

FACTOR XI DEFICIENCY

Coagulation factor XI (FXI), or plasma thromboplastin antecedent, is a coagulation protein essential to normal hemostasis and acts by cleaving factor IX (FIX) in the intrinsic blood-coagulation pathway. FXI deficiency was first described in 1953 by Rosenthal and Colleagues.[17] It is a rare coagulopathy found predominantly, in Ashkenazi Jews.[2] The estimated prevalence in the general population is 1 in a million population.[18]

Structure and Function

FXI is a plasma glycoprotein synthesized in the liver and circulates as a complex with HMWK. FXIa remains tightly bound to cell-surface HMWK.

Inheritance

In majority of the cases FXI deficiency is inherited as an AR trait, although some recent data suggests that AD pattern of inheritence may also occur.[19,20] On the basis of the concordance or discordance of FXI antigen and activity levels, the disease can be classified into the more frequent cross-reactive material negative (CRM–) and the rarer CRM positive (CRM+).

Clinical Features

Unlike severe hemophilia A or B, FXI deficiency is generally associated with a mild bleeding disorder that becomes clinically manifest after trauma or surgery, e.g. dental extractions, chronic epistaxis and menorrhagia and only rarely is associated with hemarthroses and muscle hematomas. Easy bruising is a common symptom. Factor XI indirectly increases thrombin activatable fibrinolysis inhibitor (TAFI), resulting in reduced fibrinolysis and stabilized clot formation.[21] Hence sites with higher fibrinolytic potential such as the oral cavity and genitourinary tract tend to bleed more.

Laboratory Features

An isolated prolongation of APTT with a normal prothrombin time is suggestive of FXI deficiency provided that FXII deficiency, Hemophilia A and B and forms of von Willebrand disease are ruled out.[22] Most cases of FXI deficiency represent a quantitative defect; homozygotes generally have FXI coagulant levels of <15 u/dl while heterozygoes have levels >15 u/dl but below 70 u/dl.

Confirmation of the disorder requires demonstration of reduced levels of coagulant FXI and absence of an alternate cause for the laboratory abnormality, e.g. liver disease. Family studies are recommended and may provide additional evidence of an inherited defect.

Treatment

Since spontaneous bleeding is uncommon in patients with FXI deficiency, replacement therapy is necessary only in individuals with a history of clinically significant bleeding or as hemostatic cover for major surgery. When assessing the requirement for replacement therapy, several variables should be taken into consideration, including:

- Patients coagulant FXI level
- Personal history of bleeding
- Type of surgery especially if involving tissues rich in fibrinolytic activity
- Risk of bleeding complications due to the surgical procedure itself
- Precence of inhibitors
- Presence of combined defects.

Patients with FXI deficiency can safely undergo such surgery under cover of antifibrinolytic therapy (tranexamic acid 25 mg/kg/dose, 4 times daily, administered from 1 day prior to surgery to 7 days after surgery). Concomitant aspirin use appears to be associated with clinically significant bleeding in some FXI-deficiency patients. Highly purified FXI concentrates prepared from human plasma are available. However,a major concern with the use of FXI concentrates is the potential for thrombosis.

FXI dose (units) =

$$\frac{[\text{FXI rise required (u/dl)} \times \text{body weight (kg)}]}{2}$$

The maximum single dose infused should not exceed 30 u/kg. For postsurgical maintenance, a dose of 10–15 u/kg body weight every 2–3 days is usually adequate.

Inhibitors (alloantibodies) to FXI deficiency may occasionally occur in severely deficient patients after exposure to plasma products. In these cases response to activated prothrombin complex concentrates, or activated FVII (FVIIa) may be seen.

FACTOR X (STUART-PROWER FACTOR) DEFICIENCY

Factor X deficiency was first reported in a male patient.

Structure and Function

FX is a vitamin K-dependent glycoprotein that is synthesized in the liver. The mature protein is composed of a light chain and a heavy chain that are held together by a single disulfide bond. The conversion of FX to its active form; FXa, involves the cleavage of a polypeptide from the heavy chain. The reaction is catalyzed by FIXa in the presence of FVIIIa, Ca^{2+} and a negatively charged phospholipid surface, or by FVIIa in the presence of tissue factor. Once formed, FXa catalyzes the conversion of prothrombin to thrombin, a reaction that is accelerated in the presence of FVa, $Ca^{2+}$and phospholipid.

Inheritance

FX deficiency is a rare AR coagulation disorder affecting an estimated 1 in million people. However, more recent data derived from the World Federation of Hemophilia Global Survey shows that FX deficiency afflicts 10% of patients with bleeding disorders. FX deficiency includes gene deletions, dysfunctional variants and variants that affect synthesis and/or secretion of FX.

Clinical Features

Clinical manifestations of FX deficiency vary from a severe bleeding disorder presenting early in life through a very mild bleeding tendency to asymptomatic individuals. Patients with <1% functional FX activity may experience severe bleeding; individuals with 10% or greater functional activity are only mildly affected. Bleeding sites vary according to the severity of the deficiency. Hemorrhage from the umbilical cord and later hemarthroses, severe epistaxis, menorrhagia, central nervous system hemorrhage and postoperative or post-traumatic hemorrhage have been reported in severely affected patients.[23] Mildly affected patients may experience easy bruising or menorrhagia and occasionally bleed significantly after more severe challenges to the hemostatic system, as with trauma or surgery. Epistaxis has been reported as the most common symptoms in all types of the disease.

Laboratory Features

Features of severe congenital FX deficiency include prolongation of the PT and APTT. Of note, the PT and APTT may be differentially affected in individuals with dysfunctional FX variants, reflecting the interaction of the mutant FX with the FIXa-FVIIIa-Ca–phospholipid complex (reflected in the PT). The Russell's viper venom (RVV) time is a test in which FX is directly cleaved and activated by the venom, and is usually prolonged in patients with severe FX deficiency but may be normal in some variants. The bleeding time is occasionally prolonged in severely affected patients, possibly due to defective FVa-FXa interactions on the platelet surface. For a diagnosis of FX deficiency to be made it is essential that a specific functional assay of FX be performed.

The differentiation of congenital from acquired FX deficiency should include consideration of liver disease and vitamin K deficiency. Another disorder associated with FX deficiency is primary amyloidosis, an association that reflects binding of FX to amyloid fibrils.

Treatment

The need for FX replacement should be guided by the circulating FX level, clinical severity of the hemorrhagic episode, or estimated risk of hemostatic challenge, e.g. surgery. Generally, a FX level of 10-40% is considered adequate for hemostasis.

Treatment consists of FFP or FX containing prothrombin-complex concentrates (PCCs). PCCs are preferred. It is important to remember, however, that with thromboembolic complications and occasional episodes of disseminated intravascular coagulation (DIC) may occur with PCCs. If FFP is used, a loading dose of 10-20 ml/kg is recommended. Because of the long half-life of FX (24-48 hours), the level of FX can be built up in the circulation by infusion of plasma every 12 hours. The recommended dose is 3-6 ml/kg.

FACTOR V DEFICIENCY

First defined in the year 1947. Clinically, it manifests as skin bleeding, severe and recurrent epistaxis menorrhagia and possibly an episode of hematuria. The disorder was called parahemophilia and the missing factor was later identified as Factor V (FV), also called accelerator globulin (Ac globulin) or proaccelerin.[24]

Structure and Function

Factor V is a glycoprotein synthesized by hepatocytes and megakaryocytes. It can be converted to its active form. FVa, by FXa, thrombin, meizothrombin (a reaction intermediate formed during prothrombin activation) and Russell's viper venom. The major biologic role of FV is its participation in prothrombinase assembly on the platelet surface. The prothrombinase complex consists of the serine protease FXa, the nonenzymatic protein cofactor FVa, Ca and a negatively charged phospholipid surface. FVa binds with high affinity to negatively charged phospholipids. FXa binds to both the light and heavy chains of FVa; prothrombin binds to the heavy chain of FVa.[25] Under physiologic condition FVa accelerates prothrombin activation more than 10,000 fold by:

- Increasing the catalytic activity of FXa
- Acting as a receptor that promotes the binding of FXa to negatively charged surfaces
- Promoting the interaction of prothrombin within the prothrombinase complex.

Approximately, 20% of the total FV present in healthy individuals is contained in the α-granules of platelets. Following activation of platelets by thrombin, platelet FV is released and converted into FVa which functions as a coafactor in FXa-driven prothrombin activation at the platelet surface. The generation of thrombin at the surface of activated platelets is known to be important in normal hemostasis. Inactivation of FVa is the result of limited proteolysis by activated protein C (APC), a vitamin K-dependent protease formed following activation of the zymogen protein C. The interaction of APC and FVa is stimulated by protein S and inhibited by FXa. FV also acts as a cofactor in the APC-mediated inactivation of FVIIIa, a reaction that is also stimulated by protein S.

Inheritance

FV deficiency is a rare congenital bleeding disorder with AR inheritance. The frequency of the disorder is probably <1/1, 000,000 of the general population. Homozygotes have low FV levels and manifest clinically significant bleeding while heterozygotes have FV levels between 30 and 60% and are usually asymptomatic. Both quantitative and qualitative defects have been described. Combined deficiencies of FV and FVIII (or FVII) have been reported.

Clinical Features

Individuals with severe congenital FV deficiency and levels below 10% of normal often have hemorrhagic manifestations, although they may be asymptomatic. Umblical stump bleeding is uncommon, the most common manifestation being mucosal bleeding. Common hemorrhagic manifestations include ecchymoses, epistaxis, menorrhagia, oral cavity bleeds and excessive postpartum or postabortion bleeding. Hemarthroses may occur and gastrointestinal bleeding, hematuria and bleeding into the central nervous system have been reported.

Laboratory Features

Factor V deficiency can be initially diagnosed observing a prolongation of both the prothrombin time (PT) and activated partial thromboplastin time (APTT) in association with a normal thrombin time (TT). Both PT and APTT are corrected by mixing the patient plasma with a"normal" plasma pool. Deficiency of FV should be confirmed by a PT-based FV assay. Individuals with FV deficiency should also be tested for a concurrent FVIII deficiency as the two often coexist.[26]

Treatment

Factor V replacement therapy is accomplished by FFP administration. FV levels should be raised to at least 15 IU/dl by using 15 to 20 ml/kg of FFP. The initial dose should be 15 to 20 ml/kg followed by smaller amounts, such as 5 ml/kg every 12 hours, adjusting the dosage on the basis of FV levels, PT, and APTT. Studies of FV recovery recommend maintaining a level of 20 to 25% of FV activity for surgery or in case of severe bleeding.

FACTOR VII DEFICIENCY

Inherited FVII deficiency is the most common among the rare congenital coagulation disorders and is characterized by autosomal recessive inheritance. Clinical heterogeneity is a feature of this hemorrhagic disorder, which ranges in severity from lethal to mild or even asymptomatic forms.

Clinical Features

In majority of the cases FVII deficiency tends to be mild. However, severe to very severe cases are not infrequent, characterized, by bleeding tendency in the form of hemarthrosis, muscle hematomas, or even central nervous system (CNS) and gastrointestinal (GI) bleeding. Postoperative bleeding may also occur, and clotting tests may not be helpful in predicting the inherent bleeding risk. Prolonged bleeding following dental extraction is common, although some patients with severe FVII deficiency may tolerate surgery quite well. In some newborn infants bleeding form the umbilical stump has been observed. Patients with mild FVII deficiency (levels >5%) bleed infrequently.

Laboratory Features

Severe FVII deficiency is characterized by a prolonged PT in the presence of a normal APTT, thrombin time and RVV test. Congenital deficiency must be differentiated from acquired FVII deficiency as may occur in patients with liver disease, vitamin K deficiency secondary to malabsorption or those on oral anticoagulant therapy. On rare occasions, FVII deficiency may be due to circulating inhibitor.

Treatment

A FVII level of >20% is considered hemostatic. Products that may be used to treat Factor VII-deficient individuals include FFP, a prothrombin complex concentrate (containing Factor II, VII, IX and X) and a specific Factor VII concentrate where available. A specific virus-inactivated FVII concentrate is preferred to FFP. This recommendation reflects the opinion that a single dose of a virus inactivated factor concentrate prepared from a very large plasma pool is virally safer than exposure to multiple packs of FFP which have not been virus inactivated. Recombinant Factor VII is now available (NovoSeven) which can be used.

Replacement therapy for patients with FVII deficiency should be individualized and will depend on the nature and severity of the coagulation defect, site of bleeding and type of interevention. For the treatment of bleeding or as cover for minor surgery, a single dose of FVII concentrate has generally been found to be sufficient. For surgical interventions it is recommended to maintain a plasma level of at least 20% for approximately 8-10 days. The maintenance dose should be given at intervals of 2-6 hours.

DEFICIENCIES OF THE COMMON PATHWAY PROTHROMBIN DEFICIENCY

Herditary prothrombin deficiency is one of the rarest congenital coagulation defects with a nestimated prevalence of 1 in 2 million in the general population.[27-29]

Structure and Function

Prothrombin is a vitamin K-dependent glycoprotein synthesized in the liver. During blood coagulation prothrombin is converted to thrombin by FXa mediated cleavage in the presence of FVa, Ca^{2+} and negatively charged phospholipids present on the surface of activated platelets.[30] The plasma concentration of prothrombin is 100 μg/ml and its biological half-life is around 70 hours.

Inheritance

The mode of inheritance is AR. Prothrombin defects can be classified as in other defects of clotting factors in terms of:

- True deficiency, or **hypoprothrombinemia** (homozygotes and double or compound heterozygotes)
- Dysfunctional form, or **dysprothrombinemia** (homozygotes and heterozygotes)
- **Hypo-dys** or **dys-dys** forms (compound heterozygotes).

A discrepancy between the clinical severity of the prothrombin deficiency and its antigen level/coagulant activity is often observed among prothrombin-deficient patients. Patients who are compound heterozygotes or who are homozygous for the condition are usally asymptomatic and generally have functional prothrombin levels of 50% or greater by both functional and immunologic assays. In dysprothrombinemia the functional assay for prothrombin is usually decreased with the immunologic assay showing near normal levels of prothrombin antigen.

Clinical Features

The signs and symptoms vary with the level of functional prothrombin. True deficiency of prothrombin, a condition in which plasma levels are <10% in homozygous patients, is always characterized by severe bleeding manifestations. Heterozygous individual with prothrombin levels of 40–60% have no bleeding problems. Patients with lower levels may experience easy bruising, epistaxis, menorrhagia, postpartum bleeding and hemorrhage following surgery or trauma. Hemarthroses and intracranial bleeds are uncommon but have been reported.

Laboratory Features

The diagnosis of hypoprothrombinemia or dysprothrombinemia is suggested by the binding of variable prolongation of the PT and PTT and a normal thrombin time. These screening tests are not specific since deficiencies of FV and FX result in the same abnormalities. A definitive diagnosis depends on specific assays for functional and immunologic prothrombin. The differential diagnosis of hypoprothrombinemia includes vitamin K deficiency states and inhibitors to prothrombin (as may occur in patients with systemic lupus erythematosus (SLE). Studies of family members plus measurement of vitamin K-dependent coagulation factors help to distinguish acquired from inherited prothrombin deficiencies.

Treatment

The treatment of hypoprothrombinemia or dysprothrombinemia depends on the circulating prothrombin level and on the type of bleeding. The exact level of prothrombin needed for hemostasis is not known, but 10 to 15% may suffice for preventing minor hemorrhages and 20 to 40% for major trauma or surgery.[31] Usually, treatment is performed by administering FFP, PCCs, or both.[32] FFP may be used to treat clinically significant bleeding or as preparation for major surgery. A loading dose of 10-20 ml/kg is suggested followed by 3 ml/kg every 12-24 hours. Since the biologic half-life of prothrombin is about 3 days, the need for replacement therapy is infrequent and should be monitored by specific assays and clinical response. PCCs contain Factors II, VII, IX and X. Advantages of such concentrates include a prolonged shelf life, ease of administration and the ability to achieve high levels of clotting factors without fluid overload. Importantly all currently available commercial PCCs are treated during prepration with processes known to inactivate lipid-coated viruses such as the human immunodeficiency type 1 virus and hepatitis C; these preparations are thus preferred to nonvirus inactivated preparations such as FFP. Because of the risk of thrombosis, its recommended that PCCs should not be used in patients with acute liver disease or those with other risk factors for thrombosis such as DIC or AT deficiency. The dose of infused product should not exceed 100 u/kg, and the frequency of infusion should be adjusted to maintain hemostatic, but not excessive, levels of prothrombin.

FIBRINOGEN DEFICIENCY

The normal plasma fibrinogen concentration is 150–350 mg/dl. Afibrinogenemia referes to the total absence of measurable fibrinogen, hypofibrinogenemia to decreased levels of normal fibrinogen and dysfinrinogenemia to the presence of abnormal fibrinogen molecules in the plasma. Table 13.2 summarizes the features of congenital fibrinogen disorders.

Structure and Function

Fibrinogen is a dimeric molecule consisting of 3 pairs of polypeptide chains linked by disulfide bonds. The key role of fibrinogen in the coagulation system is the

Table 13.2: Congenital fibrinogen deficiencies

	Afibrinogenemia	*Hypofibrinogenemia*	*Dysfibrinogenemia*
Prevalence	1 in 1 million	More frequent*	More frequent*
Fibrinogen	Not detectable	100 mg/dl or less	150-350 mg/dl
Symptoms	Bleeding, rare thrombosis	In general symptomatic	Asymptomatic, bleeding and/or thrombosis
Treatment	Fibrinogen	Occasional fibrinogen	Fibrinogen and/or anticoagulants

* The prevalence of hypofibrinogenemia and dysfibrinogenemia is difficult to establish because of the large number of asymptomatic cases.

formation of fibrin which together with platelets forms the hemostatic plug. *In vivo* the transformation of fibrinogen to fibrin is catalyzed by thrombin. The first step in this process involves the release of fibrinopeptides A and B with the formation of fibrin monomers; subsequent polymerization leads to the formation of an interconnected network of fibrin fibers. The mechanical strength of the fibrin clot is also enhanced by the presence of Ca^{++}. Fibrinogen is synthesized in the liver prior to its release into the circulation. The synthetic reserve of the liver is large and up to 20-fold increases in production rates have been found in patients with peripheral consumption in fibrinogen. Such observations explain why hypofibrinogenemia due to decreased synthesis is uncommon in liver disease or in most clinical states associated with increased plasma fibrinogen turnover. Fibrinogen is also present in the α-granules of platelets. The level of platelet fibrinogen may reflect both synthesis in megakaryocytes and uptake from the plasma.

Inheritance

Afibrinogenemia is a rare congenital bleeding disorder that appears to be transmitted as an AR trait. Consanguinity is common. Dysfibrinogenemia is generally inherited as an AD trait with most cases representing the heterozygous state. Over 200 cases of dysfinrinogenemia have been reported with abnormalities that affect one or more of fibrinogen's known monomer polymerization, fibrin cross-linking by FXIIIa, fibrin binding of thrombin, plasminogen binding, aceleration of tissue plasminogen activator, wound healing and binding of fibrinogen to platelet GpIIb/IIIa receptors.

Clinical Features

Patients with congenital afibrinogenemia suffer from a life-long hemorrhagic diathesis of variable severity. It usually presents in the neonatal period with 85% of the cases presenting with umblical cord bleeding[33,34] but later age of onset is also not unusual. Bleeding may occur in the skin, gastrointestinal tract, genitourinary tract, or the central nervous system, with intracranial hemorrhage being reported as the major cause of death. Joint bleeding, which is common in patients with severe hemophilia, is infrequent: in a series of 72 patients with severe fibrinogen deficiency, hemarthrosis was only observed in 25% of cases.[35] Persistent damage to the musculoskeletal system and resulting handicap is also less frequent in patients with afibrinogenemia. There is an intriguing susceptibility of spontaneous rupture of the spleen in afibrinogenemic patients.[36] Symptoms are generally present only in patients with fibrinogen levels of <50 mg/dl. Menstrual bleeding is often severe and fetal loss due to spontaneous abortion or abruptio placenta is common in pregnant women with very low fibrinogen levels.

Patients with dysfibrinogenemia are often asymptomatic. The bleeding manifestations are usually limited to epistaxis, menorrhagia and mild-to-moderate postoperative bleeding. Individuals with the lowest levels of fibrinogen measured by a functional assay are those most likely to experience significant bleeding. Of note, a number of patients with qualitative fibrinogen defects have experienced arterial or venous thromboses, or defective wound healing. These complications are consistent with fibrinolysis and wound healing being dependent on the formation of cross-linked fibrin during blood coagulation. A compilation of more than 260 cases of dysfibrinogenemia revealed that 55% of the patients had no clinical complications, 25% exhibited bleeding, and 20% displayed a tendency to thrombosis, mainly venous.[37] However, when patients with deep vein thrombosis are screened for thrombophilia, the prevalence of dysfibrinogenemia is very low (0.8% based on a review of 2376 patients), so that systematic testing for dysfibrinogenemia in patients with thrombophilia is not recommended.[38] In general, polymerization defects are more frequently associated with thromboses, whereas fibrinopeptide release defects are more common in patients with abnormal bleeding.

Laboratory Features

Absence of immunoreactive fibrinogen is essential to the diagnosis of congenital afibrinogenemia. All coagulation tests that depend on the formation of fibrin as the end point, that is, prothrombin time (PT), partial thromboplastin time (PTT), or thrombin time (TT), are infinitely prolonged. Plasma activity of all other clotting factors is normal. Some abnormalities in platelet functions tests can be observed, which are almost reversible upon addition of fibrinogen.[39] Because fibrinogen is one of the main determinants of erythrocyte sedimentation, it is not surprising that afibrinogenemic patients have very low erythrocyte sedimentation rates. When skin testing is performed for delayed hypersensitivity, there is no induration due to the lack of fibrin deposition.[40]

Hypofibrinogenemia is defined as a proportional decrease of both functional and immunoreactive fibrinogen. Coagulation tests depending on the formation of fibrin are variably prolonged, the most sensitive assay being the TT.

Dysfibrinogenemia is diagnosed by a discrepancy between clottable and immunoreactive fibrinogen. Only one defect, fibrinogen Oslo I, has been characterized by a shorter than normal thrombin time in plasma, and this defect results in a prothrombotic tendency. The reptilase time, which is based on clotting induced by fibrinopeptide A release, is often more prolonged than the thrombin time in patients with congenital dysfibrinogenemia. Unlike the thrombin time, the reptilase time is not prolonged by heparin. The gold standard for the diagnosis of dysfibrinogenemia is thus the characterization of the molecular defect, which however, is only available in specialized laboratories.

The congenital fibrinogen disorders must be differentiated from the acquired hypodysfibrinogenemias that occur in patients with liver disease or certain malignancies or in those taking drugs such as L-asparaginase. A rare cause of acquired hypofibrinogenemias that occur in neonates is due to a physiologic fibrinogen variant that results in delayed aggregation of fibrin multimers without causing a bleeding disorder. Acquired inhibitors of fibrin polymerization and fibrin stabilization have been described in patients with SLE, inflammatory bowel disease and following therapy with certain drugs, e.g. isoniazid.

Treatment

Therapy in patients with afibrinogenemia is given to achieve fibrinogen levels that are adequate for hemostasis and wound healing. FFP and cryoprecipitate have been used for replacement therapy. Each bag of cryoprecipitate contains 200-300 mg of fibrinogen. In adults, 10 bags of cryoprecipitate raise the circulating level of fibrinogen by 60-80 mg%; the recommended dose in children is 4 bags/10 kg body weight (to a maximum of 10 bags). Since the half-life of fibrinogen is about 3-4 days, replacement is needed only every other day. Fibrinogen concentrates prepared from large pools of human plasma are available in some countries and offer the advantage of specific virus inactivation during preparation. For this reason these preparations, if available, are preferred to nonvirus-inactivated FFP and cryoprecipitate as replacement therapy for patients with congenital deficiencies of fibrinogen. One commercially available product (fibrinogen concentrate [Human] vapor heated immune) is virus inactivated during preparation using a 2-step vapor-heat process. The manufacturers recommend that for hypofibrinogenemic patients with massive bleeding or who have undergone surgery or suffered major trauma that the fibrinogen concentration be increased to at least 100 mg/dl. This level should be maintained until complete wound healing has occurred, if necessary by periodic infusion of fibrinogen concentrate. Approximate initial dose to raise the fibrinogen concentration by 100 mg/dl in normal-weight adults is suggested to be 3000-4000 mg. The calculation of maintenance doses should rely on circulating fibrinogen levels obtained on a daily basis. In hypofibrinogenemic patients with lesser hemorrhagic risk, a minimum circulating fibrinogen concentration of 50 mg/dl may be adequate. In most cases minor bleeding may be managed by single infusions. The proposed single dose in adults is 1000 mg; in children 500 mg.

As the correlation between laboratory tests and clinical bleeding is poor for most of the dysfinrinogenemic defects. The individual patient's clinical history should be used to define the need for replacement therapy, taking into consideration the requirement of a basal fibrinogen level of approximately 50 mg/dl maintain hemostasis.

FACTOR XIII DEFICIENCY

Structure and Function

FXIII is also known as the fibrin stabilizing factor or transglutaminase (TGase), and it circulates in blood as a heterotetramer consisting of two catalytic A subunits (FXIII-A) and two noncatalytic B subunits (FXIII-B) A_2B_2.[41] The genes for FXIII-A and FXIII-B are localized to chromosomes 6p and 1q, respectively.

FXIII is a proenzyme converted to an active enzyme called FXIIIa by thrombin that is generated in the final stage of the blood coagulation cascade. FXIII plays an important role in hemostasis, wound healing, and maintenance of pregnancy. The enzyme promotes clot stability by forming covalent bonds between fibrin molecules and also by crosslinking fibrin with several proteins including α 2-plasmin inhibitor (α 2-PI) and fibronectin. These reactions lead to an increase in the mechanical strength, elasticity, and resistance to degradation by plasmin of fibrin clots, and promotion of wound healing by providing a scaffold for fibroblasts to proliferate and spread.

Classification of Factor XIII Deficiency

The normal range of Factor XIII in the plasma is 70-130%. Hence individuals with levels less than 70% are Factor XIII deficient. The disorder can be further subdivided into congenital and acquired types. The former is inherited in an autosomal recessive manner and is caused by defects in either the FXIII-A or FXIII-B gene.[42] However, heterozygotes of these deficiencies may manifest a mild bleeding tendency.[43,44]

The acquired form is caused by a secondary FXIII reduction mainly due to hyposynthesis and/or hyper-consumption through a primary disease, such as leukemia, myelodysplastic syndrome and liver diseases, disseminated intravascular coagulation (DIC), major surgery, or chronic inflammatory bowel diseases. FXIII deficiency can also be subclassified into hemorrhagic (symptomatic) and nonhemorrhagic (asymptomatic/laboratory) categories.

CONGENITAL FACTOR XIII DEFICIENCY

Most of the cases are secondary to a wide variety of mutations in Factor XIII-A subunit. More recently, it has been reported that FXIII-B deficiency is not uncommon, at least in the German white population.[44] The estimated prevalence is 1 in 2 milion population with 500 cases being described in literature so far.

Clinical Features

The homozygous state results in a moderate-to-severe hemorrhagic disorder. Bleeding from the umbilical stump and delayed and repeated bleeding from superficial wounds are common. Typically, a clot appears to form normally at the wound site which then breaks down 24 hours later and bleeding resumes. This cycle can be repeated many times. A similar scenario is often observed after dental extraction. FXIII-deficient patients also may experience soft tissue and joint hemorrhage after trauma but the spontaneous hemarthroses seen in hemophilia usually do not occur. The most serious form of bleeding is into the central nervous system, and FXIII-deficient patients have a high frequency of intracranial hemorrhage often resulting in death. Women with FXIII deficiency will abort spontaneously if they become pregnant. Full-term pregnancy can be achieved only if the patient is transfused throughout pregnancy. Some patients with FXIII deficiency are reported to have severe scar formation from superficial wounds, but this is not true of all cases.

Laboratory Features

In the homozygous state, the levels are <1% of functional FXIII activity. Heterozygotes are characterized by partially reduced levels of the A and B proteins; as a group they have approximately 50% of the A protein activity and about 80% the level of the B protein. A variant molecular form of FXIII has been described.

The screening test for FXIII deficiency is the solubility of the patient's recalicified plasma clot in urea or monochloracetic acid. An unambiguous diagnosis of the disorder among heterozygotes is usually possible with sensitive assays for FXIII and for the A and B protein. In the absence of an inhibitor to FXIII, there is a good correlation between FXIII activity and the immunochemical concentration of the a protein.

In acquired deficiency of FXIII, levels of approximately 50% of normal have generally been reported. Acquired inhibitors to FXIII are rare and can result in severe bleeding; reported cases have developed after prolonged therapy with certain drugs (isoniazid, phenytoin, penicillin and procainamide) or transfusions.

Treatment

The immediate goal of treatment is to stop bleeding by injecting FXIII products whenever possible. Good results have been reported with a placental concentrate of FXIII. A FXIII concentrate prepared from pools of human plasma is available (fibrinogammin P, Behringwerke, Marburg, Germany). The product is virus inactivated by pasteurization (heat treatment in aqueous solution of 60°C for 10 hours) and, if available, is preferred for FXIII deficiency. The lypohilized material is available in 4 and 20 ml doses containing not less than 250 and 1250 FXIII units, respectively. Preoperatively, it is recommended that adults receive 40 ml of FXIII intravenously with 8-12 ml on each of the following 5 days or until the wound has healed completely. In the case of severe hemorrhages and extensive hematomas the dose is 8-10 ml daily until bleeding has stopped. For prophylaxis of hemorrhages 8-12 ml should be infused at intervals of 4 weeks with the interval shortened if spontaneous hemorrhages develop. The product insert should always be consulted for specific treatment recommendations.

Treatment of FXIII deficiency is facilitated by the long half-life of FXIII (8-14 days) and by the observation that very low levels (approximately 1%) inhibit bleeding. Because of the risk of intracranial bleeding there is agreement that all injuries to the head should be treated and that children should be treated prophylatically because the probability of intracranial bleeding in children is high. Prophylatic therapy may also allow pregnant women successfully to carry fetuses to term. Dental extractions often lead to significant bleeding in FXIII-deficient patients; thus, prophylactic treatment is justified. The combination of FXIII replacement therapy and antifibrinolytic drugs (E-aminocaproic acid or tranexamic acid) has been used with success. Cryoprecipitate and FFP are other options for treatment of these patients but they contain only 1 u/ml and 3 u/ml of Factor XIII respectively.[45]

For individuals with acquired inhibitors to FXIII immune tolerance therapy may be tried. Corticosteroids are usually the first line of treatment followed by cyclophosphamide. In resistant cases, rituximab has also been tried.

ACQUIRED COAGULATION DISORDERS

Disseminated Intravascular Coagulation

Disseminated intravascular coagulation (DIC) is a relatively common problem, especially in the unwell neonate. The neonatal age group appears to be particularly susceptible. DIC always occurs as a secondary event, and a number of prenatal and neonatal problems are associated with this complication: birth asphyxia, acidosis, respiratory distress syndrome, infection, necrotizing entercolitis, meconium aspiration, aspiration of amniotic fluid, brain injury, hypothermia, giant hemangiomas, homozygous protein C/S deficiency, thrombosis, and malignancy. As in older children and adults, once established, DIC is often associated with increased mortality.

Although DIC is often regarded as a hemostatic problem, it is in fact complex systemic process involving activation and dysregulation of both coagulation and inflammatory processes. Clinically both bleeding and thrombotic problems may occur and microvascular thrombosis in particular contributes to multiorgan damage. Failure to regulate the coagulation process results in massive uncontrolled thrombin generation, with widespread fibrin deposition and consumption of coagulation proteins and platelets. DIC, particularly in the early stages, can be difficult to diagnose, and the clinical setting can be an important initial pointer. The condition is much more commonly observed in the sick neonate, who may have obvious sepsis or other complications such as necrotizing enterocolitis.

The laboratory diagnosis of DIC in older children and adults is usually based on a typical pattern of reduced platelets, prolonged coagulation variables (PT, APTT with or without TCT), reduced fibrinogen, and increased D-dimers (or other markers of fibrin or fibrinogen degradation). Although this pattern is likely to be present in a neonate with fulminating DIC, findings can vary, and a number of factors complicate the diagnosis during the neonatal period.

Thrombocytopenia can be an early manifestation of DIC, but is an extremely common hematological complication during the neonatal period, particularly in the neonatal intensive care units. Published studies suggest that thrombocytopenia develops in up to 22-35% of neonates admitted to the neonatal intensive care unit and is severe in 20%.[46] Until recently; thrombocytopenia was often attributed to the presence of a consumptive process, but it now seems more likely that many of these episodes of apparently self-limited thrombocytopenia relate to underproduction of platelets secondary to placental insufficiency. This contrasts with the development of profound, persistent thrombocytopenia a few days after delivery which is more likely to represent underlying DIC. Coagulation variables, at least initially, may be minimally deranged and there may be difficulties distinguishing what represents an abnormal result particularly in preterm infants. Similarly, there are no reliable normal ranges for D-dimers, and there is limited evidence to suggest that baseline concentrations may be higher during the neonatal period. In addition, fibrinogen concentrations normally increase slightly during the first few days of life and may initially be preserved. Early diagnosis of this condition is likely to be increasingly important in order to target management, and with this in mind scoring systems have been developed for use in adults, which may help to predict early nonovert DIC.

Treatment

As DIC is a secondary process, it follows that an important aspect of the management of this complication, i.e. prompt and effective treatment of the underlying cause. Although this is logical, once DIC is well established, it may be difficult to switch off the processes involved.

Evidence based guidelines for other specific treatment modalities are lacking, which relects the abence of recent randomoized controlled trails in this age group. There is considerable interest in the use of activated protein C which has been shown to be of benefit in sepsis associated DIC in adults, but there is only limited information on the use of this agent in the neonatal period.

Much of the management of DIC thus continues to centre on the use of supportive treatment with fresh frozen plasma, cryoprecipitate, and platelets to try to maintain adequate hemostasis. Although the use of blood products and the thresholds set for transfusion are largely empirical, it would appear reasonable to institute replacement therapy, particularly where there is an increased risk of bleeding, guidelines for the transfusion of platelets suggest that platelet count should be maintained above 50 × 10/L by the transfusion of platelet concentrates (10-15 ml/kg). Fresh frozen plasma (10-15 ml/kg) can be used to replaced hemostatic proteins, although cryoprecipitate (5-15 ml/kg) is a better source of fibrinogen, which should be kept above 1 g/L.

Heparin administration has been tried in a few cases and has shown beneficial effect especially in neonates with coagulopathy secondary to indwelling vascular catheters. However, anticoagulation of patients with DIC by administration of heparin depends heavily on plasma antithrombin levels, which can be depleted in advanced DIC by consumption.[47] This is reflected in a report on 10 newborns with DIC, in whom, after initial failure of isolated heparin therapy, fast improvement of DIC was observed after normalization of antithrombin plasma levels.[48] The increased risk of bleeding in neonates, however, precludes more widespread use of this agent.

VITAMIN K DEFICIENCY BLEEDING

Vitamin K deficiency bleeding (VKDB) refers to bleeding that occurs as a consequence of vitamin K deficiency during the first six months of life. Previously known as hemorrhagic disease of the newborn, it was renamed to emphasize that bleeding problems during the neonatal period are not confined to those arising from vitamin K deficiency and that bleeding secondary to vitamin K deficiency may occur beyond the first month of life. Concentrations of the vitamin K-dependent factors (FII, FVII, FIX and FX) are reduced in the newborn period and are functionally inactive in the absence of vitamin K.

Vitamin K deficiency bleeding (VKDB) has traditionally been classified as early, classical, and late depending on the timing of the presentation. This classification reflects the differing risk factors associated with this condition. Early VKDB is typically associated with antenatal ingestion of drugs which interfere with vitamin K metabolism, whereas classical and late forms are associated with breast feeding, malaborption and liver disease. Bleeding manifestations are variable, but there is a relatively high incidence of intracranial hemorrhage, particularly in late VKDB, which is associated with considerable morbidity and mortality.

The diagnosis of vitamin K deficiency may be suspected from the results of coagulation screening where initially there is isolated prolongation of the prothrombin time, followed by prolongation of the APTT, in association with a normal fibrinogen concentration and a normal platelet count. Confirmation of the diagnosis requires measurement of the specific vitamin K-dependent factors (II, VII, IX, X) which are corrected by the administration of vitamin K.

Once the diagnosis is confirmed, intravenous vitamin K should be administered to correct the existing deficiency. In suspected cases, vitamin K can be given while factor concentrations are pending, in the presence major bleeding, factor replacement therapy may also be required with fresh frozen plasma, prohrombin complex concentrate (FII, FIX, FX) or a four factor concentrate containing all the vitamin K-dependent factors.

Optimal methods for the prevention of VKBD have been the subject of considerable debate in recent years and remain to be fully resolved; it is generally accepted that although single intramuscular dose of vitamin K administered after birth will prevent both classical and late VKBD a single oral dose will not protect all infants against late VKDB. The safety of intramuscular vitamin K was questioned some years ago, and although the results of this study have not been confirmed, many centers have preferred to use an oral dosing schedule for prophylaxis, the optimal formulation and dosing regimen for oral vitamin K prophyaxis remains to be defined, but it is clear that regimens consisting of multiple doses are more effective; particularly for breast fed infants. Recent data have also shown that oral administration of mixed micellar vitamin K is not superior to older vitamin K preparations.

CONCLUSION

A number of different coagulation disorders may manifest with bleeding problems during the neonatal period, early recognition of abnormal bleeding together with careful use of appropriate diagnostic investigations and recognition of those features unique to the neonatal hemostatic system should facilitate prompt diagnosis and appropriate management for these infants.

REFERENCES

1. Mann KG. Thromb Haemost. 1999;82:165-74.
2. Skogen B, Husebekk A, Killie MK, Kjeldsen-Kragh J. Neonatal alloimmune thrombocytopenia is not what it was: a lesson learned from large prospective screening intervention program. Scand J Immunol. 2009;70:531-4.
3. Hancock JF, Wieland K, Pugh RE, et al. A molecular genetic study of factor XI deficiency. Blood. 1991;77:1942-8.
4. Motta M, Tincani A, Lojacono A, et al. Neonatal outcome in patients with rheumatic disease. Lupus. 2004;13:718-23.
5. Hall GW. Kasabach-Merritt syndrome: pathogenesis and management. Br J Haematol. 2001;112:851-62.
6. Ljung RC. Intracranial haemorrhage in haemophilia A and B. Br J Haematol. 2008;140:378-84.
7. Smith AR, Leonard N, Kurth MH. Intracranial hemorrhage in newborns with hemophilia: the role of screening radiologic studies in the rst 7 days of life. J Pediatr Hematol Oncol. 2008;30:81-4.
8. Nelson MD Jr, Maeder MA, Usner D, et al. Prevalence and incidence of intracranial haemonhage in a population of children with haemophilia. The Haemophilia Growth and Development Study. Haemophilia. 1999;5:306-12.
9. Chalmers EA, Brown SA, Keeling D, et al. Early factor VIII exposure and subsequent inhibitor development in children with severe haemophilia A. Haemophilia. 2007;13:149-55.
10. Gouw SC, van der Bom JG, Marijke van den Berg H. Treatment-related risk factors of inhibitor development in previously untreated patients with hemophilia A: the CANAL cohort study. Blood. 2007;109:4648-54.
11. Andrew M, Schmidt B, Mitchell L, et al. Thrombin generation in newborn plasma is critically dependant on the concentration of prothrombin. Thromb Haemost. 1990; 63:27–30.
12. Citarella F, Tripodi M, Fantoni A, et al. Assignment of human coagulation factor XII (fXII) to chromosome 5 by cDNA hybridization to DNA from somatic cell hybrids. Hum Genet. 1988;80(4):397-8.
13. Rocha E, Silva M, Beraldo WT, et al. Bradykinin, a hypotensive and smooth muscle stimulating factor released from plasma globulin by snake venoms and by trypsin. Am J Physiol. 1949;156:261-73.
14. Ghebrehiwet B, Silverberg M, Kaplan AP. Activation of the classic pathway of complement by Hageman factor fragment. J Exp Med. 1981;153:665-76.
15. DiScipio RG. The activation of the alternative pathway C3 convertase by human plasma kallikrein. Immunol. 1982; 45:587-95.
16. Spronk H, Heemskerk JW, Ten Cate H, et al. Feedback activation of factor XI by thombin is essential for haemostasis *in vivo*. J Thromb Haemost. 2009;7(s2):1-316.
17. Rosenthal RL, Dreskin OH, Rosenthal N. New hemophilia-like disease caused by deficiency of a third plasma thromboplastin factor. Proc Soc Exp Biol Med. 1953;82: 171-4.
18. Peyvandi F, Lak M, Mannucci PM. Factor XI deficiency in Iranians: its clinical manifestations in comparison with those of classic hemophilia. Haematologica. 2002;87:512-4.
19. Kravtsov DV, Wu W, Meijers JC, et al. Dominant factor XI deficiency caused by mutations in the factor XI catalytic domain. Blood. 2004;104:128-34.
20. Kravtsov DV, Monahan PE, Gailani D. A classification system for cross-reactive material-negative factor XI deficiency. Blood. 2005;105:4671-73.
21. Bouma BN, Meijers JC. Role of blood coagulation factor XI in downregulation of fibrinolysis. Curr Opin Hematol. 2000; 7:266-72.
22. Mannucci PM, Duga S, Peyvandi F. Recessively inherited coagulation disorders. Blood. 2004;104:1243-52.
23. Peyvandi F, Mannucci PM, Lak M, et al. Congenital factor X deficiency: spectrum of bleeding symptoms in 32 Iranian patients. Br J Haematol. 1998;102:626-8.
24. Owren PA. Parahaemophilia; haemorrhagic diathesis due to absence of a previously unknown clotting factor. Lancet. 1947;1(6449):446-8.
25. Mann KG, Kalafatis M. Factor V: a combination of Dr Jekyll and Mr. Hyde. Blood. 2002;101:20-30.
26. Zhang B, Spreafico M, Zheng C, et al. Genotype-phenotype correlation in combined deficiency of factor V and factor VIII. Blood. 2008;111:5592-600.
27. Girolami A, Scarano L, Saggiorato G, et al. Congenital deficiencies and abnormalities of prothrombin. Blood Coagul Fibrinolysis. 1998;9:557-69.
28. Klaus C, Plaimauer B, Studt JD, et al. Epitope mapping of ADAMTS13 autoantibodies in acquired thrombotic thrombocytopenic purpura. Blood. 2004;103:4514-9.
29. Peyvandi F, Cattaneo M, Inbal A, et al. Rare bleeding disorders. Haemophilia. 2008;14(Suppl 3):202-10.
30. Mosesson MW. Fibrinogen and fibrin structure and functions. J Thromb Haemost. 2005;3:1894-904.
31. Gill FM, Shapiro SS, Schwartz E. Severe congenital hypoprothrombinemia. J Pediatr. 1978;93:264-6.
32. O'Marcaigh AS, Nichols WL, Hassinger NL, et al. Genetic analysis and functional characterization of prothrombins Corpus Christi (Arg382-Cys), Dhahran (Arg271-His), and hypoprothrombinemia. Blood. 1996;88:2611-8.
33. Lak M, Keihani M, Elahi F, et al. Bleeding and thrombosis in 55 patients with inherited afibrinogenaemia. Br J Haematol. 1999;107:204-6.
34. Acharya SS, Coughlin A, Dimichele D. North American Rare Bleeding Disorder Study Group. Rare Bleeding Disorder Registry: deficiencies of factors II, V, VII, X, XIII, fibrinogen and dysfibrinogenemias. J Thromb Haemost. 2004;2:248-56.
35. Peyvandi F, Kaufman RJ, Seligsohn U, et al. Rare bleeding disorders. Haemophilia. 2006;12(Suppl 3):137-42.
36. Ehmann WC, al-Mondhiry H. Congenital afibrinogenemia and splenic rupture. Am J Med. 1994;96:92-4.

37. Haverkate F, Samama M. Familial dysfibrinogenemia and thrombophilia. Report on a study of the SSC Subcommittee on Fibrinogen. Thromb Haemost. 1995;73:151-61.
38. Hayes T. Dysfibrinogenemia and thrombosis. Arch Pathol Lab Med. 2002;126:1387-90.
39. Dupuy E, Soria C, Molho P, et al. Embolized ischemic lesions of toes in an afibrinogenemic patient: possible relevance to *in vivo* circulating thrombin. Thromb Res 2001;102:211-9.
40. Colvin RB, Mosesson MW, Dvorak HF. Delayed-type hypersensitivity skin reactions in congenital afibrinogenemia lack fibrin deposition and induration. J Clin Invest. 1979;63:1302-6.
41. Ichinose A. Extracellular transglutaminase: factor XIII. Prog Exp Tumor Res. 2005;38:192-208.
42. Ichinose A, Asahina T, Kobayashi T. Congenital blood coagulation factor XIII deficiency and perinatal management. Curr Drug Targets. 2005;6(5):541-54.
43. Seitz R, Duckert F, Lopaciuk S, et al. Study Group ETRO Working Party on Factor XIII questionnaire on congenital factor XIII deficiency in Europe: status and perspectives. Semin Thromb Hemost. 1996;22(5):415-8.
44. Ivaskevicius V, Biswas A, Loreth R, et al. Mutations affecting disulphide bonds contribute to a fairly common prevalence of F13B gene defects: results of a genetic study in 14 families with factor XIII B deficiency. Haemophilia. 2010;16(4):675-82.
45. Caudill JS, Nichols WL, Plumhoff EA, et al. Comparison of coagulation factor XIII content and concentration in cryoprecipitate and fresh-frozen plasma. Transfusion. 2009; 49(4):765-70.
46. Mehta P, Vasa R, Neumann L, Karpatkin M. Thrombocytopenia in high-risk infant. J Pediatr. 1980;97(5):791-4.
47. Blauhut B, Necek S, Kramar H, et al. Activity of antithrombin III and effect of heparin on coagulation in shock. Thromb Res. 1980;19(6):775-82.
48. von Kries R, Stannigel H, Go¨bel U. Anticoagulant therapy by continuous heparin-antithrombin III infusion in newborns with disseminated intravascular coagulation. Eur J Pediatr. 1985;144(2):191-4.

14 von Willebrand's Disease

Neha Rastogi, Vinita Jain, SP Yadav, Anupam Sachdeva

The most common inherited bleeding disorder in humans is von Willebrand's disease. It was originally described by Erik von Willebrand in 1926. It is caused by a deficiency, dysfunction or complete absence of von Willebrand's factor (vWF).

von Willebrand's factor is a large multimeric glycoprotein that is synthesized in megakaryocytes and endothelial cells as pre-pro-vWF. Sequential cleavage releases mature vWF which undergoes multimerization and is stored in specific cellular storage granules such as the Weibel-Palade body in endothelial cells and α-granules in platelets. It is present in normal amounts in plasma and levels can be significantly increased by administering drugs such as desmopressin (DDAVP) that induce the release of vWF from storage sites into plasma. von Willebrand's factor has two main functions in hemostasis. It is essential for platelet-plug formation as an adhesion protein that diverts circulating platelets to the sites of vascular injury, particularly through larger multimers, and it forms a noncovalent complex with coagulation factor VIII in plasma, thereby protecting it from inactivation and clearance.

The gene that encodes vWF is located on the short arm of chromosome 12. The vWF gene is a large and complex locus encompassing 175 kb of deoxyribonucleic acid (DNA) and comprising 52 exons. Most cases of types 1, 2A, 2B and 2M disease represent autosomal dominant conditions with type 1 disease exhibiting incomplete phenotypic penetrance and variable expression. In contrast, types 2N and 3 vWD are autosomal recessive conditions.

CLINICAL PRESENTATION

Patients of vWD usually have symptoms of mucocutaneous bleeding like excessive bruising, epistaxis, menorrhagia and postoperative hemorrhage, particularly after mucosal surgery, such as tonsillectomy or wisdom tooth extraction.

Menorrhagia is a common presentation but since menstrual history of a girl is evaluated in context of other family members, sometimes it is missed as other members in the family may also be affected by same disorder.

Since vWF is an acute phase reactant, its level increases in stress and that's the reason why patients of vWD do not bleed with surgeries that incur major stress as appendicectomy and child birth but may bleed during cosmetic and mucosal surgery. Levels of vWF vary with blood type (type O <A <B <AB), which can confound the clinical diagnosis of vWD.

vWD type 1 patients (10-80% of cases vWD) have very mild to moderate symptoms. In type 2, mucosal bleeding is frequent but soft-tissue bleeding is rare. Type 3 has more severe symptoms, joint bleeds, muscle hematomas, postoperative and postpartum bleeds.

LABORATORY DIAGNOSIS AND MONITORING (TABLE 14.1)

Ideally, a simple, single laboratory test could screen for the presence of vWD. Such a screening test would need to be sensitive to the presence of most types of vWD and would have a low false positive rate. However, no such test is available.

a. *Initial hemostatic laboratory evaluation:* An initial hemostatic laboratory evaluation usually includes (i) a platelet count and complete blood cell count; (ii) partial thromboplastin time (PTT); (iii) prothrombin time; (iv) and optionally either a fibrinogen level or a thrombin time.

   Historically patients with vWD were described to have a long BT and a long PTT, these findings are frequently normal in type 1 vWD. This testing neither rules in nor rules out vWD, but it can suggest whether coagulation factor deficiency or thrombocytopenia might be the potential cause of clinical bleeding.

Table 14.1: Laboratory findings in the various types of vWD

	1	*3*	*2A*	*2B*	*2M*	*2N*
vWF:Ag	↓	↓↓↓	↓	↓	↓	↴
vWF:RCo	↓	↓↓↓	↓↓	↓↓	↓↓	↴
FVIII:C	↴	0.05-0.1	↴	↴	↴	0.1-0.4
VWF:RCo/VWF:Ag ratio	>0.6	—	<0.6	<0.6	<0.6	>0.6
Multimers	N	—	Abn	Abn	N	N
RIPA	N	—	↓	↑	↓	N

b. The PFA-100 (platelet function analyzer) test result has been demonstrated to be abnormal in the majority of persons with vWD, other than those with type 2N, but its use for population screening for vWD has not been established. Persons with severe type 1 vWD or type 3 vWD usually have abnormal PFA-100 values, whereas persons with mild or moderate type 1 vWD and some with type 2 vWD may not have abnormal results.

c *vWF:Ag assay:* vWF:Ag is an immunoassay that measures the concentration of vWF protein in plasma. Commonly used methods are based on enzyme-linked immunosorbent assay (ELISA) or automated latex immunoassay (LIA).

d *vWF:RCo assay:* vWF:RCo is a functional assay of vWF that measures its ability to interact with normal platelets. The antibiotic ristocetin causes vWF to bind to platelets, resulting in platelet clumps and their removal from the circulation. Several methods are used to assess the platelet agglutination and aggregation that result from the binding of vWF to platelet GPIb induced by ristocetin (vWF:RCo). The methods include (1) time to visible platelet clumping using ristocetin, washed normal platelets (fresh or formalinized) and dilutions of patient plasma; (2) slope of aggregation during platelet aggregometry using ristocetin, washed normal platelets and dilutions of the person's plasma; (3) automated turbidometric tests that detect platelet clumping, using the same reagents noted above; (4) ELISA's that assess direct binding of the person's plasma vWF to platelet GPIb. The vWF:RCo assay has high intralaboratory and interlaboratory variation, and it does not actually measure physiological function.

e. Ristocetin induced platelet agglutination: The other test that utilizes ristocetin is the ristocetin-induced platelet agglutination (RIPA) assay that evaluates the sensitivity of a patient's platelets to low-dose ristocetin. This test is especially useful in identifying individuals with type 2B vWD in whom the platelet membranes are 'overloaded' with the high-affinity mutant vWF resulting in increased sensitivity to ristocetin concentrations below 0.6 mg/ml. Low-dose RIPA is carried out in platelet-rich plasma, using a low concentration of ristocetin. This low concentration of ristocetin does not cause vWF binding and aggregation of platelets in samples from normal persons, but it does cause vWF binding and aggregation of platelets in samples from patients with either type 2B vWD or mutations in the platelet vWF receptor. The latter defects have been termed pseudo-vWD or PLT-vWD, and they can be differentiated from type 2B vWD by vWF:PB assay. At higher concentrations of ristocetin (1.1–1.3 mg ml), RIPA is reduced in persons with type 3 vWD. However, the test is not sufficiently sensitive to reliably diagnose other types of vWD.

f. *vWF:PB assay:* The vWF:PB assay measures the binding of vWF to normal paraformaldehyde-fixed platelets using low concentrations of ristocetin. Both type 2B vWD and PLT-vWD have agglutination of platelet-rich plasma to low-dose ristocetin, but the vWF:PB assay can differentiate type 2B vWD from PLT-vWD. Only vWF from persons with type 2B vWD has increased vWF:PB, while vWF from persons with PLT-vWD has normal vWF:PB with low doses of ristocetin.

g. *vWF collagen-binding assay:* The vWF collagen binding (vWF:CB) assay measures binding of vWF to collagen. Patients who have defects in collagen binding may have a normal vWF:RCo and thus escape clinical diagnosis unless a vWF:CB assay is performed.

h. *vWF FVIII-binding assay:* The vWF FVIII-binding (vWF:FVIIIB) assay measures the ability of a person's vWF to bind added exogenous FVIII and is used to diagnose type 2N vWD.

i. *FVIII assay:* FVIII coagulant assay is a measure of the cofactor function of the clotting factor, FVIII, in plasma. In the context of vWD, FVIII activity measures the ability of vWF to bind and maintain the level of FVIII in the circulation.

j. *vWF multimer analysis:* The vWF multimer test is usually performed after the initial vWD testing indicates an abnormality. vWF multimer analysis is a qualitative assay that depicts the variable concentrations of the different-sized vWF multimers by using sodium dodecyl sulfate-protein electrophoresis followed by detection of the vWF multimers in the gel, using a radio-labeled polyclonal antibody or a combination of monoclonal antibodies. Alternatively, the protein is transferred to a membrane (Western blot), and the multimers are identified by immunofluorescence or other staining techniques.

k. *Ratio of vWF:RCo to vWF:Ag:* The vWF:RCo/vWF:Ag ratio can aid in the diagnosis of types 2A, 2B and 2M vWD and help differentiate them from type 1 vWD. For example, a vWF:RCo/vWF:Ag ratio of <0.6 has been used as a criterion for dysfunctional vWF.

l. *DNA sequencing analysis:* DNA sequencing of patient DNA has been used to make a molecular diagnosis of variants of type 2 vWD. In the common forms of type 2A vWD, in which the vWF is spontaneously cleaved by ADAMTS13, mutations cluster in the A2 domain (which contains the cleavage site). In the less common type 2A variants of vWD, in which multimer formation is inhibited, the mutations may be scattered throughout the gene. In most persons with type 1 vWD, the genetic mutations have not been established, although several studies are under way to characterize these mutations.

m. Special considerations for laboratory diagnosis of vWD. Repeated laboratory testing. Repeated testing for vWD is sometimes needed to identify low levels of vWF. Stress including surgery, exercise, anxiety, crying in a frightened child, as well as systemic inflammation, pregnancy or administration of estrogen or oral contraceptives—can increase plasma levels of vWF and mask lower baseline values. vWF levels vary with the menstrual cycle, and lowest values are detected on days 1-4 of the menstrual cycle. As noted above, anxiety may falsely elevate the vWF and FVIII levels, and the setting for phlebotomy should be as calm as possible. If a person has polycythemia or profound anemia, the amount of anticoagulant should be adjusted on the basis of nomograms designed for this purpose.

ABO blood type: Individuals who have blood type O have concentrations approximately 25% lower than persons who have other ABO blood types.

VON WILLEBRAND'S DISEASE CLASSIFICATION (TABLE 14.2)

The vWD subcommittee of the Scientific and Standardization Committee of the International Society of Thrombosis and Hemostasis proposed the currently accepted classification of vWD in 1994. This involves three major categories.

Type 1 von Willebrand's Disease

While this is clearly the most common form of the disease, it is also the most problematic to diagnose with certainty. Plasma levels of vWF (both vWF:Ag and vWF:RCo) and FVIII can range from about 0.05 to 0.45 units/ml in this condition. Recent attempts to clarify the diagnosis of this condition have focused on three factors:

- A personal history of excessive mucocutaneous bleeding
- Evidence of a family history of the condition
- Laboratory demonstration of vWF deficiency.

Table 14.2: Types of von Willebrand and their frequency

Type	*Description*	*Frequency of cases*
1	Partial quantitative deficiency of vWF	70-80%
2	Quantitative deficiency of vWF	15-20%
2A	Decreased platelet dependent vWF function with lack of LMWM*	10-20%
2B	Increased platelet dependent vWF function with lack of HMWM*	3-5%
2M	Decreased platelet dependent vWF function with normal multimeric structure	1-2%
2N	Decreased vWF affinity for FVIII	1-2%
3	Complete deficiency of vWF	1-3%

Abbreviations: LMWM: Low molecular weight multimers; HMWM: High molecular weight multimers

Patients with type 1 vWD exhibit an increase in mucocutaneous bleeding. The most common features are nosebleeds, easy bruising, bleeding from trivial cuts and excessive menstrual bleeding. Prolonged and delayed-onset bleeding following tooth extractions and oral surgery is also a common feature. Bleeding into soft tissues and joints does not occur unless provoked by trauma.

Type 3 von Willebrand's Disease

Unlike most other forms of the disease (aside from type 2N), the inheritance pattern of type 3 disease best fits that of a recessive condition Manifestations are severe, joint and soft tissue bleeds seen. In the laboratory, this condition is characterized by prolongation of the activated partial thromboplastin time (APTI) and bleeding time, undetectable levels of vWF:Ag and vWF:RCo, and FVIII levels <0.10 u/ml.

Type 2 von Willebrand's Disease

Type 2A

Type 2A disease is characterized by the presence of vWF that lacks the large- and intermediate-sized multimers of the protein. This defect appears to result from either an inherent inability to form the higher molecular-weight multimers (Group I mutations) or the synthesis of multimers that are more susceptible to ADAMTS13-mediated proteolysis (Group II mutations) type 2A disease can initially be suspected from a disproportionately low vWF:RCo level relative to the vWF:Ag (ratio <0.6). The FVIII level may be low or normal.

Type 2B

In this condition, the mutant form of vWF binds with greater affinity to the GPIb receptor on platelets, resulting in the selective depletion from the plasma of the highest multimeric forms of vWF. As with type 2A disease, in patients with type 2B vWD the vWF:RCo will likely be disproportionately low relative to the vWF:Ag, but with this subtype there is increased sensitivity to low-dose ristocetin-induced platelet agglutination.

A disorder known as platelet-type vWD (PT-vWD) exhibits identical clinical and laboratory features to those of type 2B vWD.

Type 2M

This type 2 variant form of vWD is characterized by the same disproportionate reduction in vWF:RCo levels relative to vWF:Ag seen in type 2A and 2B disease, but in type 2M vWD the plasma and platelet multimers are normal and ristocetin induced platelet agglutination is reduced.

Type 2N

This vWD subtype has low plasma FVIII level. Unlike the other type 2 forms of vWD, type 2N vWD exhibits a recessive mode of inheritance. Type 2N disease has been described as an autosomal form of hemophilia.

Acquired vWD Type 3

This is seen in lymphoma, myeloproliferative disorders, hypothyroidism, wilms tumor, hepatoma, systemic lupus erythematosis, congenital cardiac defects (VSD, ASD, aortic stenosis), cyanotic heart disease, ITP platelets, pernicious anemia, EBV, HbE—thal, scurvy, uremia TB, and drugs: Ciprofloxacin (transient vWD), and type 1 vWD occurs in 67% of children with seizure disorders treated with valproate.

Management of vWD

1. Desmopressin/DDAVP
2. High purity FVIII/vWF concentrate
3. DDAVP and IL-11
4. Cryoprecipitate
5. Fresh frozen plasma (FFP).

Desmopressin (a Vasopressin Analog)/DDAVP

In vWD, desmopressin, in a dose of 0.3 μg/kg IV induces a rise in FVIII and vWF of 3 to 5 times the basal value in 30 minutes and is sustained for 8 to 10 hours. This response is consistent for any child on different occasions. DDAVP can be given subcutaneously (0.03 μg/kg) or intranasally, 1 spray (150 μg for children).

It may cause headache and flushing, which is mild and transient. DDAVP is effective in vWD type 1 and ineffective in types 2A, 2M, 2N and 3 and may be contraindicated in type 2B because platelets are transiently decreased.

Blood Component Therapy

Treatment of vWD with blood component transfusion is required for major dental and surgical procedures, following trauma and to treat life threatening bleeding. Cryoprecipitate, the standard component used for vWD therapy during the 1970s and 1980s, is no longer the material of choice. The blood components currently used are plasma-derived, intermediate-purity FVIII concentrates that have undergone a variety of viral inactivation steps to prevent viral infection. The latest high-purity and ultra-high-purity FVIII concentrates, such as the monoclonal purified concentrates and recombinant FVIII, have a very low vWF content and are not useful in this context.

Finally, there have been successful preclinical trials of recombinant vWF and interleukin-11 preparations, but at this stage it is too early to assess the relative advantages and likely clinical application of these compounds.

Drugs to be Avoided

1. ASA, ibuprofen, antihistamines
2. Antiplatelet agents—Dipyridamole, ticlopidine
3. Antimicrobials—High dose penicillin, cephalosporin nitrofurantoin, hydroxychloroquine
4. Cardiovascular drugs—Propranolol, furosemide, Ca^{+} channel blocker, quinidine
5. Caffeine, tricyclic antidepressants, phenothiazines, valproate, heparin.

BIBLIOGRAPHY

1. David Lillicrap. von Willebrand's disease. In: Robert J Arceci, Ian M Hann, Owen P Smith (Eds). Pediatric Hematology, 3rd edn. Blackwell Publishing; pp. 598-607.
2. Mannucci PM, Chediak J, Hanna W, Byrnes J, Ledford M, Ewenstein BM, et al. Alphanate Study Group. Treatment of von Willebrand's disease with a high-purity factor VIII/ von Willebrand's factor concentrate: a prospective, multicenter study. Blood. 2002;99(2):450-6.
3. Mannucci PM. Treatment of von Willebrand's disease. N Engl J Med. 2004;351(7):683-94.
4. Nichols WL, Hultin MB, James AH, Manco-Johnson MJ, Montgomery RR, Ortel TL, et al. von Willebrand's disease (VWD): evidence-based diagnosis and management guidelines, the National Heart, Lung, and Blood Institute (NHLBI) Expert Panel report (USA). Haemophilia. 2008; 14(2):171-232.
5. Rodeghiero F, Castaman G, Tosetto A. How I treat von Willebrand's disease. Blood. 2009;114(6):1158-65.
6. Ruggeri ZM, Zimmerman TS. von Willebrand's factor and von Willebrand's disease. Blood. 1987;70(4):895-904.
7. Sadler JE. von Willebrand's disease type 1: a diagnosis in search of a disease. Blood. 2003;101(6):2089-93.

15 Management of Hemophilia

Vikram Mathews

INTRODUCTION

Hemophilia is a hereditary disorder of coagulation that results in deficiency of factor VIII (Hemophilia A) or factor IX (Hemophilia B). The disorder has an X-linked inheritance and as a result is almost exclusively seen in males.

It is characterized by recurrent spontaneous and post-traumatic bleeds usually into the joints and muscles. Recurrent bleeds into joints can lead to severe joint deformities. Mucocutaneous bleeds are rare but can occur.

Hemophilia can be classified as mild, moderate or severe depending on the factor assay:

Severe	<1%
Moderate	1-5%
Mild	6-30%

Management guidelines laid down for the developed country are often not feasible in our set-up. Significant improvisation is required within our system to accommodate for the various socioeconomic backgrounds of our patients, in an effort to offer the most cost effective therapy. Recommendations of factor support and duration of factor support for various conditions in this article varies from those laid down in international publications.

Table 15.1 summarizes some of the standard international recommendations for common acute bleeding episodes. Recommendations in this article are based on the HFI guidelines laid down for our country. Management of patients with hemophilia can be considered under the following headings:

- Products for replacement therapy
- Nonfactor pharmacological agents
- Management of acute bleeds
- Management of chronic complications
- Physical therapy and rehabilitation
- Surgical management
- Management of patients with inhibitors
- Carrier detection and antenatal diagnosis
- Recent advances.

PRODUCTS FOR REPLACEMENT THERAPY

Essential to the management of patients with hemophilia is replacement of appropriate factors. Factor replacement can be from a number of sources.

1. Wet products, e.g. fresh frozen plasma, cryoprecipitate, cryosupernatant, fresh blood
2. Factor concentrates, e.g. intermediate purity, high purity, recombinant.

Risk of transmission of viral infections is highest with blood bank products and lowest with recombinant factor concentrates. Ideally all replacement products used today should be recombinant factor concentrates only in reality this is not practical for financial constraints.

Dosage calculation is based on the principle that for:

FVIII 1 u/kg raises the factor level by 2%
FIX 1 u/kg raises the factor level by 1%

From this observation the following formula can be used to calculate the dose of factor concentrate required to achieve a certain target factor level.

FVIII dose (IU/kg) = ½ × rise in FVIII required (IU/dl)

FIX dose (IU/kg) = 1 × rise in FIX required (IU/dl)

Table 15.1: International guidelines for the management of common acute bleeding presentations (Hemophilia. 1995;1 (Suppl): 8-13)

Bleeding site	*Optimal factor level*	*Duration*
Hemarthrosis	30-50%	1-2 days
Muscle hematomas	30-50%	1-2 days
GIT bleed	30-50%	2-3 days
Intracranial bleed	60-80%	7-10 days
Hematuria	30-50%	1-2 days

NONFACTOR PHARMACOLOGICAL AGENTS

1. *Antifibrinolytic agents,* e.g. cyclocapron, tranexamic acid. These are useful in the management of mucosal bleeds. They may also be beneficial in central nervous system bleeds. They are not useful in the management of serosal bleeds and in the management of hemarthrosis. An absolute contraindication to their use is the presence of hematuria.
2. *Desmopressin (DDAVP):* The mechanism of action is by increasing the release of stored factor VIII from endothelial cells. It is useful in the management of mild and moderate hemophilia. It has no role in the management of severe hemophilia. Response to DDAVP is very variable with a 2–10 fold increase in factor levels and before using it as prophylaxis for a surgical procedure, a trial should be given prior to the procedure and an adequate response is documented.
3. *Fibrin sealant:* These are available commercially and can also be manufactured in house. It mimics the final common pathway of coagulation with application of thrombin to a source of fibrinogen on the surface of the wound to form a fibrin plug. It is useful as an adjunct in certain surgical situations, for dental extraction and for circumcision.

MANAGEMENT OF ACUTE BLEEDS

Common to the management of acute bleeding episodes in patients with hemophilia is replacement of the appropriate factor, additional red cell infusion if indicated and other nonfactor replacement measures to control the bleed. The quantity and duration of factor replacement will depend on the site and severity of the bleed.

Common sites of bleeding include joints, muscles, soft tissue, epistaxis and gum bleeds. Bleeding can also occur though less commonly in the central nervous system (CNS), gastrointestinal (GIT) and genitourinary (GUT) tract. Some common presentations and their management is addressed below.

Acute Hemarthrosis

It accounts for 70-80% of bleeding episodes in patients with hemophilia. Majority of hemarthrosis are noted in the knee joints and more than 90% of joint bleeds occur in the knee, elbow and ankle joints. Patients usually present with severe pain, limitation of joint movement, swelling and tenderness. Management involves factor replacement of 10-20% levels as early as possible with 1-2 additional doses after 12-24 hours if required. Additional measures include cold compresses with ice packs, analgesics (avoid aspirin and NSAID) and rest to the affected limb. It is very important to stress the importance of restarting physiotherapy as soon as the pain has settled. The practice of aspirating the joint is best avoided.

Muscle and Soft Tissue Bleeds

It usually involves large flexor groups of muscles, a common site is the iliopsoas muscle. For iliopsoas bleeds a factor replacement schedule as follows can be used:

	FVIII	FIX		
Immediate	20%	15%		
Day 1	10% bd	10%	×	2-3 days

All patients with iliopsoas bleeds can potentially be large volume bleeds and could result in hemodynamic compromise. The hemoglobin should be checked at admission, monitored serially and blood transfused if required. Under factor cover traction can be initiated if tolerated at the earliest. Appropriate analgesic should be administered.

Management of other muscle and soft tissue bleeds can be managed as per the guidelines used for managing an acute hemarthrosis. If there is evidence of a compartment syndrome as can occur with forearm and gastrocnemius bleeds, then an emergency surgical decompression may be required.

Gum/Oral Mucosal Bleeds

Minor oral mucosal bleeds can be managed with local application of antifibrinolytic agents alone. More severe bleeds may require factor concentrates (10-20% levels for 2–3 days) along with antifibrinolytic agents. A local etiology for the bleeding should be evaluated for and treated appropriately if found. Importance of good oral hygiene should be stressed, especially regular (2-3 times/day) use of a soft toothbrush.

Epistaxis

It usually occurs from the Little's area, often post-traumatic though it can occur spontaneously. The patient is made to sit up and firm pressure applied to both nostrils with two ice cubes wrapped in a cloth or a gauze piece for 5-15 minutes. Local anti-fibrinolytic agent is also helpful. If bleeding persists, an anterior nasal pack, factor concentrates (20–30% for 1–2 days) along with anti fibrinolytic agents may be required.

Gastrointestinal Bleed

It will require factor concentrate support urgently to achieve 20-40% levels. Priority should be given to establish the etiology (endoscopy, angiogram, etc.) of the bleed and appropriate treatment measures instituted. Factor support may need to be continued for 2–3 days.

Hematuria

It is an uncommon presentation in a hemophiliac but can occur both spontaneously and following a trauma, most often it is due to a local lesion. If mild with no significant drop in hemoglobin, then adequate hydration for 2-5 days may be adequate. If it persists or is more severe, factor replacement may be required (20-40% level for 1-2 days). A urological evaluation should be initiated to look for and treat any local etiology. Antifibrinolytics are contraindicated in this situation.

CNS Bleed

It is the most dreaded complication in hemophilia. An urgent CT scan is required to document the presence/ absence and location of a bleed. Urgent factor replacement is required to achieve a target level of 50%, this may need to be continued for 7-14 days. If surgical intervention is required appropriate factor replacement should be administered. Antifibrinolytic agents may be beneficial in this situation.

Even if a CT scan is normal the patient should be admitted and monitored for 24–48 hours if the clinical suspicion is strong.

MANAGEMENT OF CHRONIC COMPLICATIONS

Various chronic complications can occur in patients with hemophilia which include chronic synovitis, chronic deforming hemophilic arthropathy, pseudotumors, muscle wasting and debilitation. The approach to the management of these problems are usually more difficult, require a multidisciplinary approach and patience.

Chronic Synovitis

It usually presents with a grossly distended joint without significant pain and is not tense. It is often associated with a history of recurrent hemarthrosis and significant muscle wasting. Principles of management include partial immobilization with intermittent regular physiotherapy under supervision with factor prophylaxis. This can also be done with minimum factor replacement or administered on an, if required basis. If it persists or is associated with frequent bleeds, one could consider synovectomy by one of the following methods:

- Surgical
- Chemical, e.g. rifampicin
- Radioactive, e.g. Yttrium

Deforming Arthropathy

It is the end result of recurrent synovitis secondary to hemarthrosis. In it usually restriction in joint movements, progresses to fibrous ankylosis and if not corrected at these stages it will end in bony and irreversible ankylosis. In the early stages it can occasionally be managed with prolonged physiotherapy alone, with minimal factor support. Often a multidisciplinary approach involving the orthopedic surgeon, a rehabilitation unit and the hematologist is necessary.

Pseudotumor

They are large encapsulated hematomas that represent progressive cystic swelling from recurrent bleeds and incomplete resorption. As they enlarge they acquire a fibrous capsule and destroy adjacent tissue. While intensive factor replacement, high and low-dose radiotherapy has been reported to be successful, surgical excision remains the most effective treatment for pseudotumors. Depending on the size and location of the lesion, percutaneous evacuation of the cavity and subsequent introduction of sclerosing agents, fibrin sealant and cancellous bone have been reported to be successful.

PHYSICAL THERAPY AND REHABILITATION

Physiotherapy is the cornerstone of hemophilia management in the developing world. Regular physiotherapy under appropriate guidance can prevent and significantly reduce the morbidity associated deforming arthropathy. Importance of physiotherapy should be stressed to all patients with hemophilia this is especially true following surgery, prolonged immobilization and other procedures that can lead to decreased joint mobility. Physiotherapy should preferably be initiated under the supervision of trained personnel and subsequently a home training program could be provided to the patient to continue it on a regular basis. In certain situations (e.g. postoperative) it should preferably be conducted only under the supervision of a qualified physiotherapist. A common misconception among patients with hemophilia is that physiotherapy can be conducted safely only under factor prophylaxis.

SURGICAL MANAGEMENT

A surgical procedure in a patient with hemophilia is a major intervention and should preferably be carried out in a tertiary center with experience in handling it. However in emergencies and due to various other constraints this may not be possible.

The standard recommendations for factor prophylaxis, for surgery are significantly higher (Table 15.2). The low dose protocols that are mentioned here have been found to be as effective as the standard recommendations with no significant difference in the incidence of delayed bleeds.

Guidelines for the management of patients with hemophilia undergoing surgical procedures:

A. Preoperative evaluation:
   1. Baseline coagulation work-up and inhibitor screen (if positive—preferable to avoid elective surgery)
   2. Baseline weight
   3. Virology HbsAg, HCV, HIV
   4. Availability of blood products and factor concentrates for surgery.

B. Day of surgery:
   1. Infuse appropriate amount of factors one hour before the surgery
      Hemophilia A—target 80%
      Hemophilia B—target 60%
   2. Collect sample for factor assay 30 minutes after infusion of factor concentrates. Once the assay report is ready, the patient is cleared for surgery if a level of >70% is achieved for factor VIII and >50% for factor IX.

C. Postoperative factor support: Postoperative factor concentrate can be administered either as intermittent boluses or as a continuous infusion.

The theoretical advantages of continuous infusion of factors include:

Table 15.2: International guidelines for factor prophylaxis for major surgery in patients with hemophilia (Hemophilia. 1995;1 (Suppl):8-13)

Days	*Target factor levels*	
	VIII	*IX*
Preoperative	80–100	50–80
Days 1–3	80–100	50–80
Days 4–6	60–80	40–50
Days 7–10	30–60	30–40
Days 10–12	20–40	20–30

- Avoid excessive peaks in factor levels.
- Avoid dangerous troughs
- Potential to reduce factor support by 1/3 to 2/3 of standard recommendation
- Adjusted dose continuous infusion can further reduce the factors used
- Unlike in intermittent bolus replacement where factor assays have to be done at trough levels, here factor assays can be done at any convenient time
- Reduces work of the nursing staff.

For continuous infusion the target levels to be aimed for as follows:

Target levels

Time	FVIII	FIX
Preoperative	80%	60%
Days 1, 2, 3	30%	30%
Days 4, 5	20%	20%
Day 6+	10%	10%

While for intermittent bolus infusion of factors, the following peak and trough levels are recommended.

Target levels (Peak and trough levels)

Time	FVIII	FIX
Preoperative	80–100%	60–80%
Days 1–3	20–40%	15–30%
Days 4+	15–30%	10–20%

Factor support is usually continued till suture removal or day +10. In few patients it may be administered for less or more days depending on the type of surgery and site of surgery.

MANAGEMENT OF PATIENTS WITH INHIBITORS

A dreaded complication in the management of patients with hemophilia is the development of alloantibody inhibitors. This usually occurs in patients with severe hemophilia. It is seen in 10-20% of patients with hemophilia A and 1.5-4% of patients with hemophilia B. Depending on the titer of the antibody level they can be classified as low responders (<5 Bethesda units) and high responders (>10 Bethesda units). High responders are characterized by a rapid anamnestic response on exposure to factors, while low responders usually do not manifest an anamnestic response.

Management of patients with inhibitors is difficult, the options include:

A. Higher than usual doses of factors (2–5 fold higher doses) may be effective in patients who are low responders

B. Use of agents that by pass the inhibitor:
   - Prothrombin complex concentrates (PCC)
   - Activated prothrombin complex concentrates (APCC)

C. Other agents:
   - Porcine factor VIII
   - Recombinant factor VIIa
D. Temporary reduction of inhibitor:
   Extensive plasma exchange
   Immunoadsorption
E. Induction of immune tolerance:
   - High dose regimen—Bonn method (200–300 IU/kg/day for 1-3 years)
   - Low or intermediate regimens 25/50 IU/kg on alternate days for 1->12 months
   - Malmo model—Cyclophosphamide, factor VIII/IX, high-dose IVIg
   - One can also use rituximab for reducing the antibodies.

Most commonly used in our setting is PCC/APCC, most of the other options are prohibitively expensive.

The usual recommended dose of APCC is 50–75 IU/kg IV q8h for major bleeds. At high-doses a disseminated intravascular coagulation can occur, antifibrinolytic agents should not be administered along with these agents.

CARRIER DETECTION AND ANTENATAL DIAGNOSIS

It is very important in the management of patients with hemophilia to offer facilities for carrier detection and antenatal diagnosis.

A woman is a definite carrier if:
- Her father has hemophilia
- She has one son who has hemophilia and a first degree relative (brother, maternal uncle or other male relatives who have hemophilia)
- She has two or more sons with hemophilia.

A women is a possible carrier if:
- She has one or more maternal relatives with hemophilia.
- She has one son with hemophilia and no other affected relative.

Laboratory diagnosis of carrier status using factor VIII/IX assays or FVIII/vWFAg ratio's are accurate in about 60-90% of cases. These methods and their level of accuracy are not considered acceptable.

While DNA analysis using the appropriate markers can be accurate and informative in >99%.

RECENT ADVANCES

1. Improvements in development of recombinant factor VIII production, with the recent development of B domain less recombinant FVIII (BDDrFVIII). Important to note that it has been observed that one stage factor assays in patients on these products give a lower (up to 50% lower) value than compared with a two stage assay or with a chromogenic assay, a similar phenomenon has been observed with recombinant factor IX.
2. *Gene therapy:* Rapid strides are being made in the treatment of hemophilia with gene therapy. Clinical trials are on and the preliminary data is exciting.

CONCLUSION

Hemophilia is a relatively rare disorder and medical personnel are sometimes not familiar with its diagnosis and treatment, which can occasionally have disastrous consequences for the patient. This is compounded by the high-cost of replacement factors, the chronic debilitating nature of the illness and lack of a comprehensive government program to cover the cost of care of these patients. Within these constraints it is a challenge to offer quality care to these patients.

BIBLIOGRAPHY

1. Astermark J, Berntorp E, White GC, Kroner BL. MIBS Study Group. The Malmö International Brother Study (MIBS): further support for genetic predisposition to inhibitor development in hemophilia patients. Haemophilia. 2001;7: 267-72.
2. Bernstein MJ, Manco-Johnson MJ, Riske B. The Joint Outcome Study Authors Prophylaxis versus Episodic Treatment to Prevent Joint Disease in Boys with Severe Hemophilia. N Engl J Med. 2007;357:2087-8.
3. High KA. Update on Progress and Hurdles in Novel Genetic Therapies for Hemophilia. Hematology Am Soc Hematol Educ Program; 2007.pp.466-72.
4. Kitchen S, McCraw A. For the WFH Laboratory Sciences Committee. Diagnosis of Haemophilia and other Bleeding Disorders. Montreal, Canada: WFH, 2000. May be downloaded free of charge from www.wfh.org.
5. Manco-Johnson MJ, Abshire TC, Shapiro AD, et al. Prophylaxis versus episodic treatment to prevent joint disease in boys with severe hemophilia. N Engl J Med. 2007;357:535-44.
6. Negrier C, Dargaud Y, Bordet JC. Basic aspects of bypassing agents. Haemophilia. 2006;12(Suppl. 6):48-53.
7. Prabhu R, Jijina F, Shetty S, Ghosh K. Successful surgery in severe hemophilia—a two stage replacement approach in resource poor countries. Hemophilia. 2008;14:1125-6.
8. Rodriguez NI, Hoots WK. Advances in Hemophilia: experimental aspects and therapy. Pediatar Clin N Am. 2008;55:357-76.
9. Srivastava A, Chandy M, Sunderrajan GD, Lee V, et al. Low dose intermittent factor replacement for post operative hemostasis in Hemophilia. Hemophilia. 1998;4:99-801.
10. Srivastava A, Chuansumrit A, Chandy M, Duraiswamy G, Karagus C. Management of Haemophilia in the Developing World. Haemophilia. 1998;4:474.
11. Srivastava A. Factor concentrates for haemophilia in the developing world. Haemophilia; 1998.pp.481-5.
12. Verbruggen B, Meijer P, Novakova I, et al. Diagnosis of factor VIII deficiency. Haemophilia. 2008;14(Suppl 3):76-82.

16 Thrombocytopenia Other than ITP and Thrombasthenia

Sunil Gomber

Thrombocytopenia is reduction in number of platelets (<1.5 lac/cumm; normal count being 1.5-4 lac/cumm) while defective function of platelets is known as thrombasthenia. Platelets, or thrombocytes are small, irregularly shaped clear cell fragments, 1-4 μm in diameter, which are derived from fragmentation of precursor megakaryocytes. The average lifespan of a platelet is normally just 7 to 10 days. They are involved in hemostasis, leading to the formation of blood clots.

CLINICAL PRESENTATION

Bleeding may be a presenting feature of both thrombocytopenia and thrombasthenia. Bleeding typically involves skin and mucus membranes including petechiae, purpura, ecchymosis, epistaxis hematuria and gastrointestinal hemorrhage. Intracranial hemorrhage can occur rarely. The level of platelet counts typically associated with the type of bleed is shown in the Table 16.1.

Etiology

In the present article, the secondary thrombocytopenic purpura would be talked about. As mentioned in Table 16.2, the thrombocytopenia due to infections is mainly immune-mediated. In the late stages of infections, e.g. due to HIV there may be a direct marrow suppression causing anemia and leukopenia along with thrombocytopenia.

DRUG-INDUCED THROMBOCYTOPENIA

As mentioned previously, the drugs can cause thrombocytopenia either by producing marrow depression or causing platelet destruction. Thrombocytopenia usually resolves when the offending drug is eliminated. A marrow examination and/or platelet antibodies specific to an offending drug clinches the diagnosis.

Thrombocytopenia Secondary to Platelet Consumption

- *Disseminated intravascular coagulation (DIC)*: Thrombocytopenia is seen secondary to several diseases associated with DIC including purpura fulminans and fulminant sepsis. In an unusual case of thrombocytopenia, PT, PTT, fibrinogen and FDP should be determined as screening tests to exclude DIC as the cause of thrombocytopenia.
- *Hemolytic-uremic syndrome (HUS)*: This acute disease of infancy and early childhood usually follows an episode of acute gastroenteritis often triggered by *E. coli* 0157:H7. It has also occurred following typhoid fever and *Shigella* infection. Shortly after the acute illness signs and symptoms of hemolytic anemia, thrombocytopenia and acute renal failure ensue. The presence of anuria and severe azotemia indicates grave renal damage.

Table 16.1: Level of platelet counts

Platelet count ($\times 10^9$ /cumm)	*Type of bleed*	*Examples*
<75	Primary hemostasis impaired	After major surgery or trauma
<50	Spontaneous bleed mostly skin	Petechiae, purpura
<20	Noticeable bleed in skin and mucosa	Epistaxis, gingival bleed
<10	Possible life threatening hemorrhage, mucosal and CNS bleed	Acute GI hemorrhage, intracranial hemorrhage

Table 16.2: Various causes of thrombocytopenia

I. Increased platelet destruction
   A. Immune thrombocytopenias
      1. Idiopathic
      2. Secondary
         a. Infection induced, e.g. viral (HIV, CMV, EBV, rubella, etc.) or bacterial (TB, typhoid)
         b. Drug induced (Table 16.3)
         c. Post-transfusion purpura
         d. Autoimmune hemolytic anemia (Evan's syndrome)
         e. Systemic lupus erythemetosus (SLE)
         f. Hyperthyroidism
         g. Allergy, anaphylaxis
      3. Neonatal immune thrombocytopenias
         a. Alloimmune
         b. Autoimmune
         c. Erythroblastosis fetalis (Rh incompatibility)
   B. Nonimmune thrombocytopenias
      1. Due to platelet consumption
         a. Disseminated intravascular coagulation (DIC)
         b. Hemolytic-Uremic syndrome (HUS)
         c. Kasabach-Merritt syndrome
         d. Cyanotic heart disease
      2. Due to platelet destruction
         a. Drugs (e.g. protamine sulfate, bleomycin)
         b. Infections
         c. Cardiac (e.g. prosthetic heart valves, repair of intracardiac defects)
II. Disorders of platelet distribution or pooling
         a. Hypersplenism (e.g. portal hypertension, hemolytic anemia, neoplastic)
III. Decreased platelet production
   A. Hypoplasia or suppression of megakaryocytes
      1. Drugs (thiazides, ethanol, tolbutamide)
      2. Constitutional
         a. TAR syndrome
         b. Amegakaryocytic thrombocytopenia
         c. Rubella syndrome
         d. Fanconi's anemia
      3. Ineffective thrombopoiesis
         a. Megaloblastic anemias (folate, B_{12} deficiencies)
         b. Paroxysmal noctural hemoglobinuria (PNH)
         c. Familial thrombocytopenias
      4. Acquired aplastic disorders
         a. Idiopathic
         b. Drug induced (e.g. dose related: anticancer drugs, antithyroids, antidiabetics, phenylbutazone, insecticides, idiosyncratic: chloramphenicol)
         c. Radiation induced
         d. Viral infections (hepatitis, HIV, EBV)
   B. Marrow infiltrative processes
      1. Benign
         a. Osteopetrosis
         b. Storage diseases
      2. Malignant
         a. Leukemias, Langerhan's cell histiocytosis, lymphomas, neuroblastoma
IV. Hereditary platelet disorders
         a. May-Hegglin anomaly
         b. Wiskott-Aldrich syndrome

Table 16.3: Drugs causing antibody mediated immune thrombocytopenia

Analgesics	Acetyl salicylic acid, acetaminophen, phenylbutazone
Antibiotics	Antitubercular drugs (rifampicin, INH, PAS) sulfonamides, vancomycin, amphotericin B, gentamycin
Anticonvulsants	Barbiturates, carbamazepine, phenytoin, diazepam
Cinchona alkaloids	Quinidine, quinine
Miscellaneous	Methyldopa, thiazides, levamisole, cimetidine

Treatment of most cases involves institution of careful fluid management, correction of anemia by red cell transfusion and prompt appropriate dialysis.

- *Kassabach-Merritt syndrome*: The association of giant hemangioma associated with thrombocytopenia is the hallmark of this disease. Increased consumption of coagulation factors occurs in some patients. Recovery follows spontaneous regression of hemangioma by one year of age or surgical excision. Some lesions regress after treatment with corticosteroids.
- *Cyanotic congenital heart disease*: It may occur in children with severe polycythemia (hematocrit >65%) which could be due to margination of platelets in small blood vessels. These children can have prolonged bleeding time despite normal platelet count due to impairment in platelet aggregation by ADP, norepinephrine and collagen. The impairment is correlated with severity of hypoxia. The corrective surgery if successful results in an improved platelet count.
- *Hypersplenism*: Splenomegaly resulting from a variety of conditions may be associated with thrombocytopenia probably due to sequestration or destruction of platelets by the enlarged spleen. It is usually associated with neutropenia and anemia. Megakaryocytes are plentiful in the marrow. Splenectomy or splenic embolization may attenuate the thrombocytopenia in many instances even though the underlying disease is not affected.

DECREASED OR ABSENT MEGAKARYOCYTES IN THE MARROW

A variety of syndromes/diseases have been described that have in common a primary impairment of platelet production as a major cause of thrombocytopenia. Bone marrow examination usually reveals decreased number of megakaryocytes. This may be an isolated megakaryocytic hypoplasia or part of a generalized bone marrow disease such as aplasia of marrow or infiltration of the marrow by non-neoplastic or neoplastic disease.

Constitutional

These genetic disorders with various modes of inheritance may be associated with number of congenital abnormalities especially of bones, kidneys and heart. Several of these disorders may present initially with a single cytopenia and subsequently progress to pancytopenia (e.g. amegakaryocytic thrombocytopenia, Shwachman diamond syndrome). These disorders can be autosomal recessive (e.g. Fanconi's anemia, dyskeratosis congenita), X-linked or autosomal dominant (dyskeratosis congenita).

Hereditary Thrombocytopenia

These may be classified on the basis of inheritance and frequently overlap with congenital platelet function defects. The presence of normal or increased number of megakaryocytes in the bone marrow suggests that the thrombocytopenia is a result of shortened platelet survival caused by an intrinsic platelet defect.

Autosomal dominant syndromes include May-Hegglin anamoly (large platelets and large Dohle bodies in the granulocytes). Many of the syndromes are sex-linked as represented by the typical Wiskott-Aldrich syndrome and variants thereof. The clinical features consist of eczema, recurrent infections and thrombocytopenia. The infants are ill from the first few months of life and die in early childhood. Bleeding manifestations are usually mild to moderate in hereditary thrombocytopenia and treatment is symptomatic.

Neonatal Thrombocytopenia

The incidence of neonatal thrombocytopenia (platelet count <1,00,000/mm^3) is 0.12%. Most neonates who have thrombocytopenia are ill, premature and have other disorders including bacteremia and DIC. The nonimmune causes are the same as enlisted in Table 16.2.

The immune disorders would be briefly discussed.

There are two causes of immune thrombocytopenia in the newborn:

1. Neonatal alloimmune thrombocytopenia
2. Maternal autoimmune thrombocytopenia.

Neonatal alloimmune thrombocytopenia: NAIT occurs in 1 in 2,000 to 1 in 5,000 births. It should be suspected in thrombocytopenic infants born to mothers with a normal platelet count. Immunization arises from fetomaternal passage of platelets in which there is incompatibility of fetal and maternal platelet antigens.

The pathophysiology is similar to that of Rh disease. The platelet antigenic system most commonly associated with neonatal purpura is PIA. Clinically the hemorrhagic mainfestations in the form of petechiae may appear at or shortly after birth. The incidence of intracranial hemorrhage is as high as 20%. Fetal thrombocytopenia has responded to infusion of washed maternal platelets, IVIg (1 g/kg/daily for 1-3 days) or corticosteroids.

To prevent thrombocytopenia in subsequent pregnancies IVIg (1 g/kg) may be given weekly from mid-gestation until birth. Cesarean section should be recommended for all pregnancies at risk for alloimmune thrombocytopenia.

Neonatal autoimmune thrombocytopenia: Pregnant women with idiopathic thrombocytopenic purpura (ITP) are at 50% risk for delivering thrombocytopenic infants whether or not the mother is thrombocytopenic during pregnancy or at the time of delivery. This results from the transplacental passage of maternal IgG autoantibodies into the fetal circulation with destruction of fetal platelets. It is a less severe disease than alloimmune thrombocytopenia. Maternal treatment with corticosteroids for 10-14 days prior to delivery may produce a higher neonatal platelet count. Infants may be treated with IVIg, corticosteroids or exchange transfusion followed by random donor platelets.

Disorders of Platelet Function

The abnormalities of platelet function should be suspected in patients with a bleeding time inappropriately prolonged for the platelet count. Normally the bleeding time does not become prolonged until the platelet count falls below 50,000/mm^3.

In general there is a history of petechiae, ecchymosis or epistaxis of mild to moderate severity. The hemostatic screening tests except for bleeding time are normal. In many instances tests of platelet aggregation must be performed to make a specific diagnosis. The platelet aggregation is currently measured using platelet aggregometry. In the aggregometer, agonists such as collagen, ADP, ristocetin, arachidonic acid and thrombin are added to platelet rich plasma and clumping of platelets over time is measured by an automated machine.

Steps of Platelet Function

Adhesion Activation Secretion Aggregation

Normally the vessel wall serves as a barrier between the flowing blood and the extravascular space. When this barrier is disrupted, platelets can adhere to components of the subendothelium in the presence of plasma von Willebrand factor. Platelets after stimulation by ADP adhere (ADP is secreted by injured endothelial cells), by thrombin (which is formed by plasma coagulation) or by collagen the main component of subendothelium. The activation of platelets is marked by synthesis of prostaglandins such as thromboxane A2. These phenomena lead to the sequential release of granules permitting the binding of plasma fibrinogen with the extracellular calcium ions leading to platelet aggregation. Modern instruments measure the release of granular contents such as ATP from the platelets following activation. The ability of platelets to aggregate and their metabolic activity can also be assessed simultaneously. Among the thrombocytopathies every step of platelet physiology may be affected.

Acquired Disorders

A number of systemic illnesses like septicemia, liver diseases or uremia are associated with platelet dysfunction. These disorders are often associated with other abnormalities of the coagulation mechanism. Many drugs also alter platelet function, the most commonly used drug is aspirin, the other drugs include Nonsteroidal anti-inflammatory drugs (NSAIDS), valproic acid and high-dose penicillin. Therefore during evaluation it is important to exclude the presence of other exogenous agents and to study the patient after all the medications are stopped for 2 weeks.

Congenital Abnormalities

Bernard-Soulier syndrome: It is an autosomal recessive disorder of platelet adhesion which is characterized by thrombocytopenia with giant platelets and a markedly prolonged bleeding time. The cause for platelet dysfunction is the absence or severe deficiency of vWF receptor (GPIb complex) on the platelet membrane. Appropriate aggregation in response to ADP and other agents is normal.

Glanzmann thrombasthenia: It is characterized by absent platelet aggregation with all agonists like ADP, epinephrine and collagen except ristocetin. The disorder is caused by deficiency of platelet fibrinogen receptor, GPIIb/IIIa on the platelet surface. Fibrinogen binds this complex and causes platelets to aggregate. This disorder is inherited as autosomal recessive.

The treatment of platelet function defects depends on the severity of the hemorrhagic event. DDAVP 50 µg/kg IV may be used for mild to moderate bleeding episodes. It provides increased levels of vWF and factor VIII and provides normal hemostasis in mild to moderate platelet function defects. For severe bleeding episodes, platelet transfusion 1 u/5-10 kg body wt. may be life saving.

Diagnostic Evaluation

Most thrombocytopenias in children are the result of increased platelet destruction. The bone marrow in such cases responds with compensatory increase in the rate of production with increased number of immature megakaryocytes. The large young platelets, which are functionally very active, are more prominent in the peripheral blood smear. The increased mean platelet volume provides supportive evidence of the larger size.

In disorders with decreased platelet production, the decreased platelet number is associated with small sized platelets, a decreased mean platelet volume and a longer bleeding time relative to platelet number. The megakaryocytes are decreased in number or absent in bone marrow aspirate.

In the diagnostic evaluation of thrombocytopenia, it is important first to determine whether other blood components are involved. Coexisting abnormalities of the white blood cells or red cells may indicate disease involving the bone marrow or the spleen. Abnormalities in coagulation, in association with thrombocytopenia, suggest disorders of consumption including DIC.

Approach to Platelet Disorders

- The etiological list provided above is quite exhaustive, however if carefully looked into, most causes can be excluded on the basis of a good history and clinical examination (infections like HIV, rubella, tuberculosis, typhoid; drug mediated immune or nonimmune thrombocytopenia, post-transfusion, SLE, hyperthyroidism, allergy/anaphylaxis, DIC, HUS, kassabach meritt, cyanotic heart disease, prosthetic valves, portal hypertension, hemolytic anemia, neoplasia, etc.)
- If platelet count is abnormal but bleeding time is prolonged, think of thrombasthenias. Platelet aggregation studies would be most useful. (ristocetin induced platelet aggregation, RIPA would be absent in Bernard soulier while in glanzmann's thrombasthenia, RIPA would be present but aggregation with all other agonists would be abnormal.
- If hemoglobin and TLC are also low with a low platelet count, think of aplastic anemia, megaloblastic anemia or marrow infiltrative processes.
- Increased platelet size, mean platelet volume and presence of megakaryocytes on marrow suggest increased destruction of platelets, while the opposite suggests a decreased production of platelets.

17 Immune Thrombocytopenia: Diagnosis and Management

Vasant Chinnabhandar, MR Lokeshwar, Trupti Dongre

Immune thrombocytopenia (ITP) previously meant idiopathic thrombocytopenic purpura. However, with the elucidation of the immune mechanisms involved in this disorder and the absent/minimal bleeding seen in a large majority of children the modified name, immune thrombocytopenia seems more appropriate. ITP in children is an acquired hemorrhagic disorder occurring in an apparently healthy child, usually due to transient postviral autoimmune phenomenon characterized by an association of isolated thrombocytopenia (platelet count <1,00,000/µl) with normal or increased megakaryocytes in an otherwise normal marrow without evidence of concurrent abnormality or disease process that might account for the thrombocytopenia.

The traditional concept of thrombocytopenia in ITP due to autoantibody mediated increased platelet destruction has been replaced with elucidation of more complex mechanisms in which both impaired platelet production and T cell–mediated effects play a role.

Typically, ITP in adults has an insidious onset with no preceding viral or other illness and it normally follows a chronic course. Immune thrombocytopenia in children is usually short-lived with at least two-thirds recovering spontaneously within 6 months. Signs and symptoms vary widely, ranging from asymptomatic to those with life-threatening bleeding.

Recent developments have led to changes in the accepted definitions associated with ITP. We discuss these briefly in this chapter along with currently accepted recommendations for management of pediatric ITP.

WHAT ARE VARIOUS TYPES OF ITP?

The definitions and terminology proposed for standardized use by an international working group of ITP (2007) are as follow:

- *Primary ITP:* It is an autoimmune disorder characterized by isolated thrombocytopenia (peripheral blood platelet count $<100 \times 10^9/L$) in the absence of other causes or disorders that may be associated with thrombocytopenia. The diagnosis of primary ITP remains one of exclusion; no robust clinical or laboratory parameters are currently available to establish its diagnosis with accuracy. The main clinical problem of primary ITP is an increased risk of bleeding, although bleeding symptoms may not always be present.
- *Secondary ITP:* All forms of immune-mediated thrombocytopenia except primary ITP. Secondary forms include thrombocytopenias that are due to an underlying disease or to drug exposure. The name of the associated disease should follow the designation in parentheses. For example: "secondary ITP (systemic lupus erythematosus-associated or SLE-associated)".

This differentiation of ITP into primary and secondary types carries implications for management and is hence important. Management of secondary ITP would involve treatment of the underlying disorder which would lead to improvement in ITP in the majority of cases.

The term "acute" ITP which was previously used to describe the possibly self-limited form of the disease is now to be avoided. The following terms were recommended for use to describe the phases of ITP:

- *Newly diagnosed ITP:* Within 3 months from diagnosis.
- *Persistent ITP:* Between 3 and 12 months from diagnosis. Includes patients not reaching spontaneous remission or not maintaining complete response off therapy.
- *Chronic ITP:* Lasting for more than 12 months.
- *Severe ITP:* Presence of bleeding symptoms at presentation sufficient to mandate treatment, or occurrence of new bleeding symptoms requiring additional therapeutic intervention with a different platelet-enhancing agent or an increased dose.

Traditionally ITP has been divided into three subtypes—acute, recurrent and chronic. These differ especially in respect to patient's age at onset, sex, medical events preceding the onset, duration of thrombocytopenia and response to treatment. It is not possible to distinguish them at the onset of symptomatology. Acute ITP is common after the age of 3 months through childhood with a peak incidence between 2 and 5 years of age, which also is the age at which children are most susceptible to viral infections, a major etiological factor. Acute ITP is generally a benign and self-limiting condition, with 80-90% of them making an uneventful recovery within 3 weeks to 6 months with or without specific treatment. Only 10-20% of ITP cases progress to chronic ITP. In the age group above 13 years, the incidence of chronic ITP is higher. In this age group 80-90% cases continue to have active disease after 6 months to one year. The 65-95% of prepubertal children who develop ITP have the acute form of the disease. Immune thrombocytopenia occurring for the first time before the age of 10 years is predominantly acute whereas after 20 years of age chronic ITP is almost the rule, though the disease is not limited to any age. Although there is no sex predilection for ITP in childhood, in the adult form of the disease, there is 3:1 predominance in women. In recurrent ITP there is recurrence of thrombocytopenia after a sustained normal platelet count. It is precipitated each time usually following a viral infection.

PATHOPHYSIOLOGY OF ITP

Immune thrombocytopenia is probably an immune mediated increased destruction of platelets or decreased production of platelets which results in overall decrease in circulating platelet number. B and T-cells are an integral part of the cascade involved in platelet destruction. Antiplatelet antibodies opsonize the platelets which are then attached to antigen presenting cells with the help of Fcγ receptors. Opsonized platelets are finally phagocytosed by the macrophages. At the same time T-cells stimulate B-cells to produce more antiplatelet antibody and new research shows that some cryptic epitopes from platelet antigens stimulate platelet specific T-cells.

Reduced platelet production is also thought to play a significant role in the pathogenesis of this disorder. The recent elucidation of thrombopoietin (TPO) and its role in thrombopoiesis has helped us understand the role of reduced thrombopoiesis in ITP. Increase in platelet numbers after administering TPO mimetics in some study populations has consolidated the fact that TPO has a definitive role in ITP.

DIAGNOSIS OF ITP

There is no "gold standard" test that can reliably establish the diagnosis of ITP. This diagnosis is still a clinical one, based on the patient's history, physical examination and complete blood cell count as well as examination of peripheral blood smear (Table 17.1). The diagnosis is more by exclusion of other causes of thrombocytopenia. Response to ITP-specific therapy, for example, intravenous immunoglobulin (IVIg) and intravenous anti-D is supportive of the diagnosis, but a response does not exclude secondary ITP. Intercontinental Childhood ITP Study (ICIS) group found the mean age of presentation of ITP in cohort of children to be 5.7 years. Boys especially below 10 years are found to have higher incidence of ITP.

IMPORTANT FACTORS IN DIAGNOSIS

Patient History

Thrombocytopenia can be caused by a variety of conditions including systemic disease, infection, drugs, and primary hematologic disorders. Around 60% of pediatric cases have a history of a previous infection. An increased risk of ITP is also associated with measles-mumps-rubella vaccination. Inherited thrombocytopenia should be considered in patients with long-standing thrombocytopenia unaffected by treatment and in those with a family history of thrombocytopenia or bleeding disorders. The possibility of abuse must be considered by emergency department staff when dealing with a young child who presents with bruising and purpura for the first time.

Physical Examination

Physical examination should probably be normal aside from bleeding manifestations (Figs 17.1 and 17.2). Mild splenomegaly may be found, particularly in children, but moderate or massive splenomegaly suggests an alternative cause. Constitutional symptoms, such as fever or weight loss, hepatomegaly, or lymphadenopathy might indicate an underlying disorder.

American Society of Hematology in 1996 suggested no further tests in typical cases of ITP. A typical case is a child with ITP, characterized by isolated thrombocytopenia, with normal counts in otherwise healthy child without any hepatosplenomegaly, no lymphadenopathy and bony tenderness and may be preceded by viral infection 2-3 weeks earlier. However, patients with risk factors for human immunodeficiency virus (HIV) should be tested for HIV antibodies.

Peripheral Blood Counts

Immune thrombocytopenia is characterized by isolated thrombocytopenia with an otherwise normal complete blood count (Fig. 17.3). Anemia from blood loss may be present, but it should be proportional to the amount, and the duration, of bleeding. Reticulocyte counts can

Table 17.1: Recommendations for the diagnosis of ITP

Basic evaluation	*Tests of potential utility*	*Tests of uncertain benefit*
Patient history	Glycoprotein-specific antibody	TPO
Family history	Antiphospholipid antibodies (including anticardiolipin and lupus anticoagulant)	Reticulated platelets
Physical examination	Antithyroid antibodies and thyroid function	PAIgG
Complete blood count and reticulocyte count	Pregnancy test in women of child-bearing potential	Platelet survival time
Peripheral blood film	Antinuclear antibody	Bleeding time
Quantitative immunoglobulin level measurement	Viral PCR for parvovirus and CMV	Serum complement
Bone marrow examination (selected patients)		
Blood group (Rh)		
Direct antiglobulin test		
H. pylori		
HIV		
HCV		

Abbreviations: HIV: Human immunodeficiency virus; HCV: Hepatitis C virus; PCR: Polymerase chain reaction; CMV: Cytomegalovirus; TPO: Thrombopoietin; PAIgG: Platelet-associated immunoglobulin G

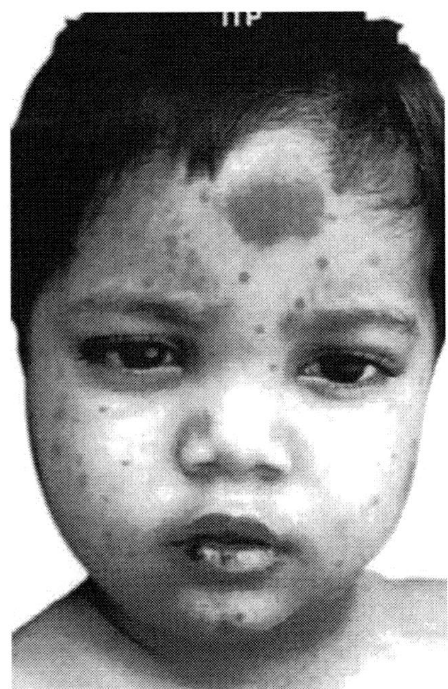

Fig. 17.1: Typical skin manifestations in a case of ITP (*Courtesy:* MR Lokeshwar) *(For color version, see Plate 2)*

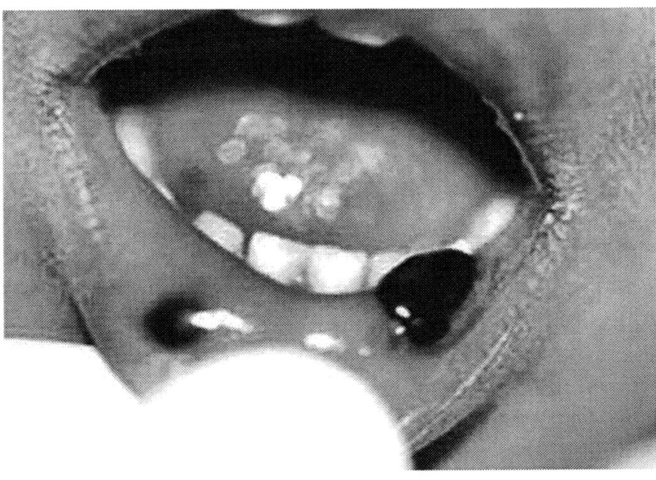

Fig. 17.2: Mucosal bleeds in the oral cavity in ITP (*Courtesy:* MR Lokeshwar) *(For color version, see Plate 2)*

help define whether anemia is the result of poor production or increased destruction of red blood cells (RBCs). If the degree of anemia is disproportionate to amount of bleeding seen, then other sinister conditions like leukemia, aplastic anemia or occult blood loss and Evan's syndrome should be kept in mind.

A platelet count of less than 100,000/µl has been established as the cut-off for diagnosis of ITP. Eighty percent of children with newly diagnosed ITP have platelet count less than 40,000/µl. In chronic ITP, platelet count at the time of presentation is usually higher (20,000 to 75,000/µl). Thrombocytopenia is evident on peripheral smear and is accompanied by bizarre shaped or giant forms of platelets. In chronic ITP

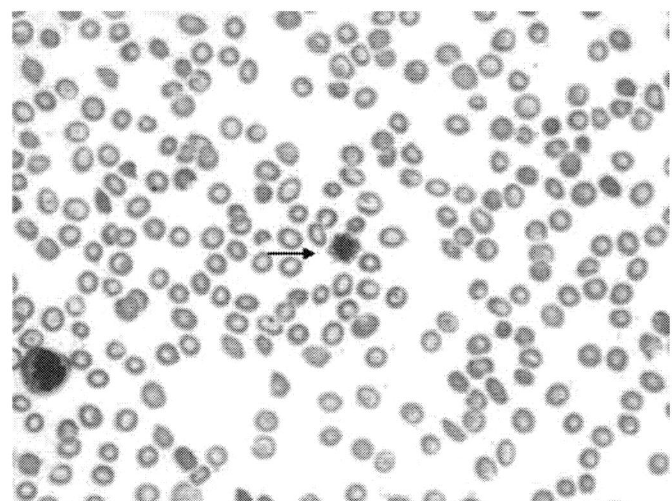

Fig. 17.3: Peripheral blood smear showing paucity of platelets and a giant platelet (arrow)
(For color version, see Plate 2)

both mean platelet volume (MPV) and number of large platelets are significantly increased compared to control values. The presence of low or normal MPV in a case of thrombocytopenia suggests aregenerative thrombocytopenia, i.e. bone marrow suppression or marrow infiltration. Platelet distribution width (PDW) may be more discriminating than MPV in detection of compensated thrombocytopenic states.

The total leukocyte count is usually normal though mild-to-moderate lymphocytosis with increased number of atypical lymphocytes may be seen especially when preceded by viral infection. Mild peripheral eosinophilia may be seen in 20% of children but is of no diagnostic or prognostic value.

Bone Marrow Examination

Is it necessary? In a typical case of ITP bone marrow evaluation is unnecessary. Thus, acute onset of bruising following a viral infection in a previously healthy child without any significant hepatosplenomegaly, anemia, bony tenderness or lymphadenopathy and appearance of megathrombocytes without any abnormal premature cells on peripheral smear does not need evaluation of bone marrow aspirate. Bone marrow evaluation in children with newly diagnosed ITP is recommended only when abnormalities are present other than isolated thrombocytopenia in the blood count/smear, if systemic features (e.g. bone pain) are apparent, or if the patient has an otherwise unexplained enlarged spleen. It is also suggested prior to the initiation of corticosteroid therapy or blood transfusion for presumed ITP (although this recommendation is still open to debate) as this may lead to a temporary remission and may mask the presence of blast cells. Bone marrow evaluation should at least be considered in cases who respond minimally or not at all to first-line therapies.

Bone marrow examination is recommended in adult patients over the age of 60 years who are considering splenectomy. However, there are anecdotal reports of apparent typical ITP in which bone marrow biopsy has revealed occult metastatic carcinoma, early aplastic anemia and unsuspected myelodysplastic syndrome (MDS).

Quantitative Immunoglobulin Level Testing

Recommendations for measuring baseline immunoglobulin (Ig) levels (IgG, IgA, and IgM) exist for adults with ITP. In pediatric practice, this may be considered at baseline in children with ITP, and measured in those children with persistent or chronic ITP as part of a reassessment evaluation. Low levels may reveal conditions such as common variable immunodeficiency (CVID) or selective IgA deficiency.

Helicobacter pylori Testing

The urea breath test or the stool antigen test for *H. pylori* is recommended in adult patients. However, current literature does not support similar testing in children except in high prevalence areas and it is yet to enter widespread use in developing countries.

Direct Antiglobulin Test

A positive direct antiglobulin test (DAT) has been reported in a significant proportion of ITP patients, especially adults, but its clinical significance is unknown. A DAT is generally appropriate if anemia associated with a high reticulocyte count is found and if treatment with anti-D immunoglobulin is being considered.

Blood Group Rh(D) Typing

This is especially important if anti-D immunoglobulin is being considered.

Other Potentially Useful Tests

Antiplatelet Antibody Assays: Glycoprotein-Specific Antibody Testing

Understanding of the pathophysiology and insight into the clinical and laboratory aspects of ITP started with a published series of observation by Harrington in 1951, which revealed transferable plasma factor mediated the disease in many patients. This was accomplished by infusion of plasma from ITP patients into healthy volunteers, which led to acute thrombocytopenia in the recipient. Platelet associated IgG antibody (PAIgG) is present in 80% of thrombocytopenic children with ITP. However, PAIgG is elevated in both immune and non-immune thrombocytopenia. Absence of PAIgG makes the diagnosis of ITP less likely. In fact American Society of Hematology guidelines indicate that serologic testing for platelet antibody is unnecessary.

Antiphospholipid Antibodies

Antiphospholipid antibodies (APLA), including anticardiolipin antibodies and lupus anticoagulant, can be found in approximately 40% of otherwise typical adult patients with ITP. The presence of APLA does not appear to affect the response to ITP treatment. Routine testing is not recommended in the absence of symptoms of antiphospholipid syndrome.

Antinuclear Antibodies

A positive antinuclear antibody (ANA) test may be a predictor of chronicity in childhood ITP.

OTHER INVESTIGATIONS

Plasma glycocalcin (a fragment of platelet membrane glycoprotein Ib) levels are significantly below the normal range (5-27%) in aregenerative thrombocytopenic conditions like aplastic anemia and amegakaryocytic thrombocytopenic purpura. The levels are above the normal range (48-261%) in thrombocytopenia associated with normal or increased megakaryocytes in bone marrow.

Over the last few years, platelet survival studies using the radioisotope chromium-51, indium-111 (In-111) have become available. There are characteristic patterns of platelet recovery and survival. Disorders like ITP have nearly normal platelet recovery but a very short platelet survival, whereas markedly reduced platelet recovery with normal platelet survival is seen in hypersplenism. Aregenerative thrombocytopenia as in aplastic anemia and amegakaryocytic thrombocytopenic purpura is characterized by normal platelet recovery with normal platelet survival. Glycoprotein specific acute antibody assay appears promising. Early studies showed encouraging results with sensitivity of 75-85% and specificity of almost 100%. Unfortunately recent large studies showed low (40-60%) sensitivity but high specificity (78-92%). However, patients with MDS and lymphoma with thrombocytopenia also tested positive. Thus these tests are specific but are not sensitive enough to be clinically useful for the diagnosis of ITP. Further studies, perhaps using new technology may give better sensitivity and specificity.

Older children are more likely to have chronic ITP. Other autoimmune diseases associated with thrombocytopenia, including SLE, CVID, and autoimmune lymphoproliferative syndrome (ALPS [although difficult to assess in some instances]) should be considered in cases with multiple autoimmune cytopenias, as should HIV infection in those with risk factors for this infection.

EVALUATION OF PATIENTS WITH PERSISTENT/ EARLY REFRACTORY ITP

For patients with an initial diagnosis of ITP and no improvement in platelet count after 3 to 6 months and who still require treatment, several evaluations are recommended, some of which are listed below in Table 17.2.

Table 17.2: Recommended evaluation for children newly diagnosed with ITP and no improvement after 3 to 6 months

1. Bone marrow evaluation (recommended if ITP persists and no prior response)
2. Tests to identify infection (HIV/HCV/*H. pylori*) if clinical suspicion or high local prevalence
3. ANA
4. Testing for APLA including ACA and LAC
5. Serum immunoglobulins (IgG, IgA, IgM)
6. Review of medication usage

MANAGEMENT OF ITP

The main strategy of treatment of ITP is to administer least amount of therapy possible. As mentioned earlier, in ITP, the child and not the platelet count should be treated. Why certain patients bleed but most do not, remains unclear. Some patients may have marked thrombocytopenia yet normal or near normal hemostasis, because of increased young platelets having better functional capacity. On the other hand, some patients (5% of all children with ITP) may have impaired platelet function as a result of antibodies and these children have prolonged bleeding time and increased bleeding tendency despite having near normal platelet count. Therefore, platelet count is an imperfect indicator for decision-making in the therapy of ITP and treatment decisions based on platelet count threshold remain controversial.

The major goal for treatment of ITP is to provide a safe platelet count (e.g. one that prevents major bleeding) rather than correcting the platelet count to normal levels. Because of the real and potential toxicity of currently available treatments, a critical concept is to avoid unnecessary treatment of asymptomatic patients with milder degrees of thrombocytopenia. Current guidelines suggest that treatment should be initiated in the presence of bleeding symptoms. The ICIS group recommended that children without bleeding may not require therapy regardless of their platelet count, with the exception of "on-demand therapy".

A Clinical Classification of Severity—Should We Treat the Child?

Classification of children with ITP by severity of bleeding is useful to guide management (Table 17.3). Most children with ITP do not have serious bleeding problems despite very low platelet counts. The severity of mucocutaneous bleeding does not predict the risk for life-threatening bleeding (e.g. ICH), and cutaneous signs alone cannot be used as guide to initiate treatment without consideration of other factors including the circulating platelet count, activity profile, and psycho-social issues.

Only 3% of children with ITP have clinically significant symptoms such as severe epistaxis or GI bleeding. Severe bleeding is more likely in children with platelet counts less than $10 \times 10^9/L$. The incidence of intracranial hemorrhage (ICH) in children with ITP is quite low at approximately 0.1 to 0.5%, but predicting with confidence which children will develop an ICH is not possible. Risk factors for ICH include head trauma and concomitant use of medications that adversely affect platelet function. In children with ITP and coexisting vasculitis or coagulopathies, as may be seen in cases with varicella-associated ITP a high degree of caution is warranted.

Therapy also depends on whether it is newly diagnosed or chronic ITP. In general, 70-80% of children with acute ITP will have complete remission and permanent recovery without sequel with or without treatment. Fifty-five to seventy-five percent of those who recover do so within the first month and 80-90% within 4-6 months of diagnosis. However, in chronic ITP only 1/3rd go into remission spontaneously, that too usually late in the course of the disease (between 1 and 10 years after the diagnosis). Children with chronic ITP whose platelet count remains within a relatively safe range (more than 10-30,000/cumm) and whose bleeding time is fairly normal need no therapy except defensive management.

At a meeting of the International Working Group organized by the European Hematology Association in 2007 a combination of platelet counts and clinical criteria has been proposed, which could be used as a measure to assess response to therapy in ITP. These proposed criteria are presented in Table 17.4.

Expectant "Watch and Wait" Policy

The majority of children with newly diagnosed ITP lack significant bleeding symptoms and may be managed without therapy directed at raising the platelet count at the discretion of the hematologist and the patient. It is essential, therefore, that parents and children with ITP understand the risks of serious or life-threatening hemorrhage, and are also aware that children for whom drug therapy is prescribed are those at substantial risk of serious hemorrhage.

During this period, restriction of physical activity and avoidance of all contact sports, playground activities and use of helmets to prevent trauma especially head injury are indicated. Restriction of contact sports (football, soccer, kabbadi, etc.) is advocated until platelet count is above 100,000/µl. Most noncontact sports can be safely enjoyed with platelet count greater than 30,000/µl. Serious athletes may need frequent platelet count measurement and treatment during their participation in sports. Certain antiplatelet drugs like aspirin, phenacetin,

Table 17.3: Grade of severity and management of patients with ITP

Bleeding/quality-of-life	*Management approach*
Grade 1: Minor bleeding, few petechiae (≤100 total) and/or ≤ 5 small bruises (≤3 cm diameter); no mucosal bleeding	Consent for observation
Grade 2: Mild bleeding, many petechiae (>100 total) and/or >5 large bruises (>3 cm diameter); no mucosal bleeding	Consent for observation/ treatment for selected children
Grade 3: Moderate bleeding, overt mucosal bleeding, troublesome lifestyle	Intervention to reach grade 1/2 in selected children
Grade 4: Mucosal bleeding or suspected internal hemorrhage	Intervention

Table 17.4: Proposed criteria for assessing response to ITP treatments

Quality of response*†
- CR: Platelet count ≥ 100 × 10^9/L and absence of bleeding
- R: Platelet count ≥ 30 × 10^9/L and at least 2-fold increase the baseline count and absence of bleeding
- Time to response: Time from starting treatment to time of achievement of CR or R‡
- NR: Platelet count < 30 × 10^9/L or less than 2-fold increase of baseline platelet count or bleeding
- Loss of CR or R: Platelet count below 100 × 10^9/L or bleeding (from CR) or below 30 × 10^9/L or less than 2-fold increase of baseline platelet count or bleeding (from R)

Timing of assessment of response to ITP treatments

Variable, depends on the type of treatment (see Table 17.3)

Duration of response§
- Measured from the achievement of CR or R to loss of CR or R
- Measured as the proportion of the cumulative time spent in CR or R during the period under examination as well as the total time observed from which the proportion is derived

Corticosteroid-dependence

The need for ongoing or repeated doses administration of corticosteroids for at least 2 months to maintain a platelet count at or above 30 × 10^9/L and/or to avoid bleeding (patients with corticosteroid dependence are considered nonresponders)

Supplemental outcomes (whenever possible)
- Bleeding symptoms measured by a validated scale (requires additional studies)
- Health-related quality of life assessment measured by a validated instrument (requires additional studies)

Abbreviations: CR: Complete remission; R: Remission; NR: No remission

*Platelet counts should be confirmed on at least two separate occasions (at least 7 days apart when used to define CR, R) or 1 day apart when used to define NR or loss of response.

†Baseline platelet count refers to platelet count at the time of starting of the investigated treatment; for postsplenectomy response evaluation, basal platelet count refers to the platelet count before patient was first treated (initial treatment).

‡Late responses not attributable to the investigated treatment should not be defined as CR or R.

§The two definitions are not mutually exclusive: the first definition, collectively represented using Kaplan-Meyer analysis, is more suitable for short-course treatments aimed at inducing prolonged remission of the disease, whereas the second one is more suitable to evaluate the overall benefit of continuous or intermittent repeated administration of agents requiring dose adjustments with anticipated temporary losses of CR or R

phenothiazines and nonsteroidal anti-inflammatory drugs should be avoided. Deep intramuscular injections should be avoided but if essential, administration must be followed by pressure over the injection site, maintained continuously for a minimum ten minutes. Immunization with live viral vaccines is preferably avoided during the period of severe thrombocytopenia.

Hospitalization

For children with an established diagnosis of ITP, hospital admission should be reserved for those who have clinically significant bleeding. Problematic psychosocial circumstances of child and family (e.g. behavioral issues, residence remote from a health care facility) should also be considered. Parents should be advised to watch for other signs of bleeding and be given a contact name and telephone number where a physician can be reached at all times. The child should not participate in competitive contact activities that have a high-risk of head trauma. Other activities need not be restricted and the child should be encouraged to continue schooling.

Most children with minor, mild, or moderate symptoms can be safely managed as outpatients with judicious use of supportive care (e.g. antifibrinolytic agents, oral contraceptives) and weekly or less-frequent outpatient visits. When severe thrombocytopenia persists, limiting activities may be an option or treatment can be initiated. During teenage years, the issues of lifestyle and self-image assume greater importance and should also be discussed and may influence treatment decisions.

General Measures for Persistent and Chronic ITP in Children

The management of children with persistent/refractory ITP is essentially the same as those with newly diagnosed ITP. Many children stabilize with an adequate platelet count (~20-30 × 10^9/L) and have no symptoms unless injured. Spontaneous remission may occur over time and expectant management can continue depending on the risk of bleeding and the degree of activity restriction of the child. The onset of menstruation may be problematic and can be managed with antifibrinolytic agents and hormonal medication. Some children with ITP will have platelet counts of 10 to 30 × 10^9/L and, although they have no serious bleeding, they are nonetheless troubled by purpura. Treatment may be beneficial in these cases. As adolescents, minors may become very conscious of their appearance and need sympathetic support.

SPECIFIC THERAPY IN ITP

Corticosteroid Therapy

The use of corticosteroids in the management of ITP is a matter of controversy. In a heterogeneous disease that usually sooner or later gets better on its own and gives rise to little morbidity and low mortality, it is difficult to evaluate the modality of treatment. A double blind randomized prospective study is more likely to give the truth and eliminate both physician and patient bias. For newly diagnosed patients many but not all authors conclude that steroids are beneficial. Normalization of platelet counts as well as reduction in prolonged bleeding time occurs earlier in the steroid treated group as compared to the untreated group. However, it takes 8-10 days before significant changes are noticed. In a randomized double blind and placebo-controlled trial, platelet counts reached a level of 30,000/µl or more (safe range) significantly earlier, with corticosteroids. Platelet survival increased in ITP after steroids. Numerous retrospective studies of steroid treatment in both children and adults in ITP have been reported. Prednisolone at a dose of 1 to 2 mg/kg/day may be effective at inducing a response in children. Higher doses (4 mg/kg/day) for 3 to 4 days have been shown to be effective in up to 72 to 88% of children (platelet count >50 × 10^9/L) within 72 hours. Complete and partial response in patients treated with prednisolone is around 65-80%, but sustained response after discontinuation of drug occurs in only 25% or fewer of patients. Platelet count increased within one week in responding patient and reach peak values by 2-4 weeks. Because of the serious side effects associated with prolonged corticosteroid treatment in children with ITP, prednisolone should be used only to maintain a hemostatic platelet count, and for as short a time as possible. It is important to taper down the dose and terminate the drug on either stoppage of bleeding or on achieving a platelet count higher than 20 × 10^9/L.

Indications for Steroids in ITP

Though there is a lot of controversy whether steroids should be given to children with newly diagnosed ITP or not, there is uniformity in the opinion that large doses of steroids for a prolonged period should not be given, since steroids may in fact suppress platelet production. Adverse effects of steroids include hyperglycemia, hypertension, fluid electrolyte imbalance, psychosis, and osteoporosis, etc.

A child with severe thrombocytopenia with a platelet count of less than 10,000 to 30,000/µl with generalized petechiae and purpura, wet purpura with mucosal bleeding, gastrointestinal hemorrhages and fundal hemorrhages and ICH should be treated with steroids. Active young children less than 3-4 years with low platelet count also may be treated with steroids, because of fear of trauma induced severe bleeds.

Effect of Steroids in ITP

The mechanism of action of steroids in treating thrombocytopenia is multiple:

1. Decreased consumption of antibody coated platelets by spleen or bone marrow (reticuloendothelial system [RES]).
2. Reduces antibody production by spleen and bone marrow.
3. Increase marrow platelet production by undetermined production.
4. Other effect of steroid on endothelial cells: Experimental evidence suggests thinning of endothelium with development of endothelial fenestration in both animal model and humans with ITP. Experimentally investigators demonstrated that three days steroid therapy in rabbits and four days in patients, the endothelial thinning reversed towards normal.

Although imperfect and only a rough guide, incidence of bleeding is often correlated with platelet count and patients with platelet count >50,000/µl rarely have spontaneous bleeding and hence may only require treatment if extensive operative procedures are planned or following trauma. Patients with platelet count <10,000 to 20,000/µl, and/or significant mucosal bleeding with platelet count <50,000/µl are usually treated.

Steroids in ICH

No proof exists that use of steroids reduces the incidence of ICH or death. Previous studies have reported no benefit in reduction of ICH with steroid use in ITP. Review of literature done in 1851 cases showed

19 cases with ICH (1.026%) and 6 cases had ICH when they were on steroid therapy. Eight children had ICH within 1 month of diagnosis and the other 10 children after 1 month of onset of ITP. Few of the precipitating factors included hypertension, aspirin ingestion, platelet count less than 20,000/µl and trauma.

Dose of Steroids

Prednisolone is used in the dose of 2 mg/kg/day for two to three weeks followed by tapering of dose over the next week irrespective of platelet count. However, as steroids are being tapered some patients may develop a drop in their platelet count. This is usually transitory and not an indication to step up the dose to previous levels since clinically purpura often improves. In severe cases, for initial 4-5 days, prednisolone may be given in a dose of 4 mg/kg followed by reduction in the dose thereafter to conventional levels. A small number of patients with chronic ITP with recurrent mucosal bleeds or severe thrombocytopenia can be managed successfully with small maintenance dose (0.5-1.0 mg/kg/alternate day or even less) of corticosteroids.

Intravenous Methylprednisolone Pulse Therapy

Intravenous high-dose methylprednisolone pulse (HDMP) therapy of few days' duration—single-dose short course of methylprednisolone 15-25 mg/kg/day on 3 consecutive days has resulted in early response lasting for 3 months or more. The HDMP (given as an oral 7 day course of 30 mg/kg/day for 3 days followed by 20 mg/kg/d for 4 days) has also been used as an alternative to IVIg. One of our patients, a 16-year-old with chronic ITP for 8 years responded well to three doses of methylprednisolone and platelet count increased from 5,000/µl to 1,50,000/µl following which tooth extraction could be done. Similar results have been reported by other authors.

INTRAVENOUS IMMUNOGLOBULIN

The major goal in the treatment of newly diagnosed ITP is to restore the platelet count to relatively safe levels as soon as possible so as to prevent ICH and life threatening hemorrhages. Intravenous immunoglobulin (IVIg) raises the platelet count in more than 80% of children and does so more rapidly than corticosteroids or no therapy. Transient side effects (fever, headache, nausea/vomiting) are highest with a dose of 1 g/kg given on consecutive days. The original IVIg dose of 0.4 g/kg daily for 2 to 5 days has been superseded by short course with a single dose of 0.8 to 1 g/kg, with possible repeat treatment based on the short-term platelet response. The effect of corticosteroids and IVIg were identical for children who responded rapidly to the treatment and IVIg does not offer a major advantage over corticosteroids. However, in steroid nonresponders, IVIg can produce better remissions. Reactions seen in 20% of children are trivial, e.g. headache, fever, vomiting, fatigue, etc. The high cost of IVIg is often a major barrier to its use. As the chance of spontaneous recovery is high and chances of ICH are very low (0-3.3%) routine administration of IVIg is not recommended. Intravenous immunoglobulin should be considered for any patient with ITP in whom rapid rise in platelet count is deemed essential such as before surgery, after significant trauma, especially a child with head injury, menorrhagia, delivery, life-threatening bleeds like gastrointestinal bleeding and ICH, and during pregnancy as steroids are contraindicated. In addition young children below the age of 5 years with severe, recurrent hemorrhage may be given IVIg to postpone/avoid splenectomy. Intravenous immunoglobulin acts by causing temporary reticuloendothelial blockade. This might be due to two separate effects, a decrease in Fc receptor affinity for platelet associated IgG and competition for Fc receptors by the increased serum IgG.

Intravenous Immunoglobulin in Chronic ITP

Intravenous immunoglobulin is effective for temporarily raising the platelet count in 70-80% of children with chronic ITP. Platelet count rises within 1-3 days of infusion. Permanent remission occurs only in minority (0-20%) of these children. A safe count however (above 10-30,000/µl) may be achieved with periodic booster doses.

ANTI-D IN ITP

Rh anti-D globulin has been recommended as an alternative to IVIg in treatment of ITP. Rh anti-D globulins have been tried in varying doses intravenously. Better responses occurred when higher doses and multiple courses were administered. Intravenous anti-D immunoglobulin can be given to Rh(D)-positive children as a short infusion and is usually effective in transiently raising platelet counts. Responses are usually slower in onset when compared to IVIg and are transient. However in some patients sustained responses have been seen, lasting for 6 months to 3 years. Splenectomized and Rh –ve blood group patients respond less well. Anti-D globulin is much less expensive than IVIg. Mild extravascular hemolysis is common and a few instances of intravascular hemolysis, disseminated intravascular coagulation, and renal failure have been reported in pediatric patients with comorbidities. Hemolysis has been observed and patient may need blood transfusions due to anemia caused by IV anti-D globulin. Intravenous anti-D appears to be useful in treatment of ITP as it is cheaper and effective in steroid-refractory patients prior to splenectomy.

Recent reports suggest that a dose of 75 μg/kg over 3-5 minutes is more efficacious than 50 μg/kg dose though the side effects are more common with higher dose. Though occasionally a complete remission has been observed after a single course of anti-D globulin, repeated booster doses at intervals of more than 3 weeks may be required to maintain platelet count at a safe level. A number of children are able to discontinue the therapy during the first year of treatment. The drug is administered slowly in 20-50 ml of saline over 1-2 hours or can be administered fast over 3 minutes. Though the peak platelet counts occur at a mean of 8 days following initial infusion, platelet counts increase significantly in 72 hours.

Emergency Treatment in Children

In organ- or life-threatening situations (as with adult patients), a larger-than-usual dose (2 to 3-fold) of platelets should be infused together with IV high-dose corticosteroids and IVIg or IV anti-D. The goal of treatment is to elevate the platelet count to a level where the risk of severe bleeding is minimized as soon as possible. In special circumstances, emergency splenectomy may need to be considered.

RITUXIMAB

Rituximab is a monoclonal antibody which acts by reducing the number of B-cells which produce autoantibodies. Rituximab is a human murine monoclonal antibody against the CD20 antigen on B lymphocytes. Most studies have used rituximab doses of 375 mg/m^2, lower doses (100 mg IV weekly for 4 weeks) may also be effective, although associated with a longer time to response. At the current time, the standard dose of rituximab for ITP patients is unknown, and, due to the potential toxicity and expense of the agent, future studies are required to identify the optimal dose. High response rates have recently been reported for a combination of rituximab with high-dose dexamethasone as initial therapy. Recent trials have also suggested good response with single dose rituximab. Rituximab has been used with success in children with chronic refractory ITP. Overall, the response rate ($>50 \times 10^9/L$ platelet count) is between 31 and 68%.

Severe side effects after rituximab therapy are fortunately rare but there is potential of neutropenia and reactivation of chronic infections like tuberculosis. Adverse events associated with rituximab are usually mild or moderate, with a low incidence of infections. There are also reports of more than 50 cases of progressive multifocal leukoencephalopathy associated with rituximab treatment for lymphoma and also in limited number of SLE and ITP patients.

THROMBOPOIETIN-RECEPTOR AGONISTS: ROMIPLOSTIM AND ELTROMBOPAG

Thrombopoietin (TPO) is the primary factor regulating platelet production. Two agents, romiplostim and eltrombopag, are FDA-approved for the treatment of ITP. Romiplostim is structurally unrelated to TPO but a potent stimulator of megakaryopoiesis *in vitro*. It is an Fc-fusion protein (also known as a peptibody), i.e. a recombinant protein composed of two domains: a carrier Fc domain and a peptide-containing domain that binds TPO-receptor and thus stimulates megakaryocytopoiesis. It is administered as a 1 to 10 μg/kg subcutaneous weekly injection. Eltrombopag is an oral nonpeptide TPO-receptor agonist administered as a 25, 50, or 75 mg daily dose. It stimulates megakaryocyte differentiation.

Long-term data with romiplostim showed that responses were sustained for up to 4 years on continuous therapy, with most patients able to decrease or discontinue concurrent corticosteroid therapy. TPO-receptor agonists have the potential to minimize morbidity and mortality in these patients.

Due to their mechanism of action, TPO-receptor agonists are considered as a maintenance therapy. Upon cessation of treatment, most patients return to lower platelet counts (~10% transiently falling below baseline platelet counts); however, a few patients are able to discontinue treatment successfully.

Although most adverse effects were mild, concerns have been raised over the increased bone reticulin found in some patients using these agents. No finalized studies in children are available to support the use of these agents in this patient population. Assuming that the long-term safety of these agents is confirmed, they could be used not only for children with chronic refractory ITP, but also in those with persistent but highly symptomatic disease resistant to usual first-line treatments.

DAPSONE (DIAMINO-DIPHENYL SULFONE)

Recently some studies have reported reversal of thrombocytopenia in 40-50% of patients taking dapsone. The dose recommended is 25 to 100 mg per day and it takes about a month for response to be noticed. The effect of this drug is expected to persist for few months before relapse occurs, which demands reinstatement of therapy again. Some researchers believe that dapsone in addition to prednisolone should be recommended for those patients who require low dose steroids for maintenance of high platelet count.

SPLENECTOMY IN ITP

The spleen is the most important site for the destruction of antibody-coated platelets. It is one of the major sites of antiplatelet antibody production. Splenectomy does appear to have a role in the management of ITP. Reported efficacy rates in regard to achieving a stable increased platelet count have varied from 40 to 86% with most reporting approximately 60% responses. Platelet count increased to normal range of 150,000 to 400,000/µl in 5-60 days.

Splenectomy is deferred for as long as possible and the postoperative risk of infection is the major deterrent to its routine use. Splenectomy with appropriate previous vaccination, followed by prophylactic antibiotics, is an effective treatment for pediatric ITP. However, it is rarely recommended in children because the risk of death from ITP in childhood is extremely low (0.5%). The comparative figure associated with post-splenectomy overwhelming sepsis is up to 3% in children. The risk of sepsis probably persists for life. In children who do undergo splenectomy, the overall effectiveness is good, but complications, primarily sepsis, remain a concern.

A few of the indications which justify splenectomy are severe menorrhagia, life-threatening hemorrhage and relentless lifestyle limitation.

SPLENECTOMY IN CHRONIC ITP

For children with bleeding symptoms whose count remains precariously low (less than 10,000/µl), with recurrent mucosal bleeds and, those who do not respond to steroids and IVIg, splenectomy is still an alternative. Response rate to splenectomy in chronic ITP is about 65-88%. There is no definite test by which one can predict response to splenectomy. But some authors have found that the initial response to steroids and thrombokinetic studies could demonstrate predictive relationship. At the time of splenectomy the surgeon should look for accessory spleens which if missed may result in relapse of ITP. Patients who fail to respond to splenectomy or who relapse after an initial response to splenectomy should be studied for the presence of accessory spleen. The incidence of accessory spleen in patients who relapse after splenectomy may be high as 50%. Administration of platelet transfusions prior to surgery usually is not required as platelet count starts rising immediately following surgery (immediately after clamping splenic pedicles) reaching as high as 3,00,000/µl in the immediate postoperative period and reaching a peak within 1-2 weeks and then gradually dropping to normal values by 4-8 months. Though platelet count can rise as high as 1-2 million, there are no reported cases of thrombosis and hence routine administration of antiplatelet drugs like aspirin is not recommended. Platelet transfusions are usually only given if patient has bleeding after the spleen has been removed.

Problems After Splenectomy

Risk of postsplenectomy infection is related to age; it is very high in early infancy and in those with underlying disorders, but an elevated risk appears to persist for life. As compared to ITP, the risk of infection is more when splenectomy is done for diseases like thalassemia major, sickle cell disease and Hodgkin's disease. A detailed review in 1973 estimated the risk of fatal sepsis following splenectomy for ITP to be 1 to 4%. *Pneumococcus* was the commonest infecting organism with adrenal hemorrhages occurring in over 25% of fatal cases. Most deaths occur within first 2-3 years following splenectomy, though deaths are reported as late as 30 years after splenectomy. Children rapidly develop progressive, overwhelming sepsis presenting initially with acute onset of fever, nausea, vomiting and then rapidly progressing with altered sensorium, confusion and leading to convulsion/coma and death within few hours. This may be associated with DIC, electrolyte imbalance and shock. Parents of splenectomized children should be educated and instructed to seek immediate medical attention whenever child develops febrile illness. Broad-spectrum antibiotics by intravenous route are recommended after collecting blood samples for cultures. Third generation cefalosporins should be administered as the first-line of therapy. Prophylactic antibiotics (penicillin), particularly during infancy, are recommended for several years after splenectomy. Pneumococcal vaccine (containing antigen for 23 sero-types) should be administered at least 2-8 weeks prior to the surgery. Revaccination after 5 years is recommended. Other vaccinations such as *H. influenzae*, meningococcal and typhoid vaccine also may be given. With the advent of newer vaccines the incidence of postsplenectomy sepsis has been brought down to less than 1%. Thus splenectomy should not be the first treatment initiated in the management of patients with ITP particularly in children. It should be performed only after all other therapeutic modalities have been exhausted. Late morbidities of splenectomy, low rate of mortality of ITP and the chance of late spontaneous remission of thrombocytopenia have led to deferment of splenectomy indefinitely, particularly in childhood ITP.

ARE IMMUNOSUPPRESSANT DRUGS USEFUL IN CHRONIC ITP?

A small percentage of children (less than 2%) with severe chronic ITP do not respond either to IVIg, steroids or splenectomy and continue to have bleeding tendencies with a platelet count of less than 10-30,000/µl. In these patients, immunosuppressive therapy maybe a useful alternative. Symptomatic patients with platelet count <10-30,000/µl with/or recurrent mucosal bleed, who had initial response to steroid may then be tapered to find the minimum dose that can maintain the patient hemorrhage free even if patients platelet count is not above 30,000/µl. If they can be maintained on minimal dose of 5-10 mg on alternate days, no additional treatment may be needed, particularly in adults.

Nonsteroidal immunosuppressive agents used are vincristine, vinblastine, azathioprine, 6-mercaptopurine, cyclophosphamide and cyclosporin. The overall effectiveness of these potent drugs has been variable and remission achieved short lived. Poor results have been reported in children. Vincristine (0.025 mg/kg not over 2 mg) or vinblastine (0.125 mg/kg) IV is given at weekly intervals for 3-4 doses. In ITP, the mechanism of action has been postulated to be inhibition of microtubular dependent events required for macrocyte-monocyte phagocytic function.

Studies using azathioprine in chronic ITP refractory to splenectomy show marked variation in the rate of remission. The dose used ranged from 1 to 4 mg/kg/day, which may cause mild neutropenia. Three to six months of treatment may be necessary before maximum response is observed. The major side effects, which are encountered relate to granulocytopenia and other features of bone marrow suppression. Cyclophosphamide has been used in ITP with variable success rates. It may be given either orally 1-2 mg/kg/day or intermittently intravenously in a dose of 750-1000 mg/m^2 every three weeks. Response occurs 2-10 weeks after the initiation of therapy and hence drugs must be administered several weeks before platelet count rises and often must be continued for an indefinite period to maintain the remission and side effects like alopecia, bone marrow suppression and cystitis, late malignancy often are significant. Cyclosporin has been recently tried in refractory ITP with transient increase in platelet counts after the treatment. It is known to modulate cell-mediated immunity or alter T-helper cell aspect of humoral immunity. It is given in the dose of 8-10 mg/kg/day in two divided doses continued over 2-3 months. The drug is usually tolerated well without major side effects but a significant rise in glutamine transpeptidase may be present. Secondary lymphomas have been reported. Nonsteroidal immunosuppressive drugs should be used with great caution in children as alkylating agents are known to be mutagenic and increase the risk of subsequent malignancy. Close monitoring of these patients, including WBC count is necessary. Plasmapheresis may be considered as an emergency measure but other measures are probably more effective. Since children with chronic ITP can have a spontaneous remission even many years after their initial diagnosis, it is important to reduce or withdraw the drugs periodically. It has been reported that approximately 0.5-3% of children with chronic ITP will eventually develop autoimmune diseases and hence it is necessary to evaluate children with chronic ITP particularly adolescent females, for evidence of concomitant autoimmune disease.

CONCLUSION

A large majority of pediatric ITP go into remission in a 1-6 months period. Very few of these children have an ICH (<1%) and morbidity is minimum, the dictum of treatment in ITP should be the too frequently forgotten maxim 'first do no harm'. In mild ITP, with cutaneous bleeding and a platelet count >50,000/µl - no drug therapy - defensive management—nonfrantic watchful waiting is the rule. In severe ITP with mucosal bleeding and platelet count of less than 20,000/µl prompt vigorous treatment with steroids should be started. In nonresponders, and during emergency, IVIg should be given. Intravenous anti-D globulin and intravenous methylprednisolone bolus dose may be tried before splenectomy. In chronic ITP treat the child and not the platelet count. No treatment is required for cutaneous purpura and ecchymosis with a platelet count above 20-30,000/µl. For platelet counts less than 20,000/µl and mucosal bleeding, 1-2 courses of steroids may be

American Society of Hematology 2011 Guidelines (for Pediatric Patients)

Diagnosis of ITP

1.1A. We recommend:

- Bone marrow examination is unnecessary in children and adolescents with the typical features of ITP
- Bone marrow examination is not necessary in children who fail IVIg therapy

1.1B. We suggest:

- Bone marrow examination is also not necessary in similar patients prior to initiation of treatment with corticosteroids or before splenectomy
- Testing for antinuclear antibodies is not necessary in the evaluation of children and adolescents with suspected ITP

Initial management of ITP

1.2A. We recommend:

- Children with no bleeding or mild bleeding (defined as skin manifestations only, such as bruising and petechiae) be managed with observation alone regardless of platelet count

Initial pharmacologic management of pediatric ITP

1.3A. We recommend:

- For pediatric patients requiring treatment, a single dose of IVIg (0.8-1 g/kg) or a short course of corticosteroids be used as first-line treatment
- IVIg can be used if a more rapid increase in the platelet count is desired
- Anti-D therapy is not advised in children with a hemoglobin concentration that is decreased due to bleeding, or with evidence of autoimmune hemolysis

1.3B. We suggest:

A single dose of anti-D can be used as first-line treatment in Rh-positive, nonsplenectomized children requiring treatment

Appropriate second-line treatments for pediatric ITP

2.1A. We suggest:

- Rituximab be considered for children or adolescents with ITP who have significant ongoing bleeding despite treatment with IVIg, anti-D, or conventional doses of corticosteroids
- Rituximab may also be considered as an alternative to splenectomy in children and adolescents with chronic ITP or in patients who do not respond favorably to splenectomy
- High-dose dexamethasone may be considered for children or adolescents with ITP who have significant ongoing bleeding despite treatment with IVIg, anti-D, or conventional doses of corticosteroids
- High-dose dexamethasone may also be considered as an alternative to splenectomy in children and adolescents with chronic ITP or in patients who do not respond favorably to splenectomy

Splenectomy for persistent or chronic ITP or ITP unresponsive to initial measures

2.2A. We recommend:

- Splenectomy for children and adolescents with chronic or persistent ITP who have significant or persistent bleeding, and lack of responsiveness or intolerance of other therapies such as corticosteroids, IVIg, and anti-D, and/or who have a need for improved quality of life

2.2B. We suggest:

- Splenectomy or other interventions with potentially serious complications be delayed for at least 12 months, unless accompanied by severe disease defined by the International Working Group as unresponsive to other measures or other quality of life considerations

***H. pylori* testing in children with persistent or chronic ITP**

2.3A. We recommend:

- Against routine testing for *H. pylori* in children with chronic ITP

Management of MMR-associated ITP

3.1A. We recommend:

- Children with a history of ITP who are unimmunized receive their scheduled first MMR vaccine
- In children with either nonvaccine or vaccine-related ITP who have already received their first dose of MMR vaccine, vaccine titers can be checked. If the child displays full immunity (90-95% of children), then no further MMR vaccine should be given. If the child does not have adequate immunity, then the child should be reimmunized with MMR vaccine at the recommended age

given for 3-4 weeks each time. Low dose maintenance may be continued in partial responders at the minimum dose required. Avoid long-term high dose steroids. Nonresponders may be treated with IVIg and booster dose if required or anti-D globulin may be given intravenously along with maintenance booster dose if required. Pulse methylprednisolone therapy is another alternative in a resource-limited setting. Avoid splenectomy in children below 5-6 years and before 1 year from onset of the disease. In 2% of cases who do not respond to above therapy, immunosuppressive drugs may be used with caution. Immune thrombocytopenia in children is generally a benign condition. Only 10-20% of children ultimately develop chronic ITP. Intravenous immunoglobulin (IVIg) or high-dose steroid may benefit some patients who have evidence of clinical bleeding and severe thrombocytopenia and splenectomy may be of value in patients with chronic ITP with recurrent manifestations of bleeding or very low platelet counts. In acute ITP with severe bleeding like intracranial hemorrhage or severe menorrhagia, splenectomy may be indicated above the age of 5 years amongst those children who cannot afford IVIg or are nonresponsive to steroids. In some children with recurrent thrombocytopenia periodic booster dose of IVIg or methylprednisolone may be required so as to keep the platelet count in the safe range. However, there is no way to predict which patients are at a high risk for the development of ICH/severe hemorrhage and which patients will respond to a particular type of therapy and hence the decision to treat the child with ITP is more often based on the clinical picture, severity of bleeding and experience of the clinician rather than only the platelet count.

BIBLIOGRAPHY

1. Blanchette VS, Imbach P, Andrew M, et al. Randomized trial of intravenous immunoglobulin G, intravenous anti-D and oral prednisone in childhood acute immune thrombocytopenic Purpura. Lancet. 1994;344:703-7.
2. Blanchette VS, Luke B, Andrew M, et al. A prospective randomized trial of high dose intravenous immune globulin G therapy, oral prednisolone therapy and no therapy in childhood acute immune thrombocytopenic Purpura. J Pediatr. 1993;123:989-95.
3. George JN, Raskob GE. Idiopathic thrombocytopenic purpura, a concise summary of pathophysiology and diagnosis in children and adults. Semin Hematol. 1998;35:5-8.
4. Harrington WJ, Minnich V, Hollingsworth JW, Moore CV. Demonstration of a thrombocytopenic factor in the blood of patient with thrombocytopenic purpura. J Lab and Clin Med. 1951;38:1-10.
5. Neunert C, Lim W, Crowther M, et al. The American Society of Hematology 2011 evidence-based practice guideline for immune thrombocytopenia. Blood. 2011;117(16):4190-207.
6. Provan D, Stasi R, Newland AC, Blanchette VS, Bolton-Maggs P, Bussel JB, et al. International consensus report on the investigation and management of primary immune thrombocytopenia. Blood. 2010;115:168-86.
7. Rodeghiero F, Stasi R, Gernsheimer T, Michel M, Provan D, Arnold DM, et al. Standardization of terminology, definitions and outcome criteria in immune thrombocytopenic purpura of adults and children: report from an international working group. Blood. 2009;113:2386-93.
8. Sartorius JA. Steroid treatment of idiopathic thrombocytopenic purpura in children. Prelimanary results of a randomized cooperative study. Am J Pediatr Hematol Oncol. 1984;6:165-9.

18 Vitamin K Deficiency Bleeding

Jagdish Chandra

INTRODUCTION

Charles Townsend, towards the last decade of nineteenth century used the term "hemorrhagic disease of newborn" to describe bleeding in early days of life. Though the exact etiology of this bleeding was not known, bleeding due to traumatic delivery, asphyxia and infection were excluded.[1] Later it became obvious that this bleeding was due to deficiency of vitamin K (VK) and consequent fall in VK dependent coagulation factors, the term was still restricted to neonatal period.

Over the last 2-3 decades, two more forms of disease were described: an early HDN manifesting within 24 hours after birth and associated with certain risk factors, and late HDN, which was described to occur in late neonatal period and early infancy.[2-4] The cases resembling the ones originally described were now labeled as classic HDN. For the reasons that bleeding in neonatal period is not always due to VK deficiency and bleeding due to VK deficiency is not restricted to neonatal period, it has been suggested that the term HDN be replaced by a more apt term vitamin K deficiency bleeding (VKDB).[2]

The tendency of the neonate to become VK deficient is in part due to the limited stores available at birth. Biochemical evidence of VK deficiency has been reported in 20-80% newborns, but fortunately, clinical bleeding is rare.[5,6]

DEFINITION AND INCLUSION CRITERIA

Vitamin K deficiency bleeding of late onset has been described as late HDN or acquired prothrombin complex deficiency (APCD), VK deficiency related hemorrhage, and late hemorrhagic disease of infancy from various parts of the world.[2,7-9] In a recent report, the perinatal subcommittee of International Society on Thrombosis and Hemostasis (ISTH), VKDB has been defined as "bleeding due to inadequate activities of VK dependent coagulation factors (II,VII,IX, X), which is correctable by VK replacement".[2]

On the basis of age of onset, ISTH has classified VKDB as: early (onset within 24 hours of birth), classical (onset first week of life, excluding first 24 hours), and late (onset day 8 of life or later). However, as regards this categorization, some discrepancies are noticed in literature. The American Academy of Pediatrics committee on fetus and newborn has used two terms—early (with onset at birth to 2 weeks, formally described as classic HDN) and late—with onset from 2-12 weeks.[10] In the Cochrane review, three categories are maintained but late disease is described with onset from 2-12 weeks.[11] ISTH in their newer guidelines on case definition and diagnostic criteria have recommended to include cases with onset beyond 7 days as late VKDB.[2]

The cut-off for upper age limit for inclusion has also been variable. Most cases of late VKDB (L-VKDB) are seen up to 12 weeks of age, but the upper age limit was extended to six months from an earlier recommendation of 12 weeks as more cases older than 12 weeks were being reported.[2,4] However, Cochrane review and American Academy of Pediatrics till recently have persisted with 12 weeks cut-off.[10,11] In the Indian series, though most cases were under six months at diagnosis, the disease occurred in infants 7 months and 12 months old as well.[5-7] We have also reported cases of L-VKDB occurring in late infancy and beyond.[12] Age restriction in the earlier diagnostic criteria appears mainly due to initial description in neonatal period and the word 'newborn' in the term HDN (as late VKDB was initially described as late HDN). Currently, with the use of the term VKDB, it may appear prudent to include all cases occurring beyond first week of neonatal period as L-VKDB that fulfil other criteria. A recent report from Germany includes cases as old as 35 weeks which further substantiates the case for doing away with upper age restriction for diagnosis.[13]

The ISTH subcommittee laid down the diagnostic criteria as follows—in bleeding infant, prolonged prothrombin time (PT) together with normal fibrinogen level and normal platelet count is highly suggestive of VKDB. Rapid correction of PT within 30-120 minutes after VK administration is confirmatory.[2] In VKDB, prolongation of a PTT is also observed. However, the diagnostic criteria for VKDB included prolongation of PT as isolated prolongation of PT is the earliest laboratory evidence of VK deficiency.[14] The sub-committee also added that circulating acarboxy proteins—PIVKA (protein included in vitamin K absence) are present but this rest may not be routinely available.

INCIDENCE

Cases of L-VKDB were first described by McNinch et al from UK in 1983.[15] In almost a decade or more before that, cases of VKDB were a rarity as prophylactic VK administration in neonatal period was widely practised. In their report on resurgence of VKDB (then HDN), McNinch et al described some cases who were older than one week, were exclusively breastfed and had not received VK prophylaxis. Following this, cases of L-VKDB appeared in Indian literature and from other countries of south-east Asia.

Incidence of classical VKDB is reported to vary between 0.01 and 1.5% while that of L-VKDB in infants without VK prophylaxis is estimated to be 4-10 per 100,000 births. Incidence in India and other developing countries is not clearly known. It is believed to be more common in south-east Asia—the higher incidence is probable related to maternal malnutrition and increased prevalence of diarrheal diseases in infants and children in these regions.[2-4]

In the countries where proper surveys have been done and meticulously recorded, a decline in prevalence with VK prophylaxis is clearly demonstrated, von Kries et al from Germany reported 1.8/100,000 prevalence rate when oral 1 mg × 3 doses of VK were used which decreased to 0.72/100,000 after oral 2 mg × 3 doses schedule was adopted.[17] In Switzerland, where mixed micellar preparation of oral VK is currently used, the prevalence has decreased from 7.2/100,000 in 1986-87 to 2.8/100,000 in 1995-98.[18] In Australia, a decline from 2.5/100,000 when oral 1 mg × 3 doses of VK was in vogue to zero has been observed after 1 mg intramuscular VK administration for prophylaxis was restated.[19]

CLINICAL FEATURES

Late VKDB is more common among boys than girls and in summer than winter months.[2,7,9]

According to etiology or presence of association factors, the disease has been described as *idiopathic*-when no risk factor other than breastfeeding is identified: and *secondary*, when additional risk factors are present.[2] L-VKDB is a disease of exclusively/ predominantly breastfed infants[2,5,7] Initial description of cases of L-VKDB was in "children who were breastfed and who never had received even a few complementary feeds of bottle milk". This is the single most common risk factor (other than not receiving VK prophylaxis) even in cases who are otherwise classified as secondary L-VKDB. Cases from developing countries have not received VK prophylaxis, as up to 80% are home delivered.[16] In countries where oral VK prophylaxis was/is in vogue, cases have occurred even in infants who had received such prophylaxis.[17,18,20] The causes of secondary L-VKDB have included cystic fibrosis, biliary atresia, hepatitis, α-1-antitypsin deficiency and chronic warfarin exposure[9,21,22] L-VKDB secondary to liver disease has accounted for 73 and 87% cases from European countries.[17,18] von Kries et al from Germany have reported cholestasis being detected in 21 of 29 patients after the bleeding episodes. Diseases included bile duct hypoplasia, bile duct atresia, Byler's disease, sclerosing cholangitis and α-1 antitrypsin deficiency.[13] Association with hepatobiliary disease has also been described as the first manifestation of disease.[22] In Indian series, almost all cases have been primary type except 15% reported to have probable liver disease in recent reports.[23,24] Association or past history of diarrheal disease has been recorded in one-third Indian patients.

Bleeding manifestations in these cases may be in the form of minor skin or mucosal bleeds, bleeding from injection sites or cuts, gastrointestinal bleeding or following surgical intervention. Severe life threatening intracranial bleeding is relatively more frequent than classical VKDB.[2,17] Indian data reveal occurrence of intracranial bleeding in 20-90% cases.[7-9,12,23,24] Corresponding Western figures are 58-73%.[17,18] Cases developing L-VKDB after receiving VK prophylaxis tend to be older and are less likely to have intracranial bleeding. Patients presenting with serious bleeds may give history of minor "warning bleeds," such as umbilical oozing, skin bruises or nasal bleeds occurring few days before the intracranial or other serious life threatening bleeds. In cases secondary to liver disease, history of pale stools and dark urine may be elicited.

DIAGNOSIS

In a child with bleeding manifestations, initial diagnostic work-up included a check on platelet count and PT and al PTT estimation. In L-VKDB, as in its classical form PT and a PTT are prolonged. In early and milder cases prolonged PT may be the only abnormality,[14] platelet count is normal. The activity of VK dependent factors (II, VII, IX and X) is decreased. Levels of fibrinogen are normal. PIVKAs are present and their presence is useful in diagnosis even after correction of coagulation defect, as they have a long half-life.[2] Fibrin degradation products (FDP) and D-dimer assay will exclude DIC. Correction of PT rapidly (within 30-120 minutes) after VK administration is diagnostic of VKDB.[2,4] Other confirmatory tests include Echis prothrombin time ratio and measurements of VK concentration, but these tests are rarely available for routine laboratory use.[14] Hereditary coagulation defects of hemophilia group are excluded, as in this groups, only a PTT is abnormal. Rare defects like factors VII deficiency will be excluded on the observation that clinical improvement and significant shortening or normalization of PT after VK L-VKDB, a careful search for associated factors particularly presence of hepatobiliary disease is warranted as many a times L-VKDB may be the only initial manifestation in such cases.

TREATMENT

As in all deficiency states, replacement is the treatment required. Replacement with VK needs to be rapidly effective as L-VKDB is often associated with potentially life threatening intracranial bleeding. In a child suspected to have L-VKDB. Intravenous or subcutaneous administration of VK is recommended. Intravenous injections can result in anaphylactoid reaction possibly due to presence of polyethoxylated castor oil triggering histamine relese.[14,25] Therefore, intramuscular administration is avoided, because of the danger of deep hematoma formation. A dose of 1 mg is usually given; however, doses as high as 2-5 mg have been recommended. VK should be used with caution in neonates with jaundice. The affected cases may require plasma, fresh frozen plasma, or prothrombin complex infusion.[14] When required,10-15 ml/kg of FFP should be infused which will increase the VK dependent factors levels to 10-20 IU/dl. Care should be taken to avoid fluid overload. Prothrombin complex concentrates are required in children with life threatening bleeds. In the absence of data in neonates, based on adult studies a dose of 50 u/kg has been suggested.[14] Packed red cell transfusion may be required in cases with anemia due to substantial blood loss. Meticulous supportive care is needed particularly in cases with intracranial bleeding.

PROGNOSIS

Cases with minor bleeds respond well to VK administration alone or in combination with plasma transfusion. The cases with intracranial hemorrhage have high morbidity and mortality. In developing countries where neurosurgical intervention is not easily available, mortality has been reported in 30-50% cases.[16-24] Survivors are left with debilitating disability.

PREVENTION

For prevention of HDN/VKDB, American Academy of Pediatrics recommends neonatal VK administration since 1961. VK is administered intramuscularly though oral route has also been found to be effective as far as prevention of classical type VKDB is concerned. In addition, oral route has an appeal of being less expensive, less traumatic. One mg VK administration as practised in USA and Sweden has completely eliminated VKDB, including the late onset type.[2,25-27]

Association of parenteral VK administration and risk of cancer in later childhood was reported in 1992. It is suggested that plasma VK concentration 12-24 hours after 1 mg VK administration are approximately 5000 fold higher than found in normal breastfed infants. Such high concentration of VK has been shown to be associated with increased sister chromatid exchange *in vitro*. Vitamin K_1 has been incriminated to have an adjuvant role in mutagenecity and carcinogenicity of certain compounds.[28-30] This report led many counties to switch to oral VK prophylaxis. Different strategies are followed in these countires—1 mg oral dose × 3 (during neonatal period), 2 mg × 3 or 1 mg in neonatal period followed by 25 μg daily oral dose of all babies till 13 weeks of age. Surveillance data on these forms of prophylaxis has revealed that 1 mg × 3 doses is not as effective as intramuscular administration for preventing L-VKDB. Daily administration is probably as effective as parenteral administration. Using 2 mg × 3 schedule has also not provided complete protection against L-VKDB. Australia lately has reverted back to intramuscular prophylaxis and has noticed almost complete disappearance of L-VKDB.[19] In Germany and Sweden, fat-soluble oral VK was replaced by a new water-soluble mixed-micellar analogue of VK1. This preparation was thought to be better absorbed in presence of liver disease, but the results are variable.[13,31] In Germany, surveillance data following use of mixed micellar oral preparation (3×2 mg doses) showed L-VKDB in 0.44/100,000 children compared to 0.76/100,000 children with use of other preparations. Mixed micellar preparation thus did not significantly improve the efficacy of 3×2 mg oral VK prophylaxis schedule. Moreover, the preparation is not being widely marketed.[19,25] AAP has reiterated its stand regarding universal administration of parenteral VK in neonatal period.[10] More data on VK and cancer has accumulated. While these studies have failed to confirm the risk, it is realized that it is difficult to prove that no risk exists.

REFERENCES

1. Townsend CW. The haemorrhagic disease of newborn. Arch Paediatr; 1894. pp. 1747-52.
2. Sutor AH, von Kries R, Marlies Conelissen EA, McNinch AW, Andrew M. Vitamin K deficiency bleeding (VKDB) in infancy. Thrombo Haemost. 1999;81:456-61.
3. Narang A. Hemorrhagic disease of newborn. Indian Pediatr. 1989;26:523-4.
4. von Kries R, Hanawa Y. Neonatal vitamin K prophylaxis. Thrombo Haemost. 1993;69:293-5.
5. Greer F, Marshall SP, Severson RR, et al. A new mixed micellar preparation for vitamin K prophylaxis. Arch Dis Child. 1998;79:300-5.
6. von Kries R, Shearer MJ, Goebel U. Vitamin K in infancy. Eur J Paediatr. 1988;147:106-12.
7. Marwaha RK, Kumar A, Garewal G, Marwaha N, Walia BNS. Vitamin K deficiency related bleeding manifestations in older neonates and infants. Indian Pediatrics. 1987;24:307-11.
8. Merchant RH, Divekar RM. Late hemorrhagic disease with intracranial hemorrhage. Indian Pediatr. 1988;25:381-4.
9. Merchant RH, Divekar R, Shah MD. Late hemorrhagic disease of infancy. Indian Pediatr. 1989;26:553-8.
10. American Academy of Pediatrics Committee on Fetus and Newborn: Controversies concerning vitamin K and the newborn. J Pediatr. 2003;112:191-2.
11. Puckett RM, Offringa M. Prophylactic vitamin K for vitamin K deficiency bleeding in neonates (Cochrane review). In The Cochrane Library, Issue 3, 2004. Chicheser UK: John Wiley and sons Ltd.
12. Chandra J, Naithani R, Chhetri A, Singh V, et al. Serious and life-threatening bleeding in late vitamin K deficiency. Ann Tropical Pediatr. 2007;27:241-2.
13. von Kries R, Hachmeister A, Gobel U. Oral mixed micellar vitamin K for prevention of late vitamin K deficiency bleeding. Arch Dis Child. 2003;88:109-19.
14. Guideline (UK). The investigation and management of neonatal hemostasis and thrombosis. Br J Haematol. 2002;119:295-309.
15. McNinch AW, L'Orme R, Tripp JH. Hemorrhagic disease of newborn returns. The lancet. 1983;1:1089-90.
16. Choo KE, Tan KK, Chuah SP, et al. Hemorrhagic disease of newborn and infants: a study of hospitalized children in Kelanatan, Malaysia. Ann Trop Pediatr. 1994;14:231-7.
17. von Kries R, Hachmeister A, Gobel U. Can 3 oral 2 mg doses of vitamin K effectively prevent late vitamin K deficiency in bleeding? Eur J Pediatr. 1999;158 Suppl 3 (6):S183-6.
18. Schubiger G, Stocker C, Banziger 0, Laubscher B, Zimmermann H. Oral vitamin K prophylaxis for newborns with a new mixed-micellar preparation of phylloquinone: 3 year experience in Switzerland. Eur J Pediatr. 1999;158: 599-602.
19. Cornelissen M, von Kries R, Loughnan P, Schubiger G. Prevention of vitamin K deficiency bleeding: Efficacy of different multiple oral dose schedules of vitamin K. Eur J of Pediatr. 1997;156:126-30.
20. Humpl T, Ruhl K, Brezinska R, Hafrier G, Coerdt W, Shearer MJ. Fatal vitamin K deficiency after oral vitamin K prophylaxis secondary to unrecognized bile duct paucity. J Pediatr Gastro Nutr. 1999;29:594-7.
21. Lane PA, Hathway WE. Vitamin D in infancy. J Pediatr. 1985;106:351.
22. Shenoi A, Marwaha RK, Singh RP, Banerjee CK. Late hemorrhagic disease: A first manifestation of neonatal hepatitis due to alpha-1-antitrypsisn deficiency. Indian Pediatr. 1989;26:838-40.
23. D'Souza IE, Subba Rao SD. Late hemorrhagic disease of newborn. Indian Pediatr 2003;40:226-9.
24. Pooni PA, Singh D, Jain BK. Intracranial hemorrhage in late hemorrhagic disease of newborn. Indian Pediatr. 2003;40: 243-8.
25. Hey E. Vitamin K- what why and when. Arch Dis Child Fetal Neonatal Ed. 2003;88:80-3.
26. Committee on Nutrition, American Academy of Pediatrics. Vitamin K compounds and water-soluble analogues: Use in therapy and prophylaxis in pediatrics. J Pediatr. 1961;26:501-7.
27. Sen S, Kumari S, Narayan S, Bains C, Dutta AK. Efficacy of oral water soluble vitamin K in neonates. Indian Pediatr. 1989;26:992-5.
28. Golding J, Greenwood R, Birmingham K, Mott M. Childhood cancer, intravascular vitamin K and pethidine given during labour. BMJ. 1992;305:341-6.
29. McNinch AW, Upton C, Samuels M, et al. Plasma concentration after oral and intramuscular vitamin K in neonates. Arch Dis Child. 1985;60:814-8.
30. Israels LG, Freissen E, Jansen AH, Israels ED. Vitamin K increases sister chromatin exchange in-vitro in human leucocytes and *in vivo* fetal cells: a possible role for 'vitamin K deficiency' in the fetus. Ped Research. 1997;22:405-8.
31. Pereira SP, Shearer MJ, Williams R, Mieli-Vergani G. Intestinal absorption of mixed micellar phylloquinolone (vitamin K 1) is unreliable in infants with conjugated hyperbilirubinemia: implications for oral prophylaxis of vitamin K deficiency bleeding. Arch Dis Child Fetal Neonatal Ed. 2003;88:113-8.

19 Neonatal Thrombocytopenia

Nivedita Dhingra, Sachin Thakur, Anupam Sachdeva

The normal platelet counts in a preterm baby are slightly lower than that in a full-term baby but are essentially in the range of 150,000/μl to 450,000/μl.[1] Thrombocytopenia in preterm and full-term infants is defined as platelet counts below 150,000/μl, same as in adults.[2] It can be classified into four groups, mild (platelet count 100-149 × 10^9/L), moderate (platelet count 50-99 × 10^9/L), severe (platelet count 30-49 × 10^9/L) or very severe (platelet count < 30 × 10^9/L), according to standard classification.[3] The significance of platelet counts between 1,00,000/μl and 1,50,000/μl is unclear in neonates, as many normal babies have counts in this range, and requires monitoring of the patient with repeat counts but a platelet count below 1,00,000 is definitely abnormal at any gestational age and needs further evaluation.

Thrombocytopenia is seen in 0.7-0.12% of newborns but the incidence increases to 0.28% if babies developing thrombocytopenia in the first few days of life are included.[2,4] Oren et al have reported an incidence of thrombocytopenia in 18.2% of the preterms and 0.8% of the term neonates admitted to the NICU.[5] It is more common in sick newborns admitted to the NICU with 35% of them having low counts.[6] Often there is no definite cause that can be found in these sick newborns for the thrombocytopenia. Some of the reasons for the low count may be:

- Lower ploidy and size of preterm and term megakaryocytes, thus producing less number of platelets
- Lower levels of thrombopoietin (TPO)
- Lesser number of megakaryocyte precursors
- Increased destruction of platelets.

The underlying cause of neonatal thrombocytopenia can often be predicted by the timing of the onset of the thrombocytopenia and its natural history[7] (Table 19.1).

Neonatal Alloimmune Thrombocytopenia

Neonatal alloimmune thrombocytopenia (NAIT) is seen in approximately 10-20% of babies with neonatal thrombocytopenia and is seen in an otherwise healthy appearing baby.[1] The pathogenesis is somewhat similar to that of erythroblastosis fetalis and is due to the maternal antibodies directed against the baby's antigens. When there is an incompatibility between the maternal and fetal platelet antigens then the mother may get sensitized to the antigens on the baby's platelets and mount an immune response. Platelet antigens appear in the fetus in early gestation and the maternal antibodies can cross into the baby in the 2nd trimester thus causing fetal thrombocytopenia in the first pregnancy itself. The

Table 19.1: Conditions causing fetal and neonatal thrombocytopenia

Fetal
- Alloimmune
- Congenital infections (e.g. *CMV*, *Toxoplasma*, Rubella)
- Aneuploidies (e.g. trisomies 18, 13, 21)
- Autoimmune (e.g. SLE, ITP)
- Severe Rh hemolytic disease
- Inherited (e.g. Wiskott-Aldrich syndrome)

Early onset neonatal (<72 hours)
- Chronic fetal hypoxia (e.g. PIH, IUGR, diabetes)
- Perinatal asphyxia
- Perinatal infection (e.g. *E. coli*, *GBS*, *H. influenzae*)
- DIC
- Alloimmune
- Autoimmune (e.g. SLE, ITP)
- Congenital infections (e.g. CMV, *Toxoplasma*, Rubella)
- Thrombosis (e.g. aortic, renal vein)
- Bone marrow replacement (e.g. congenital leukemia)
- Kasabach-Merritt syndrome
- Metabolic disease (e.g. propionic and methylmalonic academia)
- Inherited (e.g. CAMT, TAR)

Late onset neonatal (>72 hours)
- Late onset sepsis
- NEC
- Congenital Infections (e.g. CMV, *Toxoplasma*, Rubella)
- Autoimmune (e.g. SLE, ITP)
- Kasabach-Merritt syndrome
- Metabolic disease (e.g. propionic and methylmalonic academia)
- Inherited (e.g. CAMT, TAR)

Table 19.2: Platelet antigen systems

Antigen systems	*Other names*	*Antigens*
HPA-1	Zw, P1A	HPA-1aHPA-1b
HPA-2	Ko, Sib	HPA-2aHPA-2b
HPA-3	Bak, Lek	HPA-3aHPA-3b
HPA-4	Pen, Yuk	HPA-4aHPA-4b
HPA-5	Br, Zav, Hc	HPA-5aHPA-5b
HPA-6	Ca, Tu	HPA-6b
HPA-7	Mo	HPA-7b
HPA-8	Sr	HPA-8b
HPA-9W	Max	HPA-9Wb

Adapted from American Medical Association Manual of Style. Baltimore: Williams and Wilkins; 1998. p. 343.

common antigen responsible for this immune thrombocytopenia is HPA1-a (also known as PLA-1) in the Caucasian population and HPA-4 (or Yuk/ Pen) for the Asian population.[8,9] The various antigens involved in the pathogenesis are as given in Table 19.2. Studies have also described an association between the maternal HLA class II and alloimmunization against platelet specific antigens (DR52a and antibodies against HPA-1a antigens and DR6 and antibodies against HPA-5b antigens). The severity of thrombocytopenia also depends on several factors like:

1. Density of the antigen on the platelets.
2. Birth order.
3. Ability of the antibody to fix complement.

Clinical Features

Up to 81% of the affected newborns with NAIT present with petechiae, purpura or bleeding at birth. The classic patient is a healthy neonate with severe thrombocytopenia (<50,000/µl) at birth without the clinical findings of sepsis or factors that account for thrombocytopenia. Ten to fifteen percent of newborns with NAIT may also present with an intracranial bleed and in half of these the bleed is *in utero*.[10] Specific antibodies associated with severe symptoms, including perinatal intracerebral hemorrhage (ICH), are anti-HPA-1a, anti-HPA-4a, anti-HPA-3a, anti-HPA-1b, and anti-HPA-5b. Differential diagnosis also includes sepsis, maternal ITP, maternal drug exposure and other rare causes of neonatal thrombocytopenia.

Laboratory Diagnosis

Thrombocytopenia within first 3 days of life is uniformly present in babies with NAIT with normal maternal platelet counts. The diagnosis of NAIT is made by demonstrating platelet antigen incompatibility between mother and baby serologically. The monoclonal antibody-specific immobilization of platelet antigens (MAIPA) assay is the main technique used for HPA antibody detection and identification of maternal platelet-specific antibodies.[7] Up to 85% of the maternal sera thus tested will show antibodies specific for the implicated antigen, though the absence of detectable maternal antibodies does not rule out NAIT. The parents and infant are also genotyped for the HPA alloantigens. In general, there are no validated laboratory parameters (e.g. titer of antibody) which predict the severity of NAIT, and therefore, prediction of severity tends to be based on history of previously affected pregnancies and estimation of fetal platelet counts.[7] Two investigations commonly available to the clinician to test the rate of production and rate of destruction of the platelets are mean platelet volume (MPV) and the rate of fall of platelet count after a platelet transfusion, respectively. The mean platelet volume may be increased reflecting an increase in the platelet production in the marrow (younger platelets have larger MPV). This is available in the routine electronic counters but may not be very specific for reflecting the rate of platelet production and may be decreased in some instances. So the routine use of MPV is not very helpful in making clinical decisions. The rate of fall of post-transfusion platelet count is generally a good indicator that an immune process is involved in the pathogenesis of thrombocytopenia. In adults patients with ITP, mean platelet survival is 2.7 ± 0.9 days and a similarly shortened lifespan has been seen in neonates with immune mediated thrombocytopenia.

Treatment

Prevention of any bleeding complication is the goal of treating NAIT. Neonates with NAIT, or those with an unexplained platelet count below 50,000/µl and presumed NAIT, have a high-risk of ICH and should have their platelet count maintained above 50,000/µl in the first 2 weeks of life pending diagnosis. All babies with severe thrombocytopenia due to NAIT should also have a cranial USG to look for evidence of ICH. Ideally these transfusions should be with platelets that lack the specific antigen. Most common source for this is the washed maternal platelets collected via plasmapheresis, which are negative for the offending platelet antigen. Maternal platelets need to be washed thoroughly for removing any antibody in the serum, which may cause further platelet destruction in the baby. Random platelet concentrates have been used, if there is an urgent need to transfuse, and studies have shown an adequate response in up to 40% of the cases.

Table 19.3: Guidelines for platelet transfusion in neonates[7]

Platelet count 10^9/L	*Nonbleeding neonate (1st week of life)*	*Nonbleeding neonate (week 2 onwards)*	*Neonate with major bleeding*	*Autoimmune thrombocytopenia*	*NAIT (suspected case)*	*NAIT (known case)*
<30	Transfuse all patients	Transfuse all patients	Transfuse	Transfuse if bleeding present or IVIg unavailable	Transfuse using HPA-1a/5b negative platelets	Transfuse using HPA compatible platelets
30-49	Do not transfuse, if clinically stable Transfusion appropriate if: • <1000 g and <1 week of age • Clinically unstable • Previous major bleeding tendency (IVH grade 3-4) • Surgery or exchange transfusion • Concurrent coagulopathy	Do not transfuse	Transfuse	Do not transfuse, if stable and not bleeding	Transfuse using HPA-1a/5b negative platelets	Transfuse using HPA compatible platelets
50-99	Do not transfuse	Do not transfuse	Transfuse	Do not transfuse	Transfuse using HPA-1a/5b negative platelets	Transfuse using HPA compatible platelets

High dose IVIg has been successful in increasing platelet counts within 24-48 hours and may eliminate the need to transfuse platelets in milder cases and may be used as adjunctive therapy along with platelet transfusions in cases with severe thrombocytopenia. In new cases without major bleeding with an initial count >50 × 10^9/L an expectant approach is appropriate. In thrombocytopenic neonates with active bleeding (e.g. new or worsening ICH, gastrointestinal, frank hematuria) it seems reasonable to maintain the platelet count above 100 × 10^9 /L (Table 19.3).

Antenatal Management

The purpose of antenatal diagnosis is to prevent intracranial hemorrhages, which occur in 10-20% of untreated pregnancies.[11] Currently, there are no screening programs available for detecting first time mothers at risk for delivering babies with NAIT, but subsequent pregnancies can be monitored for intracranial bleeds and fetal platelet counts. The maternal and paternal platelet antigens can be typed to predict the occurrence of NAIT in subsequent pregnancies. Using percutaneous umbilical blood sampling (PUBS) at 18 weeks of gestation, a fetal blood sample can be collected to assess the platelet count and the antigen type to decide the plan of management. Affected fetus can be treated with maternal administration of high dose IVIg with or without dexamethasone and this has been shown to be effective in 75% of the cases. Repeat PUBS can be done to monitor the platelet count and to treat with intrauterine platelet transfusions if needed. Cesarean delivery may be planned, if the platelet counts are low and there is history of intracranial bleeds in previous siblings.

Thrombocytopenia remains a common finding in the NICU and 60% of the babies do not have a definitive cause for the low platelet count. Most of the thrombocytopenias improve with the improvement of the underlying cause. Neonatal alloimmune thrombocytopenia is the only category of thrombocytopenia associated with high frequency of intracranial bleeds and approximately 25% of these babies may have persistent neurological sequelae. Neonatal alloimmune thrombocytopenia has an overall mortality of 1-14% and presents in subsequent pregnancies too, though the outcome in later pregnancies is better as antenatal diagnosis and intervention improve the overall outcome.[12]

NEONATAL AUTOIMMUNE THROMBOCYTOPENIA

In the presence of maternal autoimmune thrombocytopenia (ITP or another autoimmune condition), placental transfer of IgG antibody may result in neonatal thrombocytopenia. The antibodies in this context are directed against antigens common to both maternal and fetal platelets. The estimated incidence of maternal ITP is between 1 and 5/10,000 pregnancies, however, clinically significant neonatal thrombocytopenia is relatively uncommon. Significant neonatal thrombocytopenia (platelets <50 × 10^9/L) occurs in approximately 10% of the neonates whose mothers have autoantibodies and the incidence of ICH is 1% or less.

Unlike NAIT the platelet nadir usually occurs a few days post delivery and bleeding problems *in utero* or at delivery are rare. It should be noted that the count can be normal at birth and fall subsequently, necessitating serial platelet counts. The condition is self-limiting and the count is usually normalized by 2-3 months of age. Where the platelet count is <50 × 10^9/L, treatment options include IVIg and corticosteroids. IVIg (2 g/kg over 2-5 days) is effective in the majority of cases and produces a relatively rapid response. The response to platelet transfusion is generally poor and this should only be used in infants with life-threatening hemorrhagic problems.

Management of the fetus in the presence of maternal ITP remains controversial and there is no evidence that any maternal therapy increases the fetal platelet count. In addition, there is no correlation between the maternal and neonatal platelet counts and there is currently no reliable method which can be used to predict the development of clinically significant neonatal thrombocytopenia. Fetal scalp sampling has now been abandoned in most centers due to the risk of bleeding and the inaccurate counts. Fetal blood sampling has been advocated by some authors but carries a significant procedural mortality which may be higher in the severely thrombocytopenic fetus and may not be justified by the number of infants at risk. Routine cesarean section for maternal ITP has not been shown to improve fetal outcome and, as the risk of neonatal hemorrhage is low, the route of delivery should be determined primarily by obstetric factors.

NONIMMUNE THROMBOCYTOPENIA

Thrombocytopenia in the neonatal period is most frequently secondary and nonimmune in origin. Especially in sick preterm infants, the etiology is often multifactorial with birth asphyxia, acidosis, RDS, necrotizing enterocolitis and sepsis often coexisting. The underlying mechanism in these cases is thought to relate predominantly to increased platelet destruction due to underlying DIC, and thrombocytopenia may occur alone or as part of a generalized coagulopathy.

Congenital intrauterine infections are frequently associated with thrombocytopenia. In addition to increased destruction, reduced platelet production, and splenic pooling all contribute to the thrombocytopenia in this situation. In a study looking at the platelet counts of fetuses with known congenital infections low platelet counts were found in rubella in 20%, toxoplasmosis in 26% and cytomegalovirus (CMV) in 36% of cases.[13] Thrombocytopenia in this study was most marked in cases of CMV infection. In general, however, congenital infections are an uncommon cause of severe (<20 × 10^9/L) thrombocytopenia. HIV infection can also lead to thrombocytopenia, but this is an uncommon presentation in the neonatal period.

Rare causes of thrombocytopenia caused by increased platelet consumption include giant hemangiomas (Kasabach-Merritt syndrome) and extensive thrombosis.

HEREDITARY THROMBOCYTOPENIA

A number of hereditary syndromes associated with thrombocytopenia may also present in the neonatal period.

Decreased Platelet Production

Thrombocytopenia due to decreased platelet production is uncommon, accounting for <5% of all cases of neonatal thrombocytopenia. Nevertheless, in many of these cases, thrombocytopenia is severe and affected infants are at risk of serious hemorrhage, including ICH. Chromosomal abnormalities are a well recognized but relatively uncommon cause of neonatal thrombocytopenia. The platelet count is usually only mildly reduced and clinical bleeding is uncommon. The diagnosis is almost always obvious due to the presence of characteristic associated abnormalities. The prevalence of thrombocytopenia in this setting is not known, although useful data come from a series of fetal blood samples, which found a high frequency of thrombocytopenia in association with trisomy 18 (86%) and triploidy (75%) and a lower frequency in Turner syndrome (31%), trisomy 13 (31%), and trisomy 21 (6%).[13] The mechanism of thrombocytopenia is incompletely understood but is thought to involve defects in megakarocyte maturation.

Two amegakaryocytic syndromes are recognized: thrombocytopenia with absent radii (TAR) and congenital amegakaryocytic thrombocytopenia (CAMT). TAR, which is recessively inherited, is characterized by early thrombocytopenia which may be severe, together with bilateral hypoplastic or absent radii. More than 50% have thrombocytopenia either at birth or within the first week of life, with 38% of affected infants having a platelet count of <10 × 10^9/L. More recently, TAR has been diagnosed prenatally, and it is clear that thrombocytopenia does develop *in utero*. Although deaths have been reported in infancy, the natural history of the condition is for the thrombocytopenia gradually to resolve with complete or near complete normalization of the platelet count usually occurring during the first few years of life.

Fanconi's anemia is also recessively inherited and typically with marrow hypoplasia in association with a variable pattern of coexisting sensitivity to DNA damage by alkylating agents and ionizing radiation and the diagnosis can be confirmed by performing chromosome breakage studies following exposure to clastogenic agents such as diepoxybutane (DEB) and mitomycin C. In Fanconi's anemia, although thrombocytopenia is often an early hematologic finding, it usually presents after the neonatal period.

Congenital leukemia, neuroblastoma, and histiocytosis may present with thrombocytopenia in the neonatal period as a consequence of marrow infiltration.

REFERENCES

1. Uhrynowska M, Maslanka K, Zupanska B. Neonatal Thrombocytopenia: Incidence, serological and clinical observations. Am J Perinatol. 1997;14(7):415-8.
2. Andrew M, Kelton J. Neonatal thrombocytopenia. Clin Perinatol. 1984;11(2):359-91.
3. Sola-Visner M, Saxonhouse MA, Brown RE. Neonatal thrombocytopenia: what we do and don't know. Early Hum Dev. 2008;84:499-506.
4. Burrows RF, Kelton JG. Fetal thrombocytopenia and its relation to maternal thrombocytopenia. N Engl J Med. 1993; 329(20):1463-6.
5. Oren H, Irken G, Oren B, Olgun N, Ozkan H. Assessment of clinical impact and predisposing factors for neonatal thrombocytopenia. Indian J Pediatr. 1994;61(5):551-8.
6. Mehta P, Vasa R, Neumann L, Karpatkin M. Thrombocytopenia in high-risk infant. J Pediatr. 1980;97(5):791-4.
7. Roberts I, Stanworth S, Muttay NA. Thrombocytopenia in the neonate. Blood Rev. 2008;22(4):173-86.
8. Homans A. Thrombocytopenia in the neonate. Pediatr Clin North Am. 1996;43(3):737-56.
9. George D, Bussel J. Neonatal thrombocytopenia. Semin Thromb Hemost 1995;21(3):276-93.
10. Blanchette VS. Neonatal alloimmune thrombocytopenia: a clinical perspective. Curr Stud Hematol Blood Transfus. 1988;54:112-26.
11. Ghevaert C, Campbell K, Walton J, et al. Management and outcome of 200 cases of fetomaternal alloimmune thrombocytopenia. Transfusion. 2007;47:901-10.
12. Bonacossa IA, Jocelyn LJ. Alloimmune thrombocytopenia of the newborn: neurodevelopmental sequelae. Am J Perinatol. 1996;13:211-5.
13. Hohlfeld P, Forestier F, Kaplan C, Tissot JD, Daffos F. Fetal thrombocytopenia: a retrospective survey of 5,194 fetal blood samplings. Blood. 1994;84:1851-6.

Hypercoagulable Disease in Children and its Diagnostic Approach

R Saxena

Hypercoagulability or thrombophilia is defined as an increased tendency of blood to clot, which may manifest as thrombosis. Thrombosis may be arterial or venous.[1] Manifestations of venous thromboembolism include deep vein thrombosis (DVT), pulmonary embolism, superficial thrombophlebitis, and rarely, mesenteric or cerebral vein thrombosis. Arterial thrombotic manifestations include gangrene of fingers and toes, skin necrosis or stroke due to cerebral arterial thrombosis. In a preliminary study by Lawson et al, 43% of children presenting with symptomatic thromboembolism were found to have congenital thrombophilia.[2] The manifestations of inherited thrombotic disorders occurred in less than 5% of affected children compared with about 40% of adults.[3] Neonates have been found to be at the greatest risk of childhood thromboembolic complications and the incidence decreases significantly after the first year of life.[4]

Thrombophilic states may be divided into the following categories:

1. Acquired hypercoagulable state.
2. Inherited hypercoagulable state.
3. Mixed (inherited and acquired) hypercoagulable state.

ACQUIRED HYPERCOAGULABLE STATE

Several causes may lead to thrombosis in children. Central venous line was detected as a major acquired risk factor.[5] Other associated risk factors are peripartum asphyxia, infection, dehydration and congenital heart disease.[6,7] Although various inherited prothrombotic defects have been well established as risk factors of thromboembolism in adults, the impact of inherited prothrombotic defects in neonatal thrombosis remains inadequately defined. Apart from these, several systemic diseases may be associated with hypercoagulable state (Table 20.1). Thrombosis may be secondary to reduced antithrombotic proteins (ATIII, Pr C, or S) as in nephrotic syndrome (due to excessive protein loss) liver disease (reduced synthesis) disseminated intravascular coagulation (increased consumption), drugs like L-asparginase. In patients with connective tissue disorders or antiphospholipid syndromes, associated anticardiolipin antibodies or lupus anticoagulants predispose to thrombosis.

In diabetes mellitus, vasculitis, fractures, immobilization, postsurgery, pregnancy and steroid therapy, elevated levels of von Willebrand's factor, factor VIII, VII, X, XI or fibrinogen may contribute to hypercoagulability. Impaired fibrinolytic potential, described in patients with hypertriglyceridemia, insulin resistance syndrome and obesity may predispose to hypercoagulability.

INHERITED HYPERCOAGULABLE STATES

Inherited hypercoagulable states may be secondary to deficiency of natural clotting in inhibitors (Table 20.2). Amongst these, activated protein C (APC) resistance, secondary to FV Leiden defect (replacement of arginine

Table 20.1: The secondary hypercoagulable states

- Central venous line catheter
- Abnormalities of coagulation and fibrinolysis
  - Malignancy
  - Infusion of prothrombin complex concentrates
  - Nephrotic syndrome
  - Liver diseases
- Abnormalities of platelets
  - Paroxysmal nocturnal hemoglobinuria
  - Hyperlipidemia
  - Diabetes mellitus
- Abnormalities of blood vessels and rheology
  - Condition promoting venous stasis
  - Artifical surfaces
  - Vasculitis and chronic occlusive arterial disease
  - Thrombotic thrombocytopenic purpura
- Sickle cell disease
- Megaloblastic anemia

Table 20.2: The inherited hypercoagulable state

- Antithrombin III deficiency
- Protein C and S deficiency
- Disorders of the fibrinolytic system
- Dysfibrinogenemia
- Factor XII deficiency
- Factor V Leiden defect
- P 20210
- Homocystinuria
- FVIII levels

at 506 position in FV molecule, by glycine) is the most common cause, seen in 20-50% patients with inherited thrombophilia. It has an autosomal dominant inheritance. Heterozygosity for FV Leiden mutation confers an 8-fold increased risk, whereas homozygosity confers 50-100-fold increased risk of DVT. Its prevalence in children (1-12 years age) is comparable to that in adults and may be associated with arterial or venous thrombosis.

Inherited deficiency of protein C, a vitamin K-dependent anticoagulant protein, which inactivates activated FV and VIII, constitutes 2-3% cases of inherited thrombophilia. Homozygous deficiency presents as life threatening neonatal thrombosis or purpura fulminans. Heterozygous deficiency is seen in 1-5% of general population. 50% of heterozygotes may show thrombosis. Its deficiency often causes warfarin induced skin necrosis since warfarin further reduces protein C levels causing thrombosis in skin capillaries leading to necrosis type I (qualitative), type II (quantitative), and type III (quantitative + quantitative) defects are described.

Deficiency of free protein S, another vitamin K dependent protein, which serves as a cofactor to protein C, is seen in 0.1-5% of general population and 2.3% of DVT patients. It is often associated with arterial thrombosis. As in protein C deficiency, qualitative and quantitative defects (Types I-III) are described. Deficiency of ATIII, which inactivates thrombin, is found in 0.2% general population. It has an autosomal dominant inheritance and constitutes 5-10% of DVT patients. Qualitative and quantitative defects (Types I-III) can occur. Since heparin combines with ATIII to inactivate thrombin in patients with ATIII deficiency, the antithrombotic action of heparin is markedly reduced in these patients.

FV Leiden is the most frequent molecular defect seen in thrombophilia in Caucasians children. It has been found in 31.8% children with venous thrombosis, 20.3% of children (>6 months) suffering from spontaneous ischemic stroke, 18.7% of neonatal ischemic stroke and about 4.1% of healthy Caucasians. Protein C and protein S deficiency has been found in 9.2% and 5.7% respectively in children of venous thrombosis. Protein C deficiency is found in 6.1% children of spontaneous ischemic stroke. Hyperhomocysteinemia secondary to homozygous C to T substitution at nucleotide position 677 of the 5, 10 MTHFR gene has been found in 23.6% and 16.5% of children >6 months and neonates suffering from ischemic stroke respectively and 10.5% controls. Mutation at nucleotide position 20210 of the prothrombin gene is found in 4.2% of children of venous thrombosis (controls - 1.1%), 6.1% (controls - 1.4%) and 4.4% (controls - 2.2%) of children >6 months and neonates of ischemic stroke respectively. As a result of this mutation, these patients have FII levels >115 IU/dl, which increases the risk of DVT 2 times. However this is not seen in Indians.

Hyperhomocysteinemia with homocysteine levels greater than 18.5 µmol/L increases the thrombotic risk 2.5-fold. Its prevalence has been found to be 5% in healthy Dutch population and 19% in inherited thrombophilia. This may be due to mutations in MTHFR gene or due to deficiency of vitamin B_{12}, B_6, or folic acid. Elevated FVIII levels (>150 IU/dl) confer a 6-fold increased risk of DVT. Inherited elevation of VIII or FXI have been found in 11% of Dutch population FVIII and vWF levels may rarely be secondary to vasculitis. Thrombosis in patients with elevated FVIII levels is often seen in patients with O blood group and vWF levels >150 IU/dl.

Diagnostic Approach

Diagnosis in hypercoagulable states is reached on the basis of history, evaluation of clinical status and laboratory tests. Occurrence of recurrent episodes of thromboembolism in a young individual, especially with a positive family history and no underlying predisposing cause suggests inherited thrombophilia. Laboratory evaluation of a patient with thrombosis involves evaluation of coagulation, prothrombotic factors, DNA analysis and hemogram (Flow chart 20.1).

Screening coagulogram comprising of prothrombin time (PT), activated partial thromboplastin time (APTT) provides extremely useful information in some cases. Shortened coagulation tests suggest presence of elevated coagulation factor levels, which may be confirmed by factor assays.

Isolated prolongation of APTT with normal PT may be secondary to FXII deficiency or presence lupus anticoagulants. The latter are to be confirmed by dilute Russel viper venom time (d RVVT) or kaolin clotting time (KCT) mixing tests with normal plasma and phopholipid neutralization procedure. Prolongation of

Flow chart 20.1: Laboratory approach to a patient with thrombosis

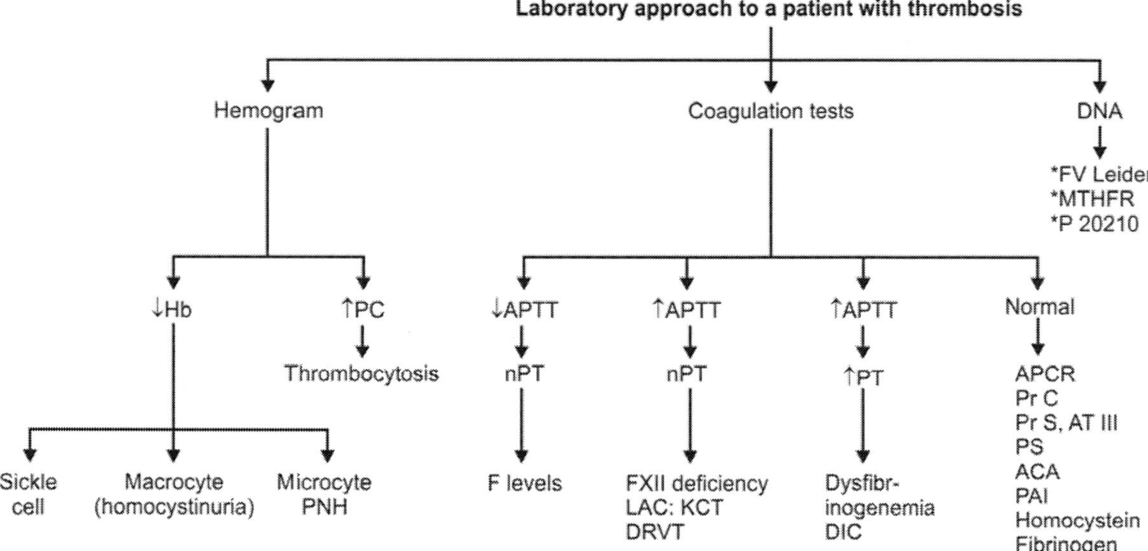

both APTT and PT suggests reduction in multiple factors as in DIC, or dysfibrinogenemia. Normal TT with mildly reduced fibrinogen suggests dysfibrinogenia. However, very low fibrinogen levels and positive D-dimer test suggests DIC.

APC of Patients

When the screening tests are normal, antigenic and clotting assays for ATIII, Pr C and S, plasminogen activator inhibitor (PAI) need to be performed. APC resistance may be looked for by calculating the normalized sensitivity ratio:

$$\text{n APC SR} = \left[\frac{\text{APC of patients}}{\text{APC of normal pool plasma}}\right]$$

n APC SR suggests the presence of APC resistance. Anticardiolipin and homocystein levels in blood may be estimated.

Sometimes hemogram analysis may provide useful information regarding the underlying cause of thrombosis. Occurrence of thrombocytosis (platelet count >10 lakhs) may be associated with iron deficiency anemia. Megaloblastic anemia may be associated with secondary hyperhomocystinuria. Sickle cell syndromes may cause sickling of blood in the capillaries leading to arterial thrombosis.

The interpretation of the above abnormal results requires a careful assessment of underlying secondary factors. DNA samples may be analysed using specific primers to look for defects in genes underlying methylene tetrahydrafolate reductase (MTHFR), FV Leiden, and P20210 defects.

It is thus concluded that ascertaining the underlying etiology in hypercoagulable state requires a good clinical assessment coupled with an extensive laboratory work-up.

REFERENCES

1. Mannucci PM, Tripoli A. Laboratory screening of inherited thrombotic syndromes. Thromb Haemost. 1987;57:247-51.
2. Lawson SE, Butler D, Enayat MS, Williams MD. Congenital thrombophilia and thrombosis: a study in a single centre. Arch Dis Child. 1999;81:176-8.
3. Andrew M. Development hemostasis. Relevance to thromboembolic complications in pediatric patients. Thromb Haemost. 1995;74:415-25.
4. Nowak Gottl-U, von Kries R, Gobel U. Neonatal symptomatic thrombo-embolism in Germany: two year survey. Archive Childhood. 1997;76:F163-7.
5. Nowak-Gottl U, Dubeers A, Kececioghe D, Koch HG, Kotthoff S, Runde J, et al. Factor V Leiden, protein C and lipoprotein (a) in catheter related thrombosis in childhood: a prospective study. J Pediatr. 1997;131:608-12.
6. Bokenkamp A, Von Kries R, Nowak Gottl U, Gobel U, Hoyer PF. Neonatal renal venous thrombosis in Germany between 1992 and 1994; epidemiology, treatment and outcome. Eur J Pediatr. 2000;159:44-8.
7. Ultenreuther-Fischer MM, Vetter B, Hellmann C, Otting U, Ziemer S, Hausdorf G, et al. Pediatric thrombo-embolism: the influence of nongenetic-genetic factor and the role of activated protein C resistance and protein C deficiency. Eur J Pediatr. 1997;156:277-81.

21 Antithrombotic Therapy in Pediatrics

ATK Rau, Shruti Patil, Anupam Sachdeva

INTRODUCTION

Antithrombotic therapy (ATT) is used for the prevention or treatment of venous and/or arterial thromboembolism (TE). In children, unlike in adults, its use is limited, owing to natural 'developmental hemostasis', in which proteins and compensatory mechanisms involved in coagulation, quantitatively and qualitatively improve with age.[1] This protects children against spontaneous thrombosis. For the same reason, insults, such as immobilization are also unlikely to trigger the development of thrombotic diseases in children. Further, inherited genetic predisposition to thrombosis is also unlikely to cause disease in childhood, as compensatory mechanisms are usually sufficient to prevent thrombosis until early adulthood. As a result, the epidemiology of TE disease differs between children and adults, with the majority of thrombotic events occurring in children being iatrogenic in nature.

In the rare event that ATT is required for the prevention and treatment of TE conditions in children, owing to the fact that the pathophysiology of thrombotic processes and the response to thrombotic agents is different in pediatric patients when compared to adults, the indications for ATT are restricted and quite specific. However, owing to the paucity of studies in children, recommendations for its use have largely been and continue to be extrapolated from recommendations in adults.

UNFRACTIONATED HEPARIN

Unfractionated heparin (UFH or standard heparin) remains a commonly used anticoagulant in pediatric patients. The advantage of using UFH in children is its short half life (4 hours), which permits rapid cessation of anticoagulation by simply discontinuing the infusion. In addition, the availability of a specific antidote (Protamine) is also a great advantage in many clinical situations.

MECHANISM OF ACTION AND PHARMACOLOGY

Unfractionated heparin is a heterogeneous glycosaminoglycan with a molecular weight ranging from 3000-30,000 kD. It catalyses and enhances the ability of antithrombin (AT) to inactivate specific coagulation enzymes, of which thrombin is the most sensitive. However, thrombin generation in the newborn and in early childhood is physiologically markedly curtailed as compared to adults and thrombin levels are noted to be similar to plasma from adults receiving therapeutic amounts of heparin. Thus, heparin needs to be used with utmost caution in this age group and children will require lower doses than adults.[2] Factors that affect the action of UFH in children are given in Table 21.1.

Table 21.1: Factors that affect the action of UFH in children

• UFH acts via antithrombin-mediated catabolism of thrombin and factor Xa	Reduced levels of antithrombin	Strong
	Reduced capacity to generate thrombin	Strong
	Age-related difference in anti-FXa: anti-IIa activity	Weak
• UFH is bound to plasma proteins, which limits free active UFH	Alterations in plasma binding	Weak
• Endothelial release of TFPI	Age-related differences in amount of TFPI release for same amount of UFH	Weak

DOSING AND ADMINISTRATION

Few randomized controlled trials regarding the dosing, route of administration or duration of therapy of UFH have been conducted in the pediatric population. The majority of evidence available is based upon a handful of cohort studies[3,4] in children at risk of or who have been diagnosed with thrombosis.

PROPHYLACTIC THERAPY

A weight-based nomogram is usually preferred to address the dosing schedule of UFH in pediatric patients where the requirement is to achieve adult therapeutic APTT values (60-85 seconds which reflects an anti-FXa level of 0.30–0.70 u/ml). Using this method, a bolus dose of 75-100 u/kg given over 10 minutes achieves therapeutic APTT value in 90% of children after 4-6 hours. Further maintenance doses are age dependent: Infants up to 2 months of age require between 25 and 28 u/kg/h and children between 2 months and 1 year of age between 20 and 24 u/kg/h. The dose of UFH required for older children is similar to the weight-adjusted requirement in adults, i.e. 18 u/kg/h. Therapy should be continued for a minimum of 5 days but 7-10 days is the norm in most institutions. Oral anticoagulant therapy may be initiated on day 1 of UHF therapy or later if a longer course is contemplated. There is little or no data to define the optimal prophylactic dose of UFH. Clinicians commonly start with a dose of 8-10 u/kg/h (continuous infusion) and titrate it with the APTT as indicated below in Table 21.2.

MONITORING

Close monitoring of UFH action is necessary due to its relatively narrow therapeutic window. The various assays used to monitor the UFH therapy are given in Table 21.3. Sub-therapeutic levels of UFH are associated with an increased risk of initiation, propagation or recurrence of TE, while supra-therapeutic UFH levels are associated with a significant risk of bleeding. The gold standard method for measuring UFH concentration in plasma is by protamine level titration.

ADVERSE EFFECTS, REVERSAL OF ACTION AND ANTIDOTE OF UHF

The three main adverse effects of UHF include bleeding, heparin-induced thrombocytopenia, and osteoporosis. Termination of UFH infusion/administration will

Table 21.2: Heparin dosing normogram

APTT	*Antifactor Xa*	*Heparin hold*	*Rate change*	*Repeat APTT after*
<50	<0.1	0	Inc 20%	4 hours
50-59	0.1-0.34	0	Inc 10%	4 hours
60-85	0.35-0.70	0	0	24 hours
86-95	0.71-0.89	0	Dec 10%	4 hours
96-120	0.90-1.20	30 minutes	Dec 10%	4 hours
>120	>1.2	60 minutes	Dec 15%	4 hours

Table 21.3: Summary of assays used to monitor UFH therapy

Assay	*Common uses*	*Advantages*	*Disadvantages*
APTT F-Clot	Coagulation screening assay Therapeutic UFH monitoring	Low cost Easy to perform Broadly available	Prolonged APTT does not indicate effective clinical anticoagulation Wide variability in reagent sensitivity Non-physiological measure of UFH effect
Anti-Xa levels F-Ch	Calibration of APTT To provide reference ranges Therapeutic UFH monitoring	Direct measure of UFH activity Can be used in the presence of FXa inhibitors Easy to perform	Not as broadly available as APTT Costs > APTT Some variability in reagent sensitivity Does not measure other mechanisms of UFH effect (e.g. Anti-IIa).
Protamine Titration Q	Cannot be used clinically Used only by reference laboratories	Only assay that directly measures UFH concentrations Inexpensive Not broadly available	Automated methods have not been validated Manual methods are labor intensive

Abbreviations: F-Clot: Functional clot-based assay; F-Ch: Functional chromogenic assay; Q: Quantitative assay

Table 21.4: Reversal of heparin therapy

Time since end of UFH infusion	*Protamine/100 units UFH*
<30 minutes	1 mg
30-60 minutes	0.5-0.75 mg
61-120 minutes	0.375-0.5 mg
>120 minutes	0.25-0.375 mg

usually suffice if mild bleeding occurs and anticoagulation needs to be discontinued. The APTT will revert back to normal 4-6 hours after cessation of therapy. However, if bleeding is severs and immediate reversal is required, protamine sulfate neutralizes heparin activity within 5 minutes. The dose of protamine is dependant on the dose of UFH received in the previous two hours and time since end of infusion (Table 21.4). The maximum dose of protamine sulfate that can be given at a time is 50 mg.

HEPARIN-INDUCED THROMBOCYTOPENIA

Heparin-induced thrombocytopenia (HIT) has been reported in children from the ages of 3 months to 15 years.[5,6] Many infants and children in neonatal and pediatric intensive care units who are exposed to heparin have multiple reasons for thrombocytopenia and or thrombosis; thus, a high index of suspicion is required for the diagnosis of HIT. During ATT with UHF therapy, the platelet count should be estimated on a daily basis and any reduction of platelet count of more than 50% from baseline with clinical suspicion of HIT, should entail immediate discontinuation of heparin therapy. Danaparoid, hirudin, and agratroban may be used as alternatives to UHF in such conditions, although there is a paucity of dosing data in children. Platelet transfusions are of limited value and at times harmful.

LOW MOLECULAR WEIGHT HEPARIN (LMWH)

Despite their as yet unproven superiority over UFH, LMWHs have rapidly become the anticoagulant of choice in many pediatric patients, both for primary prophylaxis as well as for the treatment of TE. The potential advantages of LMWH for pediatric patients include minimal monitoring requirements; lack of interference by other drugs or diet; reduced risk of HIT; and probable reduced risk of osteoporosis with long-term use when compared to UFH. However, the predictability of the anticoagulant affect with weight-adjusted doses appears to be reduced, compared to adults, presumably due to altered plasma binding.[4]

MECHANISM OF ACTION

Low molecular weight heparin is prepared by chemically or enzymatically altering UFH chains to isolate the region containing the unique pentasaccharide sequence required for binding to antithrombin. *In vitro*, thrombin generation is similar in adults and children at the same concentration of LMWH. However *in vivo*, at 25% of adult LMWH dose, thrombin generation was delayed and reduced by approximately half in newborns compared to adults.

THERAPEUTIC RANGE

Therapeutic doses of LMWH are extrapolated from adults and are based on anti-FXa levels. The therapeutic end point of LMWH therapy is an anti-FXa level of 0.50 to 1.0 u/ml in a sample taken 4-6 hours following a subcutaneous injection of LMWH.[4]

DOSING

The doses of LMWH required in pediatric patients to achieve adult therapeutic anti-FXa levels have been assessed for various preparations, e.g. enoxaparin, reviparin, dalteparin, and tinzaparine. Peak anti-FXa levels occur 2-6 hours following a subcutaneous injection of LMWH. Increased requirements are noted in children less than 2 months of age or less than 5 kg weight which is probably due to larger volume of distribution. (Table 21.5).

Anti-FXa levels are monitored every month and the dosage is adjusted accordingly. This is necessary in the pediatric population as children gain weight and outgrow current doses.

REVERSAL AND ANTIDOTE

Unless immediate reversal is necessary, withholding two doses of LMWH will suffice to reverse its effect. If immediate reversal is required, protamine sulfate

Table 21.5: Enoxaparin dosing normogram

	Age ≤ 2 months	*Age ≥ 2 months*
Initial prophylactic dose	0.75 mg/kg/dose q12h or 1.5 mg/kg/dose once daily	0.5 mg/kg/dose SC q12h or 1 mg/kg/dose daily
Initial treatment dose	1.5 mg/kg/dose q12h	1 mg/kg/dose q12h
Maximum dose	3 mg/kg/dose q12h	2 mg/kg/dose q12h

reverses 80% of the anti-FXa activity of LMWH within 4-6 hours.

SIDE EFFECTS

Low molecular weight heparin therapy is associated with bleeding and bruising and hematoma at the site of administration. Firm pressure for 3-5 minutes after administration will minimize these effects.

VITAMIN K ANTAGONISTS

Vitamin K antagonists (VKAs) function as anticoagulants by reducing the functional plasma concentration of vitamin K-dependent factors (II, VII, IX, and X). Warfarin, phenprocoumon, and acenocoumarol are the main compounds in use. As they are administered orally, treatment with these drugs is also referred to as oral anticoagulant therapy (OAT).

MECHANISM OF ACTION

Bacteria in the gut are responsible for the reduction of vitamin K to vitamin K epoxide. This is absorbed in the intestine and converted to available vitamin K by the enzyme vitamin K epoxide reductase. Available vitamin K is essential for the formation of vitamin K-dependent proteins which are subsequently converted to clotting factors II, VII, IX and X. VKA exert their action by inhibiting vitamin K epoxide reductase thereby reducing the amount of vitamin K available resulting in effective anticoagulation. The physiologically decreased levels of vitamin K-dependent proteins in neonates make the use of VKA in this age group particularly problematic.

The dose-response relationship of VKA therapy is influenced by both genetic and environmental factors. Genetic resistance to VKAs has been reported in human and animal models.[7] Environmental factors, such as coexisting disease states, concomitant medications, and diet also influence VKA response. Medications, such as aspirin and nonsteroidal anti-inflammatory drugs, although not directly influencing VKA, do increase the risk of bleeding secondary to VKA therapy by disrupting normal platelet function.

Prothrombin time (PT), reported as an international normalized ratio (INR), is the test used to monitor oral (VKA) anticoagulant therapy. The therapeutic target INR is 2.5 (range, 2.0-3.0) and the low dose prophylactic target of VKA is an INR of 1.7 (range, 1.4-1.9). The protocol for the usage of VKAs is given in Table 21.6.

MONITORING

Monitoring oral anticoagulant therapy in children is difficult. If requires close supervision and frequent dose adjustments. Approximately, only 10-20% of children can be safely monitored by monthly estimations of INR and most will require more frequent evaluations, if possible with PT/INR monitors at home.

ADVERSE EFFECTS

Bleeding is the main complication of VKA therapy which occurs in 20% of all children on VKA. The risk of serious bleeding in children receiving VKAs for mechanical prosthetic valves is <3.2%/patient/yr. Another single-center study, with a nurse-coordinated anticoagulant service, has reported bleeding rates of 0.05%/patient/year.[8] Nonhemorrhagic complications, such as tracheal calcification or hair loss have been described on rare occasions in young children. Two cohort studies have described reduced bone density in children on warfarin for >1 year.[9]

Table 21.6: Protocol for oral (VKA) anticoagulation therapy for pediatric patients to maintain INR between 2 and 3

Protocol	*Action*
Day 1: If baseline INR is 1.0-1.3	Dose 0.2 mg/kg PO
Days 2-4: Loading	
INR 1.1-1.3	Repeat initial loading dose
INR 1.4-1.9	50% of initial loading dose
INR 2.0-3.0	50% of initial loading dose
INR 3.1-3.5	25% of loading dose
INR >3.5	Hold until INR 3.5 restart at 50% of previous dose
Maintenance dose	
INR 1.1-1.4	Increase by 20% of dose
INR 1.15-1.9	Increase by 10% of dose
INR 2.0-3.0	No change
INR 3.1-3.5	Decrease by 10% of dose
INR > 3.5	Hold until INR <3.5, then restart at 20% < previous dose

REVERSAL AND ANTIDOTE

- Nonurgent reversal of VKA effects is done by withholding three subsequent doses and estimating the INR
- For urgent reversal, give vitamin K_1 0.5-2 mg orally, depending upon the weight or 0.3 mg/kg IV
- For most urgent reversal (in case of major bleed/IV procedures) administer activated FVII 50 µg/kg IV or FFP 20 ml/kg IV

A useful algorithm for the diagnosis and treatment of thromboembolic phenomenon is given in Flow chart 21.1 and the conditions in which we require antithrombotic therapy are given in Table 21.7.

ANTIPLATELET THERAPY

Despite neonatal platelets being hyporeactive to thrombin, ADP and epinephrine (all potent stimulators of platelet activity), the bleeding time is paradoxically shortened due to increased RBC size, increased hematocrit and increased levels of von Willebrand factor activity. Thus the antiplatelet drug doses in young children may be substantially different than in adults. The commonly used drugs in this category are aspirin (1-3 mg/kg/day) and dipyridamole (2-5 mg/kg/day), which are frequently used in children with Blalock-Taussig and other endovascular shunts. Clopidogrel and ticlodepine, used extensively in adults, have not been studied in children. Newer antiplatelet compounds include the newly approved GPIIb-IIIa antagonists which will play a significant role in the days to come.

THROMBOLYTIC THERAPY

Systemic thrombolytic therapy is indicated for clinical situations where there is potential loss of limb, organ

Flow chart 21.1: Algorithm for the diagnosis and treatment of thromboembolism (TE)

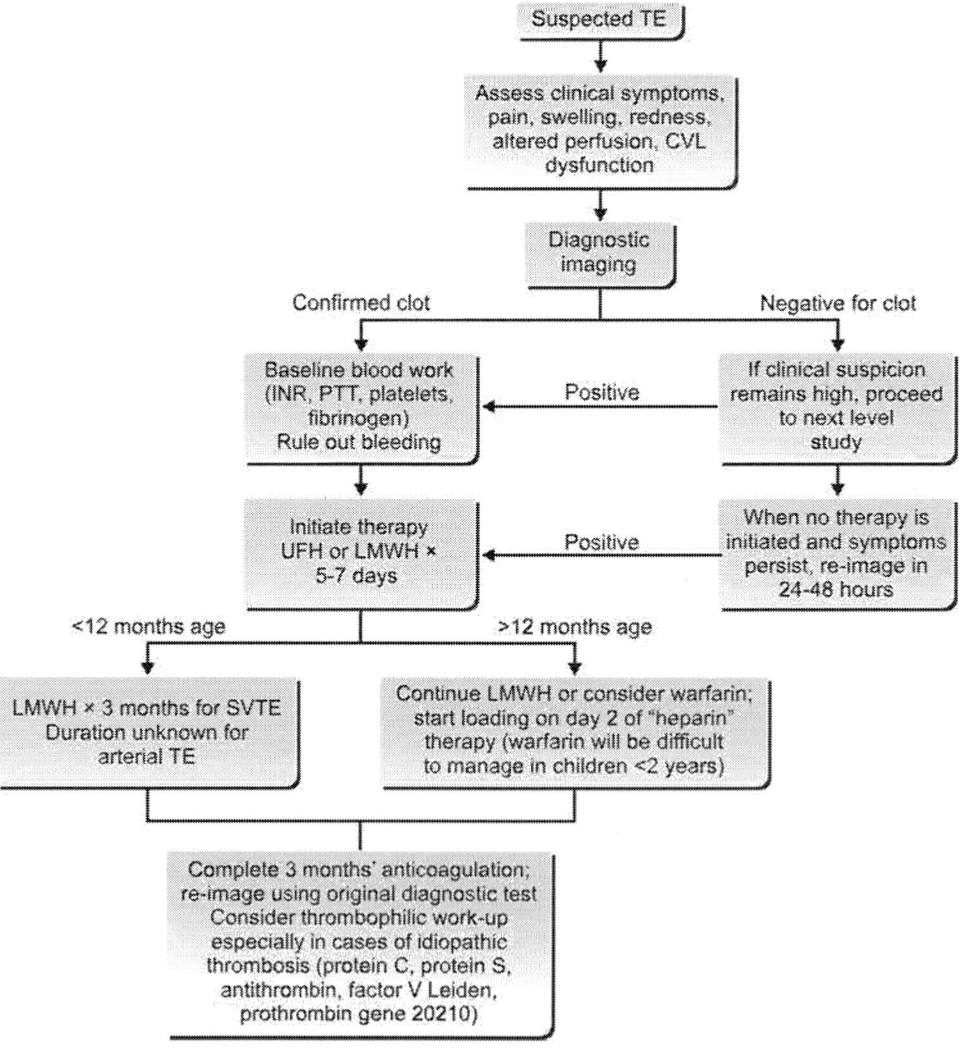

Table 21.7: Indications for antithrombotic therapy in children

- Deep vein thrombosis (DVT) related to central venous line (CVL) *in situ*
- Non-central venous line related DVT
- Prophylaxis for veno-occlusive disease
- Neonatal renal vein thrombosis
- Primary antithrombotic prophylaxis for CVLs
- Primary prophylaxis for Blalock-Taussig shunts
- Primary prophylaxis for Fontan surgery
- Primary prophylaxis for stage I Norwoods procedure
- Primary prophylaxis for Glenn or BCPS
- Primary prophylaxis for endovascular stents
- Primary prophylaxis for dilated cardiomyopathy
- Primary pulmonary hypertension
- Biological prosthetic heart valves
- Mechanical prosthetic heart valves
- Ventricular assist devices (VADs)
- Extra-corporeal membranous Oxygenation (EMCO)
- Therapy of arterial thrombosis
- Arterial catheter prophylaxis
- Primary prophylaxis for venous access related to hemodialysis
- Use of UFH or LMWH for hemodialysis
- Kawasaki disease
- Cerebral sinovenous thrombosis (CSVT)
- Arterial ischemic stroke (AIS)
- Purpura fulminans

or life, such as in arterial occlusions, massive pulmonary embolus (PE) or PE not responding to heparin therapy. A common feature of management of all the TE diseases is the desire to restore vascular patency in a timely fashion to prevent loss of tissue, organ, limb function and life.

Drugs Employed

The major reaction of the fibrinolytic (plasminogen) system involves the conversion of the inactive pro-enzyme plasminogen, to the active enzyme plasmin by tissue plasminogen activators (t-PA). Plasmin then breaks the clot by degrading fibrinogen, fibrin monomers and cross-linked fibrins into fibrin degradation products (FDPs). Most thrombolytic agents are fashioned after endogenous t-PA or urokinase. Traditional thrombolytic drugs include bacteria derived streptokinase (SK), anisoylated plasminogen SK activator complex, urokinase and recombinant t-PA. Newer thrombolytic agents include mutants of PA, chimeric PA, conjugates of PA with monoclonal antibodies and novel PA from animal and bacterial origin. Non PA thrombolytic agents which degrade fibrin and/or fibrinogen directly like microplasmin, alfimeprase and ancrod, are under investigations.

DOSING IN THROMBOLYTIC THERAPY

There is no therapeutic guideline or dosage range for thrombolytic agents. In general, the dose of t-PA given through central lines in children ranges from 0.05 - 0.6 mg/kg/hr but peripheral lines can deliver only lower doses (Tables 21.8 and 21.9).

Table 21.8: Thrombolytic therapy for pediatric patients—local instillation of tissue plasminogen activator

Treatment	Single – Lumen CVL	Double – Lumen CVL	SC port
tPA: Child's weight <10 kg	0.5 mg diluted in 0.9% NaCl to volume required to fill line	0.5 mg per lumen diluted in 0.9% NaCl to fill volume of line. Treat one lumen at time	0.5 mg diluted with 0.9% NaCl to 3 ml
tPA: Child's weight >10 kg	1.0 mg in 1.0 ml 0.9% NaCl Use amount required to fill volume of line, to maximum of 2 ml = 2 mg	1.0 mg/ml use amount required to fill mount of line, to a maximum of 2 ml = 2 mg per lumen Treat one lumen at a time	2.0 mg diluted with 0.9% NaCl to 3 ml

Systemic thrombolytic therapy*

	Load	*Maintenance*	*Monitoring*
UK	4400 U/kg	4400 U/kg/hr for 6-12 hours	Fibrinogen, TCT, PT, APTT
SK	2000 U/kg	2000 U/kg for 6-12 hours	Same
Tpa	None	0.1-6.0 mg/kg/hr for 6 hours	Same

Abbreviations: CVL: Central venous line; SC: Subcutaneous port; tPA: Tissue plasminogen activator; NaCl: Sodium chloride; UK: Urokinase; SK: Streptokinase; TCT: Thrombin clotting time; PT: Prothrombin time; APTT: Activated partial thromboplastin time.
*Start heparin therapy either during or immediately upon completion of thrombolytic therapy. A loading dose of heparin may be omitted. The length of time for optimal maintenance is uncertain. Values provided are starting suggestions, as some patients may respond to longer or shorter courses of therapy[10]

Table 21.9: General guidelines for thrombolytic therapy[11]

- During thrombolytic therapy, UFH should be administered concurrently at a dose of 20 u/kg/hr
- No IM injections should be given during therapy
- Minimal manipulation or handling of the patient is desirable
- Avoid concurrent use of warfarin or antiplatelet agents
- Urinary catheterization/arterial punctures/rectal monitoring of temperature must not be done
- Blood samples must be collected only from superficial veins/ indwelling catheters
- Monitor response q6h by PT/INR and APTT (monitor fibrinogen levels, if bleeding occurs)
- Expect a decrease in fibrinogen levels by 20-50% during therapy
- Platelet count should be maintained at 50-100 × 10^9/L
- If no change in fibrinogen concentrations is noted, estimate D-dimer levels to confirm established thrombolytic state.

ADVERSE EFFECTS

The major adverse effect is bleeding. Severe bleeding requiring treatment with packed RBC occurs in about 20% of pediatric patients, the most frequent site being where an invasive procedure has been performed. The incidence of intracranial hemorrhage is 1.5%.

TREATMENT OF BLEEDING

Clinically, mild bleeding can be treated with local pressure and supportive care. Major bleeding should be treated by stopping thrombolytic therapy, administering cryoprecipitate (usual dose of 1 bag/5 kg body weight), and administering other blood products as indicated. If the bleeding is life threatening, an antifibrinolytic agent can also be used. The choice and dose of blood product transfusion can be guided by hemostatic monitoring of which fibrinogen assay is the most sensitive parameter of thrombolytic activity and must be closely monitored in these situations.

CONTRAINDICATIONS OF THROMBOLYTIC THERAPY

- Active bleeding from any site
- Significant potential for spontaneous bleed
- Hypertension
- AV malformations
- Recent severe trauma.

TREATMENT OF PEDIATRIC VENOUS THROMBOEMBOLISM IN CHILDREN

1. Children (over 2 months of age) with DVT/PE should be treated with IV heparin sufficient to prolong the APTT to a range that corresponds to an anti-factor Xa level of 0.3–0.7 u/ml. (recommendation in adults). LMWH sufficient to achieve an anti FXa level of 0.5-1.0 u/ml 4 to 6 hours after an injection is an alternative to initial therapy with heparin.
2. It is recommended that treatment with heparin or LMWH be continued for 5-10 days and that oral anticoagulants be overlapped with heparin for at least 4-5 days. In many patients, heparin and warfarin can be started together and heparin discontinued on day 6, if the INR is in the therapeutic range on two consecutive days. For massive PE or extensive DVT, a longer period of heparin or LMWH therapy is indicated.
3. Long-term anticoagulant therapy should be continued for at least 3 months using oral anticoagulants to prolong the PT to an INR of 2.0-3.0. This is again based on recommendations for adults, a 2 cohort and a 6 case series in children. Alternatively LMWH is an option in children in whom long-term oral anticoagulant therapy is problematic. If LMWH is chosen for long-term use, bone density should be constantly monitored to detect osteoporosis at an early stage.
4. Standard dose oral anticoagulant therapy keeping the INR between 2 and 3, low dose maintenance therapy (INR < 2.0), low dose LMWH, or close monitoring should be considered for children with a first recurrence of venous TE or an initial venous TE and a continuing risk factor, such as a central venous line (CVL), AT III deficiency, protein C or S deficiency, activated protein C resistance, prothrombin gene 20210, Lupus anticoagulants in the antiphospholipid antibody syndrome or systemic lupus erythematosus. This is based on recommendations for adults and a case series in children.
5. Indefinite oral anticoagulant therapy with an INR of 2.0-3.0 should be considered for children with a second recurrence of venous/TE or a first recurrence of a venous TE and a continuing risk factor as mentioned above. In circumstances in which oral anticoagulation therapy is problematic, LMWH is an option.
6. The use of thrombolytic agents in the treatment of venous TEs continues to be highly individualized. Further clinical investigation is needed before more definitive recommendations can be made.
7. Children with known congenital prothromotic disorders should receive short-term prophylactic anticoagulation in high-risk situations such as immobility, significant surgery or trauma. The role of screening for prothrombotic disorders remains controversial.[12]

Treatment of Venous/Arterial Thromboembolism in Special Situations

In the newborn, the use of anticoagulation therapy in the treatment of newborns, with DVT, PE or arterial TEs is highly individualized and fraught with problems. Further clinical investigations are needed before more definite recommendations can be made. However, the following guidelines may help in critical situations:

1. If short-term anticoagulation therapy is deferred, the thrombus should be closely monitored with objective tests and if found to be increasing in size, anticoagulation therapy is instituted as soon as possible.
2. If anticoagulation is used, a short course (10-14 days) of UFH, sufficient to prolong the APTT to the therapeutic range that corresponds to an anti-factor Xa level of 0.3-0.7 u/ml or, alternatively a short course of LMWH, sufficient to achieve an anti-factor Xa level of 0.3-0.7 u/ml or, a short course of LMWH, sufficient to achieve an anti-factor Xa level at the low end of the adult therapeutic range (0.5-1.0 u/ml) may be used. Longer courses of anticoagulant therapy, up to 3 months, may also be considered and dependent on the location and seriousness of the thrombus. The thrombus should be closely monitored with objective tests for evidence of extension or recurrent disease. If the thrombus extends following discontinuation of heparin therapy, oral anticoagulation therapy or extended LMWH should be considered.

Prophylaxis During Cardiac Catheterization in Children and Newborns

These patients should be offered prophylactic UFH in the dose of 100-150 u/kg as a bolus. Aspirin may also be given concurrently and continued for 5-7 days after the procedure.

Mechanical Prosthetic Heart Valves in Children

1. It is strongly recommended that children with mechanical prosthetic heart valves receive oral anticoagulation therapy. This recommendation is based on recommendations for adults and 13 case series in children.
2. Levels of oral anticoagulation therapy that prolong the INR to 2.5-3.5 are recommended.
3. Children with mechanical prosthetic heart valves who suffer systemic embolism despite adequate VKA may benefit from the addition of aspirin 6-20 mg/kg/day. Dipyridamole 2-5 mg/kg/day, in addition to oral anticoagulation therapy is also an alternative.
4. When full-dose oral anticoagulation therapy is contraindicated, long-term therapy with oral anticoagulation therapy enough to increase the INR 2.0-3.0 in combination with aspirin (6-20 mg/kg/day) or dipyridamole (2-5 mg/kg/day) may be used.

TREATMENT OF KAWASAKI DISEASE IN CHILDREN

In addition to IV gamma globulin (2 g/kg as a single dose), children with Kawasaki disease should also receive aspirin, 80 to 100 mg/kg/day during the acute phase (up to 14 days) as an anti-inflammatory agent and then again at doses of 3-5 mg/kg/day for 7 weeks or longer to prevent the formation of coronary aneurysm thrombosis.

CHILDREN UNDERGOING FONTAN PROCEDURE

Further clinical investigations are needed before definitive recommendations for primary postoperative prophylaxis can be made. Current options include aspirin, or therapeutic amounts of heparin followed by oral anticoagulation therapy to achieve an INR of 2-3. The optimal duration of prophylaxis is unknown.[13]
Children undergoing Blalock-Taussig shunts procedure Further clinical investigation is needed before definitive recommendations can be made. One option is to initially treat these patients with therapeutic amounts of heparin, followed by aspirin at doses of 3-5 mg/kg/day indefinitely.

CHILDREN WITH HOMOZYGOUS PROTEIN C AND S DEFICIENCY

1. It is recommended that newborns with purpura fulminans due to homozygous deficiency of protein C or S be treated initially with replacement therapy (either fresh frozen plasma or protein C concentrate) for approximately 6-8 weeks until the skin lesions have healed.
2. Following resolution of the skin lesions, and under cover of replacement therapy, oral anticoagulation therapy can be introduced with target INR values of approximately 3 to 4.5. Treatment duration with oral anticoagulant is indefinite. Recurrent skin lesions should be treated with replacement therapy of protein C or S.

For patients with mild homozygous protein C and S deficiency with measurable plasma concentrations of either, LMWH is a therapeutic option.

SUMMARY

Unlike in adults, ATT is rarely used in neonates and children as their physiological mileu predisposes them to a preexisting mildly hypocoagulable state.

Recommendations on the therapeutic spectrum of ATT are extrapolated from adult studies and may not give the true picture in neonates and children.

Specific indications exist for initiation of ATT and must be strictly adhered to.

All children undergoing ATT must be hospitalized and monitored for any untoward effects.

The role of ATT must be reassessed promptly once the indication disappears or the clinical condition improves.

CONCLUSION

Anticoagulant therapy has been used for the last 50 years or so for specific indications in children. However, dose recommendations and therapeutic alternative are almost entirely based on studies in adults and may be inadequate in newborn and children in whom physiological responses are often immature and lacking. Therefore, it is essential to use anticoagulant therapy judiciously, if at all and to monitor children on therapy regularly and scrupulously. If this is the norm, anticoagulant therapy will be a very useful tool in the battle against thrombosis and thrombotic disorders.

REFERENCES

1. Andrew M, Paes B, Johnston M. Development of the hemostatic systems in the neonate and young infant. Am J Paediatr Hematol Oncol. 1990;12:95-104.
2. Andrew M Mitchel L, Vegh P, Ofosu F. Thrombin regulation in children differs from adults in the absence and presence of heparin. Thromb Haemostat. 1994;72:836-42
3. Bauman M, Mitchell L, Chan AK, de Verber C, Maesecotle MP. Very low dose warfarin for primary and secondary prophylaxis in children: a prospective Cohort study of 20 Children J. Thromb Haemostat. 2003;1(suppl 1)P0063.
4. Kulile S, Eulmeskian P, Massicotte PM, et al. Poor correlation between APTT, anti-Xa levels and heparin dose in children receiving therapeutic doses of IJFH. J. Thromb Haemostat. 2003;1(suppl 1):P0060.
5. Magnani HN. Heparin – induced thrombocytopenia (HIT)– an overview of 230 patients J Thromb Haemostat. 1993;70:554-61.
6. Severin T, Sutor AH. Heparin induced thrombocytopenia in paediatrics. Severin Thromb Haemostat. 2011;27:293-9.
7. Wilson SE, Watson HG, Crowther MA. Low dose oral vitamin K therapy for the management of asymptomatic patients with elevated INR: a brief review. Can Med Assoc J. 2004;170:821-4.
8. Turpie AG, Gent M, Laupacis A, et al. A Comparison of aspirin with placebo in patients treated with warfarin after heart valve replacement. N Engl J Med. 1993;329:524-9.
9. Strief W, Andrew M, Marzinotto V, et al. Analysis of warfarin therapy in paediatrics patients. A prospective cohort study of 319 patients. Blood. 1999;94:3007-14.
10. Monagle P, Michelson AD, Bovil E, et al. Antithrombotic therapy in children. Chest. 2004;119:3445-705.
11. Andrew M, Monagle P, Brooker L. Thrombolytic therapy. In: Thromboembolic complications during infancy and childhood, Hamilton, BC: Decker; 2000. pp.57-84.
12. Andrew M, David M, Adams M, et al. venous thrombo-embolic complication (VTE) in children. An analysis of the Canadian registry of VTE. Blood. 1994;83:1251-7.
13. Monagle P, Cochrane A, Mc Crindle B, Benson L, Williams W, Andrew M. Thromboembolic complications after fountan, procedures, the role of prophylactic anti-coagulation. J Thoracic cardiovasc Sur. 1998;115:493-8.

22 Stroke in Children

Vasant Chinnabhandar, Vinita Jain, SP Yadav, Anupam Sachdeva

Stroke may be defined as "an abrupt onset neurologic deficit that is attributable to a focal vascular cause"[1] or "the sudden occlusion or rupture of cerebral arteries or veins resulting in focal cerebral damage and clinical neurologic deficits that persist for longer than 24 hours."[2] Stroke is now increasingly recognized as an important neurologic disorder in pediatrics. However, delays in diagnosis are still common, leading to limitation in opportunities for timely therapeutic interventions.[3] Data from various western studies provide an estimated incidence of 2-8/100,000 children/year and, in neonates of approximately 1:4000 live births.[4,5] The reported incidence and prevalence of stroke in children has increased over time, because of improvement in imaging techniques. The mortality rate attributable to pediatric stroke (PS) has reduced but mortality in children <1 year has remained same in the last 40 years.[6] Mortality in pediatric stroke varies with the type of stroke. High morbidity and adverse long-term outcomes add to its heavy consequences and costs, both personal and social. Indeed, about half of the surviving patients develop some neurologic or cognitive impairment.[7] Although bacterial meningitis was a common cause of ischemic stroke in the past, cardiac disorders, blood disorders, vasculopathies, vascular malformations and viral infections (viz. varicella) account for a large proportion of stroke in children today.[8-10]

There are no universally accepted classification schemes for PS. As in adults, PS can be ischemic or hemorrhagic; although ischemic stroke is more common, prevalence is variable. Ischemic stroke includes arterial ischemic stroke (AIS) and cerebral sinovenous thrombosis (CSVT); hemorrhagic stroke (HS) includes intracerebral and subarachnoid hemorrhage.[11] The incidence of hemorrhagic stroke reported is 2.9/100,000 and that of ischemic stroke 7.8/100,000.[12]

Based on age at occurrence, PS may also be divided into perinatal or childhood stroke. Perinatal stroke is an under-recognized entity. It is defined as a cerebrovascular accident that occurs between 28 weeks of gestation and 29 days of life. It may be hemorrhagic or ischemic, with each occurring approximately 50% of the time. The most common cause of perinatal stroke is thrombosis secondary to a congenital coagulation disorder, although cardiac or vascular abnormalities may also lead to stroke. In addition, there are a number of fetal–maternal factors that may predispose a patient to stroke, including prematurity, preeclampsia and fetal, or maternal sepsis.[13]

Childhood stroke is defined as a cerebrovascular event occurring in patients between the ages of 30 days and 18 years, may also be ischemic or hemorrhagic, although ischemic stroke is far more common.[5] The mortality rate in males is higher than in females as also in blacks as compared with whites.[14]

ISCHEMIC STROKE

Mechanism

The cerebral vascular supply is structured to protect the cerebral hemispheres and brainstem from the consequences of blood flow cessation. Blood flow to the brain, i.e. the cerebral blood flow (50-100 ml/100 g/min) is conspicuously higher than that required for most other organs due to two synergistic factors. These being, firstly the high metabolic rate of brain and secondly the almost complete lack of energy stores in the brain. Also, neurons are very sensitive to hypoxia and as a result neuronal derangement occurs rapidly in the presence of hypoxia. As an adaptive mechanism, the brain has developed the ability to autoregulate its blood flow as per its metabolic needs. Reversal of blood flow around local obstructions is a feature of the microvascular beds of the striatum and cerebral cortex.

Arterial ischemic stroke (AIS) results from occlusion of cerebral arteries, usually via pathological thrombus or thromboembolism. Most AIS involves the middle cerebral artery (MCA) with recognizable clinical and imaging patterns, including (i) proximal M1 occlusion (entire MCA infarcted), (ii) distal M1 (basal ganglia spared), (iii) anterior or posterior trunk/M2 occlusion (frontal or parietal/temporal respectively), and (iv) lenticulostriate (basal ganglia and deep white matter only). Additional AIS patterns can be defined within the posterior circulation, which involves the brainstem, cerebellum, thalamus, occipital, and mesial temporal lobes.

When blood flow ceases in the supplying artery, the relationship between the neurons and astrocytes is altered. Increased endothelial cell permeability and endocytosis leading to edema formation, and matrix degradation is associated with hemorrhage. Autoregulation is lost. Ischemia initiates leukocyte adhesion receptor expression, promoted by cytokine generation from neutrophils and activated monocytes, and also produces swelling of the microvascular endothelium, and rapid detachment and swelling of astrocyte end-feet. Ischemic injury targets microvasculature, where the inflammatory responses are initiated and contribute to tissue injury.[15] The activation of cerebral micro-vessels by ischemia is heterogeneous, involving alterations in integrin-matrix interactions, leukocyte-endothelial cell adhesion, permeability changes, and the "no-reflow" phenomenon due to platelet activation, fibrin formation, and leukocyte adhesions. The mechanisms of ischemic cellular injury are largely due to excitotoxicity, free radical formation, and activation of the inflammatory cascade. ATP dependent calcium pump failure results in increased intracellular calcium, direct damage to the mitochondria and activation of a number of DNAses, proteases, and lipases.[16] Additionally, cellular failure results in depolarization and a release of glutamate, which activates postsynaptic N-methyl-D-aspartate (NMDA) receptors, allowing for a greater influx of calcium and further cellular injury.[16-19] Nitric oxide synthase, in combination with superoxide dismutase, forms potent reactive oxygen species (ROS) that are activated by ischemia.[16,18,19] Reperfusion results in a second wave of ROS formation that increases with time. "Preactivation" may augment the inflammatory responses to ischemia.

Defined patterns involving thrombosis of veins or major venous sinuses are seen in CSVT. The superficial venous system is more frequently involved.[20, 21] Sagittal sinus thrombosis often leads to bilateral parasagittal infarcts with hemorrhagic transformation. Deep venous thrombosis involving the internal cerebral veins, straight sinus, and/or the vein of Galen will produce venous edema and infarction of the deep white matter, basal ganglia, and thalamus. Infarction in deep locations immediately adjacent to the ventricular system can produce intraventricular hemorrhage (IVH). Almost 30% term neonates with IVH have an underlying deep CSVT.

Venous thromboembolism (VTE) in children is a rapidly increasing secondary complication in children being treated for serious, life-threatening primary disease. The incidence of VTE during childhood is estimated at 0.24% of hospital admissions in neonates and 0.53% for older children in Canada.[22] Infants in the first months of life and teenagers are at greatest risk.

Perinatal Ischemic Stroke

In the newborn period, AIS has distinct associations including acute systemic insults, maternal or obstetrical factors, and prothrombotic states definable in about two-thirds of infants.[4,23,24] The most common cause of neonatal stroke is thrombosis secondary to a congenital coagulation disorder.[13]

Consideration of three variables defines distinct perinatal stroke types: (i) presence of neonatal symptoms, (ii) timing of injury, and (iii) specific blood vessel affected. The putative risk factors are:[3]

A. Maternal
   1. Primipara
   2. Autoimmune disease
   3. Coagulopathies
   4. Preeclampsia
   5. Drug use
B. Obstetric causes
   1. Prolonged rupture of membranes
   2. Chorioamnionitis
   3. Accidental and nonaccidental maternal trauma
C. Neonatal causes
   1. Emergency CS/fetal distress/nuchal cord
   2. Sepsis/meningitis
   3. Complex congenital heart disease.

Childhood Ischemic Stroke

The commonly considered etiologies are:

A. Cardiac
   1. Congenital
   2. Acquired
   3. Iatrogenic
B. Hematologic
   1. Hemoglobinopathies—
      a. Sickle cell disease
      b. Thalassemia
   2. Thrombophilia
   3. Iron deficiency anemia
   4. Thrombocytopenia

C. Infectious
   1. Meningitis
   2. Encephalitis
D. Vasculitis
   1. Primary—Primary angitis of CNS
   2. Secondary
      a. Postinfectious—(i) Varicella (ii) Other
      b. Infectious—(i) Encephalitis (ii) Meningitis
      c. Associated with collagen vascular disease or systemic vasculitides.
E. Other vasculopathies
   1. Transient/focal cerebral arteriopathy
   2. Fabry's disease
   3. NF1
   4. Moyamoya Disease
   5. Fibromuscular dysplasia
   6. Vasospasm—
      a. Migraine
      b. Other
   7. Dissection
F. Other
   1. Trauma—
      a. Dissection
      b. Fat/air embolism
   2. Toxins/drugs—
      a. Cocaine
      b. L-asparaginase
      c. Oral contraceptives
   3. Metabolic—
      a. Shock/dehydration
      b. Homocysteinuria.

Congenital or acquired heart disease is responsible for about a quarter of the children with stroke. Acute ischemic stroke in multiple vascular territories suggests a cardiac source. Of particular concern are cyanotic heart lesions with polycythemia, which increase the risk of both thrombosis and embolism. If a right-to-left cardiac shunt is present, a venous (paradoxical) embolus can bypass the pulmonary circulation and reach the brain. Many patients are already known to have heart disease prior to the stroke, but in other instances a less obvious cardiac lesion is only discovered after a stroke. Some children with congenital heart disease seem to have an increased risk of intracranial aneurysm and arterial dissection. Surgical treatments of complex congenital heart disease confer their own risk of ischemic stroke. The Fontan procedure is the cardiac procedure most commonly associated with AIS in children.[25]

Predispositions to thrombosis due to deficiencies of the intrinsic antithrombotic factors have been described in recent years. Five of them, including deficiencies in *protein C,*[26] *protein S, and antithrombin III, and the factor V Leiden and prothrombin 20210 A mutations* have been associated with thrombosis in children.[27] *Activated protein C resistance* is the most common known hereditary predisposition to venous thrombosis. Activated protein C normally degrades activated factors V and VIII by proteolytic cleavage at specific arginine residues, thereby inhibiting coagulation. Individuals with activated protein C resistance have a mutated factor V such that it is resistant to degradation by activated protein C. More than 95% cases are due to a point mutation, known as the factor V Leiden (FVL) mutation. *Protein C deficiency* occurs in 0.14 to 0.5% of the general population. The first thrombotic event usually presents between the ages of 10 and 50 years. Protein C-deficient individuals are also at increased risk for coumadin-induced skin necrosis. Homozygous deficient patients with severely decreased protein C levels present as newborns with purpura fulminans and DIC. In this condition, therapy with protein C concentrates is instituted. At birth, protein C levels are decreased to 35% of normal adult values.[28] Levels rise to above 50% of adult values by the age of 6 months; however, protein C may remain below adult normal values until the age of 10 years.

Protein S deficiency presents like protein C deficiency. It is a cofactor for activated protein C-mediated degradation of coagulation factors Va and VIIIa. Hereditary protein S deficiency occurs in 0.7% of general population.[27] Protein S in newborns is largely in the free (active) form, because C4b-binding protein is low or undetectable in newborns.[28]

Sickle cell disease is a common cause of stroke in children. The infarction risk is greatest during the first 15 years of life. Stroke is somewhat more common during thrombotic crisis, but most infarctions occur in otherwise asymptomatic patients.[29] Sickle cell disease also promotes sinovenous occlusion and subarachnoid hemorrhage, which is caused by fragile vessels due to the disease.

Increased number of platelets can cause diffuse cerebral dysfunction, as well as sinovenous and focal arterial occlusions. Rarely complete stroke may occur. Many of the neurological signs and symptoms attributed to *thrombocytosis* resemble those of complicated migraine.

Polycythemia vera is an extremely rare condition in children and the most common cause of polycythemia is cyanotic congenital heart disease or chronic chest disease, but polycythemia in the neonatal period secondary to placental insufficiency may cause vascular occlusion and infarction. Primary thrombosis may occur in the presence of high hematocrit in cyanotic congenital heart disease. Postoperative complications of cardiac surgery are more likely in the presence of severe pre-operative hyperviscous state. Hyperviscosity is also seen in severe gastroenteritis with dehydration.

The term *moyamoya* describes progressive occlusive disease of the distal internal carotid arteries, leading progressively to intracranial arterial occlusion with distal telangiectatic collateral vessels. The posterior circulation can also be affected.[30] *Moyamoya disease* is the terminology used when the arteriopathy is idiopathic; *moyamoya syndrome* is used when the arteriopathy is secondary to an associated condition like cranial radiation or genetic syndromes such as neurofibromatosis type 1, trisomy 21, or Alagille syndrome[31,32] These vessels are visible as an angiographic bluish distal to the occluded large artery. But often the term moyamoya disease is applied to children with no defined cause of their vasculopathy.[33,34]

Arterial dissection has been recognized in children more frequently in recent years. Neurologic deficit can begin immediately or may be delayed for several hours or days. Spontaneous dissection affects carotids (mainly cervical branches) more often than the vertebral arteries. Besides spontaneous dissection carotid occlusion may occur after peritonsillar trauma. Typically, intraoral trauma results when the child falls with an icecream stick, toothbrush, pen or other such object in his mouth. Although intraoral injury may seem trivial, the severity of the neurological deficit and the eventual outcome is variable, depending on whether or not the vessel is completely occluded and the availability of collateral blood flow.[35,36] Arterial dissection accounts for 7.5% to 20% of childhood arterial ischemic strokes. In a systematic review of published studies and case reports, 118 pediatric patients with stroke caused by dissection were identified.[37] In this report, 60% of anterior circulation dissections were intracranial, particularly, if the dissection was non-traumatic. 10% of children with dissection had recurrent dissection.

Infectious causes are also associated with stroke in children. *Varicella-zoster* infection is an important cause. Children with varicella-associated acute ischemic stroke have an increased frequency of hemiparesis, basal ganglia infarcts, anterior circulation infarcts, and stenosis of proximal portions of major cerebral arteries.[38] The most plausible mechanism for varicella-associated stroke involves intraneural migration of VZ virus from the trigeminal ganglion along the trigeminal nerve to the cerebral arteries.[39, 40]

CNS vasculitis is termed primary when no other condition is present that causes blood vessel inflammation and secondary when it results from another process like intracranial infection, systemic vasculitis, collagen vascular disease, malignancy, or exposure to drugs or to certain medications. It may also be classified by size of the affected vessels: large, medium, or small vessel. It can cause ischemic or hemorrhagic stroke, and may be difficult to diagnose, particularly when small vessels are involved. CNS vasculitis should be considered in children who have one or more of the following: a protracted clinical presentation, a known risk factor for vasculitis (e.g. lupus, Kawasaki disease, Henoch–Schönlein purpura, polyarteritis nodosa, Wegener's granulomatosis, systemic lupus erythematosus, Behcet syndrome, mixed connective tissue disease, Sjögren syndrome, and inflammatory bowel diseases,[41-47] multifocal deficits and lesions, diffuse neurological deficits, or systemic symptoms like fever and weight loss.[48]

HEMORRHAGIC STROKE

Perinatal Hemorrhagic Stroke

Perinatal hemorrhagic stroke (PHS) is the least well characterized pediatric stroke subtype, evidence is limited and the disease poorly understood. Intracranial hemorrhage (ICH) in neonates is estimated to be as high as 26% when common causes like preterm intraventricular hemorrhages and vaginally term born children with mild extra-axial bleeding are included.[49] Symptomatic PHS is much less common, present in perhaps six per 100,000 live births.[49-51] Identifiable risk factors are:

1. Bleeding diathesis
   a. Neonatal thrombocytopenia due to maternal idiopathic alloimmune thrombocytopenia, salicylate consumption, and congenital von Willebrand's disease.
   b. Maternal consumption of anticoagulants or anti-epileptic medications.
2. Trauma—including birth trauma.
3. Vascular malformations.

Childhood Hemorrhagic Stroke

Hemorrhagic stroke is less common than ischemic stroke in children. It also has some significant differences from ischemic stroke. Unlike ischemic stroke, the cause is more likely to be discovered, although many cases remain idiopathic. Conditions such as moyamoya, sickle cell disease, and various vasculopathies can result in both AIS and hemorrhagic stroke (HS).[40,52,53] Treatment for HS is more likely to require neurosurgical intervention than ischemic stroke. Compared with AIS, hemorrhagic stroke is associated with an initial increased mortality, but survivors tend to have better neurological outcomes.[54] Arteriovenous malformations (AVM), cavernous malformations, and aneurysms account for the majority of childhood HS.[55,56] The majority of events are supratentorial with approximately equal involvement of left and right hemisphere. Several risk factors for hemorrhagic stroke have been identified. A probable cause for childhood HS can be found in 85-90%. The common risk factors are:

A. Hematological conditions
   a. Hemophilias
   b. Thrombocytopenia (acquired/inherited)
   c. Leukemias
   d. SCD
   e. Coagulopathies
B. Congenital malformations
   a. Arteriovenous malformations (AVM)
   b. Porencephalic cysts
   c. Sturge-Weber syndrome
   d. Tuberous sclerosis
   e. Hemimegalencephaly
C. Metabolic and toxic
   a. MELAS syndrome
   b. Marfan's syndrome
D. Tumors
   a. Gliomas
   b. PNET
   c. Lymphomas
E. Others
   a. Trauma
   b. Hypertension

ICH is a devastating complication of the hemophilias. Hemophilias A and B are the most common hereditary coagulation defects to cause ICH, especially soon after birth or in the 1st year of life.[57,58] Trivial trauma may precede the event and clinical features may not be evident until several days later. Prompt initiation of factor replacement therapy after trauma may reduce the likelihood of a severe hemorrhage. Acquired coagulation defects may occur in childhood due to hepatic disorders, malabsorption and prolonged antibiotic therapy.

Thrombocytopenia resulting from either ITP,[59] or the combined effects of leukemia and its treatment, or collagen vascular diseases, or various congenital defects such as Fanconi's anemia or thrombocytopenia-absent radius syndrome may cause HS. Multiple hemorrhagic infiltrations following treatment in leukemia, when a very high CSF leukocyte count exists, may result in hyperviscosity syndrome hence resulting in multiple infarcts. Non-traumatic brain hemorrhage due to reduced platelets usually does not occur with counts >20-30 thousand/μl, and even with lower counts spontaneous hemorrhage is uncommon.

Arteriovenous malformations are the most frequent cause of HS in children.[60] They occur due to failure in the formation of capillary beds between primitive arteries and veins in the brain during fetal life. The presentation of an AVM varies with age. Neonates may present with high output cardiac failure, hemorrhage or rarely hydrocephalus. Hydrocephalus may occur later in infancy if the AVM is in posterior fossa with secondary aneurysmal dilatation of the vein of Galen. AVM in an older child or adolescent presents with seizures or intraparenchymal or subarachnoid hemorrhage.[61]

Intracranial tumors have been identified in 3-22% of children with HS in reported series.[62,63] Around 2-15% of children with a brain tumor will develop a HS. The most common neoplasms associated with HS in children are medulloblastomas and primitive neuroectodermal tumors.[64] A glioma may rarely present with acute stroke due to hemorrhage. Malignant nodes in the neck may occasionally infiltrate carotids resulting in hemiplegia.

CLINICAL FEATURES

The signs and symptoms of cerebrovascular disorders in older children resemble those of adults, but younger children tend to have more subtle and variable findings. Size and location of the lesion may be determined by the clinical presentation. However, in some children nature of risk factors also plays an important role in clinical presentation.

Neonatal Infarction

Although much less common than germinal matrix hemorrhage in premature infants, infarctions in term neonates are more common than previously thought. Acute, symptomatic neonatal AIS typically presents with neonatal seizures without encephalopathy in the first few days.[30,65-67] MRI reveals an acute restricted diffusion lesion, usually within the MCA and involving cerebral cortex. Similarly, acute neonatal CSVT usually presents with seizures or encephalopathy in the first weeks of life, typically with evidence of venous edema or infarction on imaging that is often hemorrhagic.[17,66,68,69] The superficial venous system is most often affected in neonatal CSVT.[69] The lesion typically occurs in term babies after an uneventful pregnancy, routine delivery, normal APGAR scores and no fetal distress. It is mainly a radiographic finding after the onset of motor focal seizures and sometimes the signs and symptoms may be so subtle that it may be missed. In contrast, another 50% of perinatal ischemic strokes are asymptomatic in the neonatal period. Such presumed perinatal ischemic stroke (PPIS) typically presents as a motor asymmetry or early hand preference noted by parents at 4–6 months, though epilepsy or other delays may be the initial concern.[65,66,70]

Most neonatal infarcts probably result from emboli. Systemic emboli can occasionally be demonstrated in these neonates, and the left hemisphere predominance is more common. Interruption of aortic laminar flow by blood from the patent ductus accounts for the emboli being preferentially directed to left cerebral hemisphere. Most neonatal emboli originate from degenerating placental vessels.

The clinical presentation of PHS is similar to that of ischemic stroke, with most cases presenting acutely with encephalopathy and/or seizures.[50] Many cases, however, are diagnosed with routine prenatal ultrasound.[71]

Patients who present after the immediate perinatal period are less well characterized but may resemble PPIS populations with hemiparesis or epilepsy as well as posthemorrhagic hydrocephalus in the case of intraventricular HS.[50,71]

Cerebral Embolism

The classic pattern of sudden-onset of symptoms with immediate maximum deficit is rare in young children. Very young children present with a deficit of unknown duration. In children vessels most often occluded by an embolus are the supraclinoid internal carotid arteries and the middle cerebral arteries; hence, typical signs include hemiparesis, hemisensory loss and aphasia.[72] Stroke in the posterior circulation can present as ataxia, vertigo, and vomiting. However, nonlocalizing neurological signs, like altered mental status and seizures, occur more frequently in childhood stroke.[73,74]

Cerebral Thrombosis

The clinical picture depends on the size and location of the lesion. The maximal deficit tends to evolve over minutes or hours. It is often difficult to determine whether an infarction is the result of embolism or thrombosis, particularly in children at risk for both, such as one with cyanotic congenital heart disease. The dramatic improvement that sometimes follows embolism is not seen with cerebral thrombosis, where recovery more typically evolves over weeks or months.

Lacunar Infarction

Lacunae are small infarctions resulting from the occlusion of small penetrating arteries. They commonly occur in the deep cerebral nuclei or the pons. As in adults, in children also these lesions commonly result in pure motor paresis, monoparesis, or hemianesthesia. However, unlike adults where chronic hypertension is the most common risk factor, here its small emboli, vasculitis or unidentifiable risk factors which cause the lesion. The prognosis is usually good.

Transient Ischemic Attack

Transient ischemic attacks (TIAs) result from small emboli or local hemodynamic factors, which temporarily prevent adequate cerebral perfusion. It is not very common in children though moyamoya disease may cause an artery to artery embolism; hence, transient deficits. Recurrent AIS or TIA occurs in up to 15% of patients with arterial dissection.[75]

Sinovenous Occlusion

Symptoms of CSVT tend to develop gradually over hours to days. Symptoms in such children are most commonly diffuse and nonspecific. Diffuse symptoms include headache, confusion, vomiting, photophobia, and papilledema. Infants often present with nonspecific symptoms such as bulging fontanel, lethargy, or seizures. Venous occlusion alters cerebral metabolism locally, but tissue destruction caused is less than after arterial occlusion. Venous occlusion may be associated with a nearby infection such as chronic otitis, sinusitis or orbital abscess. It also complicates conditions like hemoglobinopathy, congestive heart failure, polycythemia and dehydration.

Intraparenchymal Hemorrhage

Older children with HS may present with the classical signs of headache, vomiting, impaired consciousness, seizures, and/or focal neurological deficits. But younger children often present with subtle signs and symptoms unless motor pathways or brainstem is involved. In posterior fossa hemorrhage, bulbar signs, ataxia, and rapid deterioration to coma are typical.

Subarachnoid Hemorrhage

The classical signs and symptoms of subarachnoid hemorrhage are less distinct in children. They may present with unexplained irritability, vomiting, photophobia or seizures. Signs of raised intracranial pressure are common, and papilledema may be found within 5 or 6 hours. Various forms of autonomic dysfunction are frequently present. Besides trauma, arterial aneurysms, AVMs, SCD and coagulopathy are the most frequent causes of subarachnoid hemorrhage.[76]

There are many different signs and symptoms of stroke as mentioned above. A basic knowledge of neuroanatomy and cerebral vascular anatomy is necessary before one can determine that the patient's problem is the result of a stroke-induced brain lesion.

There are no consensus guidelines on the evaluation of stroke in children. However, as in any other disease management, it is important to identify the cause of stroke and rule out nonvascular causes.

DIAGNOSIS

Clinical

Conditions that imitate stroke, such as hypoglycemia, postictal state, drug overdose, postconcussion states, migrainous accompaniment, encephalopathies with focal signs, hyponatremia, subdural hematoma or empyema must be ruled out. A history of head or neck trauma, unexplained fever or recent infection, developmental delay, family history of bleeding problems, associated headache, SCD, cyanotic CHD should be taken.

Information about the onset of symptoms is crucial, especially the time and speed of onset. The diagnostic possibilities increase when no history can be obtained, as in the obtunded patient. Seizures are most likely to imitate stroke as they can also accompany stroke. Thrombolytic therapy is contraindicated, if a seizure occurs at the onset of stroke symptoms.

Finding the etiology of cerebrovascular disease is particularly important in children, because their recurrence risk is determined largely by the stroke's cause and whether it is treatable. A child at risk for stroke faces decades of increased susceptibility, making the identification and treatment of risk factors relatively more important in children than adults.

Investigations

The clinical assessment of an acute stroke in a child represents a diagnostic challenge. Delays in diagnosis longer than 24 hours are unfortunately common. The following questions should always be asked during the evaluation of a child with stroke:

1. Is there a cerebrovascular lesion?
2. Is it an infarction or a hemorrhage?
3. Is it in the anterior or posterior circulation?
4. What is the cause?

Ideally the diagnostic evaluation should be done in stages, with the next step influenced by results of previous tests. Often, however, it is cheaper to do a battery of studies simultaneously, adding or deleting some studies depending on the situation. All children require measurement of coagulation parameters, complete blood counts, and routine blood work as well as a detailed prothrombotic work-up.[77] Hb electrophoresis should be done on patients at risk for hemoglobinopathy.

To assess activated protein C resistance, a PTT is performed in the presence and absence of exogenously supplied activated protein C. The ratio of the PTT with activated protein C versus the baseline PTT is calculated. Normal individuals usually have a ratio of 2.0 or greater, and individuals with factor V Leiden usually have a ratio less than 2.0. A modified form of this assay can be performed even on patients receiving anticoagulants, patients with liver disease, and those with an activated factor VIII due to acute phase reaction. But the gold standard for Factor V Leiden testing is DNA analysis using PCR methodology.

PTT is also deranged in protein C-deficiency. There are two major types of protein C assays: functional and antigenic. Functional assays measure protein C function. Antigenic assays are immunoassays that measure the quantity of protein C, regardless of the quality of its function.

Because embolism is a frequent cause of childhood stroke, a careful cardiac examination is essential. After an initial chest X-ray and ECG an echocardiography may often be indicated if any doubts persist. Transthoracic echocardiography (TTE) is usually sufficient in young children, but transesophageal echocardiography (TEE) may be necessary in adolescents with a thicker chest wall.

Lumbar puncture should be considered in nonhemorrhagic stroke without significant mass effect and when the earlier evaluation has failed to establish a cause. Chronic meningitis or early tubercular meningitis could present with stroke. Syphilis serology may be done in adolescents with infarction.

Perinatal stroke may require specific testing for metabolic disorders, thrombophilias, cardiac disease in the fetus or newborn and also maternal testing for autoimmune disorders.

Cranial ultrasound is useful for intraventricular and germinal matrix hemorrhage, but not adequate for identifying ischemic stroke.[78] Transcranial doppler (TCD), which can be performed at the bedside is useful in sickle-cell related stroke and also for evaluation of the circle of Willis.[59]

Neuroimaging is the mainstay in the diagnosis of pediatric stroke. *Computed tomography* or *magnetic resonance* imaging should be done early in the evaluation. Several new MR techniques have been used for evaluation of ischemic stroke in children, including diffusion, perfusion, gradient echo and FLAIR imaging.[60,79] MRI, especially with the integration of diffusion weighted (DWI) and perfusion-weighted (PWI) imaging, is optimal for diagnosing stroke. DWI is the most sensitive tool in the diagnosis of cytotoxic edema, so it can indicate AIS even in cases with apparently normal CT and MRI conventional sequences.[80]

The gold standard for evaluating the cerebral vascular system is the conventional four-vessel angiogram. Arteriopathies, such as dissection and vasculitis are best diagnosed with conventional angiography.[81] A youngster with a small hemorrhage must undergo angiography so that a small AVM or aneurysm is not missed.[82] MRA allows the detection and location of intracerebral arterial lesions in a noninvasive way, although the characterization of the type of lesion is the main limitation of MRA. MR spectroscopy (MRS) and DWI with MRA could also, in selected cases, increase the sensitivity of MRI in the detection of ischemia and infarction. Although CT may also be used, MRI and MRV are the preferred methods for investigation of CSVT because of their sensitivity and specificity and for the excellent anatomical correlation between venous drainage system and location of parenchymal infarcts. When MRI examination cannot be performed, unenhanced CT may detect deep venous thrombosis as linear densities in the expected locations of the deep and cortical veins. CT scan with contrast misses the diagnosis of CSVT in up to 40% of patients[83] so CTV can be a reasonable in-depth examination. MR imaging should also be done in evaluation of suspected extracranial arterial dissection. A tentative schema towards the approach for diagnosis of stroke in children is given in Flow chart 22.1.

Functional MR may be useful to ascertain changes in blood flow with motor or language dysfunction and for monitoring changes in functioning during recovery. Imaging of the cervical and proximal intracranial arterial vasculature should be performed in all children with AIS and imaging of the cervical vasculature to exclude arterial dissection should be undertaken within 48 hours of presentation with AIS.[84]

Flow chart 22.1: Evaluation of the pediatric stroke patient[2]

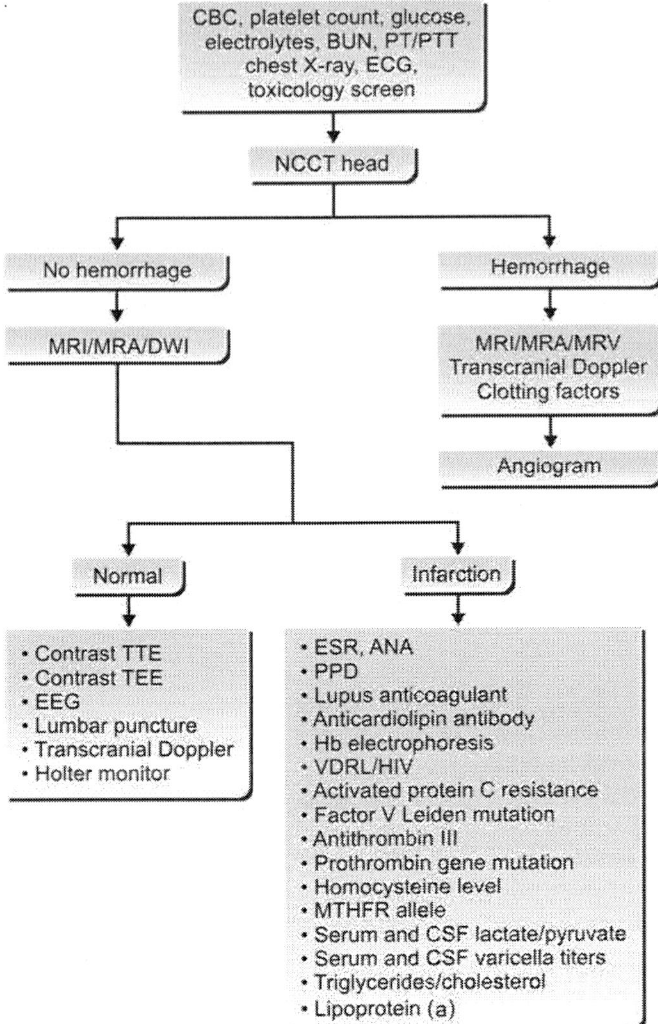

Abbreviations: ANA: Antinuclear antibody; BUN: Blood urea nitrogen; CBC: Complete blood count; CSF: Cerebrospinal fluid; CT: Computed tomography; DWI: Diffusion weighted imaging; ECG: Electrocardiogram; EEG: Electroencephalogram; ESR: Erythrocyte sedimentation rate; MRA: Magnetic resonance angiography; MRI: Magnetic resonance imaging; MRV: Magnetic resonance venography; PPD: Tuberculin purified protein derivative; PT/PTT: Prothrombin time/partial thromboplastin time; TEE: Transesophageal echocardiography; TTE: Transthoracic echocardiography; VDRL: Venereal disease research laboratory

TREATMENT

There have been no randomized clinical trials for the acute treatment or secondary prevention of AIS in children. Children with stroke require immediate, special attention and if possible should be stabilized and transferred to an institution that can offer pediatric neurovascular expertise and care.

Supportive Care and Treatment of Acute Complications

This should begin even before the diagnosis of the cerebrovascular disease has been established. A definitive benefit for the aggressive treatment of infection, fever, blood pressure, hypo/ hyperglycemia, and seizures has been demonstrated. Large lesions can generate increased intracranial pressure (ICP), and can lead to aspiration. The vital signs and neurologic status need to be monitored closely.[85] Increased ICP does not need any special measures, if the lesion is small as no significant mass effect is produced. In cases of large cerebral hemorrhage reduction of the $PaCO_2$ is the quickest way to reduce pressure. Such patients may benefit from surgical evacuation of the lesion.

Prophylactic antiepileptic treatment is not recommended but when seizures occur, a non-sedating drug like phenytoin is more useful than phenobarbital. However, children with a subarachnoid hemorrhage due to an aneurysm or AVM should receive a prophylactic anticonvulsant because a seizure might increase the risk of rebleeding. Treatment of fever is important, as hyperthermia exacerbates ischemic brain damage, and hypothermia is protective.[86] Supportive therapy and family centered treatment strategies including provisions for family support and facilitating educational testing, have a major role to play in pediatric stroke.

Definitive Treatment Strategies

In *perinatal AIS* (esp. due to cardiac disease) and more controversially CSVT existing data support the role of anticoagulation.[87,88] Correction of the underlying coagulopathy is with platelet support, coagulation factors and vitamin K is essential in *perinatal HS.* In some cases surgical evacuation of an intracranial hematoma may be indicated, if there is a raised ICP. If posthemorrhagic hydrocephalus develops, the patient may require placement of a shunt. In *childhood IS,* apart from supportive therapy anticoagulation therapy is recommended in children with stroke due to cardio-embolism or arterial dissection.[89] However, duration of therapy remains controversial and unfractionated heparin (UFH) or more recently low molecular weight heparins (LMWH) have been used. Warfarin is limited to patients requiring more long-term therapy (e.g. complex congenital heart diseases or severe prothrombotic disorders). Aspirin (ASA) is the primary antiplatelet agent for children with a well-established safety profile.[90,91] Dosing varies from 2-5 mg/kg/day, usually administered once daily. Corticosteroid or chemotherapeutic treatment may be necessary for cerebral vasculitis.[89] Surgical revascularization for specific causes of stroke, such as moyamoya disease has been shown to be effective in the pediatric population.[92] Complete MCA syndromes carry the highest risk of post-stroke edema, but MCA trunk infarcts, as well as large hemorrhagic transformations, can generate acute transtentorial herniation. Decompressive hemicraniectomy can be a lifesaving surgical intervention.[93-95]

Cases of *childhood HS* often require neurosurgical intervention, such as evacuation of a large hematoma or shunt placement, clipping or coiling of aneurysms, removal or embolization of AVM. Endovascular treatment of AVM typically involves the injection of occlusive materials into feeding arteries to diminish or potentially cure the lesion. Stereotactic radiosurgery is another option where focused irradiation (e.g. gamma knife) can obliterate small lesions or decrease the size of larger ones. A team of neurosurgeons, neuro-interventionalists, radiation specialists, and other experts is required to determine the best treatment plan. Surgical resection for cavernous malformations and aneurysms is also indicated in most cases. Medical therapies such as factor VIII replacement, antibiotics in endocarditis, vitamin K for anticoagulant reversal, immunomodulation in conditions like ITP and more controversially recombinant factor VIIa (rFVIIa) for the treatment of HS also have a role to play. The role of rfVIIa in HS remains very controversial due to an increased risk of serious thrombotic events and lack of pediatric data.[96]

Anticoagulation and Thrombolysis

Anticoagulation should be used in children with a high recurrence risk and with a minimal risk of secondary hemorrhage. The Royal College of Physicians Pediatric Stroke Working group for AIS[84] include the following: (i) children with non-sickle cell–related AIS should be started on aspirin (5 mg/kg/d); (ii) children with sickle cell-related AIS should receive emergent exchange transfusion and if not possible, blood transfusion; (iii) children with extracranial dissection-related AIS should receive anticoagulation; (iv) children with cardioembolic AIS should be treated based on recommendations from a pediatric cardiologist; and (v) children with elevated intracranial pressure and neurological worsening should be referred for neurosurgical consultation. Heparin is often used initially while the dose of warfarin is adjusted. Using this approach anticoagulation is often used in children with arterial dissection, dural sinus thrombosis, coagulation disorders, or a high risk of embolism. The loading dose of heparin is 75 U/kg intravenously followed by 20 U/kg/hour in children >1 year of age and 28 U/kg/hour in children <1 year of age. The target

APTT is 60-85 seconds. Low molecular weight heparin (LMWH) can be used in children. Enoxaparin is the most commonly used variety and typical treatment dosing is 1.5 mg/kg daily in infants under 2 months and 1.0 mg/kg daily in older children.[97] Their predictable pharmacokinetics, increased bioavailability, and longer plasma half-life allow once- or twice-a-day dosing and eliminate the need for routine laboratory monitoring. But its use in the treatment of stroke remains controversial and unproven.[98] Warfarin may be used in children with congenital or acquired heart disease, hypercoagulable states, arterial dissection, and dural sinus thrombosis. An INR of 2 to 3 is appropriate for most children.

Exchange transfusion is sometimes used after first stroke in SCD. The child is subsequently placed on a chronic transfusion regimen. The incidence of recurrent stroke can be reduced significantly with chronic transfusions to maintain the hemoglobin S concentration below 20-30%.

There is little information regarding the effectiveness or risks of thrombolytic agents in children, although extensive research has been done in adult patients. Foremost, is determining, if differences in stroke mechanisms and vascular and coagulation systems confer advantages or risks for thrombolysis. Also, the time window available for use of acute thrombolysis is very small and, if reopening of thrombosed cerebral artery is not done very early, recanalization will not reduce the size of the cerebral infarction. Urokinase and t-PA have been used occasionally in children in acute ischemic stroke.[99] Thrombolytic therapy has been recommended for childhood AIS in special situations but should only be considered at institutions able to support its complications.[2] The primary concern with thrombolytic use is hemorrhage though recent evidence suggests that younger age and careful patient selection minimize the risk in adults.[99] Tissue plasminogen activator (tPA) administered to children for non-cerebral thrombosis has shown good success in clot lysis but major bleeding in 11% and ICH in 1-2%.[100] A review by Carpenter et al[101] identified a total of 44 pediatric stroke cases in which IV or intra-arterial rt-PA was used, but only 3 of the patients who received IV rt-PA experienced clinical improvement (ped stroke-tPA). In conclusion, this treatment may be considered by emergency physicians in consultation with a pediatric neurologist, more research is required to define the role of thrombolysis in the pediatric population.

REFERENCES

1. Kirkham FJ. Stroke in childhood. Arch Dis Child. 1999;81:85-9.
2. Younkin DP. Diagnosis and treatment of ischemic pediatric stroke. Curr Neurol Neurosci Rep. 2002;2:18-24.
3. Cardenas JF, Rho JM, Kirton A. Pediatric stroke. Childs Nerv Syst. 2011;27:1375-90.
4. deVeber G. Canadian Paediatric Ischemic Stroke Study Group. Canadian Paediatric Ischemic Stroke Registry: Analysis of children with arterial ischemic stroke. Ann Neurol 2000; Ann Neurol. 2000;48(3):514. (Abstract).
5. Lynch JK, Hirtz DG, deVeber G, Nelson KB. Report of the National Institute of Neurological Disorders and Stroke workshop on perinatal and childhood stroke. Pediatrics. 2002;109:116-23.
6. National Center for Health Statistics. Health, United States, 1994. Hyattsville, MD: Public Health Service; 1995. *www.cdc.gov/nchs/hus/hus94*.
7. Lanni G, Catalucci A, Conti L, et al. Pediatric stroke: Clinical findings and radiological approach. Stroke Research and Treatment. Vol. 2011, Article ID 172168. DOI:10.4061/2011/172168.
8. Eeg-Olofsson O, Ringheim Y. Stroke in children. Clinical characteristics and prognosis. Acta Pediatr Scand. 1983;72:391-5.
9. Wiliams LS, Garg BP, Cohen M, Fleck JD, Biller J. Subtypes of ischemic strokes in children and young adults. Neurology. 1997;49:1541-5.
10. Al Sulaiman A, Badenmosi O, Ismail H, Magboll G. Stroke in Saudi children. J Child Neurol. 1999;14:295-8.
11. Lopez-Vicente M, Ortega-Gutierrez S, Amlie-Lefond C, and Torbey MT. Diagnosis and management of pediatric arterial ischemic stroke. J Stroke Cerebrovasc Dis. 2010;19(3):175-83.
12. Kramarow E, Lentzner H, Rooks R, Weeks J, Sayadah S. Health and aging chart book, Health, United States, 1999. Hyattsville, MD: National Center for Health Statistics, 1999.
13. Kirkham FJ, Prengler M, Hewes DKM, et al. Risk factors for arterial ischemic stroke in children. J Child Neurol. 2000;15:299-307.
14. Schoenberg BS, Mellinger JF, Schoenberg DG. Cerebrovascular disease in infants and children: a study of incidence, clinical features, and survival. Neurology. 1978;28:763-8.
15. Gregory J del Zoppo, John M Hallenbeck. Advances in the vascular pathophysiology of Ischemic Stroke. Thrombosis Research. 2000;98:V73-V81.
16. Doyle KP, Simon RP, Stenzel-Poore MP. Mechanisms of ischemic brain damage. Neuropharmacology. 2008;55:310-8.
17. Ferriero DM. Neonatal brain injury. N Engl J Med. 2004;351:1985-95.
18. Hossmann KA. Pathophysiology and therapy of experimental stroke. Cell Mol Neurobiol. 2006;26:1057-83.
19. Mergenthaler P, Dirnagl U, Meisel A. Pathophysiology of stroke: lessons from animal models. Metab Brain Dis. 2004;19:151-67.

20. deVeber G, Andrew M, Adams C, Bjornson B, Booth F, Buckley DJ, Camfield CS, David M, Humphreys P, Langevin P, MacDonald EA, Gillett J,Meaney B, Shevell M, Sinclair DB, Yager J. Cerebral sinovenous thrombosis in children. N Engl J Med. 2001;345:417-23.
21. Sebire G, Tabarki B, Saunders DE, Leroy I, Liesner R, Saint-Martin C, Husson B, Williams AN, Wade A, Kirkham FJ. Cerebral venous sinus thrombosis in children: risk factors, presentation, diagnosis and outcome. Brain. 2005;128:477-89.
22. Menovsky T, van Overbeeke JJ. Cerebral arteriovenous malformations in childhood: state of the art with special reference to treatment. Eur J Pediatr. 1997;156:741-6.
23. Nelson KB, Lynch JK. Stroke in newborn infants. Lancet Neurol. 2004;3:150-8.
24. Golomb MR, MacGregor DL, Domi T, Armstrong DC, Mc- Crindle BW, Mayank S, et al. Presumed pre- or perinatal arterial ischemic stroke: risk factors and outcomes. Ann Neurol. 2001;50:163-8.
25. Chun DS, Schamberger MS, Flaspohler T, et al. Incidence, outcome, and risk factors for stroke after the Fontan procedure. Am J Cardiol. 2004;93:117-9.
26. Gould RJ, Black K, Pavlakis SG. Neonatal cerebral arterial thrombosis: protein C deficiency. J Child Neurol. 1996;11:250-1.
27. Rodegheiro F, Tosetto A. The epidemiology of inherited thrombophilia: the VITA project. Thromb Hemostasis. 1997;78:636-40.
28. Fernandez JA, Estelles A, Gilabert J, et al. Functional and immunologic protein S in normal pregnant women and full term infants. Thromb Hemostasis. 1989;61:474-8.
29. Adams RJ, McKie VC, Hsu L, et al. Stroke prevention trial in sickle cell anemia ("STOP"): study results. N Engl J Med. 1998;339:5-11.
30. Roach ES, Golomb MR, Adams R, Biller J, Daniels S, deVeber G, Ferriero D, Jones BV, Kirkham F, Scott M, Smith E. Management of stroke in infants and children: a scientific statement from a Special Writing Group of the American Heart Association Stroke Council and the Council on Cardiovascular Disease in the Young. Stroke. 2008;39:2644-91.
31. Emerick KM, Krantz ID, Kamath BM, Darling C, Burrowes D, Spinner N, Whitington P, Piccoli D. Intracranial vascular abnormalities in patients with Alagille syndrome. J Pediatr Gastroenterol Nutr. 2005;41:99-107.
32. Scott RM, Smith ER. Moyamoya disease and moyamoya syndrome. N Engl J Med. 2009;360:1226-37.
33. Kurokowa T, Tomita S, Udeda K, et al. Prognosis of occlusive disease of the circle of Willis (Moyamoya diseases) in children. Pediatr Neurol. 1985;1:274-7.
34. Fukui M. Current state of study on moyamoya disease in Japan. Surg Neurol. 1997;47:138-41.
35. Gottlieb SM, Rosman NP, Stitch RA. Stroke in children after blunt intraoral trauma. Use of magnetic resonance angiography as a noninvasive diagnostic tool. J Child Neurol. 1996;11:419-22.
36. Khurana DS, Bonnemann CG, Dooling EC, et al. Vertebral artery dissection: Issues in diagnosis and management. Pedaitr Neurol. 1996;14:225-8
37. Fullerton HJ, Johnston SC, Smith WS. Arterial dissection and stroke in children. Neurology. 2001;57:1155-60.
38. Askalan R, Laughlin S, Mayank S, Chan A, MacGregor D, Andrew M. Chickenpox and stroke in childhood, A study of Frequency and Causation. Stroke. 2001;32:1257-62.
39. Sebire G, Meyer L, Chabrier. Varicella as a risk factor for cerebral infarction in childhood: a case-control study. Ann Neurol. 1999;45:679-80.
40. Danchaivijitr N, Miravet E, Saunders DE, Cox T, Ganesan V. Post-varicella intracranial haemorrhage in a child. Dev Med Child Neurol. 2006;48:139-42.
41. Belostotsky VM, Shah V, Dillon MJ. Clinical features in 17 paediatric patients with Wegener granulomatosis. Pediatr Nephrol. 2002;17:754-61.
42. Benseler S, Schneider R. Central nervous system vasculitis in children. Curr Opin Rheumatol. 2004;16:43-50.
43. Berman JL, Kashii S, Trachtman MS, Burde RM. Optic neuropathy and central nervous system disease secondary to Sjogren's syndrome in a child. Ophthalmology. 1990;97:1606-9.
44. Graf WD, Milstein JM, Sherry DD. Stroke and mixed connective tissue disease. J Child Neurol. 1993;8:256-9.
45. Morales E, Pineda C, Martinez-Lavin M. Takayasu's arteritis in children. J Rheumatol. 1991;18:1081-4.
46. Morfin-Maciel B, Medina A, Espinosa Rosales F, Berron R, Huerta Lopez J. Central nervous system involvement in a child with polyarteritis nodosa and severe atopic dermatitis. Rev Alerg Méx. 2002;49:189-95.
47. von Scheven E, Lee C, Berg BO. Pediatric Wegener's granulomatosis complicated by central nervous system vasculitis. Pediatr Neurol. 1998;19:317-9.
48. Benseler SM, Silverman E, Aviv RI, Schneider R, Armstrong D, Tyrrell P, de Veber G. Primary central nervous system vasculitis in children. Arthritis Rheum. 2006;54:1291-7.
49. Looney CB, Smith JK, Merck LH, Wolfe HM, Chescheir NC, Hamer RM, Gilmore JH. Intracranial hemorrhage in asymptomatic neonates: prevalence on MR images and relationship to obstetric and neonatal risk factors. Radiology. 2007;242:535-41.
50. Armstrong-Wells J, Johnston SC, Wu YW, Sidney S, Fullerton HJ. Prevalence and predictors of perinatal hemorrhagic stroke: results from the Kaiser pediatric stroke study. Pediatrics. 2009;123:823-8.
51. Sachs BP, Acker D, Tuomala R, Brown E. The incidence of symptomatic intracranial hemorrhage in term appropriate-for gestation-age infants. Clin Pediatr Phila. 1987;26:355-8.
52. Danchaivijitr N, Cox TC, Saunders DE, Ganesan V. Evolution of cerebral arteriopathies in childhood arterial ischemic stroke. Ann Neurol. 2006;59:620-6.
53. Schoenberg BS, Mellinger JF, Schoenberg DG. Moyamoya disease in children. South Med J. 1978;71:237-41.
54. Lo W, Zamel K, Ponnappa K, Allen A, Chisolm D, Tang M, Kerlin B, Yeates KO. The cost of pediatric stroke care and rehabilitation. Stroke. 2008;39:161-5.
55. Lin CL, Loh JK, Kwan AL, Howng SL. Spontaneous intracerebral hemorrhage in children. Kaohsiung J Med Sci. 1999;15:146-51.
56. Livingston JH, Brown JK. Intracerebral haemorrhage after the neonatal period. Arch Dis Child. 1986;61:538-44.

57. Andes WA, Wulff K, Smith WB. Head trauma in hemophilia: a prospective study. Arch Intern Med. 1984;144:1981-3.
58. Lutsch J, Vassela F. Neurological complications in hemophilia. Acta Pediatr Scand. 1981;70:235-41.
59. Woener SJ, Abildgaard CF, French BN. Intracranial hemorrhage in children with idiopathic thrombocytopenic purpura. Pediarics. 1981;67:453-60.
60. Gerosa MA, Cappellotto P, Licata C, et al. Cerebral arteriovenous malformations in children (56 cases). Childs Brain. 1981;8:356-71.
61. Ventureya ECG, Herder S. Arteriovenous malformations of the brain in children. Child's Nerv Syst. 1987;3:12-8.
62. Broderick J, Talbot GT, Prenger E, Leach A, Brott T. Stroke in children within a major metropolitan area: the surprising importance of intracerebral hemorrhage. J Child Neurol. 1993;8:250-5.
63. Meyer-Heim AD, Boltshauser E. Spontaneous intracranial haemorrhage in children: aetiology, presentation and outcome. Brain Dev. 2003;25:416-21.
64. Roach ES, Riela AR. Pediatric Cerebrovascular Disorders. 2nd ed. New York: Futura; 1995. p. 359.
65. Fitzgerald KC, Williams LS, Garg BP, Golomb MR. Epilepsy in children with delayed presentation of perinatal stroke. J Child Neurol. 2007;22:1274-80.
66. Kirton A, deVeber G. Advances in perinatal ischemic stroke. Pediatr Neurol. 2009;40:205-14.
67. Lynch JK. Epidemiology and classification of perinatal stroke. Semin Fetal Neonatal Med. 2009;14:245-9.
68. Bernard TJ, Goldenberg NA. Pediatric arterial ischemic stroke. Pediatr Clin N Am. 2008;55:323-38.
69. Ramenghi LA, Govaert P, Fumagalli M, Bassi L, Mosca F. Neonatal cerebral sinovenous thrombosis. Semin Fetal Neonatal Med. 2009;14:278-83.
70. Kirton A, Wei X. Teaching neuroimages: confirmation of prenatal periventricular venous infarction with susceptibility weighted MRI. Neurology 2010; 74:e48, DOI: 10.1212/WNL.0b013e3181d5a47a.
71. Ozduman K, Pober BR, Barnes P, Copel JA, Ogle EA, Duncan CC, Ment LR. Fetal stroke. Pediatr Neurol. 2004;30:151-62.
72. Higgins JJ, Kammermann LA, Fitz CR. Predictors of survival and characteristics of childhood stroke. Neuropediatrics. 1991;22:190-3.
73. Amlie-Lefond C, Sebire G, Fullerton HJ. Recent developments in childhood arterial ischaemic stroke. Lancet Neurol. 2008;7:425-35.
74. Hartman AL, Lunney KM, Serena JE. Pediatric stroke: do clinical factors predict delays in presentation? J Pediatr. 2009;154:727-32.
75. Fullerton HJ, Johnston SC, Smith WS. Arterial dissection and stroke in children. Neurology. 2001;57:1155-60.
76. Byard RW, Bourne AJ, Hanieh A. Sudden and unexpected due to hemorrhage from occult central nervous system lesions. A pediatric autopsy study. Pediatr Neurosurg. 1991;17: 88-94.
77. Strater R, Becker S, von Eckardstein A, Heinecke A, Gutsche S, Junker R, et al. Prospective assessment of risk factors for recurrent stroke during childhood—a 5-year follow-up study. Lancet. 2002;360:1540-5.
78. Adams R, McKie V, Nicholas F, et al. The use of intracranial ultrasonography to predict stroke in sickle cell disease. N Engl J Med. 1992;326:605-10.
79. Hunter JV. Magnetic resonance imaging in pediatric stroke. Top Magn Reson Imaging. 2002;13(1):23-38.
80. Paonessa A, Limbucci N, Tozzi E, Splendiani A, and Gallucci M, "Radiological strategy in acute stroke in children," Eur J Radiol. 2010;74(1):77-85.
81. Chabrier S, Rodesch G, Lasjaunias P, Tardieu M, Landrieu P, Sebrie G. Transient cerebral arteriopathy: a disorder recognized by serial angiograms in children with stroke. J Child Neurol. 1998;13:27-32.
82. Husson B, Rodesch G, Lasjaunias P, Tardieu M, and S´ebire G,."Magnetic resonance angiography in childhood arterial brain infarcts: a comparative study with contrast angiography," Stroke. 2002;33(5):1280-5.
83. Dlamini N, Billinghurst L, and Kirkham FJ. "Cerebral venous sinus (sinovenous) thrombosis in children." Neurosurg Clin North Am. 2010;21(3):511-27.
84. Paediatric Stroke Working Group. "Stroke in childhood: clinical guidelines for diagnosis, management and rehabilitation." Royal College of Physicians, November 2004, http://bookshop.rcplondon.ac.uk/contents/f98c6540-a541-4bed-837d-ef293- ac458bf.pdf.
85. Horowitz M, Purdy P, Unwin H, et al. Treatment of dural sinus thrombosis using selective catheterization and urokinase. Ann Neurol. 1995;38:58-67.
86. Lynch JK. Han CJ. Pediatric stroke: what do we know and what do we need to know? Semin Neurol. 2005;25(4):410-23.
87. Jordan LC, Rafay MF, Smith SE, Askalan R, Zamel KM, deVeber G, Ashwal S. Antithrombotic treatment in neonatal cerebral sinovenous thrombosis: results of the International Pediatric Stroke Study. J Pediatr. 2010;156:704-10.
88. Moharir MD, Shroff M, Stephens D, Pontigon AM, Chan A, MacGregor D, Mikulis D, Adams M, deVeber G. Anticoagulants in pediatric cerebral sinovenous thrombosis: a safety and outcome study. Ann Neurol. 2010;67:590-9.
89. Carvalho KS, Garg BP. Arterial strokes in children. Neurol Clin. 2002;20:1079-100.
90. Monagle P, Barnes C, Ignjatovic V, Furmedge J, Newall F, Chan A, De Rosa L, Hamilton S, Ragg P, Robinson S, Auldist A, Crock C, Roy N, Rowlands S. Developmental haemostasis. Impact for clinical haemostasis laboratories. Thromb Haemost. 2006;95:362-72.
91. Strater R, Kurnik K, Heller C, Schobess R, Luigs P, Nowak-Gottl U. Aspirin versus low-dose low-molecular weight heparin: antithrombotic therapy in pediatric ischemic stroke patients: a prospective follow-up study. Stroke. 2001;32:2554-8.
92. So Y, Lee HY, Kim SK, Lee JS, Wang KC, Cho BK, Kang E, Lee DS. Prediction of the clinical outcome of pediatric moyamoya disease with postoperative basal/acetazolamide stress brain perfusion SPECT after revascularization surgery. Stroke. 2005;36:1485-9.
93. Cho DY, Chen TC, Lee HC. Ultra-early decompressive craniectomy for malignant middle cerebral artery infarction. Surg Neurol. 2003;60:227-32, discussion 232-3.

94. Gupta R, Connolly ES, Mayer S, Elkind MS. Hemicraniectomy for massive middle cerebral artery territory infarction: a systematic review. Stroke. 2004;35:539-43.
95. Vahedi K, Hofmeijer J, Juettler E, Vicaut E, George B, Algra A, Amelink GJ, Schmiedeck P, Schwab S, Rothwell PM, Bousser MG, van der Worp HB, Hacke W. Early decompressive surgery in malignant infarction of the middle cerebral artery: a pooled analysis of three randomised controlled trials. Lancet Neurol. 2007;6:215-22.
96. Mayer SA, Brun NC, Begtrup K, Broderick J, Davis S, Diringer MN, Skolnick BE, Steiner T. Recombinant activated factor VII for acute intracerebral hemorrhage. N Engl J Med. 2005;352:777-85.
97. Monagle P, Chan A, Massicotte P, Chalmers E, Michelson AD. Antithrombotic Therapy in Children: The Seventh ACCP Conference on Antithrombotic and Thrombolytic Therapy. Chest. 2004;126:645S-87S.
98. Adams HP, Brott C, Crowell RM, et al. Guidelines for management of patients with acute ischemic stroke: a statement of healthcare professionals from a special working group of the Stroke Council, American Heart Association. Stroke. 1994;25:1901-14.
99. Hill MD, Buchan AM. Thrombolysis for acute ischemic stroke: results of the Canadian Alteplase for Stroke Effectiveness Study. CMAJ. 2005;172:1307-12.
100. Monagle P, Michelson AD, Bovill E, Andrew M. Antithrombotic therapy in children. Chest. 2001;119:344S–70S.
101. Carpenter J, Tsuchida T, Lynch JK. Treatment of arterial ischemic stroke in children. Expert Rev Neurother. 2007;7:383-92.

Polycythemia in Newborn

Mohammed Ramzan, Anupam Sachdeva, SP Yadav

A venous hematocrit (Hct) of over 65% or venous hemoglobin (Hb) concentration more than 22.0 g/dl any time during the first week of life is defined as polycythemia. The primary concern with polycythemia is related to hyperviscosity and its associated complications. Blood viscosity increases exponentially as the Hct level rises above 42%. This associated hyperviscosity is thought to contribute to the symptom complex observed in approximately one half of infants with polycythemia. However, only 47% of infants with polycythemia have hyperviscosity, and only 24% of infants with hyperviscosity have a diagnosis of polycythemia. Capillary blood sample should not be relied on for diagnosis of polycythemia as it varies with local perfusion and temperature. Capillary hematocrit is generally 5-10% higher than the central hematocrit.

PATHOPHYSIOLOGY

As the central Hct level increases, viscosity increases. The arterial oxygen content also increases. Changes in blood flow are observed in some organs; this is due to changes in viscosity or changes in arterial oxygen content. The change in blood flow may influence oxygenation and may influence the delivery of substances to organs that are dependent on plasma flow, such as glucose.

Many factors determine blood viscosity. The primary factor in the newborn is the Hct. As such, viscosity increases as Hct level rises. Other factors that uniquely contribute to blood viscosity in the neonate include increased RBC volume and decreased deformability of the fetal erythrocyte. Plasma proteins, platelets, WBC's, and endothelial factors also contribute to viscosity; however, they are not clinically significant in the newborn.

The central venous Hct level peaks 6-12 hours after birth and then declines until the infant is aged 24 hours, at which time it equals the Hct level in cord blood. Fewer than 40% of infants with a Hct level greater than 64% at 2 hours still have a high value at 12 hours or later.

CAUSES OF NEONATAL POLYCYTHEMIA

Important causes of polycythemia are placental red cell transfusion and placental insufficiency. Table 23.1 lists the causes of polycythemia in a newborn.

Table 23.1: Causes of neonatal polycythemia

Intrauterine hypoxia
- Placental insufficiency
  - Small for gestational age (SGA)
  - Dysmaturity
  - Postmaturity
  - Placenta previa
  - Maternal hypertension syndromes
- Severe maternal cyanotic heart disease
- Maternal smoking

Hypertransfusion
- Twin-to-twin transfusion
- Maternal-fetal transfusion
- Placental-cord transfusion

Endocrine causes
- Congenital adrenal hyperplasia
- Neonatal thyrotoxicosis
- Congenital hypothyroidism
- Maternal diabetes mellitus

Miscellaneous
- Chromosomal abnormalities
  Trisomy 13, Trisomy 18, Trisomy 21
- Beckwith-Wiedeman syndrome
- Oligohydramnios
- Maternal use of propranolol
- High-altitude conditions
- High-oxygen-affinity hemoglobinopathies

CLINICAL FEATURES

Symptoms

The clinical manifestations of polycythemia are due to consequences of the increase in blood viscosity. The most consistent symptoms are feeding problems, plethora, lethargy, tachypnea, apnea, cyanosis, jitteriness, seizures and hypotonia.

Physical Findings

a. *General:* The most obvious finding is plethora or ruddiness. Sometimes priapism may be observed in male patients.
b. *CNS:* Central nervous system (CNS) manifestations are the most common problems and include lethargy, irritability, jitteriness, tremors, seizures, and cerebrovascular accidents.
c. *Cardiopulmonary:* Manifestations include respiratory distress, tachypnea, cyanosis, apnea, and congestive heart failure. Increases in hematocrit (Hct) are associated with a decrease in pulmonary blood flow in all newborns. In those with a Hct level of 65% or more, the decrease in pulmonary blood flow may be associated with respiratory distress and cyanosis.
d. *GI:* Poor feeding is reported in more than one half of all infants with polycythemia and hyperviscosity. Necrotizing enterocolitis (NEC) is a rare but devastating complication of polycythemia or hyperviscosity. Historically, about 44% of term infants with NEC have polycythemia. More recent data suggest that polycythemia may not have a large role in the development of NEC in the term infant but may be related to partial exchange transfusion (PET) with colloid to reduce the Hct.
e. *Renal:* Manifestations include decreased glomerular filtration rates, oliguria, hematuria, proteinuria, and renal vein thrombosis.
f. *Metabolic:* Hypoglycemia is the most common metabolic derangement and is observed in 12-40% of infants with polycythemia. Hypocalcemia is the next most common metabolic derangement and is found in 1-11% of neonates with polycythemia.
g. *Coagulation:* Coagulation can be affected. Thrombocytopenia may occur. Disseminated intravascular coagulation (DIC) is rare.

Differential diagnosis such as dehydration and polycythemia vera should be kept in mind.

Lab Investigation

The central venous hematocrit (Hct) measurement is used as a surrogate for diagnosing hyperviscosity in newborns with polycythemia because it is readily available. Most clinical laboratories are not able to measure blood viscosity. Other laboratory tests include measurements of the following:

- Serum glucose, serum calcium levels, bilirubin level, arterial blood gases (ABG) and managed accordingly.
- *Platelet count:* This count may demonstrate thrombocytopenia if thrombosis or disseminated intravascular coagulation (DIC) are present.
- Chest X-ray may show prominent vascular markings.

TREATMENT

Before making a diagnosis of polycythemia, one should rule out dehydration. If this is present, then it should be treated and hematocrit should be rechecked. Once diagnosis is confirmed all polycythemic children should be monitored for hypoglycemia, hypocalcemia and hyperbilirubinemia. Therapy in newborns with polycythemia is based on both the measured central venous hematocrit (Hct) level and the presence or absence of symptoms. Treatment is either conservative or partial exchange transfusion.

Treatment of polycythemia with partial exchange transfusion (PET) remains controversial. Regarding treatment with partial exchange, the Committee of the Fetus and Newborn of the American Academy of Pediatrics states, "The accepted treatment of polycythemia is partial exchange transfusion (PET)." The group also acknowledges that no evidence suggests that exchange transfusion affects the long-term outcome.

- Treatment for asymptomatic patients
  - *Hct level of 65-75%:* Perform cardiorespiratory monitoring and monitoring of Hct and glucose levels every 6-12 hours and observe the patient for symptoms. Continue this monitoring for at least 24 hours or until the Hct level declines.
  - Hct level of more than 75% on repeated measurements: Consider PET.
- Treatment for symptomatic patients
  - *Hct level of 60-65%:* Consider alternative explanations for the symptoms. Although polycythemia and hyperviscosity may be the etiology of the symptoms, other causes for the symptoms must be excluded.
  - Hct level more than 65% with symptoms attributable to polycythemia and hyperviscosity: Consider PET or observation with intravenous fluids for added hydration. Proceed to PET if symptoms worsen.
- PET
  - Perform PET using an umbilical venous catheter to reduce the central Hct level to 50-55%. The

total blood volume to be exchanged is determined as follows: volume (patient's Hct – desired Hct)]/ (patient's Hct), where blood volume = the patient's weight in kilograms multiplied by 90 ml/kg in term infants (depends on gestational age).

– Normal saline is the replacement fluid of choice for exchange transfusions because it is effective and inexpensive. As alternatives, Plasmanate, 5% albumin, or fresh frozen plasma can be used. However, none of these is more effective than normal saline. In addition, both 5% albumin and fresh frozen plasma are blood products, and certain religious beliefs prohibit their use. Lastly, these colloid products have been associated with complications such as necrotizing enterocolitis (NEC).
– An exchange transfusion can be performed in 3 ways, depending on the type of vascular access that is available. Regardless of the method used, aliquots should not exceed approximately 5 ml/kg delivered or removed over 2-3 minutes.
    - If only a single umbilical venous catheter is in place, use a push-pull technique. With this technique, the withdrawal of blood is alternated with the administration of replacement fluid through the single catheter. Do not remove more than 5 ml/kg in any single withdrawal.
    - If both umbilical venous and arterial catheters are in place, withdraw blood from the arterial catheter while administering the replacement fluid through the venous catheter.
    - If a venous or arterial umbilical catheter and a peripheral venous catheter are in place, the former can be used for blood withdrawal, whereas the latter is used to simultaneously and continuously infuse the replacement fluid.

COMPLICATIONS OF EXCHANGE TRANSFUSION

- Apnea, arrhythmia, vasospasm, vessel perforation, air embolus, thrombosis, infarction, thrombocytopenia, hemolysis, electrolyte abnormalities, hypoglycemia, hypocalcemia, intrahepatic hematoma necrotizing enterocolitis.
- Infants are at increased risk for neurological deficits including speech abnormalities, fine-motor delays, and gross-motor delays.

BIBLIOGRAPHY

1. [Guideline] AAP. American Academy of Pediatrics Committee on Fetus and Newborn: routine evaluation of blood pressure, hematocrit, and glucose in newborns. Pediatrics. 1993;92(3):474-6.
2. Awonusonu FO, Pauly TH, Hutchison AA. Maternal smoking and partial exchange transfusion for neonatal polycythemia. Am J Perinatol. 2002;19(7):349-54.
3. Christou HA, Shannon K, Rowitch DH. Anemia. In: Cloherty JP, Eichenwald EC, Stark AR, (Eds): Manual of neonatal care. 6th edn. Lippincott Williams and Wilkins; 2008. pp. 450-4.
4. Dempsey EM, Barrington K. Short and long-term outcomes following partial exchange transfusion in the polycythaemic newborn: a systematic review. Arch Dis Child Fetal Neonatal Ed. 2006;91(1):F2-6.
5. Drew JH, Guaran RL, Grauer S, Hobbs JB. Cord whole blood hyperviscosity: measurement, definition, incidence and clinical features. J Paediatr Child Health. 1991; 27(6):363-5.
6. Jeevasankar M, Agarwal R, Paul VK, et al. Polycythemia in the newborn. Indian J Pediatr. 2008;75(1):68-73.
7. Pappas A, Delaney-Black V. Differential diagnosis and management of polycythemia. Pediatr Clin North Am. 2004;51(4):1063-86.
8. Rosenkrantz TS. Polycythemia and hyperviscosity in the newborn. Semin Thromb Hemost. 2003;29(5):515-27.
9. Schimmel MS, Bromiker R, Soll RF. Neonatal polycythemia: is partial exchange transfusion justified? Clin Perinatol. 2004;31(3):545-53.
10. Shohat M, Reisner SH, Mimouni F, Merlob P. Neonatal polycythemia: II Definition related to time of sampling. Pediatrics. 1984;73(1):11-3.
11. Werner EJ. Neonatal polycythemia and hyperviscosity. Clin Perinatol. 1995;22(3):693-710.
12. Wirth FH, Goldberg KE, Lubchenco LO. Neonatal hyperviscosity: I. Incidence. Pediatrics. 1979;63(6):833-6.
13. Wong W, Fok TF, Lee CH, et al. Randomised controlled trial: comparison of colloid or crystalloid for partial exchange transfusion for treatment of neonatal polycythaemia. Arch Dis Child Fetal Neonatal Ed. 1997;77(2): F115-8.

24 Blood Component Therapy

Vasant Chinnabhandar, VP Choudhary, Samridh Nagar, Anupam Sachdeva

Blood transfusion is an essential part of modern health care. Used correctly, it can save life and improve health. However, the transmission of infectious agents by blood and blood products has focused particular attention on the potential risks of transfusion.

Transfusion practice for the neonatal and pediatric population requires an understanding of the physiologic changes that accompany the transition from fetus through the various intermediate stages to late childhood. The most dynamic changes occur during the perinatal period and early infancy. Consequently, pediatric transfusion concerns are usually divided into two time periods:

- From birth through 4 months
- Older infants (>4 months) and children.

THE APPROPRIATE USE OF BLOOD AND BLOOD PRODUCTS

Key Points

1. The appropriate use of blood and blood products means the transfusion of safe blood products only to treat a condition leading to significant morbidity or mortality that cannot be prevented or managed effectively by other means.
2. Transfusion carries the risk of adverse reactions and transfusion-transmissible infections. Plasma can transmit most of the infections present in whole blood and there are very few indications for its transfusion.
3. Blood donated by family/replacement donors carries a higher risk of transfusion-transmissible infections than blood donated by voluntary non-remunerated donors. Paid blood donors generally have the highest incidence and prevalence of transfusion-transmissible infections.
4. Blood should not be transfused unless it has been obtained from appropriately selected donors, has been screened for transfusion-transmissible infections and tested for compatibility between the donor's red cells and the antibodies in the patient's plasma, in accordance with national requirements.
5. The need for transfusion can often be avoided by:
   - The prevention or early diagnosis and treatment of anemia and conditions that cause anemia.
   - The correction of anemia and the replacement of depleted iron stores before planned surgery.
   - The use of simple alternatives to transfusion, such as intravenous replacement fluids.
   - Good anesthetic and surgical management.

Due to advances in medical care permitting survival of extremely premature neonates, blood components tailored specifically to satisfy the needs of these very low birth weight (VLBW <1500 g) and extremely low birth weight (ELBW <1000 g) should be available.

Concerns with Cytomegalovirus

Cytomegalovirus (CMV) may be transfusion-transmitted; however current transfusion practice has made this uncommon.[1] Greatest risk of CMV is in fetuses and infants <1.5 kg, immunodeficient patients and SCT recipients. Studies in this regard have revealed:

1. Overall risk of symptomatic post-transfusion CMV infection may be inversely related to the sero-positivity in the community.
2. Risk of acquiring CMV is directly proportional to the cumulative number of different donor exposures during transfusion.
3. CMV in blood is associated with leukocytes.[2] Risk of transmission can be reduced by using seronegative donors or products which have been processed to eliminate viable CMV containing leukocytes.[2] Leukocyte reduction using highly efficient leukocyte filters appears to be effective.[3] Deglycerolized RBCs and washed RBCs (controversial) may also be useful.
4. The "Guidelines of the UK Transfusion Service" state that blood transfused in the first year of life should be CMV negative.[4] Other authorities recommend components leukodepleted to $<5 \times 10^6$/unit as they have significant reduction in risk of CMV

transmission.[5] Some clinicians also prefer CMV negative components for hematopoietic stem cell transplant (HSCT) recipients and immunodeficient individuals. However, in an emergency, transfusion of leukodepleted components is acceptable.[4, 5]

Irradiation

It is essential for blood components (especially all red cell and platelet components) to be irradiated prior to transfusion in the following cases:

1. Intrauterine transfusion (IUT)
2. Exchange transfusion of red cells after IUT.
3. Top-up transfusion after IUT.
4. When the donation is from a first or second degree relative or HLA selected donor.
5. When the child has proven or suspected immunodeficiency.

Irradiation is to prevent proliferation of T-lymphocytes, the immediate cause of GVHD. The standard dose of gamma irradiation is 2500 cGy to the central portion of the container with a minimum dose of 1500 cGy delivered to any part of the component.[5]

- *Side effects:* Erythrocyte membrane damage and increased supernatant K^+.
- The expiration date of irradiated red cells is changed to 28 days after irradiation if remaining shelf life exceeds 28 days.[5]
- There is no need to irradiate FFP, cryoprecipitate or fractionated plasma products.

WHOLE BLOOD

Description and Storage

A unit of Whole blood (WB) is collected in CPDA-1, has a volume of approximately 410 ml (350 ml WB plus 63 ml CPDA-1) and a hematocrit of 0.30-0.40, and is stored at 1-6°C and, has a shelf-life of 35 days. Within 24 hours of collection the platelets as well as the granulocytes in the unit become dysfunctional and the levels of several plasma coagulation factors (in particular Factors V and VIII) fall to suboptimal levels.[6,7]

Indications for Transfusion

Whole Blood is used in situations where a rapid, massive blood loss, has occurred. However, in most cases, the resuscitation can be achieved by the use of RBC concentrates and crystalloids or colloid solutions. Should plasma coagulation factor replacement become necessary, the levels of coagulation Factors V and VIII in stored WB are rarely sufficient to correct the deficiency of these factors. Given these considerations, most centers preparing blood components provide little or no WB but rather separate WB donations into the more commonly required blood components. WB <5-7 days old may be used for exchange transfusion in newborn infants.

Dosage and Administration

It should be ABO and Rh compatible (Table 24.1). The volume and rate of transfusion depends on the clinical situation. After an initial slow drip (to allow observation for immediate, severe transfusion reactions), the rate of infusion should be as fast as clinically indicated or tolerated and in all cases must be completed within 4 hours (to avoid bacterial contamination).

RED BLOOD CELLS

Description and Storage

RBC concentrates are prepared from WB donations. These concentrates can be further modified for use of specific clinical settings. Characteristics of the various RBC, preparations, including their contents and storage conditions, are summarized in Table 24.2.

Indications for Transfusion

Physiologic Responses to Anemia

Oxygen delivery is dependent on:

1. Cardiac Output
2. Arterial Oxygen Content

Cardiac output is dependent on heart rate and stroke volume. Thus tissue hypoxia occurs if there is: (1) Decreased Hb, (2) Cardiac insufficiency.

Physiology of Anemia

With a fall in hemoglobin there is an increase in cardiac output with increase of stroke volume in children but an increase of heart rate (primarily) in neonates. The tissue oxygen extraction ratio (ER) also increases from 25% basal but in heart and brain the ER is 55-70% under basal conditions. Increased levels of 2, 3 DPG leads to right-ward shift of Hb oxygen dissociation curve. In fact children have normally increased levels of 2, 3-DPG and thus lower hemoglobin.[9]

Indications for Transfusion

The decision to transfuse should not be based on the hemoglobin level alone, but also on a careful assessment of the child's clinical condition. Both laboratory and clinical assessment are essential. A child with moderate

Table 24.1: Possible choices of ABO blood groups for red blood cell (RBC), plasma and platelet transfusions[28]

Patient's ABO group	*ABO group of blood product to be transfused*		
	Red cells	*Platelets*	*FFP**
O			
First choice	O	O	O
Second choice	–	A or B	A or B or AB
A			
First choice	A	A	A
Second choice	O	B^	AB
Third choice	–	O#	B#
B			
First choice	B	B^	B
Second choice	O	A#	AB
Third choice	–	O#	A#
AB			
First choice	AB	AB^	AB
Second choice	A or B	A# or B^	A#
Third choice	O#	O#	B#

* Group O fresh frozen plasma (FFP) should only be given to patients of group O. Although group AB FFP can be given to people of any ABO blood group, supplies are usually limited.
# Components which test negatively for 'high titer' anti-A and anti-B should be selected. The use of group O platelets for non-O patients should be avoided as much as possible.
^ Platelet concentrates of group B or of group AB may not be available

Table 24.2: Red blood cell components

Component	*RBC recovery (%)*	*Storage*	*Indication for modified components*
RBCs in CPDA-1	>99	35 days at 1-6°C	
RBC in AS	>99	35-42 days at 1-6°C	
RBCs, buffy COAT poor	90	35 days	History of repeated febrile and/or allergic reactions
RBCs, washed	80	24 hour at 1-6°C	History of repeated febrile and/or allergic reactions unresponsive to buffy-coat poor or leukodepleted RBCs. Prevention of severe allergic reactions or anaphylaxis due to anti-IgA
RBCs, frozen deglycerolized	80	May be stored frozen for up to 10 years (depending on the glycerol concentration) After thawing: storage at 1-6°C for 24 hour	Prolonged storage of autologous units or allogeneic units with rare RBC phenotypes
RBCs, leukocyte reduced by filtration	>90	Pre-storage as for CPDA-1 or AS RBCs Post-storage: for immediate infusion	History of repeated febrile and/or allergic reactions. Prevention of HLA alloimmunization and/or CMV transmission

anemia and pneumonia may have more need of increased oxygen carrying capacity than one with a lower hemoglobin level who is clinically stable.

If the child is stable, is monitored closely and is treated effectively for other conditions, such as acute infection, oxygenation may improve without the need for transfusion.

Indications:

1. Hb concentration of 4 g/dl or less (or Hct 12%)

2. Hb concentration of 4-6 g/dl if any of the following clinical features are present:
   - Clinical features of hypoxia:
     - Acidosis (usually causes dyspnea)
     - Impaired consciousness
   - Hyperparasitemia (>20%)

Despite the large numbers of RBC transfusions administered to children, there is a remarkable paucity of scientific data on which to base RBC transfusion decisions. Recommendations for RBC transfusions in children are, therefore, for the most part based on expert opinion and experience and not on scientific studies.

Indications for RBC Transfusion <4 Months of Age[10]

- Asymptomatic with Hb <7 g/dl with low reticulocyte, or symptomatic anemia with Hb <10 g/dl
  1. On <35% hood O_2/nasal cannula
  2. CPAP/IMV with MAP <6 cm water
  3. Apnea/bradycardia, tachypnea/tachycardia
  4. Poor weight gain
- Hb <12 g/dl
  1. On >35% hood
  2. CPAP/IMV with MAP >6 to 8 cm water
- Hb <15 g/dl
  1. Cyanotic CHD
  2. ECMO

Indications for RBC Transfusion >4 Months of Age[10]

- Blood loss
  1. >15% total body volume (Table 24.3)/with hypovolemia
- Hb <8 g/dl
  1. Symptomatic perioperative anemia
  2. Chemotherapy/radiotherapy or according to protocol
  3. Chronic congenital/acquired anemia
  4. Emergency surgery with anticipated blood loss
  5. Uncorrectable preoperative anemia
  6. Severe infection
- Chronic transfusion dependent states
  1. Thalassemia and other hemoglobinopathies
  2. Bone marrow failure states
- Patient in overt or impending congestive cardiac failure due to anemia.

RBC Transfusion for Acute Blood Loss

In the presence of acute hemorrhage it is important to remember that the first priority is to correct the hypovolemia (with crystalloids and/or colloids) and to attempt to stop the bleeding. In patients with hematologic problems, the latter will often include the need to correct thrombocytopenia and/or deficiencies of coagulation factors, treatment to decrease bleeding from damaged mucosal barriers (e.g. with histamine blockers or antifibrinolytics) and or reversal of the effects of anticoagulant therapy. In patients with normal or near-normal Hb levels prior to the onset of hemorrhage, RBC transfusions are usually only necessary if the patient remains unstable following volume resuscitation. However, careful ongoing evaluation of children with acute blood loss is essential as the signs of shock may initially be subtle in the child. If acute hemorrhage totals >15% of blood volume, signs of circulatory failure (tachycardia, decrease of intensity of peripheral pulses, delayed capillary refill and cool extremities) will be observed. However, hypotension will not be present until 25-30% or more of the child's blood volume is lost.[11,12] It is also important to realize that in the setting of rapid ongoing hemorrhage with hypovolemia, the Hb concentration may not be an accurate indication of the actual RBC mass. The classification of hemorrhagic shock in children based on systemic signs is shown in Table 24.4 and guidelines for resuscitation are summarized in Figure 24.1.[13,14]

Table 24.3: Pediatric blood volumes[8]

Age	Total blood volume
Premature infants	100 ml/kg
Term newborns	85-90 ml/kg
>1 month	80 ml/kg
>1 year	70 ml/kg

RBC Transfusion for Acute Hemolysis

Unlike acute hemorrhage where the patient suffers from both hypovolemia and a decreased RBC mass, patients with acute hemolysis are usually normovolemic. The Hb concentration therefore more accurately reflects RBC mass. The decision to administer an RBC transfusion depends upon a combination of factors, including ongoing clinical evaluation, presence or absence of underlying cardiovascular disease, actual Hb concentration, and rate of decrease in Hb.

RBC Transfusion for Chronic Anemia

Factors to be considered should include:

- Presence or absence of symptom and/or abnormal physical signs and the likelihood that these are due to anemia.

Table 24.4: Classification of hemorrhagic shock in pediatric patients based on systemic signs

System	*Class I* *Very mild hemorrhage* *(<15 TBV loss)*	*Class II* *Mild hemorrhage* *(15-25% TBV loss)*	*Class III* *Moderate hemorrhage* *(26-39% TBV loss)*	*Class IV* *Severe hemorrhage* *(≥40% TBV loss)*
Cardiovascular	Heart rate normal or mildly increased Normal pulses Normal blood pressure Normal pH	Tachycardia Peripheral pulses may be diminished Normal blood pressure Normal pH	Significant tachycardia Thready peripheral pulses Hypotension Metabolic acidosis	Severe tachycardia Thready peripheral pulses Significant Hypotension Significant acidosis
Respiratory	Rate normal	Tachypnea	Moderate tachypnea	Severe tachypnea
Central nervous system	Slightly anxious	Irritable, confused combative	Irritable or lethargic diminished pain response	Coma
Skin	Warm, pink Capillary refill brisk	Cool extremities, mottling Delayed capillary refill	Cool extremities, mottling or pallor Prolonged capillary refill	Cold extremities, pallor or cyanosis
Kidneys	Normal urine output	Oliguria, increased specific gravity	Oliguria, increased BUN	Anuria

Flow chart 24.1: Approach to the treatment of hemorrhagic shock in infants and children

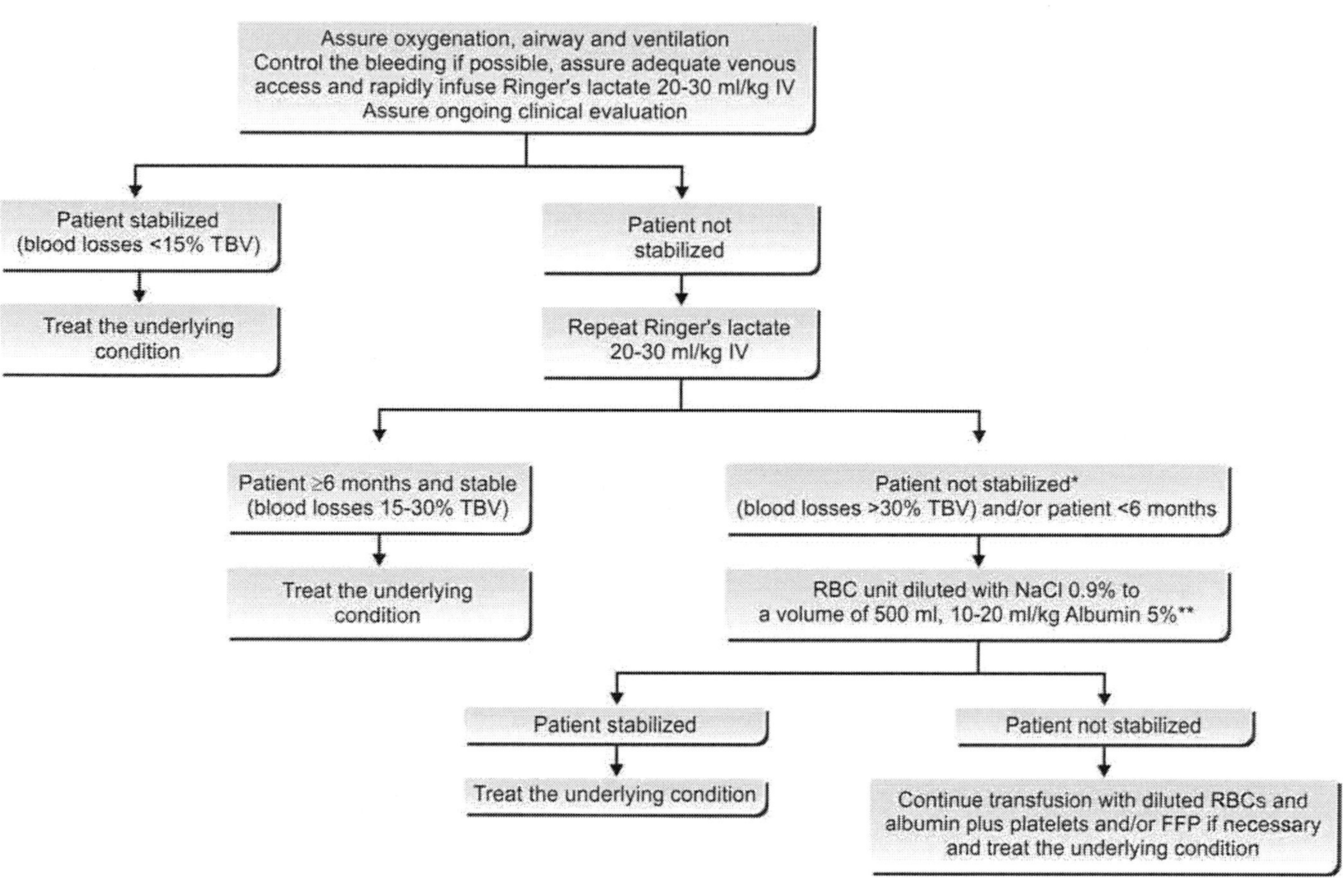

Abbreviations: TBV: Total blood volume; RBCs: Red blood cells; FFP: Fresh frozen plasma

* Patient with significant degrees of anemia prior to acute blood loss will require RBC transfusion support following smaller hemorrhagic losses.

** The use of albumin for fluid resuscitation is controversial.

- Presence or absence of underlying diseases, particularly cardiac diseases which may decrease the patient's capacity for cardiovascular compensation.
- Likely evolution of the underlying disease causing the anemia.
- Likely evolution of the anemia and its consequences with or without transfusion in both the short- and long-term.
- Possibility of using alternate, safer therapies for the treatment of the anemia.

RBC Transfusions for β-thalassemia

The hypertransfusion regimen, in which endogenous erythroid production is suppressed by maintaining a minimum pre-transfusion hemoglobin level of 9-10 g/dl, remains the commonest approach today.[15] Iron overload is a complication in these children, requiring institution of chelation therapy in early childhood. The frequency of red cell alloimmunization in chronically transfused children varies with the disease, the number of transfusions given and the ethnic background of donors and recipients. Antibodies to the common antigens of the Rh, Kell, Duff and Kidd systems are often involved. It may be desirable therefore to phenotype the patient's red cell antigens before beginning transfusion therapy, as this can be helpful in selecting compatible blood if alloimmunization occurs. Also, as these children are potential future HSCT recipients, it may be desirable to use CMV negative or at least leukodepleted products in them.

Another approach investigated during the 1980's was the possibility of decreasing transfusion exposure and increasing transfusion intervals through the use of young RBC. These "neocytes", with an average age of 12-21 days, can be collected by erythrocytapheresis or by fractionation of standard whole blood units using a cell processor. These studies caused a modest decrease of 12-16% in transfusion requirements; the use of neocyte transfusions was therefore abandoned.[16,17]

Volume of Blood for Standard Top-up Transfusion (ml)

Desired Hb (g/dl) – Actual Hb (g/dl) × Weight (kg) × 3

Current guidelines[18,19] and the new Thalassemia International Federation guidelines[20] recommend:

- Maintaining an average Hb of 12 g/dl
- Maintaining a pretransfusion Hb of 9-10 g/dl
- That transfusion should prevent marrow hyperplasia, skeletal changes and organomegaly
- Red cell requirements should be adjusted to accommodate growth and hypersplenism considered if requirements increase unexpectedly
- Chelation therapy should be considered after 10 transfusions and started once the serum ferritin is more than 1000 ng/ml.

RBC Transfusions in Sickle Cell Disease

Red cell transfusions in sickle cell disease (SCD) should not be routine but reserved for specific indications.[21,22]

1. *Simple (top-up) transfusion:*
   - Splenic or hepatic sequestration
   - Aplastic crisis

   The aim is to raise the Hb to the child's normal steady state (never to be raised acutely to >10 g/dl, as this can increase blood viscosity).
2. *Emergency Transfusion in SCD*[23,24]*:*
   - Acute chest syndrome
   - Stroke, priapism

   In such acute situations in SCD, reducing the HbS percentage in blood to <20% requires a total exchange of 1.5 to 2 times the blood volume. ET may also be used to minimize iron overload in patients on regular transfusions.[25, 26]
3. *Hypertransfusion in SCD:*
   - Patients on regular transfusion to prevent recurrence of stroke[27] – The rate of recurrent stroke has been reduced to 0-10% from ~65% by maintaining a pretransfusion Hb of 8-9 g/dl with an HbS of <30%. Due to the risk of iron overload, it may be desirable to follow several years of uneventful transfusion with a less aggressive protocol to maintain HbS between 40 and 50%.
   - Probably useful to delay or prevent deterioration in end organ failure (e.g. chronic lung disease).
   - To prevent the development of stroke in SCD with Doppler and/or MRI evidence of cerebrovascular infarction/hemorrhage in the absence of clinical evidence of stroke.

SPECIAL CONSIDERATIONS FOR NEWBORNS

Indications for RBC Transfusions

There are three major factors contributing to small volume RBC transfusion requirements in VLBW infants:

1. The rapid decline in Hb levels that occurs in the first weeks of life to a nadir at 2 months of life.[29,30] It must be remembered that concomitant with the decrease in absolute hemoglobin levels, the switch from HbF to HbA production is also occurring, so that the change in oxygen-carrying capacity is not so marked as the change in the total Hb level might suggest.
2. The associated respiratory illnesses often present in these neonates first as RDS and then as BPD. There

is necessity of maintaining hemoglobin values at a predetermined level in these neonates.[11,31]

3. Phlebotomy losses. Because of the need for laboratory monitoring of ill neonates and the relatively large volumes of blood required in relation to these tiny infants' total blood volumes, phlebotomy losses contribute significantly to the need for RBC transfusions in VLBW infants.[12] In sick neonates red cell replacement is usually considered when approximately 10% of the blood volume has been removed.

Dedicating aliquots form a single donation of red cells (or apheresis platelets) to allow sequential transfusions from the same donor for neonates and small children who are likely to be repeatedly transfused is considered good practice.

When red cells are transfused they are usually given in small volumes. A transfusion of 10 ml/kg of RBCs at a hematocrit >80% should raise the Hb by ~3 g/dl. There are 3 clinical settings in which newborns may require large volume RBC transfusion. (exchange transfusion, surgery with cardiopulmonary bypass or during treatment with extracorporeal membrane oxygenation {ECMO}).[32]

Practical Considerations

RBC units for transfusion to neonates are often chosen from a fresh (<5 days old) RBC unit at the time of his/her first small-volume RBC transfusion. In settings of large-volume RBC transfusion, replacement of plasma coagulation factors is often also required so that WB or reconstituted WB, i.e. an RBC unit mixed with a unit of fresh frozen plasma (FFP), can be used. For WB, or the RBC unit for reconstituted WB, the choice of ABO group is the same as that described above for small volume RBC transfusions. The ABO group of the FFP must also be compatible with the baby's RBC's. This may mean that the ABO groups of the RBC unit and the FFP unit are different, e.g. for a group A baby with maternal anti-A in his plasma, a unit of reconstituted WB would be prepared using a group O RBC unit and a group A FFP unit. To limit donor exposure, some experts use group O whole blood in this setting, although group O donors with high anti-A titers should be excluded.

WB units or RBC units for large volume transfusions should be relatively fresh, i.e. not >5-7 days old. The main reason for this precaution is the high potassium concentration in stored WB or RBC units.

Erythropoietin

Recombinant human erythropoietin (EPO) may reduce red cell transfusion requirements in neonates. However, its effect appears to be relatively modest and does not reduce transfusion requirements within the first two weeks of life, when sick neonates are most transfusion dependent because of frequent blood sampling. The optimal dose, timing and nutritional support required during EPO therapy has yet to be defined and currently the routine use of EPO in this patient group is not recommended as similar reduction in blood use can probably be achieved by institution of appropriate transfusion protocols (Table 24.5).[33-35]

PLASMA

Description and Storage

A typical unit of plasma has a volume of 160-250 ml if obtained from a WB donation or 400-600 ml when obtained by plasmapheresis. Immediately following collection from a normal donor, plasma contains approximately 1 unit/ml of each of coagulation factor as well as normal concentrations of other plasma proteins. Coagulation Factor V and VIII, known as the

Table 24.5: Indications for small volume red blood cell (RBC) transfusions used in the US Multicenter Erythropoietin Study[35]

Transfuse infants at hematocrit ≤20%
a. if asymptomatic with reticulocytes <100,000/μl

Transfuse infants at hematocrit <30%
a. if receiving <35% supplemental hood oxygen
b. if on CPAP or mechanical ventilation with mean airway pressure <6 cm H_2O
c. if significant apnea and bradycardia are noted (>9 episodes in 12 hours or 2 episodes in 24 hours requiring bag and mask ventilation while receiving therapeutic doses of methylxanthines)
d. if heart rate >180 beats/min or respiratory rate >80 breaths/min persists for 24 hours
e. if weight gain <10 g/day is observed over 4 days while receiving 100 kcal/kg/day
f. if undergoing surgery

Transfuse for hematocrit <35%
a. if receiving >35% supplemental hood oxygen
b. if intubated on CPAP or mechanical ventilation with mean airway pressure >6-8 cm H_2O

Do not transfuse
a. to replace blood removed for laboratory tests alone
b. for low hematocrit alone.

labile coagulation factors, are not stable in plasma stored at 1-6°C. Plasma frozen within 8 hours of donation contains at least 0.70 U/ml of Factor VIII and is referred to as fresh frozen plasma (FFP). In plasma frozen 8-72 hours after collection, referred to as frozen plasma the concentration of coagulation Factor V and VIII may be reduced by as much as 15%.[2] FFP may be stored for 12 months at -18°C or colder. Storage at -30°C or colder is recommended for optimal maintenance of Factor VIII levels.

Indications and Contraindications for Transfusion

As for RBC transfusion, the indications for FFP transfusions in children are most often generalized from observations in adult patients and/or based on expert opinion. There is broad, general consensus that the appropriate use is limited almost exclusively to the treatment or prevention of clinically significant bleeding due to a deficiency of one or more plasma coagulation factors.[36-39] Such situations potentially include the presence of:

1. A diminution of coagulation factors due to treatment with vitamin K antagonists.
2. Severe liver disease.
3. Disseminated intravascular coagulation (DIC).
4. Massive transfusion.
5. Isolated congenital coagulation factor deficiencies for which a safer and/or more appropriate product does not exist.

Not Indicated

1. Intravascular volume expansion or repletion (where crystalloids, synthetic colloids or purified human albumin solutions are preferred).
2. Correction or prevention of protein malnutrition (where synthetic amino acid solutions are preferred).
3. Correction of hypogammaglobulinemia (where purified human immunoglobulin concentrates are preferred).
4. Treatment of any other isolated congenital pro-coagulant or anticoagulant factor deficiency for which a virus-inactivated plasma-derived or recombinant factor concentrate exists.
5. As replacement fluid in therapeutic apheresis procedures for disorders other than thrombotic thrombocytopenic purpura/adult HUS unless proven to be beneficial.

Reversal of Warfarin Effect

Patients on warfarin are deficient in the functional vitamin K-dependent coagulation factors. Depending on the urgency and severity of the clinical situation, warfarin reversal may be attained by stopping or modifying warfarin therapy, by oral or parenteral vitamin K administration, by plasma transfusion or in rare situations by the administration of virus-inactivated plasma derived prothrombin complex concentrate.

Severe Liver Disease

Severe liver disease is associated with multiple abnormalities of hemostasis and coagulation including:

1. Deficient biosynthesis of antithrombin III, proteins C and S, plasminogen, antiplasmins and coagulation factors.
2. Aberrant biosynthesis of several coagulation factors.
3. Accelerated destruction of coagulation factors.
4. Deficient clearance of activated coagulation factors and plasminogen activators.
5. Thrombocytopenia and platelet dysfunction.
6. Loss or consumption of coagulation factors in ascitic fluid.[40]

The consensus is that patients who are not bleeding or not about to undergo an invasive procedure should not receive plasma merely to correct abnormal coagulation tests.[7,38,41] One exception to this may be patients with life-threatening acute fulminant hepatitis and extremely elevated INR's. Three retrospective studies found that patients with liver disease and mild coagulopathy, i.e. a PT 1.5-fold or less than the mean of the normal range (corresponding to an INR of approximately 2.2), did not have excess bleeding with liver biopsy or minor invasive procedures such as paracentesis or thoracentesis.[40,42,43] Most guidelines recommend plasma transfusion prior to invasive procedures or surgery in patients with liver disease and PT levels >1.5-fold normal or an INR >2.2, although there are no studies to support or refute these recommendations.

Disseminated Intravascular Coagulation

Acute DIC is characterized by the abnormal consumption of coagulation factors and platelets and may lead to thrombocytopenia, hypofibrinogenemia and increased PT, INR and/or activated partial thromboplastin time (APTT) with uncontrollable bleeding from wound and puncture sites. Retrospective and uncontrolled evidence suggests that the transfusion of plasma, along with other blood components, may be useful in limiting hemorrhage, provided aggressive measures are simultaneously undertaken to overcome the triggering disease. Plasma transfusion is generally not recommended in the absence of bleeding or in chronic DIC.

Massive Transfusion

Massive transfusion is usually defined as the replacement of a patient's total blood volume with stored blood in <24 hours. However, even within this definition, the degree and rapidity of blood loss can be quite variable as can the underlying etiologies and associated complications. Thus, assessment of the need for replacement of coagulation factors by FFP transfusion must be individualized. Pathologic hemorrhage in the massively transfused patient is more often caused by dilutional thrombocytopenia than by the depletion of coagulation factors.[38,41]

Past recommendations advocated routine transfusion of plasma (e.g. the administration of 2 units of plasma for every 5 units of red blood cells transfused) to reduce the risk of abnormal bleeding due to coagulation factor depletion during massive transfusion. Consequently, to the extent that it is possible, blood transfusion therapy in the setting of massive transfusion should be guided by both the ongoing clinical evaluation of the patient and laboratory measurements of hemostasis.

Congenital Coagulation Factor Deficiencies

Plasma has long been used to treat congenital deficiencies of hemostatic or anticoagulant proteins. However, more appropriate alternatives now exist for most of these disorders and, as new treatments are rapidly becoming available, recommendations for treatment are changing frequently.

Hemolytic Uremic Syndrome

Several investigators have studied the use of FFP in the treatment of pediatric HUS.[44-47] Experts have reached the consensus that plasma is not indicated for classic childhood HUS, i.e. the syndrome characterized by microangiopathic hemolytic anemia, thrombocytopenia and acute renal failure following diarrhea associated with entero-hemorrhagic *Escherichia coli* infection.[48] HUS and thrombotic thrombocytopenia purpura (TTP) may be indistinguishable pathologically, and the clinical manifestations of HUS occasionally approach those of TTP. In the absence of definitive studies, and in light of the adult TTP studies, plasma exchange seems to be a reasonable consideration in treating children with unusually complicated HUS, particularly those with neurologic complications.[49]

SPECIAL CONSIDERATIONS FOR NEWBORNS

FFP is indicated for the treatment of clinically significant bleeding, or its prevention in the case of an impending invasive procedure, due to a decrease in one or more coagulation factors, where a safer, appropriate, alternative therapy does not exist. In particular, for the neonate as for other patients, FFP is not indicated for the treatment of volume expansion or resuscitation alone.

The problems in the neonate are compounded due to:

1. Difficult to obtain blood specimens.
2. Low levels of vitamin K-dependent factors.
3. Rapid depletion of the above factors in situations like DIC. It may thus be reasonable to administer FFP transfusion relatively sooner in these situations to newborns and infants under 6 months of age than in older infants and children.

In VKDB life-threatening bleeding may require FFP treatment or in rare situations treatment with coagulation factor concentrates. The use of FFP has been advocated for prevention of periventricular-intraventricular hemorrhage (PVH-IVH) in the preterm infant, but the current evidence does not support the routine use of prophylactic FFP in preterm infants at risk for PVH-IVH. In addition to the contraindications for FFP transfusion discussed above, in the newborn FFP should not be used as a fluid for hematocrit adjustment in erythrocyte transfusions nor as a replacement fluid in partial exchange transfusion for the treatment of neonatal hyperviscosity syndrome. As discussed above FFP is used in newborns to prepare reconstituted whole blood where this product is indicated.

Dosage and Administration

Compatibility tests before plasma transfusion are not necessary. Plasma should be ABO compatible with the recipient's RBC's. Usually, Rh group need not be considered. However, when large volumes of FFP are given to RhD-negative pediatric patients or women of child-bearing age, prevention of RhD immunization by the use of Rh immune globulin should be considered.

FFP may be thawed in a waterbath at 30-37°C.

The dose of FFP depends on the clinical situation and the underlying disease process. When FFP is given for coagulation factor replacement, the dose is 10-20 ml/kg. This dose will usually raise the level of coagulation factors by 20% immediately after infusion. Post-transfusion monitoring of the patient's coagulation status (PT, APTT and/or specific coagulation factor assays) is important for optimal treatment.

PLATELETS

Description and Storage

A platelet concentrate (PC) may be prepared from a random WB donation or by apheresis procedures in which a single donor donates the equivalent of 4-8 PCs. Platelets collected by apheresis procedure are referred to as apheresis PCs. PCs contain a minimum of 5.5×10^{10} platelets/unit, approximately 50 ml of plasma, trace to 0.5 ml of RBCs and, depending upon the preparation techniques, varying number of leukocytes (predominantly monocytes and lymphocytes) up to levels of 10^8/unit. Apheresis PCs contain a minimum of 3×10^{11} platelets, approximately 250-300 ml plasma, trace to 5 ml of RBCs and, depending on the apheresis technique or instrument, 10^6-10^9 leukocytes. PCs and apheresis PCs are stored for up to 5 days at 20-24°C with continuous gentle agitation.

Indications for Transfusion

Decreased Platelet Production

1. Congenital or acquired aplastic anemia.
2. Bone marrow infiltration with leukemic or other malignant cells
3. Myeloablative chemotherapy.

Indications of using platelets in a >4-month-old child with thrombocytopenia:[10]

a. Prophylactic platelets (without bleeding) (Table 24.6)
   i. <5-10,000/cumm in a nonsick child
   ii. <20,000/cumm in a sick child with:
      1. Severe mucositis
      2. DIC
      3. Platelet likely to fall <10,000/cumm before next evaluation
      4. Associated coagulopathy/anticoagulation
   iii. Before surgery
      1. Bone marrow aspiration/biopsy can be without platelet support
      2. Lumbar puncture <30,000/cumm
      3. Other surgeries <50,000/cumm
      4. Surgery at critical sites like CNS, eyes <100,000/cumm
   iv. <50,000/cumm with acute bleeding, massive hemorrhage, head trauma, multiple trauma
b. Chronic stable thrombocytopenia only in presence of significant mucosal bleeding
c. Platelet dysfunction only in presence of significant mucosal bleeding
d. Chronic stable DIC only in presence of significant mucosal bleeding

At a Consensus Development Conference addressing platelet transfusion therapy sponsored by the National Institutes of Health in 1986, the panel concluded that patients with severe thrombocytopenia may benefit from prophylactic transfusions but that the commonly used threshold value of $20 \times 10^9/1$ may sometimes be safely lowered.[50] Slichter, in a review published in 1991, recommended that only patients with platelet counts $<5 \times 10^9/1$ should routinely be given prophylactic platelet transfusions, and for those with platelet counts $>5 \times 10^9/1$ clinical judgement should be used to assess the need for platelet therapy.[51] Prophylactic transfusions at higher platelet counts being reserved for patients in whom additional risk factors exist.[52]

While these stringent prophylactic platelet transfusion policies may be appropriate for many patients, 2 groups of leukemic patients appear to be at particularly high risk of fatal hemorrhage during induction chemotherapy, namely those with hyperleukocytosis and/or acute promyelocytic leukemia (ANLL, FAB M3).

The risk factors for hemorrhage in patients with solid tumors are similar to those in leukemic patients, although an additional consideration is the predisposition to hemorrhage associated with local tumor invasion.[53,54]

In summary, just as the indication for a RBC transfusion should not be determined solely on the basis of an Hb level, the decision to administer a platelet transfusion should also be individualized, taking into account the clinical situation as well as the platelet level. Prophylactic platelet transfusions are indicated for thrombocytopenic patients undergoing invasive procedures. At least one study suggests that major surgical procedures can be safely performed at platelet counts of 50×10^9/L.[55] Bone marrow aspiration and biopsy can be safely performed (with respect to local bleeding) at any platelet level. Suggested guidelines for prophylactic platelet transfusions for pediatric patients with thrombocytopenia due to decreased platelet production are summarized in Table 24.6.[56]

Table 24.6: Suggested guidelines for prophylactic platelet transfusions in pediatric patients with thrombocytopenia due to decreased platelet production

- Platelet count $<10 \times 10^9$/L
- Platelet count $<20 \times 10^9$/L and bone marrow infiltration, severe mucositis, DIC, anticoagulation therapy, a platelet count likely to fall below 10×10^9/L prior to next possible evaluation, or risk of bleeding due to local tumor invasion
- Platelet count $<30\text{-}40 \times 10^9$/L and DIC (e.g. during induction therapy for promyelocytic leukemia), extreme hyperleukocytosis, or prior to lumbar puncture or central venous line insertion
- Platelet count $<50\text{-}60 \times 10^9$/L and major surgical intervention.

Abbreviation: DIC: Disseminated intravascular coagulation

Massive Transfusion

Thrombocytopenia is frequently associated with massive transfusion. Depending on the underlying etiology of the bleeding, the thrombocytopenia may be dilutional from platelet loss through hemorrhage and/or due to platelet consumption. Platelet transfusion therapy should be based on a consideration of several factors including platelet count, an assessment of the role of the thrombocytopenia in the observed bleeding and the estimated hemostatic platelet count necessary for the patient's given clinical situation.

Platelet Dysfunction

Platelet dysfunction possibly requiring platelet transfusion is most commonly encountered in 2 situations: patients taking platelet inhibitory drugs and following surgery with cardiopulmonary bypass pump (CBP). Platelet dysfunction due to platelet inhibitory drugs is unlikely to contribute to bleeding if the platelet count is $>50 \times 10^9/L$. Treatment with desmopressin acetate has been shown to prevent bleeding complications in patients who have taken aspirin within 7 days of a surgical intervention.[57,58]

Platelet dysfunction lasting 4-6 hours post-CBP has been well-documented.[59,60] These patients are usually thrombocytopenic too. Nevertheless, studies have not shown a benefit for the use of prophylactic platelet transfusions for patients undergoing CBP.[61] Platelet transfusions should be reserved for those patients, who following CBP, have excessive bleeding thought to be due to platelet function abnormalities and/or thrombocytopenia.[39,50,62]

Special Considerations for Newborns (Table 24.7)

Newborns should receive platelet transfusions in the same clinical settings as described above for older children. However, since newborns frequently manifest thrombocytopenia and since preterm infants are at risk for PVH-IVH, it is possible that the platelet level at which prophylactic platelet transfusions should be administered to newborns is higher than that recommended for other patients. The platelet levels at which prophylactic platelet transfusions were given to neonates varied tremendously: from $<20 \times 10^9/L$ to $> 50 \times 10^9/L$ in stable preterm infants and $<20 \times 10^9/L$ to $> 80 \times 10^9/L$ in sick preterm infants.[63] The non-bleeding premature infants with platelet counts higher than $60 \times 10^9/L$ should not receive prophylactic platelet transfusions.[64]

Table 24.7: Suggested guidelines for platelet transfusion support of neonates

- Prophylactic platelet transfusion
- Stable preterm neonates with platelet counts $<30 \times 10^9/L$
- Stable term neonates with platelet counts $20 \times 10^9/L$
- Sick preterm neonates with platelet counts $<50 \times 10^9/L$
- Sick term infants with platelet counts $<30 \times 10^9/L$
- Preparation for an invasive procedure, e.g. lumbar puncture or minor surgery in neonates with platelet counts $<50 \times 10^9/L$ and for major surgery in neonates with platelet counts $<100 \times 10^9/L$
- Platelet transfusions in neonates with clinically significant bleeding
- Neonates with platelet counts $50 \times 10^9/L$
- Neonates with conditions that increase bleeding (e.g. DIC) and platelet counts $<100 \times 10^9/L$
- Neonates with documented significant platelet functional disorders (e.g. Glanzmann thrombasthenia) irrespective of the circulating platelet count

Abbreviation: DIC: Disseminated intravascular coagulation

Neonates with thrombocytopenia due to maternal platelet alloantibodies require special consideration with respect to the indications for platelet transfusion. These neonates require HPA-compatible platelets in addition to high-dose IVIg. In these patients, a minimum platelet count of $30 \times 10^9/L$ is recommended.

Dosage and Administration

ABO-incompatible platelets (i.e. platelets with A and/or B antigens given to a donor with a corresponding antibody) are usually clinically effective. However, in some patients particularly those receiving multiple platelet transfusions, there may be a poor post-transfusion response than that obtained with ABO-compatible platelets, and some studies have suggested that the transfusion of ABO-incompatible platelets is associated with the development of platelet refractoriness.[65,66] Also, there are reports of acute intravascular hemolysis following the transfusion of platelet concentrates containing ABO antibodies incompatible with the recipient's RBCs.[67,68] Therefore, it would seem prudent, particularly in small children where the volume of plasma maybe relatively large with respect to the patient's total blood volume, to try to use ABO-matched platelets. If these are not available, units with plasma compatible with the recipient's RBC's should be chosen. If this is also not possible, units with low titers of anti-A or B should be selected or platelets may be volume reduced. Testing of

PCs for RBC compatibility is not necessary unless red cells are detected by visual inspection.

Platelets do not carry Rh antigens.[69] However, the quantity of RBC's in platelet concentrates is sufficient to induce Rh sensitization even in immunosuppressed cancer patients.[70, 71] Rh sensitization caused by platelet transfusions in Rh-negative patients can be prevented by the administration of Rh immunoprophylaxis.[72,73] A dose of 25 mg (125 IU) of anti-D immunoglobulin will protect against 1 ml of RBCs.[74] If available, it is preferable to use of preparation of anti-D which can be administered intravenously.

A suitable starting platelet dosage that can be expected to raise the platelet level by 50 × 10^9/L is 1 PC/10 kg body weight. PCs may be pooled before administration or infused individually. An equivalent dose for apheresis platelets is approximately 5 ml/kg. Patients with increased platelet consumption (e.g. with septicemia or DIC) or splenomegaly may require larger amounts of platelets.

PC or apheresis platelets may be volume reduced prior to infusion. However, this extra manipulation leads to platelet loss and if not carefully performed might potentially adversely affect platelet function and/or be a cause of bacterial contamination. Volume reduction should therefore be limited to patients who require severe volume restriction or situations where ABO-incompatible platelets are the only available PC's for a neonate or child.

The corrected count increment (CCI) is a calculated measure of patient response to platelet transfusion that adjusts for the number of platelets infused and the size of the recipient, based upon body surface area (BSA).[28]

$$\text{CCI} = (\text{post-count} - \text{pre-count}) \times \text{BSA}/\text{platelets transfused}$$

where post-count and pre-count are platelet counts (/µl) after and before transfusion, respectively; BSA is the patient body surface area (m^2); and platelets transfused is the number of administered platelets ($\times 10^{11}$). The CCI is usually determined 10 to 60 minutes after transfusion. In the clinically stable patient, the CCI is typically greater than 7500 at 10 minutes to 1 hour after transfusion and remains above 4500 at 24 hours. Both immune and nonimmune mechanisms may contribute to reduced platelet recovery and survival. Along with supportive serologic test results, a CCI of less than 5000 at 10 minutes to 1 hour after transfusion may indicate an immune-mediated refractory state to platelet therapy. With nonimmune mechanisms, platelet recovery within 1 hour may be adequate, although survival at 24 hours is reduced.

GRANULOCYTES

Description and Storage

To assure clinical efficacy, granulocytes concentrates should contain a minimum of 10^{10} polymorphonuclear cells (PMN's)/unit. Recently, there have been reports of leukapheresis collections of >4 × 10^{10} PMN's/unit following donor stimulation with G-CSF.[48,75] However, the use of G-CSF in normal donors, and the characteristics of granulocyte concentrates following G-CSF stimulation, require further study before this approach can be recommended for routine use.

There is a recent report of the preparation of granulocytes by pooling buffy coat layers separated from 4-8 units of fresh whole blood. In pediatric patients (ages 2 to 13 years), the mean leukocyte dose transfused was 0.6 × 10^9/kg.[76] Granulocyte function deteriorates rapidly during storage. Thus, granulocytes should be transfused as soon as possible following collection and should not be given if stored for >24 hours. For the time between collection and infusion, granulocyte concentrates should be kept at 20-24°C, with little or no agitation.[77]

Indications for Transfusion

Currently, granulocytes transfusions are reserved for patients with profound neutropenia not expected to recover within a week, or severe forms of congenital neutrophil dysfunction, in whom a severe bacterial infection has been documented and who are clinically deteriorating despite optimal antimicrobial therapy.[78,79] The granulocyte transfusion should be separated from Amphotericin B infusion by 10-12 hours.

Special Considerations for Newborns

Newborns normally have a transient neutrophilia in the first week of life with mean normal absolute neutrophils counts ranging from 11.0 × 10^9/L at birth to 5.5 × 10^9/L at 1 week of life.[80] Septic newborns frequently develop neutropenia, defined in the newborn as an absolute neutrophils count below 3.0 × 10^9/L. Between 1981 and 1992, 5 controlled trials of granulocytes transfusions for septic newborns with neutropenia were reported and have recently been reviewed.[81] The data suggest a beneficial role for granulocyte transfusion provided an adequate dose is administered. Nevertheless, the use of granulocyte transfusions for neonatal sepsis has not become widespread, possibly because of the difficulty of obtaining granulocytes as rapidly as would be required in this setting. More recently, investigators in the field have begun to study the role of G-CSF in the treatment of neonatal sepsis.[82]

Dosage and Administration

Once the decision to administer granulocytes transfusions has been made, they are administered daily until there is evidence of recovery of peripheral neutrophil counts or clinical evidence of recovery from the infection. For neonates and small children, a daily infusion of 1×10^9 PMNs/kg should be given and for larger patients, $2\text{-}3 \times 10^{10}$ PMNs. As there is significant RBC contamination, units must be ABO compatible and if possible RhD negative for RhD-negative recipients and must undergo the usual compatibility testing. Alloimmunization frequently occurs in patients receiving granulocyte transfusions and may render the transfusions ineffective and/or be associated with adverse reactions including respiratory distress.[83] For patients, with HLA- and/or granulocytes-specific alloantibodies, only granulocytes from HLA-and/or neutrophil antigen-compatible donors should be used. The transfusion is usually administered over 2-3 hours. Do not administer using leukocyte reduction filters. Because most patients receiving these products are severely immunosuppressed, apheresis granulocytes are usually irradiated to prevent TA-GVHD. (AABB guidelines)

CRYOPRECIPITATE

Description and Storage

Cryoprecipitate is the precipitate formed when FFP is thawed at 4°C. The precipitate is then refrozen within 1 hour in 10-15 ml of the donor plasma and stored at –18°C or less for a period of up to 1 year. Cryoprecipitate contains 80-100 units of Factor VIII, 100-250 mg of fibrinogen, 40-60 mg of fibronectin and 40-70% of the von Willebrand factor and 30% of the factor XIII present in the original unit of plasma.

Indications for Transfusion

1. Hemophilia A
2. von Willebrand disease
3. Congenital deficiencies of fibrinogen
4. Factor XIII.

Dosage and Administration

Compatibility testing of cryoprecipitate units is unnecessary. However, cryoprecipitate contains anti-A and –B so the use of ABO-compatible units is preferable. Rh group need not be considered. The number of units of cryoprecipitate required is usually based on the amount necessary to obtain a hemostatic level of fibrinogen, i.e. a fibrinogen level >0.8-1.0 g/L. If the units are carefully pooled this can usually be accomplished by the transfusion of 1 unit/5-10 kg recipient weight.

Cryoprecipitate is prepared for transfusion by thawing at 30-37°C and mixing the thawed precipitate with 10-15 ml of sodium chloride 0.9% if necessary, according to the amount of plasma in the cryoprecipitate unit. The required number of units is then pooled.

Thawed cryoprecipitate should be stored at room temperature and transfused immediately after thawing or within 6 hours after thawing if used as a source of Factor VIII. All pooled cryoprecipitate units must be used within 4 hours of pooling.

ALBUMIN

Preparation and Storage

Albumin is derived from pools of donor plasma obtained either from whole blood or from plasmapheresis. It is prepared by the cold alcohol fractionation process (Cohn fractionation) followed by heat treatment at 60°C for 10 hours. Its composition is 96% albumin and 4% other plasma proteins. Albumin is available as a 25% solution in distilled water or as a 5% solution in saline. Plasma protein fraction (PPF) is a similar product except that it is subject to fewer purification steps in the fractionation process. PPF is a 5% protein solution composed of approximately 85% albumin and 15% other plasma proteins. All three preparations have a physiologic pH and a sodium content of about 145 mmol/L (145 mEq/L). The 5% solutions are osmotically and oncotically equivalent to plasma, while the 25% solution is osmotically and oncotically 5-fold greater than plasma. These products can be stored for up to 5 years at 2-10°C.

Indications for Transfusion

The indications for the use of albumin (or PPF) are controversial and many transfusion medicine specialists believe this product is overused.[84,85] In particular, controversy remains concerning these of albumin versus crystalloids or nonblood colloids for intravascular volume expansion.[84] The 25% solution should not be used in dehydrated patients unless it is supplemented by the infusion of crystalloid solutions.

Dosage and Administration

Albumin and PPF do not need to be administered through a filter. Dosage and rate of infusion depend upon the patient's clinical condition. In shock the usual dosage of 5% albumin is 500 ml in adults and 10-20 ml/kg in children.

IMMUNOGLOBULINS

Plasma-derived immunoglobulins are available in 2 forms: intramuscular and intravenous preparations. Intramuscular immunoglobulin, commonly known as human immune serum globulin (ISG), is prepared from large pools of donor plasma by cold alcohol fractionation (Cohn fractionation). ISG is 95% IgG with the remaining 5% consisting of other plasma proteins. It is prepared as a sterile solution with a protein concentration of 16.5 g/1. ISG is for intramuscular use; it must not be administered intravenously as it contains aggregated IgG complexes which can activate complement causing adverse reactions if administered intravenously. The commonest use of ISG is for hepatitis A or measles prophylaxis. Several special human immune globulins are available. They are identical to ISG except that they have high titers to an infectious agent or the RhD antigen. The most commonly used preparations are hepatitis B immune globulin and varicella zoster immune globulin for the prevention of hepatitis B and varicella zoster infections, respectively, and immunization. An RhD human immune globulin for intravenous injection is also available.

Human ISG may be further treated to prepare intravenous immunoglobulin (IVIg), a product virtually free of immunoglobulin complexes and therefore safe for intravenous infusion. Several IVIG preparations are commercially available. They differ in their mode of preparation, pH, use of additives, etc. but for practical purposes are generally therapeutically equivalent. Some contain less IgA than others and are therefore preferentially chosen if treating an IgA-deficient patient. IVIG is used as replacement therapy in primary immuno-deficiency states and a wide variety of secondary immunodeficiency states. It can also be used as an immunomodulation agent to treat selected patients with autoimmune thrombocytopenia purpura or other autoimmune disorders. The efficacy of IVIg in various clinical settings was assessed in 1990 at a consensus development conference of the National Institutes of Health in the USA and has recently been reviewed.[86,87]

An IVIg preparation with specificity for respiratory syncytial virus (RSV-IGIV) has been developed and studied and was recently approved in the United States for use in the prevention of severe RSV infections in selected patients.[88,89]

DISCUSSION ON SPECIAL TOPICS

Compatibility Testing in Neonates and Young Infants

As neonates and young infants are immunologically immature, alloimunization to RBC antigens is rare during this period.[90] AABB standards[91] require only limited pre-transfusion serologic testing for infants below 4 months of age. Initial testing must include ABO and Rh typing of red cells and a screen for red cell antibodies. If an unexpected red cell antibody is detected in the infant's specimen or the mother's serum contains a clinically significant red cell antibody, the infant should be given either red cell units tested and found to lack the corresponding antigen(s) or units compatible by antiglobulin cross-match; this should continue for as long as maternal antibody persists in the infant's blood. It is unnecessary to test the infant's serum for anti-A and/or anti-B unless there will be transfusion of non-group-O cells.

A positive DAT on the neonate's red cells or an atypical red cell antibody in maternal or neonatal serum suggests possible hemolytic disease of the newborn (HDN). In such cases, special serological procedures will be necessary to allow selection of appropriate blood group.

Exchange Transfusion in Neonates

Exchange transfusion (ET) may be used to manage severe anemia at birth, particularly in the presence of heart failure, and to treat severe hyperbilirubinemia, usually caused by HDN. Controversial indications such as metabolic disease, septicemia and DIC have not been subjected to adequate clinical evaluation. It is a specialist procedure associated with a potential for serious adverse events. While there is no consensus amongst neonatologists, plasma reduced red cells with a hematocrit (Hct) of 0.50-0.60 should be suitable for both hyperbilirubinemia and severe anemia.

Exchanging the estimated volume of the baby's blood in a "single volume exchange" will remove 75% of red cells, while a "double volume exchange" (160-200 ml/kg, depending on gestation) removes 90% of the initial red cells. A double volume exchange can remove 50% of available intravascular bilirubin.

Red cells for ET should be:

- Group O or ABO compatible with maternal and neonatal plasma, RhD negative (or RhD identical with neonate)

- Negative for any red cell antigens to which the mother has antibodies
- IAT- cross-match compatible with maternal plasma
- 5 days old or less
- Collected into CPD anticoagulant
- CMV seronegative
- Irradiated and transfused within 24 hours of irradiation.

Calculations for Neonatal Exchange Transfusion

- Two-volume red cell exchange transfusion for treatment of Sickle cell crisis and neonatal hyperbilirubinemia
- Replace calculated blood volume with whole blood or red cells suspended in 5% human albumin
- Volume to be exchanged (ml):
  [Estimated blood volume × (Patient's hematocrit (%) × 2]/Hematocrit of transfused unit (%).*

Intrauterine Transfusion[28]

Intrauterine transfusions (IUTs) are usually administered only in specialized units. Red cell IUT is indicated to correct fetal anemia caused by red cell alloimmunization (most important antigen- RhD followed by RhC and K) or, less commonly, for fetal parvovirus infection. Platelet IUTs are indicated to correct fetal thrombocytopenia caused by platelet alloimmunization. The aims of IUT are (i) to prevent or treat fetal hydrops before the fetus can be delivered and (ii) to enable the pregnancy to advance to a gestational age that will ensure survival of the neonate (in practice, up to 36-37 weeks) with as few invasive procedures as possible (because of the risk of fetal loss). This is achieved by (i) starting the transfusion program as late as safely possible but before hydrops develops and (ii) maximizing the intervals between transfusions, by transfusing as large a volume of red cells as is considered safe.

COMPONENT AND PROCEDURE SPECIFICATION

Red Cell Preparations

Red cells preparations for IUT should

- be group O (low titer hemolysin) or ABO identical with the fetus (if known) and RhD negative. K-negative blood is recommended to reduce additional maternal alloimmunization risks. In exceptional cases, e.g. for hemolysis because of maternal anti-C, it may be necessary to give RhD positive, C-negative blood;
- be IAT-cross-match compatible with maternal serum and negative for the relevant antigen(s) determined by maternal antibody status.
- be <5 d old and in citrate phosphate dextrose (CPD) anticoagulant.
- be CMV seronegative.
- be irradiated.
- have a hematocrit (packed cell volume, PCV) between 0.70 and 0.85.
- not be transfused straight from 4°C storage. Any active warming must be carried out with great care and the blood product not exposed to temperatures higher than 30°C. Active warming may not be necessary if the infusion is conducted carefully and at an appropriate rate (see below).
- (Desired PCV-Fetal PCV/Donor PCV-Desired PCV) × Fetoplacental BV; where BV is blood volume.
- be transfused at a rate of 5–10 ml/min.

Platelet Preparations

Platelet preparations for IUT should

- be group O RhD negative and test negatively for high-titer anti-A or anti-B (i.e. have a low titer hemolysin) or group specific/compatible with maternal antibody.
- be human platelet-specific alloantigen (HPA) compatible with maternal antibody.
- preferably be collected by apheresis. A platelet concentrate derived from whole blood donations is less preferred.
- be irradiated as above.
- be concentrated to a platelet count of at least 2000 × 10^9/l.
- be warmed, if warmed at all, with extreme care. As the ambient temperature for storing platelet concentrates is 22°C, and as the recommended rate of infusion (see below) is slower than that for red cells, active warming may not be needed. If it is conducted, it should not be beyond 30°C.
- be in a volume calculated from the formula: (Desired platelet increment/Platelet count of concentrate) × Feto-placental BV.
- be transfused at a rate of 1–5 ml/min (transfused more slowly than red cells because of the increased risk of fetal circulatory stasis and asystole).

Compatible platelets should be available at the time of diagnostic fetal sampling for alloimmune thrombocytopenia, even if the primary purpose is not that of transfusion, because in the presence of severe

---

* Hematocrit
Whole blood 35–45%
Red cell concentrates 55–75%
Red cell suspension 50–70%

fetal thrombocytopenia, fetal hemorrhage can be prevented by platelet transfusion.

REFERENCES

1. Tegtmeier GE. The use of cytomegalovirus screened blood in neonates. Transfusion. 1988;28:201-3.
2. Sayers MH. Cytomegalovirus and other herpes viruses. In Petz LD, Swisher SN, Kleinman S, et al. (Eds). Clinical practice of transfusion medicine, 3rd edn. New York: Churchill Livingstone; 1996. pp. 875-89.
3. Goldman M, Delage G. The role of leukodepletion in the control of transfusion-transmitted disease. Transfus Med Rev. 1995;9:9-19.
4. The Stationary Office (2002) Guidelines for the Blood Transfusion Services in the UK, 6th edn. The Stationary Office, UK.
5. American Association of Blood Banks (AABB) (2000). Standards for Blood Banks and Transfusion Services, 20th edn. AABB Bethesda.
6. Baldini M, Costea N, Dameschek W. The viability of stored human platelets. Blood. 1960;16:1669-92.
7. Rapport SI, Ames SB, Mikkelsen S. The level of antihemophilic globulin and proaccelerin in fresh and bank blood. Am J Clin Pathol. 1959;31:297-304.
8. WHO - Clinical uses of blood products, 2002.
9. Card RT, Brain MC. The "anemia" of childhood: Evidence for a physiologic response to hyperphosphatemia. N Engl J Med. 1973;288:388-92.
10. Indian Academy of Pediatrics (IAP), National Guidelines 2006.
11. Hume H. Red blood cell transfusions for preterm infants: The role of evidence-based medicine. Semin Perinatal. 1997;21:8-19.
12. Shannon KM, Keith JF, Mentzer WC, et al. Recombinant human erythropoietin stimulates erythropoiesis and reduces erythrocyte transfusions in very low birth weight preterm infants. Pediatrics. 1995;95:1-8.
13. Guay J, Hume H, Gauthier M, Tremblay P. Choc hemorrhagique. In: Lacroix J, Gautier M, Beaufils F (Eds) Urgences et soins intensif pediatriques. Montreal: Les Presses de l'Universite de Montreal; 1994. pp. 73-87.
14. Soud T, Pieper P, Hazinski MF. Pediatric trauma In: Hazinski MF (Ed). Nursing care of the critically ill child. St. Louis, MO: Mosby Year Book. 1992.
15. Piomelli S. Management of Cooleys' anemia. Bailliere's Clin Haematol. 1993;6:287-98.
16. Cohen AR, Schmidt JM, Martin MB, et al. Clinical trial of young red cell transfusions. J Pediatr. 1984;104:865-8.
17. Marcus RE, Wonke B, Bantock HM, et al. A prospective trial of young red cells in 48 patients with transfusion-dependent Thalassemia. Br J Haematol. 1985;60:153-9.
18. Cazzola M, Borgna-Pignatti C, Locatelli F, Ponchio L, Beguin Y, De Stefano P. A moderate transfusion regimen may reduce iron loading in thalassemia major without producing excessive expansion of erythropoiesis. Transfusion. 1997;37:135-40.
19. Pratti D. Benefits and complications of regular blood transfusions in patients with beta-thalassemia major. Vox Sanguinis. 2000;79:129-37.
20. Olivieri NF. The thalassemias. New England Journal of Medicine. 1999;341:99-109.
21. Ohene-Frempong K. Indications for red cell transfusion in sickle cell disease. Seminars in Hematology. 2001;38:513.
22. Telen MJ. Principles and problems of transfusion in sickle cell disease. Seminars in Hematology. 2001;38:315-23.
23. Emre U, Miller ST, Gutierez M, Steiner P, Rao SP, Rao M. Effect of transfusion in acute chest syndrome of sickle cell disease. Journal of Pediatrics. 1995;127:901-4.
24. Schmalzer EA, Lee JO, Brown AK, Usami S, Chien S. Viscosity of mixtures of sickle and normal red cells at varying hematocrit levels: Implications for transfusion. Transfusion. 1987;27:228-33.
25. Cohen AR, Martin MB, Silber JH, et al. A modified transfusion program for prevention of stroke in sickle cell disease. Blood. 1992;79:1657-61.
26. Kim HC, Dugan NP, Silber JH, Martin MB, Schwartz E, Ohene-Frampong K, Cohen AR. Erythrocytopheresis therapy to reduce iron overload in chronically transfused patients with sickle cell disease. Blood. 1994;83:1136-42.
27. Pegelow CH, Adams RJ, McKie V, Abboud M, Berman B, Miller ST, Olivieri N, Vichinski E, Wang W, Brambilla D. Risk of recurrent stroke in patients with sickle cell disease treated with erythrocyte transfusions. Journal of Pediatrics. 1995;126:896-9.
28. Guidelines for the Administration of Blood Products: Transfusion of Infants and Neonates; British Committee for Standards in Haematology 2004 (Modifications in 2005).
29. Strauss RG. Red blood cell transfusion practices in the neonate. Clin Perinatol. 1995;22:641-55.
30. Oski FA. Neonatal Hematology: The erythrocyte and its disorders. In: Nathan DG, Oski FA (Eds). Hematology of Infancy and Childhood, 4th edn. Philadelphia, PA: WB Saunders Co. 1993. pp. 18-43.
31. Hume H, Bard H. Small volume red blood cell transfusions for neonatal patients. Transfusion Med Rev 1995;9:187-99.
32. Luban NLC. Massive transfusion in the neonate. Transfusion Med Rev. 1995;9:200-14.
33. Maier RF, Obladen M, Kattner E, Natzschka J, Messer J, Regazzoni BM, Speer CP, Fellman V, Grauel EL, Groneck P, Wagner M, Moriette G, Salle BL, Verellin G, Scigalla P. High versus low dose erythropoietin in extremely low birth weight infants. The European Multicenter rhEPO Study Group. Journal of Pediatrics. 1998;132:866-70.
34. Franz AR, Pohlandt F. Red blood cell transfusion in very and extremely low birth weight infants under restrictive transfusion guidelines: Is exogenous erythropoietin necessary? Archives of Disease in Childhood, Fetal and Neonatal Edition. 2001;84:F96-100.
35. Shannon KM, Keith III JF, Mentzer WC, Ehrenkranz RA, Brown MS, Widness JA, Gleason CA, Bifano EM, Millard DD and Davis CB. Recombinant human erythropoietin stimulates erythropoiesis and reduces erythrocyte transfusions in very low birth preterm infants. Pediatrics. 1995;95:1-8.

36. Crosby E, Ferguson D, Hume HA, et al. Guidelines for red blood cell and plasma transfusion for adults and children. Can Med Assoc J. 1997;156(Suppl 11):SI-12.
37. Stechling L, Luban NLC, Anderson KC, et al, Guidelines for blood utilization review. Transfusion 1994;34:438-48.
38. Consensus Conference. Fresh-frozen plasma: Indications and risks. JAMA. 1985;253:551-3.
39. American Society of Anesthesiologists. Task Force on Blood Component Therapy. Practice guidelines for blood component therapy. Anesthesiology. 1996;84:732-47.
40. Zalusky R, Furie B. Hematologic complications of liver disease and alcoholism. In: Hoffiman R, Benz EJ Jr, Shatti SJ, Furie B, Cohen HJ, Silberstein Leukemia (Eds) Hematology: Basic Principles and Practice, 2nd edn. New York: Churchill Livingstone; 1995. pp. 2096-103.
41. Contreas M, Ala FA, Greaves M, et al. Guidelines for the Use of Fresh Frozen Plasma. British Committee for Standards in Haematology. Working Party of the Blood Transfusion Task Force. Transfusion Med. 1992;2:57-63.
42. McVay PA, Toy PT. Lack of increased bleeding after paracentesis and thoracentesis in patients with mild coagulation abnormalities. Transfusion. 1991;31:164-71.
43. Friedman EW, Sussman II. Safety of invasive procedures in patients with the coagulopathy of liver diseases. Clin Lab Haematol. 1989;11:199-204.
44. Loirat C, Sonsino E, Hinglias N, et al. Treatment of the childhood hemolytic uraemic syndrome with plasma. Pediatr Nephrol. 1988;2:279-85.
45. Rizzoni G, Claria-Appiani A, Edefonti A, et al. Plasma infusion for hemolytic-uremic syndrome in children. Results of a multicenter controlled trial. J Pediatr. 1988;112:284-90.
46. Ogborn MR, Crocker JF, Barnard DR. Plasma therapy for severe hemolytic-uremic syndrome in children in Atlantic Canada. Can Med Assoc J. 1990;143:1323-6.
47. Frishberg Y, Obrig TG, Kaplan B. Hemolytic uremic syndrome. In: Holiday MA, Barratt TM, Avner (Eds), Pediatric Nephrology, 3rd edn. Baltimore: Williams and Wilkins; 1994. pp. 871-89.
48. Bensinger WI, Price TH, Dale, et al. The effects of daily recombinant human granulocytes colony-stimulating factor administration on normal granulocytes donors undergoing leukapheresis. Blood. 1993;81:1883-8.
49. Fitzpatrick MM, Walters MDS, Trompeter RS, et al. Atypical (non-diarrhea-associated) hemolytic-uremic syndrome in childhood. J Pediatr. 1993;122:532-7.
50. National Institutes of Health, Consensus Development Conference. Platelet transfusion therapy. JAMA. 1987;257: 1777-80.
51. Slichter SJ. Platelet transfusions: a constantly evolving therapy. Thromb haemostas. 1991;66:178-88.
52. Beutler E. Platelet transfusions: The 20,000/μl trigger. Blood. 1993;81:1411-3.
53. Belt RJ, Leite C, Haas CD, Stephens RL. Incidence of hemorrhagic complications in patients with cancer. JAMA. 1978;239:2571-4.
54. Dutcher JP, Schiffer CA, Aisner J, et al. Incidence of thrombocytopenia and serious hemorrhage among patients with solid tumors. Cancer. 1984;53:557-62.
55. Dutcher JP, Schiffer CA, Aisner J, et al. Surgery in leukemia: A review of 167 operations on thrombocytopenic patients. Am J Hematol. 1987;26:147-55.
56. Hume H. Transfusion support of children with hematologic and oncologic disorders. In: Petz LD, Swisher SN, Kleinmans, Spence RK, Strauss RG (Eds) Clinical Practice of Transfusion Medicine, 3rd edn. New York: Churchill Livingstone; 1996. pp. 705-32.
57. Flordal PA, Sahlin S. Use of desmopressin to prevent bleeding complications in patients treated with aspirin. Br J Surg. 1993;80:723-4.
58. Sheridan DP, Card RT, Pinilla JC, et al. Use of desmopressin acetate to reduce blood transfusion requirements during cardiac surgery in patients with acetylsalicylic-acid-induced platelet dysfunction. Can J Surg. 1994;37:33-6.
59. Harker LA, Malpass TW, Branson HE, et al. Mechanism of abnormal bleeding in patients undergoing cardio-pulmonary bypass: acquired transient platelet dysfunction associated with selective a-granule release. Blood. 1980;56:827-34.
60. Buerling-Harbury C, Galvan CA. Acquired decrease in platelet secretory ADP associated with increased postoperative bleeding in post cardiopulmonary bypass patients and in patients with severe valvular heart disease. Blood. 1978;52:13-23.
61. Simon TL, Akl BF, Murphy W. Controlled trial of routine administration of platelet concentrates in cardiopulmonary bypass surgery. Ann Thorac Surg. 1984;37:359-64.
62. Development Task Force of the College of American Pathologists. Practice parameter for the use of fresh-frozen plasma. British Committee for Standards in Haematology, Working Party of the Blood Transfusion Task Force. Transfusion Med. 1992;2:57-63.
63. Strauss RG, Levy GJ, Sotelo-Avila C. National survey of neonatal transfusion practices: II. Blood component therapy. Pediatrics. 1993;91:530-6.
64. Andrew M, Vegh P, Caco C, et al. A randomized, controlled trial of platelet transfusion in thrombocytopenic premature infants. J Pediatr. 1993;123:285-91.
65. Brad A Sintnicolaas K, Class FHJ, Ernisse JG. ABH antibodies causing platelet transfusion refractoriness. Transfusion. 1986;26:463-6.
66. Carr R, Hutton JL, Jenkins JA, Lucas GF, Amphlett MW. Transfusion of ABO mismatched platelets leads to early platelet refractoriness. Br J Haematol. 1990;75:408-13.
67. Pierce RN, Reich LM, Mayer K. Hemolysis following platelet transfusions from ABO-incompatible donors. Transfusion. 1985;25:60-2.
68. Reis MD, Coovadia AS. Transfusion of ABO-incompatible platelets causing severe hemolytic reaction. Clin Lab Haematol. 1989;11:237-40.
69. Dunstan RA, Simpson MB, Rosse WF. Erythrocyte antigens on human platelets. Absence of the Rhesus, Duffy, Kell, Kidd and Lutheran antigens. Transfusion. 1984;24:243-6.
70. Goldfinger D, McGinnis MH. Rh incompatible platelet transfusion risks and consequences of sensitizing immuno-suppressed patients. N Engl J Med. 1971;284:942-4.
71. Baldwin ML, Ness PM Scott D, et al. Alloimmunization to D antigen and HLA in D-negative immunosuppressed oncology patients. Transfusion. 1988;28:330-3.

72. Heim BU, Bock M, Kold HJ, et al. Intravenous anti-D gammaglobulin for the prevention of rhesus isoimmunization caused by platelet transfusion in patients with malignant disease. Vox Ang. 1992;62:165-8.
73. Zeiler T, Wittmann G, Zingsem J, et al. A dose of 100 IU intravenous anti-D gammaglobulin is effective for the prevention of RhD immunization after RhD immunization after RhD-incompatible single donor platelet transfusion. Vox Sang. 1994;66:243.
74. National Blood Transfusion Service Immunoglobulin Working Party: Recommendations for the use of anti-D immunoglobulin. Prescribers J. 1991;31:137.
75. Caspar C, Reinhard A, Burger J, et al. Effective stimulation of donors for granulocytes transfusions with recombinant methionyl granulocytes colony stimulating factor. Blood. 1993;81:2866-71.
76. Saarinen UM, Hovi L, Vilinikka L, et al. Reemphasis on leukocyte transfusions: induction of myeloid marrow recovery in critically ill neutropenic children with cancer. Vox Sang. 1995;68:90-9.
77. Technical Manual, 12th edn. Bethesda, MD: American Association of Blood Banks; 1996. p. 121.
78. Strauss RG. Granulocyte transfusion therapy. In: Mintz PD (Ed). Transfusion Medicine I. Hematol Oncol Clin North Am. 1994;8:1159-66.
79. Chanock SJ, Gorlin JB. Granulocytes transfusions. Time for a second look. Infect Dis Clin North Am. 1996;10:327-43.
80. Nathan DG, Oski SH. Hematology of Infancy and Children, 5th edn. Philadelphia: WB Saunders; 1997. Appendix 28, p. XV.
81. Sweetman RW, Cairo MS. Blood component and immunotherapy in neonatal sepsis. Transfusion Med Rev. 1995;9:251-9.
82. Rosenthal J, Healey T, Ellis R, et al. A two-year follow-up of neonates with presumed sepsis treated with recombinant human granulocytes colony-stimulating factor during the first week of life. J Pediatr. 1996;128:135-7.
83. Stroncek DF, Leonard K, Eiber G, et al. Alloimmunization after granulocytes transfusions. 1996;36:1009-15.
84. Margarson MP, Soni N. Serum albumin touchstone or totem? Anaesthesia. 1998;53:789-803.
85. Hillyer CD, Berkman EM. Transfusion of plasma derivatives: fresh frozen plasma, cryoprecipitate, albumin and immunoglobulin. In: Hoffman R Bentz EJ, Shattil SJ, Furie B, Cohen HJ, Silberstein, Leukemia (Eds). Hematology: Basic Principles and Practice, 2nd edn. New York: Churchill Livingstone; 1995. pp. 2011-9.
86. NIH consensus development conference. Intravenous immunoglobulin: Prevention and treatment of disease. JAMA. 1990;264:3189-93.
87. Stiehn R. Appropriate therapeutic use of immunoglobulin. Transfusion Med Rev. 1996;10:203-21.
88. Meissner HC, Welliver RC, Chartrand SA, et al. Prevention of respiratory syncytial virus infection in high risk infants: consensus opinion on the role of immunoprophylaxis with respiratory syncytial virus hyperimmune globulin. Pediatr Infect Dis J. 1996;15:1059-68.
89. Harlsey NA, Aramson JS, Chesney PJ, et al. Respiratory syncytial virus immune globulin intravenous: Indications for use. Committee on Infections Diseases 1996 to 1997. Pediatrics. 1997;99:645-50.
90. Strauss RG. Transfusion therapy in neonates. Am J Dis Child. 1991;145:904-91.
91. Klein HG. Standards for blood banks and transfusion services, 17th edn. Bethesda, MD, American Association of Blood Banks; 1996.

Transfusion Transmitted Infections

Deepak Bansal, RK Marwaha

Transmission of various infectious agents remains the most significant concern for any individual receiving blood products. Prevention of transfusion related infections and maintenance of safe blood supply is a daunting task, especially in a developing country like India. With a large population, underutilization of blood components and reluctance for voluntary donations, there is a large gap between supply and demand of blood in India. Under these situations, quantity often takes precedence over quality. The developed countries on the other hand have been able to reduce risks of transfusion related infections to a miniscule level through extensive screening of donors.

The acquired immunodeficiency syndrome (AIDS) pandemic has heightened the public awareness of risks of transfusion. Post-transfusion-hepatitis is the biggest risk that a recipient faces today. With transfusion a part and parcel of many fields of medicine, it is important for the physician to be well informed of the risks associated with transfusion and measures of prevention. This chapter attempts to provide an overview of common infectious agents transmitted by transfusion, their epidemiology and prevention in the Indian context.

HEPATITIS B VIRUS

Hepatitis B virus (HBV) is a member of the hepadina virus family, a noncytopathogenic hepatotropic group of DNA viruses. It has a lipoprotein shell, in which the hepatitis B surface antigen (HBsAg) is found and an inner core. The HBsAg in serum can be identified by serological methods. People who have acute viral hepatitis or who are HBsAg carriers transmit HBV. It is transmitted parenterally, sexually or perinatally from infected mothers to their infants.

HBV is endemic throughout the world, especially in tropical and developing countries. More than 2 billion people worldwide have evidence of past or current HBV infection and 350 million are chronic carriers.[1] The virus causes 60-80% of all the primary liver cancers. India falls in the intermediate zone for HBV seroprevalence. There are estimated 43-45 million HBsAg carriers in India. The mean carrier rate in general population in India is found to be 4.7%.[2] Seroprevalence of HBV in Indian blood donors as reported by various blood banks is illustrated in Table 25.1.

HBV is thus a major public heath problem in India and a major cause of transfusion associated hepatitis (TAH).[6] TAH is a serious complication of transfusion and a common cause of morbidity and mortality. TAH is suspected when a transfusion recipient has two elevated readings of alanine transaminase (ALT), at least 5 days apart, 14-180 days after the transfusion. There should be no other obvious cause for the hepatitis.[7]

The incubation period varies and ranges from 4-12 weeks. Thirty to forty percent of individuals acquiring HBV will be symptomatic; 0.2-0.5% develop fulminant and fatal hepatitis. The remainder, develop transient subclinical hepatitis, detectable only by laboratory tests. A variable proportion of these will recover from the clinical/sub-clinical infection and develop immunity. The ominous feature is the development of a carrier state, the risk of which is inversely related to age. More than 90% of infants infected during the first year of life become carriers compared with a rate of 5-10% among older children and adults. Insidious progression to chronic hepatitis and its attendant sequelae of cirrhosis and hepatocellular carcinoma (HCC) is what makes the prevention of HBV infection a subject of paramount importance.

Thalassemics and hemophiliacs, who receive multiple transfusions of blood/plasma derivatives, are at considerably greater risk of acquiring HBV. This is because the donor plasma may be infected with undetectable levels of viruses and pooling of plasma leads to greater infectivity. This is obvious from the fact that 2-10% of hemophiliacs are identified to be HbsAg carriers; an additional 75% have evidence of past

Table 25.1: Seroprevalence of HBV in Indian blood donors[3-5]

Center	No. of donors	% Prevalence total (voluntary replacement)
AIIMS, Delhi	94,716	1.43
PGIMER, Chandigarh	33,384	(0.7/0.98)
GB Pant, Delhi	5,801	(0/4.5)
Indian Red Cross, Delhi	46,215	2.4
NRS Medical College, Kolkata	100	2.0

infection (anti-HBc or anti-HBs positive).[8,9] A study from Mumbai revealed HBsAg positivity in 45% of transfusion dependent thalassemics.[10] Similarly, in a study conducted on thalassemic children in Delhi, 72% of 75 patients had present or past evidence of HBV infection.[11]

During the course of symptomatic infection, a well-detailed sequence of serologically detectable changes occurs. HBsAg is the first serological marker to appear, often before the development of symptoms. Concentration of viral antigen rises until symptoms develop and persists for 1-5 months. In most patients who are not destined to become chronic carriers, HBsAg disappears, to be relapsed by antibody (anti-HBs), indicating immunity. The HBc antigen is not found in serum but antibody to HBc develops in all HBV infections. IgM anti-HBc develops after appearance of HBsAg and persists for 6-12 months; it is replaced by IgG anti-HBc, which persists indefinitely. It is mandatory to test blood donations for the presence of HBsAg.

The sensitivity of HBsAg screening assays has significantly improved over time reaching 0.1 IU/ml. However, the tests are unable to detect the pre-seroconversion window period or samples with very low viral load following decades of chronicity or clinical recovery.

HBV-DNA screening is the only means of covering the window period. This is the main concern of countries where infection occurs sexually or through IV drug abuse after age 15, at which people become blood donors. In contrast, anti-HBc screening can eliminate nearly all HBV present in chronically infected or recovered individuals, although only a small fraction of anti-HBc-positive donations also carries detectable HBV-DNA. However, in areas where anti-HBc prevalence is >2-5%, the deficit in blood donations that would be created by deferring anti-HBc-positive donors is considered too high to maintain sufficient blood supply. In these areas, HBV-DNA screening is the main option, although the generally very low viral load of the potentially infectious units forces to screen in very small pools (<10 plasmas) or in individual units.[11a] Unlike hepatitis C virus (HCV) and HIV testing, nucleic acid testing (NAT) HBV-DNA testing has not eliminated the necessity for serological testing for HBV carrier donors.

The value of anti-HBc for HBV prevention is limited to situations in which the donor is infectious but HBsAg is not detected. This occurs in:

1. Acute resolving HBV infection in the window period.
2. Low-level HBV infections with undetectable HBsAg, either with or without low titer anti-HBs.
3. Infections, by rare HBV mutant variants, detected by some HBsAg assays.[12]

Studies have been conducted among HBsAg-negative, anti-HBc-positive donors. Reports from high HBV prevalent areas such as Japan, China and India have reported that a signification proportion (<5% to up to 50%) of such donors are positive for HBV DNA by polymerase chain reaction (PCR).[13] In contrast, most studies from low prevalence areas have found low or undetectable rates of HBV-DNA in the serum of such donors. This suggests that most 'anticore-only' donors have false positive anti-HBc results. Extraordinary rates of HBV-DNA positivity have also been reported among HBsAg negative low risk donors. These discrepant results probably reflect differences in sensitivity and specificity of HBV-DNA assays. Thus it is clear that anti-HBc can detect some HBV infectious donations missed by HBsAg screening. Unfortunately, in high endemicity regions, where yield would be higher, cannot tolerate the high donor loss rates associated with anti-HBc screening. In a survey 14% of Indian blood banks reported testing the donor for anti HBc.[3] Whether this should be done routinely is an issue that needs to be addressed.[3,14,15]

Thus far, the consensus is that NAT should be used in conjunction with serological testing to identify low-level infections as well as infections that are at the ends of the window periods of detection. There is no consensus either on whether single-donor NAT or what size pool NAT is optimal, and it may depend on the prevalence of HBV in the country. Additionally, HBV infectivity may depend upon the immunosuppressive state of the recipient of the blood component.[15a]

Highly efficacious and safe vaccine is available. Till developing countries like India can enforce universal immunization with the HBV vaccine, the population at risk should at least be immunized.

Table 25.2: Prevalence of HCV antibody in Indian blood donors[4,14,18,19,25b]

Center	*No screened*	*% Positive*
AIIMS, Delhi	94,716	0.57
CMC, Vellore	22,245	0.77
GB Pant, Delhi	1,383	1.66
Indore	280	1.78
PGIMER, Chandigarh	16,250	0.44

HEPATITIS C VIRUS

It is now well recognized as the cause of almost all the parenterally acquired cases of what was previously known as non-A non-B hepatitis. Hepatitis C virus (HCV) is an enveloped, single stranded RNA virus of the flaviviridae family. Mainly blood/blood products, intravenous drug abuse and sexual contact transmit it. It is the most likely hepatitis virus to cause chronic infection: about two-thirds of post-transfusion infections become chronic. Chronic HCV, progresses to cirrhosis in about half, or about 25% of all those initially infected. Primary HCC can develop in patients with cirrhosis but HCV is less likely to cause primary HCC than HBV.[16]

World health organization (WHO) has estimated that 3% of the worlds population is infected with HCV and around 170 million individuals are chronic carriers, at risk of developing cirrhosis and liver cancer.[17] In the USA, an estimated 4 million people have acquired the disease, four times more than HIV infection. It has also become a leading cause for liver transplantation.[1] The efficiency of transmission of HCV through transfusion of a reactive unit is about 90%. The risk of post-transfusion HCV infection per unit transfused varies from 1:288,000 to 1:28,000 with an average of 1:103,000 using 3rd enzyme-linked immunosorbant assay (ELISA).

The global seroprevalence of HCV among blood donors varies from 0.4-19.2%. The seroprevalence of HCV in voluntary blood donors in India is between 0.12-4% (Table 25.2). The prevalence is expectedly higher in multitransfused individuals. In a study of 188 hemophiliacs from Mumbai, 24% were found to be positive for HCV.[20] Positivity in children with thalassemia has been reported to be 25% from Indore and 68% from Delhi.[11,18] Lai et al have shown that among thalassemic patients acquiring HCV through transfusion, resolution of infection is seen in 20% of cases, recurrent or chronic infection in 80% and cirrhosis in 11%.[21]

The specific diagnosis of HCV infection requires serological and/or molecular-based (NAT) assays. In rare instances, anti-HCV may not develop; in these cases, a definitive diagnosis of HCV requires molecular-based (NAT) assays.[15a] With the introduction of 1st generation assays, the incidence of TAH dropped by approximately 80% and by another 10% by the 2nd generation assay.[22] NAT of plasma intended for fractionation and of blood donations for HCV-RNA began in the late 1990s when methodologies became available. With the use of anti-HCV antibody testing only, before HCV-NAT testing, the risk of transfusion transmission of HCV was reduced considerably. The window period for HCV was approximately 70 days. With the introduction of NAT, the window period has been reduced to approximately 12 days. NAT-HCV testing is mandated in many industrialized countries.[15a]

In India, mandatory screening for HCV was introduced as late as 2002. Pool testing was performed in the past for economical reasons; it cannot be justified in well-funded transfusion centers, as there is a residual risk of false negative reactions that may occur with samples containing low titer antibody.[24,25]

The impact of screening for hepatitis C in India was shown in a cross-sectional study from Kolkata that looked at three groups of patients, the first group comprised multiple transfused patients who received transfusion before 1995, the second group of patients had received transfusions only since 1995 and the third group had control patients who had never been transfused.[25a] The HCV antibody positivity rate was 16%, 6% and 2% respectively. The differences were significant between the first and the other two groups suggesting that the prevalence had indeed fallen after HCV screening in blood banks.

To ensure transfusion of safe blood to the recipient, not only mandatory screening of blood for such infections markers is necessary, it is also important to study the prevalence, age distribution and risk factors for causing HCV infection among the donor population. In India, percutaneous exposure through minor routes of transmission like sharing of shaving kits or visit to a road side barber, surgery and multiple unsafe intravenous injections have played an important role in HCV transmission.[25b] India's blood-banking system has serious shortcomings. Professional blood donation continues to flourish despite a law condoning this. Another malaise in our health system is the reuse of improperly sterilized needles. Both these factors are potential sources for the spread of hepatitis C in India.

HEPATITIS D VIRUS

Hepatitis D virus (HDV) is the smallest known animal virus. It is considered defective, as it cannot produce infection without a concurrent HBV infection. This agent is transmitted with blood products in association with the HBV, resulting in an episode of acute viral hepatitis similar to hepatitis B virus, although with an increased risk of fulminant or chronic disease. Co-infection with HBV and HDV occurs most frequently in areas of high prevalence. In a study from Kolkata, only 2 out of 60 (3.3%) HBsAg positive jaundiced patients were positive for HDV antigen, indicating a low rate of prevalence of infection.

As HDV can be transmitted only with HBV, the testing of all blood donations for the presence of HBV will exclude virtually all transmissions of HDV. HDV is not an independent risk factor; so specific testing is not warranted.[22]

HEPATITIS A VIRUS

Hepatitis A virus (HAV) is much less significant than other hepatitis viruses in blood transfusion practice. It is spread by person-to-person contact, usually by feco-oral route. The fatality is very low and chronic hepatitis and carrier states do not occur. The viremia lasts for only a few days before symptoms appear. Although infrequent, the transmission of HAV by transfusion has been reported. As the possibility of transfusion transmitted HAV is very low and it does not have carriers state, it is inappropriate to consider donor testing for this virus.

HEPATITIS E VIRUS

Its spread is similar to HAV, in that it is enterically transmitted. There is no evidence of a chronic carrier state. Very occasionally, especially in endemic areas, transfusion associated hepatitis E is possible.[27]

HEPATITIS GB VIRUS C/HEPATITIS G VIRUS

The genome of this virus was found independently by two different groups of investigators in 1995.[28] They designated it differently as GB virus C and hepatitis G virus (HGV). Association of HGV with cases of fulminant hepatitis, post-transfusion hepatitis and sporadic hepatitis has been suggested.[29] The prevalence of HGV in blood donors in developed countries ranges from 1-5%, but these numbers correspond to HGV RNA positive persistent infections. Preliminary data suggests that 3-4 times more donors have been infected with HGV and have recovered from it.[30] In a recent study from Delhi, 4% of voluntary blood donors and 47% of professional blood donors were found to be HGV positive.[31] In another study from Delhi, HGV RNA was detected in 40% of multitransfused thalassemic children.[32] The pathogenic role of this virus is yet to be precisely defined.

TT VIRUS

A sequence suggestive of a novel DNA virus was identified in the serum of a patient with post transfused hepatitis in Japan in 1997.[33] The TT virus (TTV) positive patient was one of the five patients with non-A-G hepatitis with raised liver enzymes after transfusion. Approximately 50% of non-A-G chronic hepatitis cases in Japanese patients were found to be TTV DNA positive. In India a group from Pune has shown TTV DNA positivity of 6.7% in patients with chronic hepatitis, 24% in hemophiliacs and 7.4% in voluntary blood donors.[34] Till the association of TTV with liver disease is definitely proven, no action on the part of blood banks is warranted.[23]

HUMAN IMMUNODEFICIENCY VIRUS TYPES 1 AND 2 (HIV1 AND HIV2)

The acquired immunodeficiency syndrome (AIDS) is a fatal illness caused by the retrovirus, HIV. It breaks down the body's immune system, leaving the victim vulnerable to a host of life-threatening opportunistic infections, neurological disorders or unusual malignancies. Among the specific features of HIV infection are that once infected, it is probable that a person will be infected for life. The AIDS pandemic has brought into focus the importance of safe blood transfusion.

The incubation period, i.e. the time interval from introduction of HIV infection to development of AIDS is uncertain and varies from a few months to many years. There is no cure; antiretroviral drugs can delay the onset of AIDS but are prohibitively expensive.

According to estimates, at the end of 1999, about 34.4 million were living with HIV/AIDS, worldwide. Estimates at the national level indicated that about 3.7 million people were suffering from HIV infection at that time. Serosurveillance findings from the states show that by June 2000, out of 36,62,969 persons screened for HIV, 98,451 were HIV positive with seropositivity of 21.88 per thousand.[35]

Contaminated blood is highly infective when introduced in large quantities directly into the blood stream. The risk of acquiring HIV from transfusion of a single unit of infected blood is estimated to be over 95%. Since the likelihood of HIV transmission through blood depends on the 'dose' of virus injected, the risk of getting infected through a contaminated needle or any other skin-piercing instrument is very much lower than with transfusion. AIDS is first and foremost a sexually transmitted disease and transfusion of blood and blood products has played a less important role in its spread.[35]

Unlike adults where the primary route of transmission of HIV is sexual, majority of infected children acquire the disease from their mother at the time of birth. In India, a small population of children continues to acquire the infection through transfusion of blood/blood products. This proportion is likely to decline considerably over the next few years as blood bank screening procedures are further refined.[36]

Shortly after exposure to the virus, the patient may develop mild viral type symptoms. At this time, the p24 antigen becomes detectable. This is followed by the development of an antibody to both the envelope and core proteins. The first generation ELISA tests for anti-HIV were able to detect the great majority of asymptomatic HIV carriers, but the window period (time to seroconversion) in newly infected individuals was approximately 56 days. Second and third generation anti-HIV tests reduced the window to 33 and 22 days, respectively. The HIV p24 antigen test was introduced in 1996 with the hope of further reducing the window period.[15a]

HIV IgG ELISA is the usual screening test. Currently available tests detect both HIV 1 and 2 and the sensitivity is over 99.5%. Detection of HIV-1 p24 antigen shortens the window period to less than 20 days.[22] HIV minipool NAT–negative units have transmitted HIV, as recently as 2007; likely, these transmissions would have been prevented with single-unit NAT testing.[15a] NAT testing is out of reach, as is pooled NAT testing, in many developing countries, where the incidence of HIV in the general population is unfortunately high.

HUMAN T-LYMPHOTROPIC VIRUS I AND II

Human T-Lymphotropic virus (HTLV) I and II were the first retroviruses identified in humans in 1980 and 1982, respectively.[37,38] HTLV-1 infection is endemic in Japan, Caribbean, Couth and Central America and Africa. HTLV-II is endemic in amerindians, pigmy tribes and is commonly found in HTLV infected intravenous drug users.

Most of the HTLV infected subjects remain asymptomatic. HTLV-I has been implicated in a lymphoproliferative malignancy called the adult T-cell leukemia and a chronic demyelinating neurological disorder called tropical spastic paraparesis or HTLV-I associated myelopathy. HTLV-II has also been implicated in the latter.[39] The virus is transmitted by breastfeeding, sexual transmission, intravenous drug use and by the transfusion of infected cellular blood components. Acellular blood components, e.g. plasma do not generally transmit HTLV. The efficiency of transmission has been evaluated to be 30-60%, as compared to over 90% for HBV, HCV and HIV. In HTLV seropositive individuals there appears to be a 2.5% lifetime risk of developing adult T-cell leukemia and 0.25% risk of developing tropical spastic paraparesis.

Many western nations started routine screening for HTLV by EIA during the late 80's and early 90's. Prevalence of HTLV in blood donors in countries where routine screening is done is: USA: 0.043%, France: 0.004% and Spain: 0.02%.[39] Reports of seroprevalence of HTLV from different regions of India are variable. However all reports have one thing in common: prevalence is higher in high-risk groups, indicating common route of transmission. In a study from Delhi, 32% of 100 HIV seropositive blood donors were found to be positive for HTLV-I.[40] In a study from Vellore, 3.7% of 376 HIV positive cases compared to 0.3% of 934 HIV negative patients attending STD clinic were found positive for HTLV I/II.[41] None of the 946 adults belonging to ten different population groups of Uttar Pradesh and West Bengal were positive for HTLV I, in a study from north India.[42] In India at present, HTLV screening seems to be a distant goal.

CYTOMEGALOVIRUS

Cytomegalovirus (CMV) is a large DNA virus of the herpes family. It is one of the common infectious agents transmitted by transfusion. Like the other herpes viruses, it becomes latent in infected people. Although most of the primary infections are asymptomatic in normal persons, there may be mononucleosis like picture. CMV antibody positive subjects may infect others by sexual contact, breastfeeding, transplacental transmission or transfusion. The virus may be reactivated and cause disease, especially in the immunosuppressed host. Alternatively, through rarely, there may be reinfection with a third strain.

In most transfused patients, CMV transmission is a benign complication. Patients at risk for more severe CMV infection are the immunocompromised individuals. These include newborns, particularly those with very low birth weight and recipients of solid organ and bone marrow transplant. The frequency of subject with anti-CMV-antibody varies widely in different populations. It is lower (30-80%) in developed than in developing countries, where the figure may reach 100%.[43] In a study of prevalence of CMV from southern India, over 90% of individuals acquired CMV-IgG by four years of age.[44]

Transfusion of anti-CMV positive blood leads to clinically significant CMV infection in newborn infants only when the infant is premature, low birth-weight (especially < 1330 g) and when the mother lacks anti-CMV-antibody. CMV infection (mainly pneumonitis) is a common cause of death following the transplantation of allogeneic marrow. Renal transplant recipients are also at high-risk of primary or recurrent CMV infection. For such situation, selection of anti-CMV negative donors is an effective method to reduce transmission. Another approach is the removal of leukocytes from red cells and platelet concentrates by leukocytes filters. It is based on the fact that leukocytes transmit CMV. There is no indication for leukocyte depleted products in anti-CMV positive recipients.

The prevalence of anti-CMV (IgG) in Indian subcontinent is about 95%. About 5% of screened donor population have IgM antibody which carries eminent threat of transmitting CMV infection to immune-compromised and newborn patients. Due to the wide prevalence of CMV infection in this population, it is not possible to screen blood donors for this infection. The practical solution is to supply leukoreduced (by 3rd/4th generation filters) blood products to the needy patients.

EPSTEIN-BARR VIRUS

Epstein-Barr virus (EBV) is also a herpes virus and is endemic worldwide. In most countries, more than 90% of blood donors have neutralizing anti-EBV antibodies. In a study of prevalence of EBV from southern India, over 90% of individuals acquired EBV-IgG by four years of age.[44] Post-transfusion EBV infection is a rare occurrence and symptomatic infection is even rarer. Due to the rarity of clinically important EBV infection and in view of the high carrier rate, screening of blood donors for EBV antibodies is not recommended.

SYPHILIS

Transfusion acquired syphilis, once a serious problem, is a declining hazard now. The chief reasons are:

1. Almost universal practice of storing blood at low temperature before using it for transfusion; in citrated blood, stored for >72 hours at 4-6°C, spirochetes are unlikely to survive.
2. Decline in the prevalence of syphilis in many countries since the advent of penicillin.
3. Administration of antibiotics to a large proportion of patients requiring transfusion.[43]

Commonly used tests for screening are the VDRL (Veneral Disease Research Laboratory) and RpR (Rapid Plasma Reagin) tests. Both these tests give high proportion of biological false positive. Positive tests should be crosschecked with more specific tests. Serological tests cannot prevent all cases of transfusion syphilis: serological tests are often negative in early primary syphilis when spirochetemia is most prominent. Incubation period in transfusion syphilis varies from 4 weeks to 4 months, averaging 9-10 weeks. The recipient usually exhibits typical secondary eruption.

In the survey of Kapoor et al, 94% of Indian blood banks were found to be testing blood for syphilis.[3] Seroprevalence of syphilis in Indian blood donors is about 0.5%.[14]

MALARIA

Malaria can be transmitted by the transfusion of any blood component likely to contain even a small number of red cells; platelet concentrates, fresh plasma and cryoprecipitate have all been incriminated. Asymptomatic carriers are the source of transfusion-transmitted infection. Such people may harbor the parasites for many years without developing any symptoms. Malarial parasites (MP) can remain viable in stored blood for at least a week. The incubation period of transfusion malaria is between one week and one month for *P. vivax* and *P. falciparum*. Transfusion transmitted malaria usually responds to conventional drug therapy; primaquine is not indicated as parasites remain confined to circulating red cells.[43] In most endemic areas the frequency of post-transfusion malaria is unknown due to lack of reporting.

Preventive strategies are variable. Nonendemic areas, like USA, rely solely on the deferral of subject who have been in endemic areas, whereas, in Europe, deferral and testing for MP is combined. In endemic areas like India, blood smear examination is the most popular method of screening. In the survey of Kapoor et al, 67% of Indian blood banks screened for MP.[3] In a revealing study from SGPGIMS, Lucknow, smear examination by Geimsa and Acradine orange staining was compared with antigen detection by specific monoclonal antibody. Blood smear examination failed to reveal MP in 92% of antigen positive blood donors. The investigators concluded that antigen detection by monoclonal antibody should be adopted as a routine screening method by the blood transfusion services.[45]

CREUTZFELDT-JAKOB DISEASE

Creutzfeldt-Jakob disease (CJD) is a rapidly progressive fatal infection of the nervous system caused by an agent called prion.[22] Disease has been shown to be transmitted through administration of infected human tissues such as human growth hormone derived from the pituitary, corneal and dura mater transplants. There is a familial type of CJD too. Transmission through blood has not been proven. In view of the potential risk, people who have received any of the mentioned therapies/human growth hormone or have family history of CJD are deferred from donating blood. There are few case reports of CJD from India.[46]

BACTERIAL CONTAMINATION OF BLOOD

Despite meticulous collection techniques, organisms from either the skin or air contaminate a small proportion of blood units. As fresh blood is bactericidal, these contaminants normally die. Therefore, when blood is collected with standard aseptic precautions and refrigerated, the chances of it becoming clinically infected are rare. However, if blood is taken out from the refrigerator and left at room temperature, any organism, that is present, can multiply. Platelet concentrates are implicated more often, as they are stored at room temperature. Gram-negative organisms are more frequently recovered from RBC's whereas gram-positive organisms are more frequently recovered from platelet concentrates.[47]

Septic transfusion reactions can be acute and devastating. The manifestations often mimic those of febrile nonhemolytic reactions and are frequently not recognized. High fever, rigors, abdominal pain with cramps, diarrhea, shock, hemoglobinuria, renal failure and DIC are usual features. Contamination of blood may be suggested by gross observation. All bags prior to transfusion should be examined for hemolysis, clots, and unusual color or air bubbles. In suspected cases, cultures are taken from the donor bag, the patient and from any IV solution that may be concurrently running. Management has to be prompt and aggressive. The measures include administration of broad-spectrum antibiotics, intravenous fluids and treatment of hypotension/shock. Renal failure and DIC are potential complications that need appropriate management.

RARELY TRANSMITTED PARASITES

Babesiosis, trypanosomiasis (Chagas disease) and Leishmaniasis can be transmitted through blood component transfusion.[43]

INACTIVATION OF VIRUSES IN BLOOD PRODUCTS

Despite donor screening and testing, there is always a small risk of transmission of viruses, particularly with products obtained from large pools of plasma. Inactivation or removal of viruses can further increase the safety of transfusion and may protect against yet undiscovered organisms. Several methods are being used or in development to reduce infectivity of blood products, including solvent-detergent processing of plasma and nucleic acid cross-linking via photochemical reactions with methylene blue, riboflavin, psoralen and alkylating agents. Leukopheresis is used for removal of viruses like CMV and HTLV that are transmitted only by leukocytes. A rapid quantitative immunoassay is now available to test for the presence of lipotechoic acid and lipopolysaccharide bacterial products prior to platelet transfusion.

Technology of pathogen inactivation (PI), although not approved worldwide, has been shown to reduce the rate to near zero with the potential of eliminating extensive testing of all units. As PI does not rely on specific disease testing, it allows elimination of risk for yet unknown emerging infections. Furthermore, PI has been shown not to affect protein composition or clotting capacity. A major limitation on this technology, however, is that it is not available for use in red blood cells, although it has been suggested that treatment of whole blood before fractionation could assist in resolving this issue.[15a]

THE INDIAN SCENARIO

In India, screening is mandatory for HIV, HBV, HCV, syphilis and malaria. The Supreme Court of India took up the issue of blood safety by banning paid donations by the end of 1997. There are still a number of blood banks operating without license. While India collects three million units of blood, barely 10% is available as blood components.[48] A nation wide questionnaire based study was conducted by Kapoor et al to assess functioning of Indian blood banks. The researchers concluded that testing for transfusion-transmitted infections was unsatisfactory and poorly regulated in India.[3] Screening at district zone or regional supervising centers is especially questionable. Majority of donors being replacement rather than voluntary remains disturbing, as possibility of significant proportion of them, being paid cannot be ruled out.[23]

It is now internationally recognized that blood from non remunerated regular voluntary donors is the safest blood supply. The principles of quality assurance and GMP have now become necessary in blood transfusion services for adhering to regulations and accreditations. However, there is a long way to go to achieve 100% voluntary donation. It will require comprehensive efforts from all quarters to achieve this goal. Encouragement of voluntary donations, recipient surveillance program, quality control, legislation and development of cheap indigenous screening methods would go a long way in making transfusions safer in India.

REFERENCES

1. WHO, World Health Report 1998, Life in the 21st century, A vision for all WHO, Geneva, 1988.
2. Thygarajan SP, Jayaram S, Mohan Valli B. Prevalence of HBV in the general population in India. In: Sarin SK, Singhal AK (Eds). Hepatitis B in India. New Delhi: CBS Publishers; 1996. pp. 5-16.
3. Kapoor D, Saxena R, Sood B, Sarin SK. Blood transfusion practices in India: results of a national survey. Indian J Gastroenterol. 2000;19:64-7.
4. Meena M, Jindal T, Hazarika A. Prevalence of hepatitis B virus and hepatitis C virus among blood donors at a tertiary care hospital in India: a five-year study. Transfusion. 2011;51:198-202.
5. Bhattacharya S, Dala BS, Lahiri A. Hepatitis D infectivity profile among hepatitis B infected hospitalized patients in Calcutta. Indian J Pub Health. 1998;42:108-12.
6. Tandon BN, Gandhi BM, Joshi YK. Etiological spectrum of viral hepatitis and prevalence of markers of hepatitis A and B virus infection in North India. Bull WHO. 1984;62:67-73.
7. Kapoor D, Sarin SK. Transfusion associated hepatitis: the Indian scenario. Indian Pediatr. 1997;34:1069-74.
8. Mannuccii PM, Capitanio A, Del Ninno E, Colombo M, Pareti F, Ruggeri M, et al. Asymptomatic liver disease in hemophiliacs. J Clin Pathol. 1975;28:620-4.
9. Nebbia G, Moroni GA, Simoni L, Belli M, Carnelli V. Hepatitis B virus infection in multitransfused hemophiliacs. Arch Dis Child. 1986;621:580-4.
10. Amarapurkar DN, Kumar A, Vaidya S, Murti P, Bichile SK, Karo RH, et al. Frequency of hepatitis B, C and D and HIV infections in multi-transfused thalassaemics. Indian J Gastroenterol. 1992;11:80-4.
11. Thakur V, Guptan RC, Motwani J, Chopra K, Sarin SK. High frequency of HBV and HCV dual infection in thalassaemic children in India. Indian J Gastroenterol. 1995;14(Suppl 1):A94.

11a. Allain JP, Stramer SL, Carneiro-Proietti AB, et al. Transfusion-transmitted infectious diseases. Biologicals. 2009;37:71-7.

12. Busch MP. Prevention of transmission of hepatitis B, hepatitis C and human immunodeficiency virus infections through blood transfusion by anti-HBc testing. Vox Sang. 1998;74(Suppl 2):147-54.
13. Saraswat S, Manerjee K, Chaudhury N, Mahant T, Khandehar P, Gupta RK, Naik S. Post transfusion hepatitis type B following multiple transfusions of HBsAg negative blood. J Hepatol. 1996;25:639-43.
14. Kapoor D, Sarin SK. What is safe blood? JAPI. 2000;48:335-42.
15. Saxena R, Thakur V, Sood B, Guptan RC, Gururaja S, Sarin SK. Transfusion-associated hepatitis in a tertiary referral hospital in India. Vox Sang. 1999;77:6-10.

15a. Dwyre DM, Fernando LP, Holland PV. Hepatitis B, hepatitis C and HIV transfusion-transmitted infections in the 21st century. Vox Sang. 2011;100:92-8.

16. Snyder JD, Pickering LK. Hepatitis A through E. In: Behram RE, Kliegman RM, Arvin AM (Eds). Nelson's Textbook of Pediatrics, 15th ed. Bangore: WB Saunders Co, Prism Books; 1996. pp. 909-14.
17. Park K. Park's textbook of preventive and social medicine, 17th edn. Jabalpur: M/s Banarsidas Bhanot; 2000. pp. 162-3.
18. Jaiswa SP, Chitnis DS, Naik G, Artwani KK, Pandit CS, Salgia P, et al. Prevalence of anti-HCV antibodies in central India. Indian J Med Res. 1996;104:177-81.
19. Das PK, Harris VK, Sitaram U, Baidya S, Jacob D. Hepatitis C virus prevalence among blood donors from South India. Vox Sang. 2000;78:254-5.
20. Ghosh K, Joshi SH, Shetty S, Pawar A, Chipkar S, Pujari V, et al. Transfusion transmitted diseases in hemophiliacs from western India. Indian J Med Res. 2000;112:61-4.
21. Lai ME, De Virgiis S, Argiolu F, Farci P, Mazzoleni AP, Lisci V, et al. Evaluation of antibodies to hepatitis C virus in a long term prospective study of post transfusion hepatitis among thalassemic children: Comparison between first and second generation assay. J Pediatr Gastroenterol Nutr. 1993;16:458-64.
22. Schroeder ML. Principles and Practice of Transfusion Medicine. In: Lee GR, Foerster J, Lukens J, Paraskevas F, Greer JP, Rodgers GM (Eds). Wintrobe's Clinical Hematology; 10th edn. Baltimore: Williams and Wilkins; 1998. pp. 817-74.
23. Arankalle VA. Current bood transfusion practices in India. Indian J Gastroenterol. 2000;19:51-2.
24. Neill AG, Conradie JD. Low-cost anti-HCV screening of blood donors. Lancet. 1992;340:1096.
25. Mujeeb SA, Hafiz A. Low-cost screening of blood for HCV infection in the developing world. Vox Sang. 1998;74:210.

25a. Hazra SC, Chatterjee S, Das Gupta S, Chaudhuri U, Jana CK, Neogi DK. Changing scenario of transfusion-related viral infections. J Assoc Physicians India. 2002;50:879-81.

25b. Thakral B, Marwaha N, Chawla YK, et al. Prevalence and significance of hepatitis C virus (HCV) seropositivity in blood donors. Indian J Med Res. 2006;124:431-8.

26. Nishioka K. Transfusion associated hepatitis due to hepatitis B and C in Japan. Vox Sang. 1996;70(Supp 3):4-8.
27. Arankalle VA, Chobe LP. Hepatitis E Virus: can it be transmitted parenterally? J Viral Hepatitis. 1999;6:161-4.
28. Simons JN, Piot-Mathias TJ, Leary TP, et al. Identification of two flavivirus-like genomes in the GB hepatitis agent. Proc Natl Acad Scie. 1995;92:3401-5.
29. Heringlake S, Osterkamp S, Trautwein C, et al. Association between fulminant hepatic failure and a strain of GB Virus C. Lancet. 1996;348:1626-9.
30. Tacke M, Kiyosawa K, Strak K, et al. Detection of antibodies to putative hepatitis G virus enveloped protein. Lancet. 1997;349:318-20.

31. Kar P, Bedi P, Berry N, Chakravorty A, Gupta RK, Saha R, Das BC. Hepatitis G virus (HGV) infection in voluntary and commercial bood donors in India. Diagn Microbiol Infect Dis. 2000;38:7-10.
32. Panigrahi AK, Saxena A, Acharya SK, Panda SK. Hepatitis G virus in multitransfused thalassaemics from India. J Gastroenterol Hepatol. 1998;13:902-6.
33. Nishizawa T, Okamoto H, Konishi K, et al. A novel DNA virus (TTV) associated with elevated transaminase levels in posttransfusion hepatitis of unknown etiology. Biochem Biophys Res Commun. 1997;241:92-7.
34. Arankale VA, Gandhe SS, Deshmukh TM, Chadha MS, Walimbe AM. Prevalence and phylogenetic anaysis of TT virus DNA in western India. Clin Diagn Lab Immunol. 2000;7:845-9.
35. Park K. Park's textbook of preventive and social medicine, 17th edn. Jabalpur: M/s Banarsidas Bhanot; 2000. pp. 257-66.
36. Surjit S. Human Immunodeficiency virus infection: personal practice. Indian Pediatr. 2000;37:1328-40.
37. Poiesz BJ, Ruscetti FW, Gadzar AF, Bunn PA, Minna JD, Gallor RC. Detection and isolation of type C retrovirus praticles from fresh and cultured lymphocytes of a patient with cutaneous T-cell lymphoma. Proc Natl Acad Sci, USA. 1980;77:7415-9.
38. Kalyanaraman VS, Sarngadharan MG, Poiesz B, Ruscetti FW, Gao RC. Immunological properties of a type-C retrovirus isolated from cultured human T lymphoma cells and comparison to other mammalian retroviruses. J Virol. 1981;38:906-15.
39. Courouce AM, Pilonel J, Emaire JM, Saura C. HTV testing in blood transfusion. Vox Sang. 1998;74(Suppl 2):165-9.
40. Malhotra V, Lakshmy A. HTLV-1 in HIV seropositive Indian blood donors. J Commun Dis. 1996;28:270-2.
41. Babu PG, Ishida T, Nesadoss J, John TJ. Prevalence of HTLV-I/II antibodies in HIV seropositive and HIV seronegative STD patients in Vellore region in southern India. Scand J Infect Dis. 1995;27:105-8.
42. Roy M, Das MK, Ishida T, Das SK, Dey B, Banerjee S, Majumdar PP. Absence of HTLV-I infection in some Indian populations. Indian J Med Res. 1994;100:160-2.
43. Moison PL, Engelfriet CP, Contreras M. Bood transfusion in clinical medicine, 10th edn. London: Blackwell Science; 1996. pp. 509-57.
44. Venkataraman AR, Seigenurin JM, Lenoir GM, John TJ. Infections due to the human herpes viruses in southern India: a seroepidemiological survey. Int J Epidemiol. 1986; 15:561-6.
45. Choudhury N, Jolly JG, Ganguly NK, Mahajan RC, Dubey ML. Plasmodial antigen detection by monoclonal antibody as a screening procedure for blood donors in transfusion medicine. J Indian Med Assoc. 1991;89:334-6.
46. Satischandra P, Shankar SK Creutzfeldt-Jakob disease in India (1971-1990). Neuroepidemiology. 1991;10:27-32.
47. Jenner PW, Holland PU. Diagnosis and management of transfusion reactions. In: Petz LD, Swisher SN, Kleinman S, Spence RK, Strauss RG (Eds). Clinical Practice of Transfusion Medicine, 3rd edn, New York: Churchill Living Stone; 1996. pp. 905-29.
48. Ray VL, Chaudhary RK, Choudhury N. Transfusion safety in developing countries and the Indian scenario. Dev Biol Stand. 2000;102:195-203.

26 Supportive Care in Children with Cancer

Mohammed Ramzan, Anupam Sachdeva, SP Yadav

Supportive care is an 'umbrella' term for all services, both generalist and specialist, that may be required to support people with cancer and their carers. It includes self-help and support, information, psychological support, symptom control, social support, rehabilitation, spiritual support, palliative care and bereavement care.[1] In the context of cancer, supportive care needs include:

- Physical needs
- Psychological needs
- Social needs
- Information needs
- Spiritual needs.

WHO PROVIDES SUPPORTIVE CARE?

To meet needs across all domains of supportive care in the context of cancer, supportive care needs are provided by generalist and specialist health services as well as community services. All members of the multidisciplinary team have a role in the provision of supportive care. In addition support from family, friends, support groups, volunteers and other community-based organizations make an important contribution to supportive care.

PREVENTION AND MANAGEMENT OF INFECTION IN IMMUNOCOMPROMISED HOSTS[2]

Infectious diseases represent a major cause of morbidity and mortality in immunocompromised patients. Infectious complications are often predictable and may be preventable. Children being treated for cancer are rendered significantly immunocompromised because of chemotherapy.

Factors leading to the susceptibility to infections in cancer patients are given below.

Underlying Disease

Patients with leukemia, advanced-stage lymphoma and uncontrolled tumors are more prone to infections.

Type of Therapy

Dose-intensive therapies, high-dose cytosine arabinoside and stem cell transplantation render patients more susceptible to infections.

Degree and Duration of Neutropenia

The most important determinant of susceptibility to bacterial and fungal infections is the number of circulating neutrophils. Patients who are neutropenic (absolute neutrophil count [ANC] $<500/mm^3$) are more susceptible to infection. Neutropenia can be secondary to disease (leukemia, aplastic anemia) or chemotherapy. Neutrophil function may also be impaired by disease and by chemotherapy.

Disruption of Normal Barriers

The normal mechanical barriers to infection in the skin, respiratory, gastrointestinal and genitourinary systems are disrupted.

Nutritional Status

Malnutrition affects the function of lymphocytes, neutrophils, mononuclear cells and the complement system.

Humoral Immunity

Defects in humoral immunity result in susceptibility to encapsulated bacteria including *Streptococcus pneumoniae, Haemophilus influenzae* type B and *Neisseria meningitides*.

Cell-mediated Immunity

Defects in cellular immunity produce susceptibility to viruses, fungi and intracellularly multiplying bacteria (e.g. *Listeria, Salmonella* and *Mycobacterium tuberculosis*). Patients with Hodgkin disease and non-Hodgkin lymphoma have impaired cell-mediated immunity.

Chemotherapy, radiation and corticosteroids induce defects in lymphocyte function. Lymphopenia may persist after completion of chemotherapy.

Colonizing Microbial Flora

Most bacterial infections arise from endogenous microflora.

Foreign Bodies

Indwelling central vascular catheters, ventriculo-peritoneal shunts.

The net state of immunosuppression is determined by the interaction of several variables including: (i) the underlying disease and the patient's age, (ii) the dose and duration of immunosuppressive therapy, (iii) the state of humoral and cellular host defenses, (iv) the integrity of the skin and mucosal surfaces of the body, (v) metabolic factors such as malnutrition, uremia, hyperglycemia, and hepatic dysfunction, (vi) abnormalities of the reticuloendothelial system, most notably the absence of splenic function, and (vii) the presence or absence of immunomodulating infections such as those caused by HIV, cytomegalovirus, hepatitis viruses, and Epstein-Barr virus. The net state of immunosuppression best determines a patient's risk for infection.

Febrile Neutropenia[3,4]

Fever is defined as a temperature greater than or equal to 38.3°C (101°F) occurring once or a temperature greater than or equal to 38°C (100.4°F) occurring twice during a 24-hour period. Patients with an ANC of less than 500/mm^3 and those with an ANC of less than 1,000/mm^3 and decreasing are considered neutropenic. Because of the high risk of morbidity and mortality in the febrile neutropenic patient, the workup should be thorough and expeditious and empiric broad-spectrum antibiotics should be started as soon as possible.

MANAGEMENT

1. Management includes careful history and physical examination with special attention to important sites of infection in the neutropenic patient:
   - Oral mucosa and periodontium
   - Pharynx
   - Lower esophagus
   - Lungs
   - Skin including sites of vascular access, bone marrow aspiration sites, tissue around the nails
   - Perineum and anus.
2. In the neutropenic patient, signs of inflammation may be remarkably minimal but pain is usually preserved. Accordingly, even subtle signs of inflammation or a complaint of localized pain without physical findings must be considered as a potential source of infection and the site should be evaluated and cultured as appropriate.
3. Obtain a complete blood count, serum chemistries, urinalysis and urine culture.
4. Obtain blood cultures from all lumens of indwelling catheters and from a peripheral vein.
5. Obtain a chest radiograph.
6. Start broad-spectrum antibiotic therapy. Broad-spectrum therapy is required in the neutropenic patient even if a single source or pathogen is isolated, because the occurrence of infection with a second pathogen during continuing neutropenia is not infrequent.
7. These patients should be reassessed daily including an assessment of new symptoms, a meticulous daily physical examination, review of previous culture results, examination of the status of vascular catheters, additional cultures and diagnostic imaging of any organ suspected of having infection.

The prompt initiation of antibiotic therapy in febrile neutropenic patients has reduced the mortality rate for gram-negative infections significantly. Every empiric initial antibiotic regimen should include drugs with antipseudomonal activity. Because gram-positive, gram-negative and mixed infections occur, broad-spectrum coverage must be provided. The choice of antibiotics should be influenced by the predominant organisms and antibiotic susceptibility patterns at the local hospital. Acceptable initial regimens include:

Monotherapy

With cefepime, ceftazidime, imipenem, or meropenem (generally, imipenem or meropenem should not be prescribed routinely as empiric therapy for neutropenic patients in order to minimize the development of antimicrobial resistance to these broad-spectrum agents).

Two-drug Regimen

Ticarcillin/clavulanate, piperacillin/tazobactam, cefepime, or ceftazidime and gentamicin (or tobramycin or amikacin). Many febrile neutropenic patients have no identifiable cause for their fever. A number of risk factors have been identified in febrile neutropenic children that correlate with their risk of serious or life-threatening infection. Risk assessment of patients with fever of unexplained origin helps further define treatment options. Patients may be divided into two groups, low-risk and high-risk, based on the granulocyte count, anticipated duration of neutropenia, degree of fever, remission status and initial physical examination.

Low-risk Patients[5]

The definition of low risk is variable but has included patients with an ANC of 100 neutrophils/mm^3, an anticipated length of neutropenia less than 10 days, a nontoxic appearance, no identifiable source of fever, a normal chest radiograph, no comorbidities and a malignancy in remission status. In these patients, antibiotics may be stopped when the absolute neutrophil count reaches 500/mm^3. For patients with the availability of close ambulatory follow-up, physicians may consider discontinuing antibiotics when the absolute neutrophil count rises for two consecutive days.

High-risk Patients

Patients with neutropenia that is expected to persist for more than 10 days and there is no evidence of bone marrow recovery. If the patient is afebrile but remains granulocytopenic, antibiotics should be continued until absolute neutrophil count reaches 500/mm^3. If the patient is continuously febrile for 5 days, antifungal treatment should be added.

In a select group of low-risk patients oral therapy with amoxicillin/clavulanate plus ciprofloxacin has demonstrated equal efficacy to therapy with IV cephalosporin with or without aminoglycoside coverage. Early discharge of low-risk neutropenic patients with oral antibiotic coverage or with observation alone may be appropriate in a select group of low-risk patients. Amoxicillin/clavulanate may be valuable for the patient in palliative or end-of-life situations. Antibiotic therapy may need to be modified according to the patient's clinical status, focus for infection, or results of cultures and susceptibility testing. Empiric antifungal coverage should be initiated for patients with neutropenia and fever that persists for 3-7 days despite broad-spectrum antibacterial therapy. Institution of empiric antifungal therapy has been found to decrease the risk for mortality significantly.

FEBRILE SPLENECTOMIZED PATIENTS

The spleen acts both as a mechanical filter and as an immune effector organ. Immune functions of the spleen are as follows:

- Production of antibodies to polysaccharide antigens
- Removal of damaged cells and opsonin-coated organisms from the circulation

Splenectomized patients are immunocompromised in the following ways:

- They are deficient in antibody production when challenged with particulate antigens
- They have decreased levels of immunoglobulin M (IgM) and properdin
- They are deficient in the phagocytosis-promoting protein tuftsin. They are at risk for fulminant and rapidly fatal septicemia due to encapsulated bacteria, including *S. pneumoniae, H. influenzae* type B and *N. meningitidis*. Other pathogens which may cause septicemia are *Salmonella* species, *Capnocytophaga canimorsus* and intraerythrocytic parasites such as *Babesia microti* and *Plasmodium falciparum*.

Overwhelming postsplenectomy infection is a serious complication of asplenia. Infection may rapidly progress to bacteremic septic shock, accompanied by hypotension, anuria and disseminated intravascular coagulation.

Management

To decrease the risk of overwhelming postsplenectomy infection, the following measures are recommended:

- *Vaccination:* Two weeks or longer before splenectomy, *Haemophilus influenzae* type B vaccine, the 23-valent pneumococcal polysaccharide vaccine and quadrivalent meningococcal conjugate vaccine should be administered. If pneumococcal conjugate vaccine has not been given as part of early childhood immunization then the age-related appropriate number of doses should be given followed by the 23-valent pneumococeal polysaccharide vaccine. If the splenectomy is elective, administration of indicated vaccines should be completed 2 weeks before surgery to increase the likelihood of eliciting an optimal antibody response. Unimmunized patients who have had splenectomy should be immunized as soon as possible. A second dose of pneumococcal polysaccharide vaccine is recommended 5 years after the initial dose.
- *Antibiotic prophylaxis:* Oral penicillin (125 mg twice daily for children under 3 years; 250 mg twice daily for children 3 years of age and older) should be prescribed at least until the child is 5 years of age for children with functional asplenia due to sickle cell disease. For asplenic children the appropriate duration of prophylaxis has not been established.

For patients 5 years of age or older who have undergone splenectomy due to trauma, discontinuation of prophylaxis can be considered at least 1 year after splenectomy. For children postsplenectomy who have underlying disorders (e.g. thalassemia) prophylaxis should be continued long term and perhaps lifelong. Amoxicillin is an alternative to penicillin.

- If the splenectomized patient becomes febrile:
  - Obtain two blood cultures.
  - Start broad-spectrum IV antibiotic therapy (the currently recommended drug is ceftriaxone 2 g IV every 24 hours for adults or 75 mg/kg IV every 24 hours plus vancomycin until infection with ceftriaxone-resistant pneumococcus is ruled out). Diagnostic evaluation should not delay the initiation of antibiotic therapy.
  - Continue antibiotic therapy until the blood cultures are negative for 72 hours and the patient is afebrile for 24-48 hours.
  - If the patient is febrile and neutropenic, manage as for the febrile neutropenic patient, but include an antibiotic with excellent activity against pneumococci.

BACTERIAL INFECTIONS

Table 26.1 shows the common pathogens and treatment of various infections in children with cancer.[3] Table 26.2 shows the dose, route of administration and schedule of frequently used antibiotics.[4] Both the penicillin/beta-lactamase inhibitor drugs, ticarcillin/clavulanate and piperacillin/tazobactam and the carbapenems, imipenem and meropenem, provide broad-spectrum activity for gram-positive pathogens, gram-negative pathogens and anaerobic bacteria and are good choices for empiric therapy of patients with suspected intra-abdominal sepsis, with or without administration of an aminoglycoside. However, neither imipenem nor meropenem should be prescribed routinely in order to minimize the development of antimicrobial resistant to these very broad-spectrum agents. Vancomycin is not recommended routinely for empiric therapy because its use promotes the emergence of resistant strains such as vancomycin-resistant enterococci. Vancomycin should only be added to the initial regimen if any of the following is present:

- Suspected central venous catheter-related infection
- Patients with acute myeloblastic leukemia because of the increased risk of infection with alpha hemolytic *Streptococcus* such as *Streptococcus mitis*
- Prior history of alpha hemolytic *Streptococcus* bacteremia
- Patients colonized with resistant organisms that are treatable only with vancomycin
- Patients with a recent history of bacteremia or venous catheter-related infection requiring treatment with vancomycin
- Intensive chemotherapy causing mucositis (such as high-dose cytosine arabinoside)
- Hypotension
- Patients who have developed fever despite quinolone prophylaxis.

If vancomycin is prescribed and cultures do not grow a pathogen requiring vancomycin, it should be discontinued within 48-72 hours.

Table 26.1: Predominant pathogens in cancer patients

Gram-positive bacteria
- Staphylococci (coagulase-negative, *Staphylococcus aureus* including methicillin-resistant *S. aureus*)
- Streptococci (α-hemolytic) especially *Streptococcus mitis*
- Enterococci
- Corynebacteria
- *Listeria* sp.

Gram-negative bacteria
- Enterobacteriaceae (*Escherichia coli, Klebsiella, Enterobacter, Serratia*)
- *Pseudomonas aeruginosa, Stenotrophomonas maltophilia* (and other oxidase-positive multiresistant Gram-negative bacteria)

Anaerobic bacteria
- *Clostridium difficile*
- *Bacteroides* sp.
- *Propionibacterium acnes*

Fungi
- *Candida* sp.
- *Aspergillus* sp.
- *Zygomycetes*
- *Cryptococci*
- *Pneumocystis jiroveci* (formerly *P. carinii*)

Other
- *Toxoplasma gondii*
- *Strongyloides stercoralis*
- *Cryptosporidium*

Viruses
- Herpes simplex virus
- Varicella-zoster virus
- Cytomegalovirus
- Epstein-Barr virus
- Respiratory syncytial virus
- Adenovirus
- Influenza virus
- Parainfluenza virus
- Papovaviruses BK and JC

Table 26.2: Frequently used antibiotics in oncology and stem cell transplantation patients

Drug	Dose	Route	Schedule
Aminoglycosides			
Amikacin	22 mg/kg/day	IV	Divided q8h
Gentamicin	6.0-7.5 mg/kg/day	IV	Divided q8h
Tobramycin	6.0-7.5 gm/kg/day	IV	Divided q8h
Penicillin-related drugs			
Nafcillin	100-200 mg/kg/day	IV	Divided q4–8h
Piperacillin/tazobactam	300 mg/kg/day of piperacillin component	IV	Divided q6h
Ticarcillin/clavulanate	300 mg/kg/day (maximum 24 g/day)	IV	Divided q4–6h
Cephalosporins			
Ceftazidime	100-150 mg/kg/day	IV	Divided q8h
Cefazolin	50-100 mg/kg/day (maximum 6 g/day)	IV	Divided q8h
Cefepime	150 mg/kg/day (maximum 2 g)	IV	Divided q8h
Carbapenems	50 mg/kg/day (maximum 4 g/day)	IV	Divided q6–8h
Imipenem/cilastatin			
Meropenem	60-120 mg/kg/day (maximum dose 6 g/day)	IV	Divided q8h
Other			
Vancomycin	45 mg/kg/day (maximum 2 g/day)	IV	PO Divided q6–8h
Linezolid	30 mg/kg/day (<2 years of age)	IV	PO Divided q8h
	20 mg/kg/day (>2 years of age maximum dose 1.2 g/day)	IV	PO Divided q12h
Anaerobic drugs			
Clindamycin	40 mg/kg/day	IV	Divided q6–8h
Metronidazole	30 mg/kg/day (loading dose initially 15 mg/kg)	IV	Divided q6h

FUNGAL INFECTIONS[2,6]

The risk of fungal infections is related to the cytotoxicity of the chemotherapeutic regimen as well as the duration of neutropenia. The major causative fungi are *Aspergillus* and *Candida* with a mortality approaching 30-60% with documented invasive fungal infections (IFIs) and is even higher among posthematopoietic stem cell transplantation patients. Prompt diagnosis and treatment is paramount to improving outcomes in these patients. Difficulty in diagnosing fungal infections is caused by the frequent absence of localizing signs and symptoms and high likelihood of negative blood cultures. Notwithstanding these limitations, empiric antifungal coverage must be initiated for patients with neutropenia and fever that persists for 3-7 days despite broad-spectrum antibacterial therapy. Institution of empiric antifungal therapy has been found to decrease the risk for mortality significantly. In certain situations, e.g. stem cell transplantation recipients, antifungal prophylaxis results in a significant reduction in the risk for fungal-related death and documented IFIs and a larger relative risk reduction when used in conjunction with antibacterial prophylaxis in contrast to antibacterial prophylaxis alone. Currently available antifungal therapy belongs to three classes of agents: polyenes, azoles and echinocandins.

Polyenes

- Amphotericin B deoxycholate
- Liposomal amphotericin B (Ambisomes)
- Amphotericin B lipid complex (Abelcets)

Polyenes are fungicidal by increasing fungal cell membrane permeability. Traditionally, amphotericin B deoxycholate has been the standard drug for antifungal therapy since it offers broad-spectrum coverage and is inexpensive. However, adverse reactions such as nephrotoxicity and hypokalemia and infusion-related reactions such as fever and chills limit its use. Lipid preparations of amphotericin, e.g. liposomal amphotericin, are now more frequently prescribed because they are less nephrotoxic and some result in fewer infusion-related adverse effects.

Azoles

Fluconazole, itraconazole, voriconazole and posaconazole

- Fluconazole is a first-line drug for *Candida* infections but lacks activity against *Aspergillus*.

- Voriconazole is the drug of choice for *Aspergillus* infections because it has been shown to be more effective than amphotericin B for *Aspergillus* pulmonary infections. Voriconazole is available in intravenous and oral formulations and has excellent oral bioavailability. Oral voriconazole is an effective and relatively inexpensive agent for empiric antifungal therapy in patients with persisting fever and neutropenia despite broad-spectrum antibacterial therapy. In addition, voriconazole may also play a role in treating central nervous system disease.

  Posaconazole is a broad-spectrum azole effective against many yeasts and fungi including *Histoplasma* and *Zygomycetes*. It is available only for enteral administration. Food substantially enhances the bioavailability of posaconazole and the rate and extent of absorption, thereby limiting its utility in cases where oral intake is not feasible.

Echinocandins

Caspofungin and micafungin. Echinocandins inhibit beta-1,3-D-glucan synthetase in the fungal cell wall. They are fungicidal for yeasts and fungistatic for molds such as *Aspergillus*. They are generally well-tolerated and are not nephrotoxic.

Caspofungin has been found to be equally efficacious as amphotericin B against systemic *Candida* infection and demonstrates activity against *Aspergillus*. Hepatotoxicity with concomitant use of cyclosporin has been reported, which may limit its use in some HSCT patients.[7]

Micafungin has a similar spectrum of activity to micafungin but experience in the pediatric age group is limited and it is not currently FDA-approved for use in children.

Antifungal Agents for Empiric Therapy of Patients with Prolonged Fever and Neutropenia[8]

First-line antifungal agents include:
- Liposomal amphotericin (Ambisomes)
- Voriconazole
- Caspofungin
- Amphotericin B deoxycholate.

Second-line agents include:
- Fluconazole
- Posaconazole
- Itraconazole
- Micafungin (micafungin may be considered a first-line agent when FDA-approved for children).

Antifungal Prophylaxis in Hematopoietic Stem Cell Transplantation Patients

1. Autologous HSCT
   a. Micafungin/caspofungin
   b. Fluconazole
2. Allogeneic HSCT
   a. Micafungin/caspofungin
   b. Liposomal amphotericin
   c. Voriconazole
   d. Fluconazole
3. Postengraftment, GVHD, AML, MDS
   a. Posaconazole if eating well and tolerating oral fluids
   b. Voriconazole
   c. Fluconazole if no longer neutropenic and liver function tests are normal.

Antifungal Prophylaxis of *Candida* Infection

1. Nystatin oral swish and swallow; 2 ml twice daily in infants, 5 ml twice daily in children and adults.
2. Clotrimazole troche one bid.
3. Fluconazole 2 mg/kg/day; maximum 200 mg.

Practical Use of Current Anticandida Agents

For patients with serious *Candida* infections, caspofungin or one of the amphotericin B formulations is most appropriate, providing proven efficacy against practically all *Candida* species. Safety considerations give an edge to caspofungin over amphotericin B, including the lipid formulations. Once the infection is stabilized, then fluconazole can be substituted for continued therapy, provided the *Candida* species is a fluconazole susceptible species. For less serious *Candida* infections due to fluconazole-susceptible species, fluconazole is appropriate, especially in nonneutropenic patients.

Practical Use of Current Antiaspergillus Agents

Voriconazole is currently the drug of choice for first-line therapy. For allergic, intolerant, or nonresponsive patients, one of the lipid formulations of amphotericin B is an excellent alternative. Caspofungin is yet another option for salvage therapy.

Combination Therapy

Few controlled trials of combination therapy have been performed, despite this approach being evaluated in numerous *in vitro* and animal model studies. Combination antifungal therapy (amphotericin B plus flucytosine) is well established for cryptococcal meningitis. In a recent trial, the combination of fluconazole and amphotericin B was compared to fluconazole in high doses (800 mg/ day) as therapy for candidemia[9] overall, the response rate was higher and time to bloodstream clearance was shorter in the group receiving the combination. This advantage was offset by greater nephrotoxicity in the combination arm. Despite considerable interest in this concept, there are no controlled trials for aspergillosis. Although several case series[10] suggest benefit, the majority of *Aspergillus* cases in which combination therapy was evaluated were only "possible" infections. There are pitfalls with the use of combination therapy including potential antagonism, greater toxicity, and cost.[11] Thus, controlled trials are clearly needed.

Adjunctive Measures

For catheter-related candidemia, removal of a central venous catheter, if possible, should be strongly considered.[9] More rapid clearance of fungemia with catheter removal has been seen in several studies. For *Aspergillus* infections, consideration should be given for surgical excision of infarcted tissue, especially if the patient faces additional antineoplastic therapy. The role of cytokines such as myeloid growth factors and interferon gamma are supported by preclinical data, but there is a paucity of clinical trial data. Similarly, the use of granulocyte transfusions for neutropenic patients not responding to antimicrobial therapy is intuitively sensible, but this strategy is not without complications, is difficult to implement, and lacks convincing clinical data.

Duration of Therapy

The duration of therapy has not been defined in clinical trials but generally lasts for several weeks to months. In general, treatment of *Candida* infections should continue for at least 2 weeks beyond the time when cultures become negative, signs and symptoms of infection have improved, and preferably host defenses have improved.[9] For *Aspergillus* infections, treatment should continue until resolution of symptoms and signs, clearance of cultures at previously culture-positive sites, improvement and stabilization of radiological findings, and improvement of underlying host defenses and control of the hematologic malignancy. In the largest trial[12] to date, the planned course of therapy was 12 weeks.

Prophylaxis

Fluconazole, itraconazole, and low doses of amphotericin B have been shown in randomized trials to be effective as prophylaxis. In general, from meta-analyses of randomized trial data, the benefit appears to be meaningful when the risk of IFI is at least 15% in the patient group treated.[13] Most of the antifungal benefit seen in clinical trials has been in the prevention of *Candida* infection. Trials of itraconazole during neutropenia have been mostly conducted in patient groups at low risk for aspergillosis, and thus no clear benefit against aspergillosis has been shown. A recent meta-analysis[14] showed that itraconazole given in oral solution at adequate doses (at least 400 mg/ day) was associated with fewer *Aspergillus* infections. High rates of recurrence of IFI occur if the once infected patient is subjected to subsequent antineoplastic treatment cycles or undergoes hematopoietic stem cell transplantation, and thus "secondary" prophylaxis or chronic maintenance is necessary until the underlying disease is controlled and the full treatment course is completed. Several published case series indicate that hematopoietic stem cell transplantation can be successfully performed in patients given secondary prophylaxis.[15] After completion of therapy the patient should be observed to monitor for possible exacerbation.

Empirical Therapy for Neutropenic Patients with Persistent Fever[16]

Early trials demonstrated that rates of IFIs were 15-30% in neutropenic patients with fever persisting 4-7 days despite antibiotics; fungal morbidity could be reduced by empirical amphotericin B. Subsequent trials with lipid formulations of amphotericin B, itraconazole, voriconazole and caspofungin have been performed. In each study, the test agent was compared with either amphotericin B or liposomal amphotericin B. Since all patients had an active agent, the rates of IFIs in both groups were anticipated to be small and thus a surrogate endpoint of "success" was used as the primary endpoint. Success was judged by defervescence, resolution of an IFI if found at baseline, absence of breakthrough IFI, survival to neutrophil recovery, and no toxicity that necessitated withdrawal of study drug. None of these agents were found to be superior to amphotericin B in the primary endpoint.

Pneumocystis Jiroveci (Formerly *P. carinii*)

Pneumocystis jiroveci has been reclassified as a fungus and for this reason it has been included in the section of this chapter dealing with fungal infections. It is a ubiquitous organism that causes severe or fatal pneumonitis in immunocompromised patients.

Clinical Features

1. Rapid onset of symptoms with fever and tachypnea.
2. Progressive respiratory distress with nasal flaring and intercostal retractions.
3. Absence of rales on physical examination.
4. Hypoxemia on arterial blood gas.
5. Development of bilateral pneumonitis on chest radiograph.
6. Rapid progression of respiratory distress/respiratory failure over a few days; usually fatal if untreated.

Diagnosis

1. Typical clinical syndrome.
2. Demonstration of the organism in sputum or material from endobronchial washing or percutaneous needle biopsy or open lung biopsy.
3. Identification of organism by Gomori methenamine silver stain.

Treatment

1. Start treatment as soon as the patient develops tachypnea and hypoxemia, even if there is no laboratory confirmation of the organism.
2. Trimethoprim/sulfamethoxazole (TMP/SMX) 20 mg/kg/day of TMP component IV divided into four doses is the treatment of choice. Treatment should continue for 21 days. TMP/SMX causes myelosuppression.
3. If TMP/SMX is not tolerated, treat with pentamidine 4 mg/kg/day IV; TMP 5 mg/kg PO every 6 hours and dapsone 100 mg/ day PO for 21 days is another alternative.
4. Monitor carefully for hypotension. Pentamidine is recommended if patients fail to respond to TMP/ SMX in 72 hours or if they develop pneumocystis in spite of TMP/ SMX prophylaxis.
5. Concomitant administration of corticosteroids, e.g. 1 mg/kg methylprednisolone or prednisone given 2-4 times per day for 5–7 days followed by a taper over the next 1–2 weeks, is indicated for patients with moderate or severe infection proven to be caused by PCP.

Prophylaxis

1. TMP/SMX 5 mg/kg/day (150 mg/m^2/day), maximum dose 320 mg/day (based on TMP) divided into two daily doses for three consecutive days per week. TMP/SMX may cause rash, neutropenia and GI symptoms.
2. Alternative drugs for *Pneumocystis* PCP prophylaxis for use in patients 1-2 months old, allergic to TMP/ SMX, with G6PD deficiency, or excessive myelosuppression with TMP/SMX are dapsone, pentamidine, or atovaquone.
3. Dapsone 2 mg/kg/day PO once daily, maximum dose 100 mg/day; may be preferred agent in children under the age of 2 months who may have liver immaturity and be at risk for methemoglobinemia if TMP/ SMX treatment is used.
4. *Pentamidine aerosolized formulation for children old enough to cooperate:* Infant dose: 2.27 mg/ kg nebulizer output (L/minute) wt (kg) divided by alveolar ventilation (L/minute); Children <5 years: a dose of 8 mg/kg is recommended, children >5 years: 300 mg/dose.
5. *Pentamidine intravenous:* For children unable to cooperate with inhaled formulation, may receive 4 mg/kg administered intravenously every 4 weeks.
6. Atovaquone 30 mg/kg/day once daily in children 1-3 months and those older than 2 years of age. The recommended dose is 45 mg/kg/day for children between 3 and 24 months of age. Atovaquone is used for pentamidine breakthrough or intolerance to other agents.

VIRAL INFECTIONS[2,6]

Children on chemotherapy can tolerate many common viral infections, but defects in cellular immunity predispose them to unusually severe infections with certain viruses, particularly of the herpes virus group. The community-acquired respiratory viruses (CRVs) are well known for their ability to cause misery during the winter cold and flu season. SP such as the influenza viruses, parainfluenza viruses, and respiratory syncytial virus (RSV), however, may be fatal for patients with hematologic malignancies, particularly those who are recipients of allogeneic hematopoietic cell transplantation (HCT). Though most clinicians believe that mortality after incident CRV infection is chiefly mediated via viral pneumonitis and acute pulmonary failure, accumulating data suggest that even upper respiratory tract infections (URIs) with some of these viruses may be associated with increased long-term mortality after HCT. Moreover, the application of PCR-based diagnostics now allows a wider variety of potential pathogens to be identified, including those that are difficult to cultivate (e.g. human rhinoviruses and coronaviruses) and/or newly discovered (e.g. human metapneumovirus [hMPV]). Thus, it is likely that the full spectrum of disease associated with these potent pathogens remains to be elucidated. Primary varicella infection, in particular, can produce serious morbidity, including encephalitis and pneumonitis and mortality in 7% of patients. In stem cell transplantation recipients the herpes virus cytomegalovirus (CMV) is an important cause of interstitial pneumonitis, bone marrow aplasia and other infections. Infection with an influenza virus can cause significant morbidity in children on chemotherapy. Stem cell transplant recipients can develop life-threatening pneumonitis due to RSV, parainfluenza and rhinoviruses. Adenoviruses and papovaviruses BC are important causes of hemorrhagic cystitis.

Antiviral drugs are indicated only if there is clinical or laboratory evidence of viral infection or for prophylaxis of herpes simplex infection or for prophylaxis or pre-emptive therapy of cytomegalovirus infection in stem cell transplant recipients.

Antiviral Prophylaxis

Acyclovir prophylaxis 750-1,500 mg/m^2/day IV divided every 8 hours or 600–1,000 mg/day PO divided every 8 hours during the risk period. It is prescribed to prevent reactivations of HSV infection in seropositive stem cell transplant or high-dose chemotherapy patients.

RSV

Uncontrolled cohort studies[17] performed at the Fred Hutchinson Cancer Research Center suggest that aerosolized ribavirin given alone (2 g over 2 hours 3 times daily or 6 g continuously over 16-18 hours) improves the survival of HCT recipients with RSV pneumonia from 0% (without therapy) to 60-70%. Others have attempted to improve upon these outcomes by adding pooled immunoglobulins, high-titered RSV-IG, or RSV specific monoclonals (palivizumab). The latter two approaches may improve survival to 80-90% (particularly if applied prior to the requirement for mechanical ventilation)[18,19] Given the reasonably high rate of progression from RSV URI to pneumonia (~40%), some have advocated the use of aerosolized ribavirin to prevent pneumonia from developing. A multicenter randomized trial designed to determine whether this practice is effective was also recently closed after slow accrual. Due to the expense and inconvenience of this practice, we currently apply pre-emptive ribavirin to those with extremely high risks (i.e. among those with profound lymphopenia). The orally active fusion inhibitors are currently under-development.

Influenza

Active and easily administered agents are available for the treatment of patients with influenza. Currently preferred are the neuraminidase inhibitors (oral oseltamivir and inhaled zanamavir) given activity against both influenza A and B; M2 inhibitors (oral amantadine and rimantadine) are only active versus influenza A and also are associated with emergent antiviral resistance on therapy.[20] Small, uncontrolled studies suggest that pre-emptive therapy with any of these agents may prevent progression to lower tract disease.[21]

Parainfluenza

Unfortunately, effective therapy for PIV pneumonia has yet to be identified. Therapy with aerosolized ribavirin with or without pooled IVIG appeared unsuccessful in the largest series of HCT recipients with pneumonia performed to date. Since progression to pneumonia appears highly correlated with dose of corticosteroids given to treat GVHD, efforts to decrease the level of immunosuppression at the time of incident CRV infection are warranted. Whether the earlier application of aerosolized ribavirin (i.e. for URI) would improve outcomes is speculative.

Human Metapneumovirus

No human or animal studies are available to inform the treatment of patients with hMPV infection. Both polyclonal IVIG and ribavirin appear to be active *in vitro*, and combination therapy with these agents could thus be envisaged for the patient with hMPV pneumonitis. Monoclonal antibody preparations (such as palivizumab for RSV) are underdevelopment.

Prevention

Stringent infection control practices are critical for decreasing the morbidity and mortality associated with incident CRV infection in the at-risk host. Focus should first be directed toward the prevention of nosocomial infections during the period of highest risk (i.e. during the periods of profound lymphopenia that follow conditioning or induction chemotherapy, when progression to pneumonia appears most likely). Incident infections still may occur later after patients have returned to the community, but these are associated with lower direct mortality. Since large droplets are the most important means of viral transmission, frequent hand washing (or use of alcohol-based hand sanitizers) cannot be overemphasized; targets for this teaching include healthcare workers, close patient contacts, and the patients themselves. Recommendations for screening and isolation of patients with CRV infections have been summarized by the Centers for Disease Control and Prevention (CDC) and the American Society for Blood and Marrow Transplantation (ASBMT).[22] Hematopoietic cell transplantation (HCT) recipients and those at high risk for CRV-related complications should refrain from contact with individuals with symptomatic CRV infections; symptomatic healthcare workers or visitors should thus be restricted from access to wards where these patients are housed. Whether masks for patients or asymptomatic healthcare workers (prior to patient contact) add value to hand hygiene and the restrictions above is debatable. Inactivated influenza vaccine is an effective means to prevent this important CRV infection and should be offered yearly to nearly all patients with hematologic malignancies (patients in their first year after transplant are the possible exception due to poor antibody responses). Healthcare workers and close patient contacts should also receive the inactivated vaccine to reduce transmission to patients. Live attenuated influenza vaccine cannot currently be recommended for patients or their close contacts (including healthcare workers) due to concerns of vaccine strain transmission and resulting clinical illness in these immunocompromised hosts.

PROTOZOAN INFECTIONS

Toxoplasma gondii is the one protozoan infection that occurs relatively frequently. HIV infected and other immunocompromised patients may develop reactivation of latent infection that most frequently presents as a focal encephalitis. The first-line therapy is pyrimethamine (with folinic acid) and sulfadiazine. Clindamycin can be substituted for sulfadiazine in patients intolerant of sulfadiazine. Prophylaxis for PCP with trimethoprim and sulfamethoxazole is effective for prevention of toxoplasmosis.

G-CSF AND GRANULOCYTE INFUSIONS

Therapy with G-CSF at a dose of 5 µg/kg/day subcutaneously is recommended under certain conditions in which worsening of the clinical course is predicted and there is an expected long delay in the recovery of the marrow. It should also be considered for patients who remain severely neutropenic and have documented infections that do not respond to appropriate antibiotic treatment. There are no specific indications for standard use of granulocyte transfusions. Granulocyte transfusions may be useful in patients with profound neutropenia, in whom the infection progresses despite optimal antibiotic treatment and G-CSF and in cases of severe uncontrollable fungal infection. When granulocyte transfusions are given concomitantly with amphotericin B preparations, respiratory insufficiency may occur as a side effect. Most neutropenic patients are treated with G-CSF to shorten the period of neutropenia. Occasionally however patients are treated with granulocyte transfusions. Granulocyte transfusions are becoming more readily available.

Indications

1. Serious bacterial (particularly gram-negative) or fungal infection with persistent (48 hours or more) positive cultures despite appropriate antibiotic coverage in severely neutropenic patients (ANC 200/mm^3).
2. The ANC is not expected to increase to more than 500/mm^3 for 5-7 days.
3. Prolonged survival of the patient is reasonably expected if the infection is controlled.
4. In addition, patients with severe granulocyte dysfunction (e.g. chronic granulomatous disease) who have severe infection.
5. There is no role for prophylactic administration of granulocytes.

Risks

1. CMV infection.
2. Graft versus host disease.
3. Respiratory distress with pulmonary infiltrates (particularly in patients concurrently receiving amphotericin).
4. Alloimmunization and platelet refractoriness.
5. Hemolytic reactions.

Precautions

1. Use granulocytes from an ABO-Rh compatible donor.
2. Use CMV-seronegative donor, if available, for CMV seronegative recipients.
3. If the patient is on amphotericin, wait 4-6 hours between amphotericin and granulocyte transfusion.
4. Do not administer with a leukocyte-depleting filter.
5. Administer granulocytes as soon as possible after collection to maximize effectiveness. If not used immediately, store at room temperature.

6. Premedicate with diphenhydramine and hydrocortisone.
7. Granulocytes must always be irradiated with 2,500 cGy to prevent transfusion associated GVHD.

Dose and Duration

1. The dose of granulocytes should be as close to $0.75–1.0 \times 10^{10}$ as possible.
2. The transfusion is administered through a 170-µm filter at a rate of 150 ml/m^2/hour.
3. Granulocytes are usually administered for 5–7 days or until the ANC has risen to more than 500/mm^3.

HEMATOPOIETIC GROWTH FACTORS: BASIC BIOLOGY OF GROWTH FACTORS[23]

Hematopoietic cells are derived from self-renewing, pluripotent stem cells. Pluripotent stem cells are able to differentiate into committed progenitor cells. The most primitive form of committed progenitor is termed a colony-forming unit granulocyte, erythrocyte, macrophage and megakaryocyte (CFU-GEMM). This cell is capable of producing colonies containing neutrophils, macrophages, erythrocytes, megakaryocytes, eosinophils and basophils. The CFU-GEMMs appear to have a limited capacity for self-renewal and therefore, are not true "stem cells." The committed hematopoietic progenitors (erythroid burst-forming unit [BFU-E], erythroid colony-forming unit [CFU-E], granulocyte macrophage colony-forming unit [CFU-GM], granulocyte colony-forming unit [CFU-G], macrophage colony-forming unit [CFU-M], eosinophil colony-forming unit [CFU-Eo], basophil colony-forming unit [CFU-Ba] and megakaryocyte colony-forming unit [CFU-Meg]) are capable of giving rise to colonies containing cells of only one or two types. The hematopoietic growth factors and interleukins are cytokines that regulate the growth, differentiation and functional activities of progenitor cells in peripheral blood, bone marrow and placental-cord blood. A second important action of many of these factors is augmentation of the function of mature cells. Some growth factors are specific for one type of progenitor, whereas others affect many types of progenitors.

Uses of Hematopoietic Growth Factors

1. Enhances hematopoietic recovery, lowers hospital cost, permits increased cytotoxic drug dose.
2. Early hematopoietic recovery reduces non-hematologic toxicity (e.g. infection, mucositis, pneumonia).
3. Mobilizes peripheral-blood progenitor cells.
4. Augments transplantation using smaller number of hematopoietic cells.
5. Expands hematopoietic cells.

Clinical Use of G-CSF, GM-CSF, Erythropoietin and IL-11: Recombinant Human G-CSF

Indications for Use

1. Prophylactic use in patients in whom the expected incidence of neutropenia following chemotherapy is greater than or equal to 40%. It accelerates myeloid recovery when the expected duration of severe neutropenia is seven or more days.
2. After a prior episode of febrile neutropenia.
3. After high-dose chemotherapy with autologous progenitor stem cell support to accelerate myeloid recovery.
4. Mobilization of peripheral blood progenitor cells for harvesting prior to autologous stem cell transplant.
5. To increase granulocyte count in patients with aplastic anemia, myelodysplastic syndromes, congenital neutropenia and other congenital neutropenic disorders.

Contraindication

Hypersensitivity to G-CSF or to *E. coli*-derived proteins.

Dose and Duration

1. Start with a dose of 5 µg/kg/day SC or IV. When given intravenously, it is diluted with albumin and given over 15-30 minutes. The dose is 10 µg/kg/ day SC or IV for peripheral blood stem cell mobilization in preparation for autologous transplant. A Pegylated form of G-CSF (pegfilgrastim) is used at a dose of 6 mg SC once per chemotherapy cycle in patients over 45 kg. There is no experience with pegfilgrastim in pediatrics.
2. Continue until the ANC is greater than 10,000/mm^3.
3. Start G-CSF 24 hours after the last dose of chemotherapy.
4. Do not resume chemotherapy until 24-48 hours after discontinuing G-CSF.

Adverse Effects

1. *Common:* Bone pain, elevation of uric acid, lactate dehydrogenase and alkaline phosphatase.
2. *Uncommon:* Fever, nausea, vomiting, rash, diarrhea, splenomegaly, erythema at injection site, hypotension, exacerbation of psoriasis, allergic

reaction, acute respiratory distress syndrome, splenic rupture.

Recombinant Human GM-CSF

Indications

1. To accelerate myeloid recovery following stem cell transplantation.
2. To accelerate myeloid recovery in a neutropenic patient with fungal infection, because it also accelerates macrophage recovery.

Contraindications

1. Excessive myeloid blasts in bone marrow or peripheral blood (10%).
2. Juvenile chronic myeloid leukemia or monosomy 7 syndrome.
3. Hypersensitivity to GM-CSF or yeast-derived proteins.

Dose and Duration

1. The starting dose is 250 μg/ m^2/day SC or IV over 2 hours.
2. When given to prevent engraftment delay, the first dose should be given 2-4 hours after stem cell transplantation and continued for 21 days or until the ANC is greater than 10,000 cells/ mm^3.
3. Do not give within 24 hours of last chemotherapy or 12 hours of last radiation dose.

Adverse Effects

1. *Common:* Bone pain, reaction at injection site.
2. *Uncommon:* Fluid retention (peripheral edema, pleural effusion, pericardial effusion), leukocytosis, diarrhea, rash, malaise, fever, asthenia, headache, chills, arthralgias, chest pain, dyspnea, thrombocytopenia, thrombophlebitis, thrombosis, eosinophilia, weight gain, respiratory distress syndrome, bundle branch block, supraventricular arrhythmias. The first dose of GM-CSF may be followed within hours by a characteristic reaction involving skin flushing, tachycardia, hypotension, musculoskeletal pain, dyspnea, nausea and vomiting and arterial oxygen desaturation.

Use of G-CSF or GM-CSF and Risk of Leukemia

1. Numerous clinical studies have not shown detectable adverse effects of G-CSF on stimulation of myeloid leukemic cell growth.
2. In aplastic anemia, the risk of myelodysplastic syndrome (MDS) or leukemia is increased in children treated with immunosuppressive therapy and G-CSF.
3. Seven percent of patients with severe chronic neutropenia treated for more than 8 years with G-CSF develop AML or MDS. Patients with cyclic neutropenia treated with G-CSF have not developed a secondary malignancy.

Recombinant Human Erythropoietin[24]

When planning to use recombinant human erythropoietin (rHuEPO), the following points must be considered:

1. If the degree of anemia is disproportionate to the degree of thrombocytopenia and neutropenia, this may be due to other causes of low hemoglobin such as hemorrhage, iron deficiency, or hemolysis and these will not be resolved by rHuEPO.
2. Not all patients respond to rHuEPO because of "end-organ" problems, such as myelodysplastic syndrome and some anemias of chronic illness.
3. Patients on cisplatin-containing regimens who suffer renal damage may respond well to rHuEPO.

Indications

Thrombotic events have been associated with the use of the various forms of recombinant erythropoietin. In addition, especially in adults, there are data showing a shortening of progression to relapse in patients with various cancers including lymphoma. Any decision to use these drugs should take these factors into account. There are no proven indications for the use of recombinant human erythropoietin in pediatric oncology and concerns exist about appropriate dosing schedule, cost and risk of thrombovascular events. Possible indications in pediatrics include:

- Anemia secondary to renal failure
- Anemia of chronic illness, such as human immunodeficiency virus and juvenile rheumatic arthritis.
- Anemia secondary to chemotherapy (to decrease the need for blood transfusions, particularly in children with solid tumors)
- Anemia associated with radiation therapy
- Anemia after allogeneic stem cell transplantation
- Anemia secondary to myelodysplastic syndromes when the serum erythropoietin is low.

Contraindications

1. Anemia secondary to nutritional deficiencies, hemorrhage, or hemolysis.

2. Uncontrollable hypertension.
3. Hypersensitivity to mammalian-cell-derived products or to human albumin.

Dose and Dose Modification Schedule

1. Obtain baseline serum erythropoietin and ferritin levels prior to starting therapy.
2. If ferritin is low, prescribe ferrous sulfate 6 mg elemental iron/kg/day divided into three daily doses.
3. Start rHuEPO at a dose of 50-100 units/kg/day subcutaneously (SC) three times a week. Darbepoetin alpha is an analog of erythropoietin with a longer plasma half-life and can be used once every 2-4 weeks. The starting dose is 2.25 µg/kg/dose.
4. If there is no response within 2–4 weeks, increase dose up to 300 Units/kg/day three times a week or the darbepoetin dose to 4.5 µg/kg/week.
5. If the hemoglobin reaches 13 g/dl, discontinue rHuEPO until the hemoglobin is 12 g/dl; then resume at 25% dose.
6. If the hemoglobin increases very rapidly (1 g/dl in 2 weeks) or hemoglobin reaches 12 g/dl, reduce the dose by 25%.
7. Give rHuEPO concurrently with chemotherapy.
8. Continue rHuEPO until the patient no longer requires red cell support.

Early initiation (prior to the need for transfusions), a low observed or predicted erythropoietin level (0.825) and evidence of early response (more than 1 g/dl rise in hemoglobin within the first 4 weeks) are all associated with increased likelihood of response. Patients meeting all three of these criteria show an 85% chance of significant response (more than 2 g/dl rise in hemoglobin). Almost all of these patients have renal-failure-associated anemia and were treated with subcutaneous erythropoietin.

Adverse Reactions

1. *Common:* Hypertension, pain at the injection site, headache, fever, diarrhea.
2. *Uncommon:* Nausea, malaise, seizures, thrombosis. There are reports of pure red cell aplasia due to neutralizing antibodies during erythropoietin treatment.

Interleukin-11[25]

Interleukin-11 (IL-11) acts synergistically with IL-3 and thrombopoietin (TPO) to stimulate various stages of megakaryocytopoiesis and thrombopoiesis. Interleukin-11 (IL-11) has been evaluated in several human clinical trials and is currently approved for the prevention of severe chemotherapy-induced thrombocytopenia in patients with non-myeloid malignancies. Low dose IL-11 has also been shown to be effective in patients with bone marrow failure.

Indications

Prevention of severe thrombocytopenia after myelosuppressive chemotherapy.

Contraindications

1. Hypersensitivity.
2. Children younger than 12 years of age.
3. Myeloid malignancies.
4. In patients with heart failure, atrial arrhythmias, thromboembolic disorders, major organ dysfunction, papilledema, or CNS tumors, IL-11 should be used with caution.

Dose and Dose Modification Schedule

The dose is 50 µg/kg/day in adults. A dose of 50-75 µg a day has been suggested for children. Interleukin-11 (IL-11) has not been commonly employed because of the side effects, especially capillary leak. No large pediatric trials are available.

Adverse Reactions

1. *Common:* Edema, tachycardia, headache, fatigue, dizziness, anorexia, nausea, conjunctivitis and papilledema in children, dyspnea, skin rashes, arthralgia, myalgia.
2. *Uncommon:* Atrial arrhythmia, thrombosis, cerebral infarction, syncope.

Thrombopoietin[26]

Thrombopoietin is a hematopoietic factor that controls platelet production and levels of thrombopoietin rise 24 hours after the onset of thrombocytopenia. Studies using recombinant thrombopoetin have led to the development of antithrombopoietin antibodies in normal subjects which raises the issue of safety of its use in treating chemotherapy-related thrombocytopenia.

Interest has been increasing for the thrombopoietin mimetic agents or thrombopoietin receptor agonists that have proven their value in clinical trials of ITP. Trials are underway to assess their usefulness in the prevention of thrombocytopenia as well as in reversal of thrombocytopenia in myelodysplastic syndromes and bone marrow failure states.

PREVENTION OF ORGAN TOXICITY[27]

Prevention of Cardiac Toxicity

A baseline EKG, echocardiogram and/or multigated acquisition scan (MUGA) scan should be obtained before anthracycline treatment or thoracic radiotherapy. Cardiac toxicity is seen in patients receiving chemotherapy with anthracyclines (doxorubicin, daunorubicin, idarubicin) as well as thoracic radiotherapy. Toxicity is anticipated in patients receiving a cumulative dose exceeding 450 mg/ m^2 for doxorubicin and daunorubicin and exceeding 125 mg/ m^2 for idarubicin. Toxicity may also occur in patients receiving radiation to the heart with doses exceeding 1,000 cGy. During therapy, echocardiogram or radionuclide cardiac cineangiocardiography (RNA) should be performed regularly. If the planned cumulative dose of daunomycin/ doxorubicin is less than 300 mg/ m^2, testing is repeated after half the cumulative dose has been given. After the cumulative dose reaches more than 360 mg/ m^2, testing is repeated before each cycle. If an abnormality is detected in either the echocardiogram or MUGA is appreciated, the other test should be performed as confirmation of the abnormality. The following are criteria for progressive deteriorating cardiac function:

- A decrease in the fractional shortening (FS) by an absolute value of 10% from the previous test
- FS less than 29%
- A decrease in the RNA-left ventricular ejection fraction (RNA-LVEF) by an absolute value of 10% from the previous test
- RNA-LVEF less than 5%
- A decrease in the RNA-LVEF with stress
- Development of arrhythmia.

If there is a documented infection or development of arrhythmia during therapy, anthracyclines should be discontinued and a cardiology consultation should be obtained.

Modification of Anthracycline Therapy

1. If both the FS and the LVEF are abnormal, anthracycline therapy should be discontinued unless there is a recovery of FS and RNA LVEF to normal on two serial tests taken 1 month apart.
2. If one of the preceding test modalities is abnormal, while the other is normal, anthracyclines should be temporarily discontinued. Both tests should be repeated after 1 month. If one remains normal and the other becomes normal or does not deteriorate further, therapy should be resumed. Therapy should be discontinued if further deterioration occurs in either tests. Patients who receive anthracyclines and/ or thoracic radiotherapy should be evaluated by EKG and echocardiogram every year for 5 years.

Low-dose Radiotherapy with Combination Chemotherapy

1. Appropriately lowered cumulative dose of anthracycline should be employed when radiotherapy is administered over the heart.
2. Use of less than 450 mg/ m^2 cumulative dose for both doxorubicin and daunomycin and 125 mg/ m^2 for idarubicin and 160 mg/ m^2 for mitoxantrone. Patients who have received a cumulative dose of doxorubicin of more than 450 mg/ m^2 should not receive mitoxantrone. The recommended cumulative dose of mitoxantrone for patients who have received prior treatment with doxorubicin is 120 mg/ m^2.
3. Use of cardioprotective agents such as dexrazoxane (ICRF-187, Zinecard, DZR). The dose of dexrazoxane is 300 mg/ m^2 (10 times the doxorubicin dose) IV bolus over 15 minutes followed by doxorubicin or daunomycin IV over 15 minutes, that is, before the elapsed time of 30 minutes (from the beginning of the dexrazoxane). This drug is not standard of care and is still investigational.
4. Cardiac tissue damage serum marker (e.g. determination of cardiac Troponin T [cTnT] levels, creatinine kinase [CK]-MB isozyme). cardiac Troponin is a thin-filament contractile protein that is released from damaged cardiomyocytes. Unlike CK-MB, cTnT is not found in the serum of a healthy person.
5. ECHO/MUGA surveillance studies as recommended.
6. Use of new anthracyclines with decreased potential for cardiotoxicity is being investigated.

Prevention of Renal Toxicity

1. Maintain hydration at 125 ml/ m^2/h (i.e. twice maintenance) for a minimum of 2 hours prior to start of chemotherapy with agents such as high-dose methotrexate, moderate-to-high dose of cyclophosphamide, cisplatin, or ifosfamide to increase urine output to more than 3 ml/kg/h and decrease urinary specific gravity below 1.010.
2. During infusion of these agents, maintain hydration at 125 ml/ m^2/h and urinary output at 5 ml/kg/h.
3. After infusion, continue hydration at 90-125 ml/ m^2/h.

4. Strict monitoring of intake, output and daily weights is critical. Maintain isovolemic fluid balance. When needed, use furosemide 0.5–1 mg/ kg IV or mannitol 6 g/m^2 (200 mg/kg) in at least 25 ml of fluid over 15-60 minutes.
5. Use mesna for its uroprotective effect to prevent hemorrhagic cystitis caused by high dose cyclophosphamide and ifosfamide. A total mesna dose equal to the total dose of cyclophosphamide (0.8 mg of mesna per 1 mg of cyclophosphamide) is recommended.
6. Adjust the doses of chemotherapy according to the glomerular filtration rate (GFR).
7. During infusion of cisplatin, add mannitol 15 g/m^2 (10-24 g/m^2/L) and $MgSO_4$ in a dose of 20 mEq/L to the hydrating solution to prevent hypomagnesemia.
8. Continue postchemotherapy hydration with 5% dextrose/0.45% NaCl 120 mEq/L, KCl 120 mEq/L, $MgSO_4$ 120 g/L mannitol.
9. Measurement of renal function and electrolytes prior to and during each cycle. Correct metabolic derangements in a timely manner.

Prevention of Neurotoxicity

Neurotoxicity ranges from peripheral neuropathy following vincristine and cisplatin to acute encephalopathy following intrathecal chemotherapy or high-dose methotrexate. Following administration of vincristine, patients may complain of jaw pain, constipation, foot drop, lid lag and/or tingling and numbness in the distal extremities. Supportive care includes frequent neurologic examinations, pain management and oral laxatives to prevent constipation. If neurologic deficits persist, dose modifications or discontinuation of medications may be necessary.

PAIN MANAGEMENT[28,29]

Pain is a common symptom and a major problem during different phases of cancer treatment in children and is one of the over-riding concerns of families. At diagnosis, or during the active treatment phase, about 50% of children experience cancer-related pain. In one survey, approximately 50% of the patients assessed in hospital, and 25% of the patients assessed in the outpatient clinic were found to be experiencing some degree of pain. In the advanced stage of disease these figures are much higher, the incidence of pain requiring regular pain medication being as high as 89%. Unrelieved pain may have major consequences for the care of children. The occurrence of severe pain and adverse effects of treatment for it, as well as a desire for better and less painful interventions, were the principal determinants of parental decisions about whether or not to continue anticancer treatment for childhood cancer patients. Unrelieved pain interferes with sleep, leads to fatigue and a sense of helplessness, and may result in increased morbidity and mortality. Children who die of cancer receive aggressive treatment at the end of their lives and many have substantial suffering unrelieved in the last month of life. Yet many children with cancer do not receive the benefit of current knowledge or innovative techniques in pain management. In one study approximately 20% of consultations for psychiatric symptoms in hospitalized children with cancer resulted in a primary recommendation for improved pain control. Suitable drugs are now available for children but inexperience and unfounded fears may still result in reluctance to use appropriate potent analgesics. The need for opioid therapy is frequent and the doses required can be as high as those used in adults, in some circumstances. Although the vast majority of children with cancer need regular pain medication in the terminal phase, cancer pain in children is still not managed optimally. Children frequently receive no treatment, or inadequate treatment for pain, especially for painful procedures. Moreover, worldwide there are marked geographic and economic variations in the incidence of cancer, and also the possible therapeutic success of oncological treatment: between 30% and 50% of the world's population are below the age of 20 and about 90% of children live in developing countries, where access to medical care is inadequate and poverty and illiteracy often stifle all efforts to fight childhood cancer. Many children withdraw or deny their pain in an attempt to avoid yet another terrifying and painful experience, such as intramuscular injections. Exaggerated concerns regarding the risk of opioid addiction and respiratory depression associated with opioids, lack of advocacy, and poor understanding of the basic pharmacokinetic principles of common analgesic agents are also causal factors in the undertreatment of pediatric pain in cancer (Table 26.3). The effective relief of pain in terminally ill pediatric patients has incalculable benefits to patients and their families. Management can be dramatically improved by increasing staff sensitivity and using an integrated program of drugs, techniques and psychological approaches. Parents identified the benefits of pain management teams for the child, for themselves and also the stress associated with managing pain at home. Parents wanted more information about pain and pain treatment, and thought themselves

Table 26.3: Guidelines for opioid therapy for persistent cancer pain

Comprehensive assessment
- Define pain etiology, pathophysiology and syndrome
- Clarify status of disease
- Determine impact of the pain and comorbid physical and psychosocial disturbances

Drug selection
- Consider age and whether major organ failure is present, especially renal, hepatic, or respiratory
- Consider drug-selective differences in side effect or toxicity profile
- Consider the effects of concurrent drugs with possible pharmacokinetic and pharmacodynamic interactions
- Consider individual differences (note prior treatment outcomes) and patient preference
- Be aware of available preparations for route (e.g. oral, IV, subcutaneous injection, topical) and formulation (e.g. immediate or controlled-release)
- Be aware of cost differences

Route selection
- Use least invasive route possible
- Consider patient convenience and compliance

Dosing
- Consider previous dosing requirements and relative analgesic potencies when initiating therapy
- Start with low dose and increase until adequate analgesia occurs or dose-limiting side effects are encountered
- Consider dosing schedule (e.g. around-the-clock or as needed) depending on the anticipated time course of pain
- Consider "rescue medication" for breakthrough pain
- Recognize that tolerance is rarely the driving force for dose escalation; consider disease progression when increasing dose requirements occur

Treat side effects
- Give laxatives prophylactically
- Be prepared to treat nausea, itch and somnolence
- Trial of alternative opioids

Monitoring

Monitor treatment efficacy and pain status over time and consider modification if necessary

able to judge their child's pain better than professionals. Thus, understanding the pain experience from the perspective of family caregivers and their role in pain management can assist healthcare providers in relieving pain in children with cancer. Parents' cultural differences may explain the higher levels of anxiety in Hispanics compared with Anglo-Saxon families. Common causes of failing pain treatment are anxiety of parents when parents are not sufficiently confident to comfort their child, anxiety in children, loneliness and lack of information. Pain is not reported at times because it is thought to be an inevitable part of the malignant disease. Home-based palliative care may be an effective program for many children after adequate support for the child and family has been established. A home care team may allow for shorter hospital stays and support parents in achieving a better use of opioids at home. At diagnosis, pediatric oncology patients have tumor-related pain. As the treatment evolves, treatment-related pain predominates.

We can divide the causes of pain in a child with cancer mainly in three groups:

1. **Cancer-related pain:** Bone pain, compression of central or peripheral nervous system structures, etc.
2. **Procedure-related pain**: Venipuncture, bone marrow aspiration and biopsy, lumbar puncture, pleural tap, etc.
3. **Treatment-related pain**:
   - *Chemotherapy:* Mucositis, peripheral neuropathy, aseptic necrosis of bone, steroid induced myopathy, G-CSF induced myalgias, etc.
   - *Radiation:* Mucositis, radionecrosis, myelopathy, brachial/lumbar plexopathies.
   - *Postsurgical:* Acute postoperative pain, phantom pain.

Pain management can be attained by two ways:
1. Nonpharmacological.
2. Pharmacological.

Nonpharmacological Methods

- Preparation of the child prior to a procedure
- *Physical:* Massage, heat and cold, electrical nerve stimulation, acupuncture
- *Behavioral:* Art and play therapy, exercise, relaxation, bio-feedback, desensitization, operant conditioning
- *Cognitive:* Distraction, imagery, attention, hypnosis, music therapy, psychotherapy
- Complementary and alternative medicine.

Pharmacological

Drugs are the mainstay of pain management.

A therapeutic management plan is dependent on understanding of the causes of pain, on pain assessment, and on the myriad of drug and non-drug strategies that are essential in pain treatment. A longstanding problem in pediatric pain management has been the difficulty of objectively assessing pain. Assessment in infants before they can speak or express themselves is particularly challenging.

The type and severity of pain experienced by children with cancer varies from acute short-term, procedure-related pain to the progressive chronic pain associated with the evolution of cancer or sequel of treatment. Treatments should be individualized for each patient and family, monitored and adjusted in conformity with rigorous guidelines in order to obtain the best analgesic efficacy with the lowest adverse effect level.

The dosage and frequency of the analgesics are adjusted to the patient's pain and are gradually increased as needed to maintain the patient free of pain. The next dose should be given before the previous dose has worn off fully to erase the memory and fear of pain.

Simplest dosage schedule and least-invasive pain management modality should be used first. Medications for persistent cancer-related pain should be administered on an around-the-clock basis, with additional "as needed" doses because regularly scheduled dosing maintains a constant level of drug in body. With ongoing administration of narcotic analgesics, tolerance builds up and increasing doses must be given to maintain the same level of analgesia. Tolerance and physical dependence are expected with long-term use and should not be confused with psychological dependence ("addiction") combining a narcotic with tricyclic antidepressants, anticonvulsants, amphetamines, steroids, or topical agents may potentiate its analgesic activity.

GENERAL GUIDELINES FOR MANAGEMENT OF PAIN IN ONCOLOGY PATIENTS[30-37]

Determine the class of drug based on severity of pain:

1. *Mild to moderate:* NSAID or acetaminophen, unless contraindicated.
2. *Moderate at outset or persistent mild pain:* Opioid should be added (not substituted), i.e. codeine, oxycodone, hydrocodone. May be used in fixed-dose combinations but if pain persists, recommend separate dosages to avoid excessive doses of NSAIDs or acetaminophen.
3. *Moderate-to-severe pain at outset or persistent moderate pain:* Increase opioid potency or dose, i.e. morphine, hydromorphone, methadone, fentanyl.
4. *Severe, chronic pain:* Best managed with immediate-release and long-acting morphine.

Patient-Controlled Analgesia

Patient-controlled analgesia (PCA) is a method of opioid administration using a computer controlled pump that enables the patient to deliver small boluses as needed up to a preset maximum. It can be used with a baseline continuous infusion.

The advantages of PCA are:

- It permits titrated dosing to compensate for individual variation in pharmacokinetics and pain intensity
- It permits the patient to exercise control and diminishes anxiety
- It allows the patient to balance analgesia against its side effects such as sedation
- It helps determine conversion to oral regimen once steady level of appropriate analgesia is attained
- It is safe for home and hospital use.

The usual starting dose is 0.01–0.02 mg/kg of morphine every 6–10 minutes with or without a basal infusion of 0.01-0.02 mg/kg/h.

Anesthesia for Painful Procedures[38]

Painful or invasive procedures are a major source of anxiety for the child undergoing therapy for cancer. These procedures include insertion of intravenous lines, accessing of mediports, spinal taps, bone marrow aspirations and pleural and peritoneal taps. Adequate local or general anesthesia, if indicated, can significantly reduce the child's fear.

Local Anesthesia

Local anesthesia is adequate for inserting intravenous lines, for accessing mediports and for performing spinal taps and bone marrow aspirations on some children. Local anesthesia can be provided via:

- EMLA (Eutectic mixture of local anesthetics) cream (lidocaine 2.5%, prilocaine 2.5%) applied topically to the skin and covered with an occlusive dressing 1 hour prior to the procedure
- Lidocaine 2% injected superficially into the area of the procedure
- Skin cooling with ice or fluorocarbon cooling sprays.

General Sedation/Anesthesia

General sedation/anesthesia is required for more painful procedures, such as bone marrow biopsies and for lesser procedures in the young child who is extremely fearful. The following agents may be used:

- Propofol
  - Sedative hypnotic, not analgesic
  - May produce respiratory depression and hypotension
  - Supplied in an emulsion with egg lecithin; avoid use in patients with egg allergies
  - Short-acting anesthetic; patients awaken when infusion is terminated
  - *Dosage:* 2 mg/kg IV bolus followed by continuous infusion of 40–200 μg/kg/minute; reduce dose by half for patients with neurologic, cardiac, or respiratory disease

- Some patients develop tolerance and require higher doses.
- Brevital (methohexital)
  - Very short-acting anesthetic, barbiturate
  - May produce respiratory depression, hypotension
  - *Dosage:* 1-2 mg/kg/dose IV or 5-10 mg/kg/dose IM.
- Ketamine
  - Rapid-acting anesthetic with profound analgesia
  - Produces fugue-like state, disorientation, delirium, bizarre dreams
  - Can be given along with midazolam dose to cause amnesia of the dreams
  - *Dosage:* 2 mg/kg IV; increments of one half to the full dose may be repeated as needed.
- DPT (this combination is rarely used and should be avoided in very young children because of reports of life-threatening toxicity from phenergan)
  - Demerol 2 mg/kg IV, phenergan 1 mg/kg IV, thorazine 1 mg/kg IV
  - Sedative, analgesic and anesthetic
  - Produces sedation for 3-4 hours.

The current American Academy of Pediatrics Committee guidelines for pediatric patients undergoing conscious sedation require the presence of medical personnel trained in the administration of medications used for procedural sedation and management of complications associated with these medications. Management requires the medical staff to identify when the level of sedation has exceeded the intended effect and be skilled in rescue methods to reverse such effects. Anesthiologists and other physicians trained in the skilled management of airway problems are the preferred practitioners for procedural sedation. When an anesthesiologist is present, propofol is preferred because it is extremely short acting and the dose can be titrated as needed.

MANAGEMENT OF NAUSEA AND VOMITING[39]

In most cases, nausea and vomiting can be prevented. Every effort should be made to provide adequate antiemetic coverage. The receptors for nausea and vomiting should be blocked before treatment starts and should continue as long as the effect is likely to occur. Scheduled doses should be administered regardless of symptoms.

Vomiting is mediated by the vomiting center located in the medullary lateral reticular formation. This center gets input from five sources:

1. Chemoreceptor trigger zone.
2. Vagal and sympathetic afferents from viscera.
3. Midbrain receptors that detect changes in intracranial pressure.
4. Labyrinthine apparatus.
5. Limbic system.

Chemotherapeutic agents may stimulate vomiting by direct effect on the vomiting center or through the chemoreceptor trigger zone. Serotonin (5-HT) receptors and substance P play a role in mediating emesis. The emetogenic potential of chemotherapeutic agents[40] is listed in Table 26.4.

The etiology of vomiting should be identified before therapy is initiated. Unusual severity, timing, or duration should alert the physician to a diagnosis other

Table 26.4: Emetogenic potential of chemotherapeutic agent

Acute Symptoms

Highly emetogenic
- Actinomycin-D
- Cisplatin (40 mg/m^2)
- Cyclophosphamide (1 g/m^2)
- Cytarabine (1 g/m^2)
- Dacarbazine
- Ifosfamide
- Mechlorethamine

Moderately emetogenic
- Anthracyclines (daunorubicin, doxorubicin, idarubicin)
- Carboplatin
- Cisplatin (40 mg/m^2)
- Cyclophosphamide (1 g/m^2)
- Cytarabine (IV, 1 g/m^2, or IT)
- Mercaptopurine (IV)
- Methotrexate (IV 1 g/m^2)
- Nitrosoureas (carmustine, lomustine)

Mildly emetogenic
- Bleomycin
- Epipodophyllotoxins (etoposide, teniposide)
- Paclitaxel
- Procarbazine
- Topotecan
- Vinblastine
- Nonemetogenic Asparaginase
- Mercaptopurine (PO)
- Methotrexate (low-dose IV, IM, PO, IT)
- Steroids
- Thioguanine
- Vincristine

Delayed Symptoms

Severe
Cisplatin

Moderate
Cyclophosphamide

than chemotherapy induced nausea and vomiting. Chemotherapy-induced nausea and vomiting (CINV) is divided into:

- *Anticipatory:* Prior to chemotherapy administration–results from learned or conditioned response
- *Acute:* Within 24 hours following chemotherapy
- *Delayed:* 24 hours after chemotherapy
- *Breakthrough:* Despite the administration of antiemetics.

Chemotherapy agents are classified into four categories of emesis risk without use of antiemetics:

1. High (>90%)
2. Moderate (30-90%)
3. Low (10-30%)
4. Minimal (10%).

There are five classes of antiemetic available:

1. Serotonin antagonists
2. Neurokinin antagonists
3. Cannabinoids
4. Dopamine antagonists
5. Corticosteroids.

Serotonin (5-HT$_3$) Receptor Antagonists

1. Ondansetron (zofran).
2. Granisetron (kytril).
3. Palonosetron (Aloxi) novel 5-HT$_3$ receptor antagonist has 100-fold greater binding affinity for the serotonin receptor and a longer half-life (40 hours longer).
   a. Used for prevention of acute and delayed CINV with moderately and highly emetogenic chemotherapy for patients >18 years
   b. Palonosetron in combination with dexamethasone provides complete response of 40.7% compared to ondansetron plus dexamtheasone which has a 25.2% response rate.

Neurokinin-1 Antagonists Aprepitant (Emend)

1. Aprepitant blocks neurokinin receptor and enhances activity of 5-HT$_3$ receptor antagonists. It is metabolized by CYP34A enzyme.
   a. Used in patients—40 kg and >12 years.
   b. When combined with ondansetron and dexamethasone provides complete response rate of 72.7% on days 1-5 however, aprepitant alone or in combination with dexamethasone does not control acute emesis as well as ondansetron and dexamethasone.
   c. It is an inducer of CYP2CP and can therefore react with many drugs. The dose of steroid given concomitantly as antiemetics should be decreased by 25% if given IV or 50% if given orally. Doses of benzodiazepine may also need to be decreased. Aprepitant should be used with caution when administering with etoposide, ifosfamide, imatinib, irinotecan, paclitaxel, vincristine or vinblastine.

Cannabinoids

1. *Physiology:* Tetrahydrocannabinol (THC) activates:
   a. CB-1 receptor found in large quantities in cerebellum, basal ganglia, brainstem and hypothalamus.
   b. CB-2 on cells of the immune function.
2. Drugs available.
   a. Dronabinol (Marinol).
   b. Nabilone (Cesamet)—side effects include drowsiness, sedation, euphoria, heightened sensation, dizziness.

Dopamine Antagonists

1. Inhibits dopaminergic function.
2. Metoclopramide (Reglan).

Corticosteroids

1. Dexamethasone preferred agent.
2. Methylprednisone.

Antiemetic agents can be given in combination to increase their efficacy. For patients receiving chemotherapy with high emetic risk, there is no role for using antiemetic drugs of lower antiemetic potential and attempting to escalate the antiemetic drugs once emesis has begun. Agents of lower antiemetic potential should only be used in high-emetic-risk situations when patients are intolerant of or refractory to 5-HT$_3$ serotonin receptor antagonists, NK1 antagonists and dexamethasone. Commonly used effective regimens include: 5-HT$_3$ receptor antagonist in combination with dexamethasone and Emend on day 1, followed by dexamethasone on days 2-4 and Emend on days 2 and 3. For moderate-emetic-risk agents: Two-drug regimen consisting of a 5-HT$_3$ receptor antagonist in combination with dexamethasone on day 1 followed by either dexamethasone alone on days 2–4 or in combination with 5-HT$_3$ antagonist for delayed CINV.

For Low-emetic-risk Agents

- Dexamethasone alone is recommended when appropriate or 5-HT$_3$ antagonist alone on day 1

- No routine preventive use of antiemetics for delayed emesis is suggested.

For minimal-emetic-risk agents: Prescribe only as required.

If vomiting and nausea continue despite recommended prophylaxis:
- Conduct a careful re-evaluation of emetic risk
- Review disease status
- Consider concurrent illness and medications
- Confirm that the best regimen is being given based on emetic risk
- Consider adding lorazepam or alprazolam to regimen.

The following drugs could be used on an ambulatory basis when breakthrough occurs:
- Prochloraperazine (Compazine) 0.1 mg/kg PO every 6 hours
- Metoclopramide (Reglan) 1-2 mg/kg PO every 4 hours to be given with diphenhydramine
- Dronabinol (Marinol) 5-10 mg PO q3–6h.

*For anthracyclines: 5HT3 antagonists, dexamethasone and aprepitant, followed by aprepitant alone for days 2 and 3. Otherwise the use of aprepitant in this category is optional and based on individual response.
- Promethazine (Phenergan) 0.25–1 mg/kg PO every 6 hours (do not use in children less than 2 years of age)
- Scopolamine patch
- 1/2 patch every 3 days in infants 8–15 kg body weight
- 1 patch every 3 days if 15 kg body weight
- Hydroxyzine (Vistaril, Atarax) 0.02-0.05 mg/kg PO every 4–6 hours
- Lorazepam (Ativan) 0.02-0.05 mg/kg PO every 6 hours.

Radiation-induced Emesis

1. *High emetic risk (total body irradiation):* 5-HT_3 antagonist alone or in combination with corticosteroid before each fraction and for at least 24 hours after.
2. *Moderate emetic risk (upper abdomen, hemi body irradiation, abdominal-pelvic, mantle, craniospinal irradiation, cranial radiosurgery):* 5-HT_3 antagonist before each fraction.
3. *Low emetic risk (lower thorax, cranium and craniospinal):* 5-HT_3 antagonist before each fraction.
4. *Minimal emetic risk (radiation of breast, head and neck, cranium and extremities):* Medication as required.

Anticipatory Emesis

1. Use of the most appropriate antiemetic regimens based on chemotherapy being administered to prevent acute or delayed emesis.
2. Ativan 0.025 mg/kg PO in morning before chemotherapy.
3. Cognitive therapy and behavioral modification.
4. Hypnosis with desensitization procedures.

NUTRITIONAL SUPPORT[41]

Progressive weight loss, protein energy malnutrition (PEM) and cachexia occur in advanced malignancies in children. Cachexia leads to decreased strength, impaired immune function, decreased pulmonary function, increased disability and death. The clinical features of cachexia include:
- Wasting
- Anorexia
- Weakness
- Anemia
- Hypoalbuminemia
- Hypoglycemia
- Lactic acidosis
- Hyperlipidemia
- Impaired liver function
- Glucose intolerance
- Skeletal muscle atrophy
- Anergy.

The following factors interact to produce cachexia in pediatric oncology patients:
- Decreased intake secondary to mucositis
- Anorexia and altered taste perception (dysgeusia)
- Nausea and vomiting
- Decreased absorption secondary to the effects of chemotherapy, radiation therapy, or surgery
- Protein-losing nephropathy
- Steroid-induced diabetes
- Increased metabolic expenditure secondary to rapid tumor growth and metastases
- Endogenously produced cytokines such as TNF, IL-1, IL-6 and γ-interferon
- Hepatotoxicity with impaired liver synthetic capacity and altered protein, carbohydrate and lipid metabolism
- Psychosocial factors such as depression and anticipatory vomiting.

The net result of these factors is failure of nutritional intake to meet increased metabolic demands as a result of which, tissue wasting occurs.

Treatment

It is crucial to increase nutritional intake both to improve quality of life and to increase survival from the underlying malignancy. Methods of nutritional support include:

- Oral feeding with high-calorie supplements
- Nasogastric tube feeding
- Total parenteral nutrition (intravenous hyper-alimentation).

Oral Feeding

If the child tolerates oral intake and can absorb nutrients, oral feeding is the treatment of choice. Supplemental diet formulas and elemental diets are helpful in these children.

Tube Feeding

Oral feeding may not be adequate or may not be tolerated. Adequate nutrition may have to be supplied via nasogastric intubation if the patient has adequate blood counts and does not have mucositis. In cases where chronic tube feeding will be required, a gastrostomy tube may have to be placed. If bolus feeds are not tolerated, continuous low-volume infusions can be utilized to maximize caloric intake.

Intravenous Hyperalimentation or Total Parenteral Nutrition

Total parenteral nutrition (TPN) is indicated when enteral feeds cannot be tolerated. It is the most intensive modality of nutritional supplementation and requires a central intravenous device. Full nutritional requirements can usually be met. Total parenteral nutrition (TPN) should be continued until oral feedings can be resumed. Complications of TPN are hypoglycemia, hyperglycemia, fatty liver and cholestatic jaundice.

Indwelling intravenous catheters with ongoing therapy, it is difficult to find adequate peripheral venous access in pediatric oncology patients. In addition, chemotherapeutic agents produce venous sclerosis, further aggravating the problem of finding peripheral venous access. To alleviate this problem, permanently indwelling right atrial catheters are used. These catheters are recommended for:

- All young children and infants receiving chemotherapy
- Most older children and adults receiving chemotherapy if the protocol is prolonged and of moderate to high intensity
- Patients requiring TPN.

Types of Catheters and Methods of Insertion

Two major types of long-term indwelling tunneled catheters are in use:

1. External tunneled catheters that lead to tubing that exits the skin. They can be single, double and occasionally triple lumen. The most frequently used types are the Broviac catheter and the Hickman catheter
2. Total implantable venous access devices or "ports" are right atrial catheters that lead to reservoirs totally embedded under the skin, replacing the external portion of the catheter The device is accessed using a special nonboring needle that traverses the skin and enters the device. Such devices are more cosmetically satisfactory to older children and adolescents and have a lower infection rate than external tunneled catheters. Catheters are inserted via the subclavian, internal, or external jugular vein with a subcutaneous tunnel to the anterior or lateral chest wall. Alternatively, catheters can be placed via the femoral vein to the inferior vena cava with a tunnel to the abdominal wall.

Maintenance

1. Broviacs (or Hickmans) require daily or every-other-day heparin flushes, in addition to dressing changes three times a week.
2. Mediports require heparin flushes only once every 3-4 weeks and do not require dressing changes.
3. In both cases, completely sterile technique must be used in accessing the catheters.

Complications

The major complications are:

- *Infection:* Episodes of catheter-related bacteremia occur and are most commonly due to coagulase-negative staphylococci. Management consists of appropriate intravenous antibiotic therapy. Antibiotic therapy without catheter removal is successful in approximately 75% of episodes and higher if antibiotic lock therapy is used. If the bacteremia fails to resolve, the patient develops uncontrolled clinical sepsis, or if there is infection overlying the subcutaneous tunnel, then the catheter must be removed. Occasionally, catheter-related fungal infection occurs and, in these cases catheter removal is necessary.
- *Thrombosis:* Thrombosis may be cleared by instilling tPA 0.5-1 mg and leaving it in for 30–60 minutes. If the catheter remains occluded after two doses, a

continuous infusion of tPA is indicated. The dose is 0.01 mg/kg/hour for 6 hours. The dose may be increased to 0.02 mg/kg/hour for 6 hours, then to 0.03 mg/kg/hour for 6 hours if there is no resolution. The fibrinogen level should be monitored every 6 hours. If the line is still occluded, it should be removed. Most patients develop the preceding complications from time to time. In the majority of cases, however, the morbidity associated with these complications is outweighed by the advantages of reliable, adequate venous access.

IMMUNIZATIONS

Current CDC recommendations for immunizations are as follows:

- Immunocompromised patients should not be administered live vaccines
- Oral polio vaccine should not be administered to any household contact of a severely immunocompromised person. Measles–mumps–rubella (MMR) vaccine is not contraindicated for the close contacts (including health-care providers) of immunocompromised persons and should be given to susceptible household members
- Patients with leukemia in remission status who have not received chemotherapy for at least 3 months are not considered severely immunosuppressed and can receive live virus vaccines.
- When chemotherapy or immunosuppressive therapy is being considered vaccination ideally should precede the initiation of chemotherapy or immunosuppression by greater than or equal to 2 weeks
- Vaccination during chemotherapy or radiation therapy should be avoided
- Patients vaccinated while on immunosuppressive therapy or within 2 weeks before starting therapy, should be considered unimmunized and should be revaccinated at least 3 months after discontinuation of therapy
- When exposed to a vaccine-preventable disease such as measles, severely immunocompromised children should be considered susceptible regardless of their history of vaccination.

Measles

Severely immunocompromised patients who are exposed to measles should receive immune globulin (IG), regardless of prior vaccination status. The recommended dose of immune globulin for measles prophylaxis of immunocompromised patients is 0.5 ml/kg of body weight intramuscularly (maximum dose, 15 ml). The immunogenicity of measles vaccine is decreased if vaccine is administered within 6 months of immunoglobulin. For immunocompromised patients receiving immunoglobulin for measles prophylaxis, measles vaccination should be delayed for 6 months following immunoglobulin administration. For patients receiving immunoglobulin for replacement of humoral immune deficiencies (320 mg/kg intravenously), measles vaccination should be delayed until 8 months following immunoglobulin administration.

Varicella

Leukemic children who are in remission status and do not have evidence of immunity to varicella should be vaccinated with antiviral therapy being available should complications arise. Patients with leukemia, lymphoma, or other malignancies whose disease is in remission and whose chemotherapy has been terminated for at least 3 months can receive live virus vaccines. When immunizing persons in whom some degree of immunodeficiency might be present, only single-antigen varicella vaccine should be used rather than MMRV. Because varicella vaccine is recommended for all healthy children and adults without evidence of immunity, household contacts of immunocompromised persons should be vaccinated routinely. Vaccination of household contacts provides protection for immunocompromised patients by decreasing the likelihood that wild-type VZV will be introduced into the household. Vaccination of household contacts of immunocompromised persons theoretically poses a risk for transmission of vaccine virus to immunocompromised patients. However, no cases have been reported of transmission of vaccine virus to immunocompromised persons. Vaccine recipients in whom vaccine-related rash occurs, particularly household contacts of immunocompromised persons, should avoid contact with susceptible persons who are at high risk for severe complications. If the susceptible, immunocompromised person is inadvertently exposed to a person who has a vaccine-related rash, postexposure prophylaxis with varicella-zoster immunoglobulin is not needed because disease associated with this type of virus is expected to be mild.

Varicella Exposure

Patients who had household exposure to active varicella, or have been in the same room with an individual in the contagious state of varicella (1-2 days before and 5 days after eruption of vesicles) for at least 1 hour should receive varicella-zoster immune globulin (available in the United States as investigational Varizig) 1 vial/10 kg IM (maximum dose, 5 vials) within 96 hours of exposure. Children who have been vaccinated and have positive titers do not need to receive varicella-zoster immune globulin after exposures.

Pneumococcal Vaccine

In addition to pneumococcal conjugate vaccine that is routinely administered to all children with doses at 2, 4, 6 and 12-15 months of age, 23-valent pneumococcal polysaccharide vaccine is recommended for use in children 2 years of age or older with chronic illnesses associated with increased risk of pneumococcal disease or its complications (e.g. anatomic or functional asplenia [sickle cell disease], nephrotic syndrome, cerebrospinal fluid leaks and conditions associated with immunosuppression). Vaccination in these high-risk individuals includes two doses of pneumococcal conjugate vaccine if not previously completed and the pneumococcal polysaccharide vaccine should be given at least 2 months after the completion of the PCV-7 vaccines. A second dose of pneumococcal polysaccharide vaccine should be administered 5 years later for children at highest risk of infection, i.e. those with asplenia or sickle cell disease.

Meningococcal Vaccine

Routine immunization with the quadrivalent meningococcal conjugate vaccine is recommended for all children starting at 11 years of age and for certain high-risk children at age 2 through 10 years including children with terminal complement component deficiencies and those with anatomic or functional asplenia.

Influenza Vaccine

Because influenza may result in serious illness and complications for immunocompromised persons, annual vaccination with inactivated vaccine is recommended. However, response to this vaccine may be suboptimal in immunocompromised patients. In an attempt to decrease the exposure of such persons to influenza, all household members and all healthcare personnel should be immunized with influenza vaccine (inactivated or live, attenuated nasal vaccine) annually.

PSYCHOSOCIAL SUPPORT AND END-OF-LIFE CARE

Throughout the course of the disease, children with cancer and their families will face a number of psychological issues. In addition to the oncologist's skills in this area, specially trained psychologists, psychiatric social workers, psychiatrists and pastoral care practitioners can be helpful in dealing with these matters as they arise.

Blood Component Therapy

Has been discussed in a separate chapter in this book.

REFERENCES

1. National Institute for Clinical Excellence, 2004, Guidance on Cancer Services – Improving Supportive and Palliative Care for Adults with Cancer. The Manual, National Health Service, London, United Kingdom.
2. Supportive Care of Patients with Cancer. In: Philip Lanzkowsky (Ed). Manual of Pediatric Hematology and Oncology, 5th edn. Elsevier; 2011. pp. 857-920.
3. Alexander SW, Walsh TJ, Freifeld AG, Pizzo PA. Infectious complications in pediatric cancer patients. In: Pizzo PA, Poplack DG (Eds). Principles and Practice of Pediatric Oncology, 4th edn. Philadelphia: Lippincott, Williams and Wilkins; 2002.pp.1239-84.
4. Wolff LJ, Altman AJ, Berkow RL, Johnson FL. The management of fever and neutropenia. In: Altman AJ (Ed). Supportive care of children with cancer. Current therapy and guidelines from the Children's Oncology Group, (3rd edn). Baltimore: The Johns Hopkins University Press; 2004. pp. 200-20
5. Freifeld A, et al. A double-blind comparison of empirical oral and intravenous antibiotic therapy for low risk febrile with neutropenia during cancer chemotherapy. New Engl J Med. 1999;341:305-11.
6. Wingard JR, Nichols WG, McDonald GB. Supportive Care American Society of Hematology. Hematology; pp. 372-89.
7. Koo, et al. Efficacy and safety of caspofungin for the empiric management of fever in neutropenic children. Pediatr Infect Dis. DOL:10.1097 ISSN 0891-3668. Lippincott Williams and Wilkins, 2007.
8. Michallet M, Ito J. Approaches to management of invasive fungal infections in hematological malignancy and hematopoietic stem cell transplantation. J Clin Oncol. 2009;27(20): 10.
9. Pappas PG, Rex JH, Sobel JD, et al. Guidelines for treatment of candidiasis. Clin Infect Dis. 2004;38:161-89.
10. Kontoyiannis DP, Hachem R, Lewis RE, et al. Efficacy and toxicity of caspofungin in combination with liposomal amphotericin B as primary or salvage treatment of invasive aspergillosis in patients with hematologic malignancies. Cancer. 2003;98:292-9.
11. Johnson MD, MacDougall C, Ostrosky-Zeichner L, et al. Combination antifungal therapy. Antimicrob Agents Chemother. 2004;48:693-715.
12. Herbrecht R, Denning DW, Patterson TF, et al. Voriconazole versus amphotericin B for primary therapy of invasive aspergillosis. N Engl J Med. 2002;347:408-15.
13. Kanda Y, Yamamoto R, Chizuka A, et al. Prophylactic action of oral fluconazole against fungal infection in neutropenic patients. A meta-analysis of 16 randomized, controlled trials. Cancer. 2000;89:1611-25.

14. Glasmacher A, Prentice A, Gorschluter M, et al. Itraconazole prevents invasive fungal infections in neutropenic patients treated for hematologic malignancies: evidence from a metaanalysis of 3,597 patients. J Clin Oncol. 2003;21:4615-26.
15. Fukuda T, Boeckh M, Guthrie KA, et al. Invasive aspergillosis before allogeneic hematopoietic stem cell transplantation: 10-year experience at a single transplant center. Biol Blood Marrow Transplant. 2004;10(7):494-503.
16. Wingard JR. Empirical antifungal therapy in treating febrile neutropenic patients. Clin Infect Dis. 2004;39(1):S38-S43.
17. Nichols WG, Gooley T, Boeckh M. Community-acquired respiratory syncytial virus and parainfluenza virus infections after hematopoietic stem cell transplantation: the Fred Hutchinson Cancer Research Center experience. Biol Blood Marrow Transplant. 2001;7 Suppl:11S-15S.
18. Small TN, Casson A, Malak SF, et al. Respiratory syncytial virus infection following hematopoietic stem cell transplantation. Bone Marrow Transplant. 2002;29:321-7.
19. DeVincenzo JP, Hirsch RL, Fuentes RJ, Top FH, Jr. Respiratory syncytial virus immune globulin treatment of lower respiratory tract infection in pediatric patients undergoing bone marrow transplantation - a compassionate use experience. Bone Marrow Transplant. 2000;25:161-5.
20. Englund JA, Champlin RE, Wyde PR, et al. Common emergence of amantadine- and rimantadine-resistant influenza A viruses in symptomatic immunocompromised adults. Clin Infect Dis. 1998;26:1418-24.
21. Johny AA, Clark A, Price N, Carrington D, Oakhill A, Marks DI. The use of zanamivir to treat influenza A and B infection after allogeneic stem cell transplantation. Bone Marrow Transplant. 2002;29:113-5.
22. Guidelines for preventing opportunistic infections among hematopoietic stem cell transplant recipients. Biol Blood Marrow Transplant. 2000;6:659-713;715;717-27.
23. Rogers ZR, Aquino VM, Buchana GR. Hematologic supportive care and hematopoietic cytokines. In: Pizzo PA, Poplack DG, (Eds). Principles and Practice of Pediatric Oncology (4th edn). Philadelphia: Lippincott, Williams and Wilkins; 2002.pp.1205-38.
24. Feusner J, Hastings C. Recombinant human erythropoietin in pediatric oncology: a review. Med Pediat Oncol. 2002;39: 463-8.
25. Goldman S, et al. Feasibility study of IL-11 and granulocyte-stimulating factor after myelosuppressive chemotherapy to mobilize peripheral blood stem cells from heavily pretreated patients. J Pediatr Hematol Oncol. 2001;23(5):300-5.
26. Rizzo JD, Lichtin AE, Woolf SH, et al. Use of epoetinin patients with cancer: evidence-based clinical practice guidelines of the American Society of Clinical Oncology and the American Society of Hematology. Blood. 2002;100(7):2303-20.
27. Barnard DR, Friedman DL, Landier W, et al. Monitoring and management of drug toxicity. In: Altman AJ (Ed). Supportive Care of Children with Cancer. Current Therapy and Guidelines from the Children's Oncology Group, 3rd edn. Baltimore: The Johns Hopkins University Press; 2004.pp.100-48.
28. Mercadante S. Cancer pain management in children Palliative Medicine. 2004;18:654-62.
29. Zempsky WT, Schechter NL, Altman AJ, Weisman SJ. The management of pain. In: Altman AJ (Ed). Supportive Care of Children with Cancer. Current Therapy and Guidelines from the Children's Oncology Group, 3rd edn. Baltimore: The Johns Hopkins University Press; 2004.pp.200-20.
30. Zernikov B, Lindena G. Long-acting morphine for pain control in paediatric oncology. Med Pediatr Oncol. 2001; 36:451-8.
31. Mercadante S, Di Silvestre G, Fulfaro F. Assistenza domiciliare a bambini nella fase terminale della malattia neoplastica. Riv Ital Cure Palliat. 2000;2:85-8.
32. Collins JJ, Dunkel IJ, Gipta SK, et al . Transdermal fentanyl in children with cancer pain: feasibility, tolerability, and pharmacokinetic correlates. J Pediatr. 1999;134:319-23.
33. Hunt A, Goldman A, Devine T, Philips M. Transdermal fentanyl for pain relief in a paediatric palliative care population. Palliat Med. 2001;15:405-12.
34. Noyes M, Irving H. The use of transdermal fentanyl in pediatric oncology palliative care. Am J Hosp Palliat Care. 2001;18:411-6.
35. Schechter NL, Weisman SJ, Rosenblum M, et al . Sedation for painful procedures in children with cancer using the fentanyl lollipop: a preliminary report. In: Tyler D, Krane E (Eds). Advances in pain research therapy. New York Raven Press, 1990.pp.209-13.
36. Shir Y, Shvelzon V, Rosen G. Treating hospitalized children in severe pain with oral methadone. Harefuah. 1998;134: 438-41.
37. Sabatowski R, Kasper SM, Radbruch L. Patient-controlled analgesia with intravenous L-methadone in a child with cancer pain refractory to high-dose morphine. J Pain Symptom Manage. 2002;23:3-5.
38. Guidelines for Monitoring and Management of Pediatric Patients During and After Sedation for Diagnostic and Therapeutic Procedures: An Update. Pediatrics 2006;118(6): 2587-602.
39. Schwartzberg LS. Chemotherapy-induced nausea and vomiting: which antiemetic for which therapy? Ncbi.nlm. nih.gov 2007;21(8):946-53.
40. Barnard DR, Friedman DL, Landier W, et al. Monitoring and management of drug toxicity. In: Altman AJ (Ed). Supportive Care of Children with Cancer. Current therapy and guidelines from the Children's Oncology Group, 3rd edn. Baltimore: The Johns Hopkins University Press; 2004.pp. 100-48.
41. Bechard LJ, Adiv OE, Jaksic T, Duggan C. Nutritional supportive care. In: Pizzo PA, Poplack DG (Eds). Principles and Practice of Pediatric Oncology, 4th edn. Philadelphia: Lippincott, Williams and Wilkins; 2002.pp.1285-300.

Hematological Manifestations of Systemic Diseases

Himani Manchanda, SP Yadav, Anupam Sachdeva

A varied spectrum of diseases affects the hematological system, ranging from simple nutritional deficiencies to the more sinister malignancies. This is an overview of the common systemic disorders and their hematological manifestations.

Hematological manifestations are due to a variety of causes. These include:

1. Bone marrow dysfunction
   - Anemia or polycythemia
   - Thrombocytopenia or thrombocytosis
   - Leukopenia or leukocytosis
2. Hemolysis
3. Immune cytopenias
4. Alterations in hemostasis
   - Acquired inhibitors to coagulation factors
   - Acquired von Willebrand's disease
   - Acquired platelet dysfunction
5. Alterations in leukocyte function.

CHRONIC ILLNESS

Chronic illnesses such as cancer, connective tissue disease, and chronic infections are associated with anemia. This anemia of chronic disease (ACD) has the following characteristics:

- Normochromic, normocytic, occasionally microcytic
- Usually mild, characterized by decreased plasma iron and normal or increased reticuloendothelial iron
- Impaired flow of iron from reticuloendothelial cells to the bone marrow
- Decreased sideroblasts in the bone marrow.

Small molecules, such as hepcidin, appear to play a key role in the development of the anemia of chronic disease through interference with iron absorption from the gut, as well as impairing iron release from macrophages.

Anemia of chronic disease is the most common anemia (more common than iron-deficiency anemia) in hospitalized patients. It occurs in those with chronic infection, chronic inflammation or malignancy. A similar anemia has recently been recognized in congestive heart failure and type 1 diabetes without significant renal failure (Table 27.1).

ACD presents as normocytic, normochromic anemia associated with low serum iron and reduced transferrin saturation (reduced total iron-binding capacity) and normal or elevated serum ferritin. It is not caused by bleeding, marrow replacement by tumor or deficiency of vitamin B_{12} folate or iron, though over time the anemia may become hypochromic and microcytic as a result of impaired release of iron from the reticuloendothelial system. In malignancy, other causes of anemia such as tumor infiltration of bone marrow and bleeding may further reduce hemoglobin levels.

The severity of the anemia correlates with the activity and severity of the underlying chronic disease. Successful therapy of this leads to a reduction in the levels of the mediator cytokines, increased Epo production and reduced inhibition of erythropoiesis. Correction of the anemia may take weeks or months. Pharmacological doses of recombinant Epo have been used successfully to improve anemia in patients with rheumatoid arthritis, cancer and myeloma. This observation suggests that inadequate Epo production and its reduced action are more important than

Table 27.1: Conditions associated with anemia of chronic disorders

- Chronic infections
- Especially osteomyelitis, bacterial endocarditis, tuberculosis, abscesses, bronchiectasis, chronic urinary tract infections
- Other chronic inflammatory disorders
- Rheumatoid arthritis, juvenile rheumatoid arthritis, polymyalgia rheumatica, systemic lupus erythematosus, scleroderma, inflammatory bowel diseases, thrombophlebitis
- Malignant diseases
- Carcinoma (especially metastatic or associated with infection), lymphoma, myeloma
- Others
- Congestive heart failure, ischemic heart disease, AIDS

disturbed iron metabolism in the pathogenesis of ACD. It further suggests that the suppressive action of various cytokines can be overcome by use of pharmacological doses of Epo. Iron therapy should be reserved for patients who have genuine iron deficiency.

CONNECTIVE TISSUE DISORDERS

Connective tissue disorders are a known to have varied hematological manifestations (Table 27.2). Some disorders are often brought to notice due to hematological symptom.

Systemic Lupus Erythematosus

Hematological involvement is common in systemic lupus erythematosus (SLE). Whilst anemia is most often due to chronic disease, other causes such as autoimmune hemolytic anemia and hypoplastic anemia need to be considered. The increased risk of infection in patients with SLE is due in part to changes in the white blood cells though treatments do not yet aim to modify these. Thrombocytopenia occurs frequently and is almost invariably autoimmune. It is often of little consequence, but may occasionally be severe and serious, requiring aggressive treatment. Patients with SLE have an increased risk of thrombosis, increased further in the presence of antiphospholipid antibodies (aPL). Changes in the hemostatic system and new insights into the nature of aPL are described elsewhere.

Table 27.2: Hematological changes in connective tissue damage

Anemia
- Anemia of chronic disease
- Iron deficiency (drug-induced blood loss)
- Folate deficiency
- Sideroblastic anemia
- Pure red cell aplasia (PRCA), especially in systemic lupus erythematosus (SLE)
- *Hemolytic anemia:* Immune (especially SLE)/non-immune

White cells
- Neutropenia (e.g. Felty's syndrome)
- Neutrophilia
- Eosinophilia (e.g. Churg-Strauss syndrome, polyarteritis nodosa)

Platelets
- Thrombocytopenia: Immune/nonimmune
- Platelet dysfunction
- Thrombotic thrombocytopenic purpura
- Thrombocytosis

Pancytopenia
- SLE

Coagulation
- Lupus inhibitor
- Specific factor deficiencies
- Disseminated intravascular coagulation

Others
- Myelofibrosis
- Drug related changes (e.g. aplastic anemia due to gold phenylbutazone; PRCA due to penicillamine)
- Cryoglobulinemia
- Amyloidosis

Rheumatoid Arthritis

The majority of patients with rheumatoid arthritis have a normochromic normocytic anemia of chronic disease. However, some patients may also be deficient in iron, folic acid, or vitamin B_{12}. Felty's syndrome occurs most commonly in patients in whom seropositive nodules develop. It is characterized by the triad of chronic and often quiescent rheumatoid arthritis, neutropenia, and splenomegaly, sometimes with lymphadenopathy, thrombocytopenia, and leg ulcers. Large granular lymphocytes can be seen in the peripheral blood and bone marrow in a subset of patients with rheumatoid arthritis.

Active rheumatoid disease is generally associated with an elevated erythrocyte sedimentation rate (a nonspecific indicator of inflammation). However, a number of investigators believe that C-reactive protein is a better measure of disease activity than the routine erythrocyte sedimentation rate. Other laboratory abnormalities include thrombocytosis (a reflection of acute and chronic inflammation), polyclonal or monoclonal hypergammaglobulinemia, and a positive antinuclear antibody assay.

In patients with Sjögren's syndrome, results positive for anti-SS-A or anti-SS-B antibodies may also be found. Patients with rheumatoid arthritis and concomitant autoimmune thyroiditis have antithyroglobulin or antithyroperoxidase antibodies.

The risk of lymphoma in patients with rheumatoid arthritis is independent of immunosuppressive therapy and is two to three times that of the general population. There is no association between rheumatoid arthritis and nonlymphoid malignancies.

INFECTIONS

Anemia

Chronic infections like tuberculosis are associated with ACD. Acute infections, particularly viral infections, can produce transient bone marrow aplasia or selective transient erythrocytopenia (Table 27.3). Parvovirus B19 infection in people with an underlying hemolytic disorder (such as sickle cell disease, hereditary spherocytosis) can produce a rapid fall in hemoglobin and an erythroblastopenic crisis marked by anemia and reticulocytopenia. There may be an associated

Table 27.3: Hematological changes in viral infection

Red cells
Anemia
Autoimmune
- Measles
- Epstein-Barr virus (EBV)
- Hepatitis
- Cytomegalovirus (CMV)
- Human immunodeficiency virus (HIV)
- Others including herpes viruses, varicella, influenza

Non-immune
Microangiopathic hemolytic anemia

Reduced red cell production
- Marrow hypoplasia
- EBV (especially in X-linked lymphoproliferative syndrome) hepatitis viruses
- HIV
- CMV (especially postrenal or bone marrow transplantation)
- Others (rare) include toga viruses epidemic hemorrhagic fevers, dengue

Red cell aplasia
B19 parvovirus, especially with hemolytic anemia

White cells
Neutrophilia
Especially HIV, influenza, hepatitis, rubella, adenoviruses, measles, mumps, CMV and EBV as part of nearly all viral infections

Neutropenia
- Aplasia (see above)
- Complicating myalgic encephalitis
- (Enteroviruses, EBV)

Lymphocytosis
- Wide variety, especially early in course of infection malignant transformation
- HTLV-1
- EBV
- HIV
- *Platelets*
- *Thrombocytosis* (e.g. Kawasaki disease)
- *Thrombocytopenia*
- Often history of viral prodromal in childhood immune thrombocytopenic purpura
  Autoimmune: EBV, hepatitis, rubella, CMV, HIV
  ↓ *Production:* Aplasia (see above), measles, dengue, CMV, others
  ↑ *Consumption:* Disseminated intravascular coagulation (DIC)/hemolytic uremic syndrome (HUS) (see below)
  Coagulation changes
- DIC, especially varicella, vaccinia, rubella, arbovirus with/without microangiopathy, epidemic hemorrhagic fevers
  Hemolytic-uremic syndrome: Coxsackie virus, mumps, echoviruses
- *Hemophagocytosis:* Herpes viruses, adenoviruses, cytomegalovirus

neutropenia. Many viral and bacterial illnesses may be associated with hemolysis.

White Cell Alterations

Viral and bacterial infections can produce leukopenia and neutropenia. Neutrophilia with an increased band count and left shift frequently results from bacterial infection. Neonates, particularly premature infants, may not develop an increase in white cell count in response to infection. Eosinophilia may develop in response to parasitic infections. Bacterial, fungal and protozoal infections can cause a lot of hematological manifestations (Table 27.4).

Table 27.4: Hematological changes in bacterial/fungal/protozoal infections

Anemia
- Anemia of chronic disorder
- *Hemolytic*
- *Immune:* Mycoplasma, malaria, syphilis (PCH), listeriosis
  Nonimmune: Clostridium perfringens (toxin related)
  Bartonella bacilliformis (Oroya fever)
- Malaria, trypanosomiasis with microangiopathy/ disseminated intravascular coagulation (DIC), septicemia
- *Hemolytic-uremic syndrome:* Verotoxin-producing *Escherichia coli* and *Streptococcus pneumoniae*
- *Dilutional*
- Splenomegaly (e.g. malaria, schistosomiasis)
- *Blood loss*
- *Helicobacter pylori*
- Ancylostoma

White cells
- *Neutrophilia*
- Virtually any bacterial/fungal infection
- *Neutropenia*
- *Salmonella, Rickettsia,* brucellosis, pertussis, disseminated tuberculosis (TB)
- Overwhelming septicemia
- *Neutrophil function* defects
- Rare (e.g. Bacteroides, endocarditis)
- *Lymphocytosis*
- Whooping cough *(Bordetella pertussis),* Rickettsia
- *Lymphopenia*
- TB, acute bacterial infections, brucellosis
- *Eosinophilia*
- *Aspergillosis,* Coccidioidomycosis, *Chlamydia,* streptococcal infections, *Ancylostoma*
- *Eosinopenia*
- Common in acute bacteroides infections
- *Monocytosis*
- Subacute/chronic infections (e.g. disseminated TB, listeriosis) pancytopenia
- Bone marrow suppression (e.g. disseminated TB, listeriosis)
- *Hemophagocytosis:* Septicemia
- Peripheral destruction (e.g. DIC)

Clotting Abnormalities

Severe infections, especially gram-negative sepsis, can produce disseminated intravascular coagulation (DIC).

Thrombocytopenia

Infection can produce thrombocytopenia through:
- Decreased marrow production
- Immune destruction
- DIC

VIRAL ILLNESSES WITH MARKED HEMATOLOGIC SEQUEL

Parvovirus

Parvovirus B19 is associated with transient erythroblastopenic crisis, particularly in individuals with an underlying hemolytic disorder. In addition, it can produce thrombocytopenia, neutropenia, and a hemophagocytic syndrome. In immunocompromised individuals, parvovirus B19 infection can produce prolonged aplasia.

Epstein-Barr Virus

Epstein-Barr virus (EBV) infection is associated with the following hematologic manifestations:
- Atypical lymphocytosis
- Acquired hemolytic anemia
- Agranulocytosis
- Aplastic anemia
- Lymphadenopathy and splenomegaly
- Immune thrombocytopenia

Epstein-Barr virus infection also has immunologic and oncologic associations:

X-linked lymphoproliferative syndrome is associated with fatal EBV infection, acquired hypogammaglobulinemia, and lymphoma. EBV has also been associated with clonal T-cell proliferations. EBV can produce an acquired hemophagocytic syndrome. EBV is associated with the endemic form of Burkitt's lymphoma in Africa.

Human Immunodeficiency Virus

The main pathophysiology of human immunodeficiency virus (HIV) infection is a constant decline in CD4+ lymphocytes, leading to immune collapse and death. The other bone marrow cell lines also decline in concert with CD4+ cell numbers as HIV disease (acquired immunodeficiency syndrome [AIDS]) progresses. HIV infection has the following hematologic manifestations:

1. *Thrombocytopenia:* Thrombocytopenia occurs in about 40% of patients with AIDS. Initially, the clinical findings resemble those of immune thrombocytopenic purpura (ITP). Some degree of splenomegaly is common and the platelet-associated antibodies are often in the form of immune complexes that may contain antibodies with anti-HIV specificity. Megakaryocytes are normal or increased and production of platelets is reduced in the bone marrow. Thrombotic thrombocytopenic purpura is also associated with HIV disease. This occurs in advanced AIDS.
2. *Anemia and neutropenia:* HIV-infected individuals develop progressive cytopenia as immunosuppression advances. Anemia occurs in approximately 70-80% of patients and neutropenia in 50%. Cytopenias in advanced HIV disease are often of complex etiology and include the following:

   A production defect appears to be most common. Antibody and immune complexes associated with red and white cell surfaces may contribute. Up to 40% have erythrocyte-associated antibodies. Specific antibodies against i and U antigens have occasionally been noted. About 70% of patients with AIDS have neutrophil-associated antibodies. The pathogenesis of the hematologic disorders include.

   Infections: Myelosuppression is frequently caused by involvement of the bone marrow by infecting organisms (e.g. mycobacteria, cytomegalovirus [CMV], parvovirus, fungi, and rarely, *Pneumocystis carinii*).

   Neoplasm: Non-Hodgkin's lymphoma (NHL) in AIDS patients is associated with infiltration of the bone marrow in up to 30% of cases. It is particularly prominent in the small noncleaved histologic subtype of NHL.

   Medication: Widely used antiviral agents in AIDS patients are myelotoxic, e.g. zidovudine (AZT) causes anemia in approximately 29% of patients. Gancyciovir and trimethoprim sulfame-thoxazole or pyrimethamine I sulfadiazine cause neutropenia. In general, bone marrow suppression is related to the dosage and to the stage of HIV disease. Importantly, the other nucleoside analogues of anti-HIV compounds (dideoxycytidine [ddC], dideoxyinosine [ddl], stavudine [d4T], or lamivudine [3TC], are usually not associated with significant myelotoxicity.
3. *Coagulation abnormalities:* The following abnormalities occur:

   Dysregulation of immunoglobulin production may affect the coagulation cascade. The dysregulation of immunoglobulin production may also occasionally result in beneficial effects, as in the resolution of antifactor VIII antibodies in HIV-infected hemophiliacs. Lupus-like anticoagulant (antiphospholioid antibodies) or anticardiolipin antibodies occur in 82% of patients. This is not associated with thrombosis in AIDS patients. Thrombosis may occur secondary to protein S deficiency. Low levels of protein S occur in 73% of patients.

Role of hematopoietic growth factors in acquired immunodeficiency syndrome

Erythropoietin: Recombinant human erythropoietin (rHuEPO) results in a significant improvement in hematocrit and reduces transfusion requirements while the patient is receiving zidovudine. rHuEPO therapy should be initiated if the erythropoietin threshold is <500 IU/L.

Neutrophil growth factors: Granulocyte colony-stimulating factor (G-CSF) in a dose of 5 μ/kg/day SC is the most widely used growth factor in neutropenia. Granulocytic-macrophage colony-stimulating factor (GM-CSF) improves neutrophil counts in drug-induced neutropenia. The effects of GM-CSF are seen within 24-48 hours with relatively low doses of (GM-CSF (0.1 μg/kg/day). Interleukin-3 (IL-3) given in doses of 0.5-5 mg/kg/day increases neutrophil counts.

4. *Cancers in children with human immunodeficiency virus infection:* Malignancies in children with HIV infection are not as common as those in adults. Table 27.5 shows the malignancies occurring in children with HIV infection in the order of frequency.

Non-Hodgkin's Lymphomas

Non-Hodgkin's lymphoma (NHL) is the most common malignancy secondary to HIV infection in children. It is usually of B-cell origin as in Burkitt's (small non-cleaved cell) or immunoblastic (large cell) NHL. The mean age of presentation of malignancy in congenitally transmitted disease is 35 months, with a range of 6 to 62 months. In transfusion-transmitted disease, the latency from the time of HIV seroconversion to the onset of lymphoma is 22-88 months. The CD4 lymphocyte count is less than 50/mm^3 at the time of diagnosis of the malignancy.

Table 27.5: AIDS-related neoplasms in children

- Non-Hodgkin's lymphoma
- Burkitt's lymphoma (B-cell, small noncleaved)
- Immunoblastic lymphoma (B-cell, large cell)
- Central nervous system lymphomas
- Mucosa-associated lymphoid tissue (MALT) type
- Leiomyosarcoma and Leiomyoma
- Kaposi's sarcoma
- Leukemias

The presenting manifestations include fever, weight loss, extranodal manifestations (e.g. hepatomegaly, jaundice, abdominal distension, bone marrow involvement, or central nervous system [CNS] symptoms).

Some patients will already have had lymphoproliferative diseases such as lymphocytic interstitial pneumonitis or pulmonary lymphoid hyperplasia. These children usually have advanced (stage III or IV) disease at the time of presentation.

Central Nervous System Lymphomas

Children with CNS lymphomas present with developmental delay or loss of developmental milestones or encephalopathy (dementia, cranial nerve palsies, seizures, or hemiparesis). Differential diagnosis include infections such as toxoplasmosis, cryptococcosis, or tuberculosis. Contrast-enhanced computed tomography (CT) studies of the brain show hyperdense mass lesions that are usually multicentric or periventricular. CNS lymphomas in AIDS are fast growing and often have central necrosis and a "rim of enhancement" as in an infectious lesion. A stereotactic biopsy will give a definitive diagnosis.

Treatment of HIV Infection-related Lymphomas

Treatment consists of standard protocols as described for non-Hodgkin's lymphoma.

Treatment of CNS lymphomas is more difficult. Intrathecal therapy is indicated even for those without evidence of meningeal or mass lesions at diagnosis of NHL. Radiation therapy may be a helpful adjunct for CNS involvement. The following are more favorable prognostic features in NHL secondary to AIDS:

CD4 lymphocyte count above 100/mm^3:

- Normal serum LDH level
- No prior AIDS-related symptoms
- Good Karnofsky score (80-100)

Proliferative Lesions of Mucosa-related (Associated) Lymphoid Tissue

Mucosa-related (associated) lymphoid tissue (MALT) shows reactive lymphoid follicles with prominent marginal zones containing centrocyte-like cells, lymphocytic infiltration of the epithelium (lymphoepithelial lesion), and the presence of plasma cells under the surface epithelium. These lesions may be associated with the mucosa of the gastrointestinal tract, Waldeyer's ring, salivary glands, respiratory tract, thyroid, and thymus. Proliferative lesions of MALT can be benign or malignant (such as lymphomas).

The proliferative lesions arising from MALT form a spectrum or a continuum extending from reactive to neoplastic lesions. The neoplastic lesions are usually low grade but may progress into high-grade MALT lymphomas (as shown in following table). MALT lymphomas characteristically remain localized, but if dissemination occurs, they are usually confined to the regional lymph nodes and other MALT sites. MALT lesions represent a category of pediatric HIV-associated disease that may arise from a combination of viral etiologies, including HIV, EBV, and CMV. Children have a different spectrum (Table 27.6) as compared to adults.

Alpha-interferon: 1,000,000 units/m^2 SC 3 times a week (continued until regression of disease or severe toxicity occurs). Rituximab (monoclonal antibody-against CD20) 375 mg/m^2 IV weekly for 4 weeks (courses may be repeated as clinically indicated). Some patients may not require any treatment because of the indolent nature of the disease.

Kaposi's Sarcoma

Kaposi's sarcoma (KS) is rare in children and constitutes the third most common malignancy in pediatric AIDS patients; it occurs in 25% of adults with AIDS. KS occurs only in those HIV-infected children who were born to mothers with HIV. The lymphadenopathic form of KS is seen mostly in Haitian and African children and may represent the epidemic form of KS unrelated to AIDS. The cutaneous form is a true indicator of the disease related to AIDS. Visceral involvement has not been pathologically documented in children with AIDS.

Table 27.6: Spectrum of systemic lymphoproliferation in children with AIDS

- Follicular hyperplasia (lymph nodes, gastrointestinal tract) lymphoid follicles/nodular (liver, thymus)
- Thymitis and multilocular thymic cyst
- PLH/LIP complex, typical and atypical
- Polyclonal polymorphic B-cell lymphoproliferative disorder
- Myoepithelial sialoadenitis
- Myoepithelial sialoadenitis with lymphoma
- MALT lymphoma (involving lungs, tonsils and salivary glands)
- Non-MALT lymphoma (involving nodal and extranodal sites)

Leukemia

Almost all leukemias are of B-cell origin. They represent the fourth most common malignancy in children with AIDS. The clinical presentation and biologic features are similar to those found in non-HIV children. Treatment involves chemotherapy designed for B-cell leukemia and lymphomas.

Miscellaneous Tumors

There is no increase of Hodgkin's disease in children with AIDS as compared to adult patients. Children with AIDS rarely develop hepatoblastoma, embryonal rhabdomyosarcoma, fibrosarcoma, and papillary carcinoma of the thyroid. The occurrence of these tumors is probably unrelated to the HIV infection.

Bone Marrow Infiltration

The bone marrow may be infiltrated by non-neoplastic diseases (storage diseases) or neoplastic diseases. In storage diseases, a diagnosis is established on the basis of the clinical picture, enzyme assays of while cells or cultured fibroblasts and bone marrow aspiration revealing the characteristic cells of the disorder. Neoplastic diseases may arise *de novo* in the marrow (leukemias) or invade the marrow as metastases from solid tumors (neuroblastoma or rhabdomyosarcoma). Following table lists the diseases that may infiltrate the marrow (Table 27.7).

Table 27.7: Diseases invading bone marrow

- Non-neoplastic
  A. Storage disease
    1. Gaucher's disease
    2. Niemann-Pick disease
    3. Cystine storage disease
  B. Osteopetrosis (Marble bone disease)
  C. Langerhans' cell histiocytosis
- Neoplastic
  A. Primary
    1. Leukemia
  B. Secondary
    1. Neuroblastoma
    2. Non-Hodgkin's lymphoma
    3. Hodgkin's lymphoma
    4. Wilms' tumor (rarely)
    5. Retinoblastoma
    6. Rhabdomyosarcoma

HEMATOLOGIC CHANGES ASSOCIATED WITH SPECIFIC INFECTIONS IN THE TROPICS

Malaria

Malaria is the most important parasitic illness of humans. It has been estimated that it has a global incidence of about 200 million cases per year with over 1 million deaths. Because of failure of eradication programs and increasing drug resistance, the problems of both treatment and control are becoming increasingly complex, and this condition remains one of the major unsolved world health problems.

Severe Malaria

Life-threatening complications are estimated to occur in about 1% of episodes of *P. falciparum* infection in children. They include profound anemia, cerebral malaria (a syndrome of unarousable coma, often accompanied by severe convulsions), hypoglycemia, jaundice, renal failure, pulmonary edema, and coagulation abnormalities. There are important and as yet largely unexplained differences in the clinical parts of the world. In Southeast Asia, all the aforementioned complications are commonly seen, whereas in Africa, where cerebral malaria and severe malarial anemia together account for over 1 million deaths a year and hypoglycemia with malaria are surprisingly rare. The burden of malarial illness falls mostly on children in Africa, whereas adults are more commonly affected in some other parts of the world; it has been suggested that much of the variation in clinical symptomatology is age related.

Malarial Anemia

The pattern of hematological changes in malaria varies considerably, depending of the type of patient. During an acute attack of *P. falciparum* malaria in a nonimmune person, the hematocrit starts to fall after antimalarial treatment has been given subsequently, there is usually a steady rise, although it may take several weeks before the hematologic picture is back to normal. The anemia, which is not usually life threatening is characterized by both hemolysis and an ineffective erythropoiesis.

From the perspective of tropical child health, the most important hematological problem is the child chronically infected with *P. falciparum*, whose anemia is debilitating and sometimes fatal. Although this is most commonly seen in areas of high malarial transmission, it is a growing problem in regions of lower transmission because of the rise in antimalarial drug resistance, which has served to prolong the average duration of infection. Attempts to investigate the problem of chronic malarial anemia are often hampered by the coexistence of iron or folate deficiency and by the hemoglobinopathies. In a study in which these were carefully excluded, the most striking pathophysiologic findings were hemolysis, hypersplenism and a suboptimal bone marrow response.

Role of Hemolysis

Normal children living in rural Africa typically have extremely low levels of haptoglobin that rise significantly after malaria prevention programs, providing some indication of the burden of chronic hemolysis that malaria imposes on many tropical communities. The mechanisms of red cell destruction in falciparum malaria are complex and not fully understood. Clearly, erythrocytes are destroyed when schizonts rupture to release their progeny, and, depending on the state of immunity, a proportion of parasitized erythrocytes are destroyed by the host before schizont rupture can occur. Both mechanisms can have devastating consequences if the patient is hyperparasitemic (sometimes more than 50% of erythrocytes are infected), but such cases are rare. In most infections less than 1% of erythrocytes are infected, a loss that is important in the context of chronic infection but which would not account for the severity of anemia that is commonly observed. It is likely that uninfected erythrocytes are also destroyed, because cross-transfusion experiments clearly indicate that their survival is shortened both in the acute phase of malaria and in convalescence. Evidence is increasing that the spleen may play an important role in such nonspecific destruction of erythrocytes.

Role of the Spleen

Some degree of splenomegaly is a normal feature of malarial infection, and the prevalence of splenomegaly in regions of malarial transmission is used as a major indicator of the level of malarial endemicity. The importance of the spleen in host defense against malaria has been demonstrated in experimental systems, and individuals whose spleens have been surgically removed are more susceptible to severe infection. It is thought that the phenomenon of parasitic sequestration, discussed earlier strategy whereby the mature parasite can avoid passing through the spleen.

Several studies have attempted to define the pathophysiologic changes in the spleen during acute malaria. The available evidence all points to increased reticuloendothelial clearance in *P. falciparum* malaria, persisting long after recovery. Although these changes are presumably a host defence mechanism, serving to maximize the clearance of parasitized erythrocytes, it is clear that the survival of uninfected red cells is reduced in the process.

These observations in patients are consistent with findings at the cellular level. Active erythrophagocytosis is a conspicuous feature within the bone marrow during *P. vivax* and falciparum malaria, have high circulating levels of interferon-γ and TNF, a synergistic combination of cytokines that activate macrophages. With relatively nonspecific effector mechanisms such as erythrophagocytosis within the spleen, anemia is part of the price the host has to pay for protection against overwhelming parasitemia.

Massive Intravascular Hemolysis

A peculiar example of malaria-associated hemolysis is *blackwater fever*. This syndrome, which was frequently reported in colonial times among Europeans living in Africa, was characterized by massive intravascular hemolysis with low or absent parasitemia, leading to renal failure and was associated with a high mortality. It was suspected that intermittent quinine ingestion might have led to a drug induced immune hemolysis, although this was never proved. Classic blackwater fever seems to have largely disappeared, but massive intravascular hemolysis with hemoglobinuria remains an important complication of *P. falciparum* malaria in Southeast Asia, affecting both children and adults. This is sometimes associated with high parasitemia or destruction of G6PD-deficient red cells by oxidant antimalarial drugs. However, follow-up studies in patients who survived episodes of this type have shown that many of them do not have any definable red cell enzyme deficiency, and it has not been possible to obtain any evidence for a quinine-induced immune hemolysis. It is conceivable that hemolysis is caused simply by the rupture of a large number of sequestered parasites, but the possibility of another hemolytic process has yet to be ruled out.

Immune-mediated Hemolysis

Considerable interest has developed regarding the possibility that at least some of the hemolysis in *P. falciparum* malaria might have an immune basis. This followed the observation that some patients with malaria develop a positive Coombs direct antiglobulin test (DAT).

The little evidence exists for immune destruction of red cells in *P. falciparum* malaria in nonimmune adults. Although a varying proportion of children with chronic malaria in Africa have a positive DAT, it is only quite exceptionally that there is evidence of genuine immune destruction of the red cells. It is possible, of course that a sensitized red cell population is very rapidly destroyed and that subsequent serologic studies have missed this event. However, the persistence of a shortened red cell survival of nonparasitized cells in the absence of any consistent serologic abnormalities suggests that there must be another factor involved in shortening the red cell survival in malaria. This appears to be nonspecific "over activity" of the monocyte/macrophage populations of the spleen and liver.

Defective Marrow Response

As well as the hemolytic components to be the anemia of falciparum malaria, there is undoubtedly an inappropriate marrow response. It has been noted for many years that the reticulocytosis in response to the fall in hematocrit is often inappropriate low and delayed. Work over the past few years has suggested that this also has a complex multifactorial basis.

Some of the features of iron metabolism and bone marrow morphology and function in acute malaria resemble those of other acute infections. Thus the serum iron level rapidly falls and iron appears to be sequestrated into the storage compartments of the marrow. Serum ferritin levels are extremely high during the acute phase, although studies of isoferritins suggest a complex source, in many cases it appears that much of the ferritin is released as a consequence of liver damage.

During acute malarial infections there may be quite marked dyserythropoietic changes in the bone marrow. Although these are most marked in African children with chronic relapsing malaria, they have also been observed in nonimmune Thais and in travelers returning to the United Kingdom. These morphologic abnormalities, which have been studied by both light and electron microscopy, consist of erythroblast multinuclearity, karyorrhexis, incomplete and unequal amitotic nuclear divisions, and cytoplasmic bridging. On electron microscopy, binucleate or multinucleate erythroblasts bizarre myelination with loss of parts of the nuclear membrane and widening of the space between the two layers of the nuclear membrane have been observed, there appears to be some degree of iron loading of the mitochondria and a reduction of the electron density of the cytoplasmic matrix together with paucity of ribosomes. In addition, in acute cases, sequestration of erythrocytes in the sinuses of the bone marrow is widespread.

By using tritiated thymidine autoradiography it is clear that there is a significant abnormality of red cell proliferation in the bone marrow in acute malaria. Changes include an increased proportion of red cell precursors in G2 and arrest in progress of cells during the S phase. These findings are nonspecific and have been observed in other conditions associated with ineffective erythropoiesis.

In addition to these dyserythropoietic changes, erythrophagocytosis is particularly common in the bone marrow in *P. falciparum* malaria. This phenomenon is not restricted to the marrow and may be seen in the spleen and other organs and, as mentioned earlier, may play an important role in the hemolytic component of the disease.

Although the mechanism of these dyserythropoietic changes in unknown, it is possible that they are an exaggerated example of the bone marrow suppression that occurs in other situations of chronic infection. An important factor may be the high levels of TNF production that occur during malarial infection, because this cytokine has been strongly implicated in the anemia of chronic infection. TNF suppresses proliferation of erythroid progenitor cells in human marrow cultures, although this declines as the cells differentiate. Chronic malaria has nonspecific features that might augment these effects, because huge numbers of pigment particles are ingested by the resident macrophages of the spleen and marrow, providing a sustained stimulus for TNF production at the site of erythropoiesis.

Coagulation Abnormalities

Thrombocytopenia is a common finding during acute *P. falciparum* attacks, and occasionally the platelet count falls as low as 10,000 to 20,000/ ml, the mechanism has not been determined, although experimental studies in mice suggest that platelets sequester in venules during malarial infection. The adherence of platelets to epithelium appears to be mediated through a specific receptor-ligand interaction involving leukocyte function associated antigen (LFA-1). Some patients with severe falciparum malaria may develop a severe bleeding diathesis during the acute phase of the illness. It has been suggested that this results from disseminated intravascular coagulation although studies in Thailand have not substantiated this. Rather, the bleeding appears to reflect gross thrombocytopenia together with liver damage. However, it is becoming apparent that some patients with severe falciparum malaria and shock have coexistent gram-negative septicemia, a setting in which disseminated intravascular coagulation may be found.

HYPER-REACTIVE MALARIAL SPLENOMEGALY SYNDROME

Although splenomegaly is a feature of many tropical disorders, there is increasing evidence, particularly from work in East, West Africa and New Guinea, that there is a specific entity, formerly known as the tropical splenomegaly syndrome that occurs widely through Africa, India and Southeast Asia. This condition is characterized by gross splenomegaly a high level of malaria antibody titers, and serum IgM levels, at least 2 standard deviations above the local mean. The classic syndrome regresses after prolonged antimalarial prophylaxis with proguanil, a dihydrofolate reductase inhibitor.

Etiology and Pathophysiology

Evidence is increasing that malaria plays an important role in this syndrome. Epidemiologic studies indicate that its prevalence is related to patterns of malarial transmission, and affected individuals have higher malarial antibody titers than those who live in the same environment and are unaffected; this seems to involve IgM rather than IgG. These observations, together with' the partial clinical response to treatment with anti-malarials and the fact that individuals with the sickle cell trait seem to be partially protected, suggest that the condition probably results from an unusual form of immune response to chronic malarial infection. For this reason it is now commonly referred to as hyper-reactive malarial splenomegaly (HMS).

With progressive splenomegaly there is pooling of the formed elements of the blood; in patients with particularly large spleens one-third to one-half of the total circulating red cell mass may be sequestered. This produces a dilutional anemia that is made worse by an absolute increase in the plasma volume. There is also pooling of neutrophils and platelets so that the hematologic picture is characterized by a pancytopenia. No characteristic changes are seen in the bone marrow.

Some evidence exists of genetic predisposition to HMS. For some years researchers have debated whether it is premalignant, because it sometimes becomes refractory to antimalarial treatment, and it can also be associated with a lymphocytosis resembling chronic lymphocytic leukemia. Clonal rearrangements of the jH region of the immunoglobulin gene have been noted in some patients whose clinical syndrome appeared intermediate between HMS and chronic lymphocytic leukemia, suggesting HMS has premalignant potential.

CLINICAL FEATURES

The clinical picture of HMS is typical, with massive splenomegaly, weight loss, and a variable degree of anemia. Serum IgM levels is high, and there may be a relative increase in T-lymphocytes in the peripheral blood. The serum also may show increased cold agglutinin titers and an increase in rheumatoid factor, antibodies to thyroglobulin and antinuclear factor, and circulating immune complexes.

This condition has a remarkably poor prognosis, with up to 50% mortality in some populations. It is managed by long-term antimalarial prophylaxis, most commonly with proguanil.

Visceral Leishmaniasis (Kala-azar)

Leishmaniasis is an infection caused by intracellular protozoan parasites transmitted by various species of sandflies. Human infections can result in three main forms of disease: cutaneous, mucocutaneous and visceral (kala-azar).

The important hematologic manifestations of leishmanial infections are found in the visceral forms.

The generalized form of leishmanial disease involves the liver, spleen, bone marrow, and lymph nodes and is caused by organisms belonging to tile *Leishmania donovani* complex. The parent species, *L. donovani* is found throughout Asia and Africa and can affect individuals of all ages. There is a variety, which affects children more often than adults and is known as *L. donovani* infantum. Although visceral leishmaniasis is primarily a disease of indigenous populations, it may be contracted on short-term visits.

Although the incubation period is usually 1 to 3 months, it can be as short as a few weeks. The onset is usually insidious with fever, sweating, malaise and anorexia, although a much more acute onset may occur. As the disease progresses the acute symptoms abate, but there is gradual enlargement of the spleen and anorexia. Generalized lymphadenopathy is also present.

The hematologic findings in the later stages of the illness are characterized by anemia, neutropenia, and thrombocytopenia, a picture characteristic of hypersplenism. The bone marrow is hyperplastic with dyserythropoietic changes, and the diagnosis can usually be made by finding Leishman-Donovan bodies, (Fig. 35.2 from the book *Advances in Pediatrics*) which are macrophages containing intracellular organisms with characteristic staining properties. The diagnosis can also be made from splenic or lymph node punctures.

Red cell survival studies and ferrokinetic analyzes have suggested that hemolysis is the major cause of anemia in leishmaniasis but that there may also be plasma volume expansion associated with the massively enlarged spleen. Surprisingly, ferrokinetic studies have shown very little evidence of ineffective erythropoiesis, but a reduced plasma iron level in the presence of greatly increased iron stores suggests that the reticulo-endothelial hyperplasia is accompanied by abnormal iron detention by macrophages, typical of the anemia of chronic disorders. This may limit the marrow response to hemolysis.

In infants or young children with acute visceral leishmaniasis, the clinical and hematologic findings may differ from those described earlier. For example, in Mediterranean populations it is very common to observe a very rapid onset of anemia with severe hemolysis. Occasionally, IgG is found on the red cells, but this is not consistent and its significance remains to be determined. In most cases there is no evidence of immune hemolysis and it appears that nonsensitized red cells are destroyed in the macrophages that are recruited to the spleen and liver as part of the inflammatory response to the parasite. Severe neutropenia may also occur in young children, and this, together with dyserythropoietic changes in the marrow, marked erythrophagocytosis, and bizarre mononuclear infiltrates, may cause the disease to be confused with leukemia.

Dengue

The dengue viruses are four antigenically related but distinct organisms that are transmitted to humans by mosquitoes of the species *Aedes aegypti*. The clinical manifestations of this very common infection vary in different parts of the world. In American, African, and Indian populations the disease is characterized by classic dengue fever, but in Southeast Asia many children with dengue infections develop a much more serious condition, dengue hemorrhagic fever/dengue shock syndrome (DHF/DSS). The latter develops in infants born to dengue-immune mothers during initial infections or in children over the age of 1 year during secondary infections. It appears that this curious paradox reflects enhancement of dengue viral infection in mononuclear phagocytes mediated by sub-neutralizing concentrations of dengue antibody.

The pathophysiology of DHF/DSS is remarkable. Dengue viruses appear to be parasites of mononuclear phagocytes. Furthermore, they use antibody as a specific receptor for gaining entry to these cells. Such antibodies are known as infection-enhancing antibodies. Epidemiologic studies have shown that children 1 year old or older always have detectable dengue antibody before acquiring a subsequent infection that results in DHF/DSS. It is also clear that infants who acquire dengue antibody passively form their mothers are at risk of developing the syndrome. The syndrome of DHF/DSS is characterized by the simultaneous activation of the complement and hemostatic systems together with a marked increase in vascular permeability. It appears that complement activation follows both the classical and alternative pathways. The hemostatic abnormalities include gross thrombocytopenia, prolonged bleeding time, elevated prothrombin time, and a reduction in factors II, V, VII, and IX together with marked hypofibrinogenemia and an increase in fibrin degradation products. The vascular permeability abnormalities are characterized by an elevated hematocrit, normal or low serum protein levels due to selective loss of albumin, and variable serous effusions.

Precisely what triggers these remarkable events is not clear. However, it seems likely that the mediators are the product of dengue virus-infected mononuclear phagocytes. Studies in Thailand have suggested that low levels of heterotypic neutralizing antibodies from a single previous infection prevent the illness in those who acquire dengue type 2 infections. On the other hand, children with circulating dengue-enhancing antibodies but with no neutralizing antibodies are at high-risk.

However, once DHF has been triggered, the immune disturbance is not confined to antibodies. Both the CD4+ and CD8+ subpopulations of T-lymphocytes are more intensively activated in DHF than in uncomplicated dengue fever. High levels of TNF and other procoagulant cytokines may also contribute to the pathology. A further factor may be antibodies to plasminogen that are found in a significant proportion of dengue infections, particularly if hemorrhage is present. These antibodies are thought to arise because of structural homology between plasminogen and the dengue envelope glycoprotein.

The clinical picture of DHF/DSS is characterized by fever, malaise, and anorexia and about 2 to 5 days later by a second phase in which there are widespread hemorrhagic phenomena, including purpura, large spontaneous ecchymoses, and bleeding from previous venipuncture sites. These children may then pass into a phase of profound shock. The hematologic findings are characterized by a high hematocrit (due to hemoconcentration) associated with gross thrombocytopenia and evidence of disseminated intravascular coagulation.

The fact that the most serious pathophysiologic mechanism in this disease is fluid loss rather than hemorrhage has directed attention toward the development of treatment regimens rather similar to those used in the management of severe diarrheal illnesses in children in the tropics. When hemorrhage is a major problem, it is best managed with fresh blood transfusion and platelet replacement. Clinical trials of heparin to counteract disseminated intravascular coagulation have not given impressive results.

Hookworm

It has been estimated that more than 900 million people are infected with hookworms. There are two main species, *Ancylostoma duodenale* and *Necator americanus*, sometimes called the Old and New World hookworms, respectively. Both species are widely distributed in tropical and subtropical Asia and Africa. The prevalence of infection varies from 80 to 90% in rural areas in the moist parts of the tropics, such as West Bengal, to 10 to 20% in relatively dry countries, such as those of the Middle East and Pakistan.

Both species of hookworm produce enormous numbers of eggs, in the region of 20,000 per day per female. The eggs are discharged into the intestinal lumen where they undergo a number of cell divisions before being passed in the stools. Given appropriate conditions the eggs develop further and hatch, liberating larvae. These free-living stages go through a series of developments, designated L1 to L3, after which they penetrate the skin and the infective filarial larval forms migrate to the intestinal tract through the circulation lung, and respiratory tract. The final larval stage, L4, and the adult worms are found in the small intestine.

Hookworms attach to the mucosa of the upper intestine by their buccal capsules. Although they are found mainly in the jejunum, in very heavy infections they may be distributed as low as the ileum. Attachment of the worms results in bleeding into the gastrointestinal tract.

The worms change their attachment site every few hours. Continuous or intermittent suction causes tissue and blood to be drawn into the worm's intestinal tract. Direct recordings of blood loss have given values on the order of 0.03 ml/day per worm for *N. americanus* and up to 0.26 ml/day per worm for *A. duodenale*. Only about 50% of the iron lost as hemoglobin into the gut may be reabsorbed. Therefore, the marked increase in fecal iron is related directly to the worm load. The latter is assessed by the fecal egg count.

The hematologic findings in children or adults with heavy hookworm infections are characteristic. Because the disease is usually chronic, anemia is the major clinical feature. In severe cases, hemoglobin and a normal reticulocyte count. There is a low serum iron level, and iron is absent from the bone marrow stores. Because of associated protein loss, affected children are often hypoalbuminemic. There may be a mild eosinophilia in established cases, although very high eosinophil counts may occur during the phase of the illness in which the worms are migrating from the skin to the gastrointestinal tract.

The diagnosis is made by analysis of the stools for eggs. In heavy infections it is only necessary to examine a fecal film directly after mounting the sample in saline or iodine solution. Lighter infections require concentration by zinc sulfate flotation.

As well as treatment with antihelminthics, affected children require oral iron treatment to restore the iron stores. Although many of these children are severely anemic, they have had chronic anemia for many years and rapid restoration of the hemoglobin level is not usually required. However, in profoundly anemic children with high output failure and associated hypoalbuminemia, it may be necessary to administer red cells slowly, together with appropriate diuretics. These children may have greatly increased blood volumes and it is easy to precipitate circulatory overload and cardiac failure. If there is severe heart failure, it is sometimes helpful to exchange transfuse by removing blood from one arm while infusing red cells into the other. Whatever method is chosen, it is essential to monitor the patient's central venous pressure.

Tropical Eosinophilia

After anemia, eosinophilia is probably the most common hematologic abnormality in children in the developing world. An increase in eosinophils in the bone marrow and peripheral blood, as well as in the tissues, is a major feature of infections caused by worms that migrate through extraintestinal organs. There is a strong association between eosinophilia and infections with tissue nematodes, trematodes, or cestodes. In contrast, however, there is no well-documented evidence that worms do not invade tissues or that protozoal infections are associated with elevated eosinophil counts.

The term tropical eosinophilia syndrome was first used in the 1940's to describe patients who present with a paroxysmal cough and wheezing, particularly at night; scanty sputum production; weight loss; low-grade fever; lymphadenopathy; and an extreme blood eosinophilia (greater than 3000/μL). It was discovered later that this syndrome is due to filarial infection.

The hypereosinophil syndrome is seen in children or young adults and is found most commonly in India, Indonesia, Sri Lanka, Pakistan, and Southeast Asia, although it may occur in any area where human filariasis is common. In addition to these typical clinical and hematologic findings, these patients have very high levels of serum IgE together with increased levels of specific antifilarial antibodies. Although it is usually easy to make this diagnosis in tropical countries, other conditions that cause eosinophilia have to be considered. These include chronic eosinophilic pneumonia, allergic aspergillosis, vasculitic syndromes, and the idiopathic hypereosinophil syndrome. The major distinguishing features that identify the tropical hypereosinophil syndrome are the marked elevation of antifilarial antibody together with the very high IgE levels. It may be possible to identify filarial organisms on blood films. Traditionally, it is better to prepare these from blood samples taken at night, although some studies suggest that this may not be necessary.

What is the best approach to arriving at a diagnosis in a child who presents with a persistent eosinophilia? A careful respiratory history should be taken. Detailed studies of stools for cysts and ova should be carried out on a number of occasions by an experienced observer. Serologic studies for Filaria, *Toxocara*, and *Trichinella* infection should be carried out, and immunoglobulin levels should be determined. If these investigations fail to reach a diagnosis it is important to exclude non-tropical causes of eosinophilia, including collagen vascular disease, allergy, drug reactions, lymphoma, and leukemia associated with an eosinophil response. It may be necessary to initiate a trial of the antifilarial drug diethylcarbamazine as part of the diagnostic work-up.

Endocrinal Disorders and Hematological Manifestations

A variety of hematological manifestations are seen with endocrinal disorders. Most are due to disease process, may be due to drug treatment or associated conditions. Table 27.8 lists the manifestations and probable suggested causes of the hematological manifestations in common endocrinal dysfunctions.

Hematologic Aspects of Liver Diseases

Liver diseases are second only to bone marrow diseases in causing hematological changes. Liver, as we all know, is an important source of Epo in fetus. It is the prominent in utero hematopoietic organ in first 4-5 months of life. In *ex utero* life, it is a principal organ of extramedullary hematopoiesis. Hematological manifestations of a varied spectrum are seen in acute as well as chronic liver

Table 27.8: Hematological changes in endocrine disease

Red cells
- Anemia
- Thyrotoxicosis (normochromic, normocytic or microcytic)
- Hypothyroidism (normochromic, normocytic, occasionally macrocytic)
- Diabetes mellitus (usually when complicated by infection, cardiac disease, renal failure, enteropathy)
- Hyperparathyroidism (normochromic, normocytic)
- Hypoadrenalism (normochromic, normocytic)
- Hypogonadism (normochromic, normocytic)
- Hypopituitarism (normochromic, normocytic)
- Polycythemia (pseudo)
- Pheochromocytoma
- Cushing's syndrome

White cells

Cushing's syndrome Pheochromocytoma	Neutrophil leukocytosis
Hyperthyroidism	Lymphocytosis
Leukopenia	Antithyroid drugs
Diabetes mellitus	Impaired polymorph function

Platelets

Diabetes mellitus Hyperthyroidism	Abnormal platelet function

Coagulopathy

Diabetes mellitus	↑ Platelet aggregability, ↓ prostacyclin, ↑ factor VIII, ↓AT
Estrogen therapy	↑ Factor VIII, ↑vWF
Cushing's syndrome	↑ Factors II, IV, IX, XI, XII

disorders. Table 27.9 lists the common dysfunctions seen and their probable causes.

Hematologic Aspects of Kidney Diseases

Kidney is the major site of EPO production and hence kidney disorders, especially chronic kidney diseases are associated with a varied spectrum of hematological disorders.

Anemia is the most important hematological abnormality and its management has been revolutionized by the availability of recombinant human erythropoietin (rEPO). Patients with acute or chronic renal failure develop a normochromic, normocytic anemia, with the presence of ecchinocytes (burr cells) in the blood film. The reticulocyte count is normal or slightly low, and the bone marrow shows normoblastic erythropoiesis without the erythroid hyperplasia expected at that level of anemia. Patients who have undergone nephrectomy tend to be more severely anemic than patients with polycystic disease. Reduced Epo levels occur in renal failure and this is the dominant cause of anemia.

Table 27.9: Hematological changes in liver disease

Red cells
Anemia
- Anemia of chronic disease
- Folate deficiency
- Iron deficiency (blood loss)
- Aplastic anemia (viral hepatitis, rare)
- Sideroblastic (alcohol)
- Hypersplenism
- Microangiopathy/disseminated intravascular coagulation (DIC) (rare)
- Autoimmune (rare)
- Zieve's syndrome (rare)#
- Polycythemia
- Hepatocellular carcinoma (rare)
- Infectious hepatitis (rare)

White cells
- *Neutrophilia*
- Infection
- Hemorrhage
- Malignancy
- Hemolysis
- *Neutrophil function*
- Impaired chemotaxis (due to lowered complement levels)
- *Neutropenia*
- Hypersplenism
- Eosinophilia
- Parasitic infestation
- Chronic active hepatitis (rare)

Platelets
- *Thrombocytopenia*
- Hypersplenism, hepatic sequestration
- DIC
- Autoimmune (e.g. associated with viral hepatitis, primary biliary cirrhosis)
- Postliver transplantation
- *Thrombocytosis*
- Hepatoma (rare)
- Impaired platelet function
- Inhibitory factors (including high-density lipoprotein and apolipoprotein E)

Other
- Benign monoclonal gammopathy (biliary + other cirrhosis)
- Cryoglobulinemia (hepatitis B, hepatitis C, alcohol)

Zieve's syndrome hemolytic anemia with hypertriglyceridemia in alcoholic liver disease

Red cell survival is diminished in renal failure, but this is also a minor factor. Iron deficiency can arise through blood loss (exacerbated by hemodialysis). Folate deficiency arises in dialyzed patients but is now prevented by prophylactic folic acid therapy.

Recombinant EPO therapy can fully correct anemia in renal failure. It can be administered intravenously, subcutaneously or intraperitoneally. The subcutaneous route is effective at lower doses, and it is usual to commence 5-75 U/kg per week, given in two or three divided doses. Anemia is corrected up to a level of 10 -12 g/dl at a rate of 1 g/dl per month. Subclinical iron deficiency and impaired mobilization of storage iron are often present, so concomitant iron therapy is usually required. An impaired response to rEPO should prompt a suspicion of iron, cobalamin or folate deficiency, hemolysis, infection, occult malignancy, aluminium toxicity and hyperparathyroidism. Hypertension occurs in about one-third of rEPO-treated patients and is dose dependent; the risk of thrombosis of an arteriovenous fistula is also increased. In acute renal failure, anemia is commonly due to the drug or condition causing the renal failure, e.g. hemolysis due to sepsis or TTP.

Hematologic Aspects of Malabsorption in the Tropics

One of the major difficulties in discussing the problem of malabsorption in the tropics is its definition. A large proportion of people in tropical climates, both the indigenous populations and expatriates who have lived and worked in rural areas, have mild abnormalities of the intestinal mucosa, often associated with impairment of absorption. These structural and functional alterations of the gut have been called tropical enteropathy. It is likely that they reflect an adaptation to life in the contaminated environment of the tropics with its frequent enteric infections and differences of diet. Interestingly, similar morphologic lesions have been demonstrated in the colon of otherwise healthy residents of Southern India. Once expatriates return to temperate climates these changes revert to normal.

The more severe malabsorption syndromes, called sprue and postinfective malabsorption, are associated with chronic diarrhea, wasting and a variety of hematologic changes.

The English physician Manson while working in China first coined the term sprue; it is an Anglicization of the Dutch term Indische sprouw. During the 19th and 20th centuries tropical sprue was thought to be a disease of expatriates, but during World War II it became apparent that similar syndromes occur frequently in indigenous populations. Severe malabsorption syndromes are not distributed evenly in the tropical world. They are particularly common in the Indian subcontinent, Burma, Malaysia, Vietnam, Borneo, Indonesia, and the Philippines. They are also seen in the West Indies, in parts of Central America (Particularly Puerto Rico, Cuba, and the Dominican Republic), and in northern parts of South America. There are a few reports from the Middle East and from temperate areas. Tropical Africa seems to be spared.

It is believed that these syndromes have an infective origin. They usually present as an acute attack of diarrhea, which then becomes chronic. Many well-documented epidemics of sprue have been reported both in South India and in American military personnel in the Philippines. But despite a vast amount of work and the establishment of units specifically to study the problem, no organism has been isolated that would meet Koch's postulates. It may well be that these disorders can follow a variety of infective agents, but the reason for the peculiar geographic distribution remains unexplained. Remarkably, genetic factors have been almost totally ignored in the investigation of this disease.

Tropical malabsorption syndromes can occur in individuals of any age. They are characterized by intermittent diarrhea, weight loss, and anemia. Varying degree of mucosal damage is found on biopsy of the small intestine, although an absolutely flat mucosa, as seen in gluten-induced enteropathy, is rare. The hematologic findings in the tropical malabsorption syndromes vary considerably. In more advanced cases megaloblastic anemia is common. It is usually caused by folate deficiency but may also be complicated by vitamin B_{12} deficiency. Often bizarre pictures of iron and folic acid deficiency are found.

Interestingly, although much of the data are uncontrolled, it appears that many of the symptoms and hematologic changes associated with these syndromes can be reversed by a course of oral tetracycline. However, recovery is much more rapid if folate or vitamin B_{12} treatment is given.

It should be remembered that in a tropical setting malabsorption could also result from colonization of the small bowel by specific parasites, including *Giardia lamblia, Strongyloides stercoralis, Cryptosporidium,* and others. Furthermore, abdominal tuberculosis with malabsorption is particularly common, and in Africa HIV infection may be an important cause underlying the severe wasting that can occur with HIV infections.

It should be emphasized, particularly for hematologists without tropical experience, that the clinical and hematologic picture of tropical malabsorption syndromes could be extreme. Particularly in young children there may not always be a good history of diarrheal illness, and in many tropical populations this is the norm anyway. Folate deficiency, as well as anemia, may give rise to severe neutropenia and thrombocytopenia with associated infection or bleeding.

If there is intercurrent infection, as is often the case in severely affected children, the bone marrow appearances may be deceiving, although there is nearly always some megaloblastic changes even if the overall picture is much less hyperplastic than is usually observed with folate or vitamin B_{12} deficiency in Western settings.

A major diagnostic problem that is often encountered in children returning from the tropics with persistent diarrhea and malabsorption is whether they have postinfective malabsorption or celiac disease. If symptoms do not settle, it may be necessary to initiate a trial of a gluten free diet and then to reintroduce gluten at a later date and to monitor progress with repeated small bowel biopsies.

BIBLIOGRAPHY

1. Dallalio G, Fleury T, Neans RT. Serum hepicidin in clinical specimens. British Journal of Haematology. 2003;122:996-1000.
2. Delamore IW, Liu Yin JA. Haematological Aspects of Systemic Disease. Baillière Tindall, London, 1990.
3. Gransvswsky MO, Mueller BU, Nicholson HS, Rosenberg PS, Rabkin CS. Cancer in human immunodeficiency virus-infected children: a case series from the Children's Cancer Group and the National Cancer Institute. J Clin Oncol. 1998; 16:1729.
4. Hoffbrand AV, Pettit JE. Essential Haematology, 4th edn. Oxford: Blackwell Science, 2001.
5. McClain KL, Joshi VV. Cancer in children with HIV infection. Hematol Oncol Clin N Am. 1996;10:1189.
6. Means RT. Advances in the anaemia of chronic disease. International Journal of Haematology. 1999;70:7-12.
7. Scadden DT. Hematologic disorders and growth factor in HIV infection. Hemato Oncol Clin N Am. 1996;10:1149.
8. Spivak, JL. The blood in systemic disorders. Lancet 2002;355:1707-12.
9. Stockman J, Ezekowitz A. Hematologic manifestations of systemic diseases. In: Nathan D, Orkin S (Eds). Nathan and Oski's Hematology of infancy and childhood, 6th edn. Philadelphia, Saunders; 2003. pp. 1760-829.

28 Disseminated Intravascular Coagulation

Mir Sadaqat Hassan Zafar, SP Yadav, Vinita Jain, Anupam Sachdeva

INTRODUCTION

The hallmark of normal hemostasis is the exquisite regulation of a focussed event, i.e. the formation of a hemostatic plug, at the site of injury to a blood vessel. The antithesis of this is what occurs in disseminated intrvascular coagulation (DIC).

Disseminated intravascular coagulation is an acquired syndrome characterized by the intravascular activation of coagulation with loss of localization arising from different causes. It can originate from and cause damage to the microvasculature, which if sufficiently severe, can produce organ dysfunction. DIC is described as inappropriate response to a hemostatic challenge threatening the viability of the individual. The activation of the fibrinolytic system is initially directed at clearing the vasculature of unwanted deposits of fibrin, due to the lack of specificity of plasmin and the consequent proteolytic degradation of essential cofactors of coagulation such as factors V and VIII, it may eventually compromise hemostasis.[1]

Consumption and subsequent exhaustion of coagulation proteins and platelets, due to the ongoing activation of the coagulation system, may induce severe bleeding complications. Derrangement of the fibrinolytic system further contributes to intravascular clot formation, but in some cases accelerated fibrinolysis (e.g. due to consumption of α2-antiplasmin) may cause severe bleeding. Hence, a patient with DIC can present with simultaneous thrombotic and bleeding problem, which obviously complicates treatment (Fig. 28.1).[2] With possibly the only exception of venom, DIC is a secondary response to a pre-existing primary pathology, i.e. it is an intermediary mechanism of disease.[3]

In DIC the demonstration of increased plasma levels of coagulation activation markers, e.g. an increase of the prothrombin fragment 1+2 (F1+2) or thrombin-antithrombin (TAT) complexes, indicates an activation of the coagulation system and should have, preferably, been called "hypercoagulable state". This should not be termed DIC but may, under certain conditions, be a prodromal state of DIC. Equally well, an increase in fibrinopeptide A (FPA) may be indicative of DIC but it does not prove its existence because proteolysis of fibrinogen by thrombin could have occurred in the extravascular space.

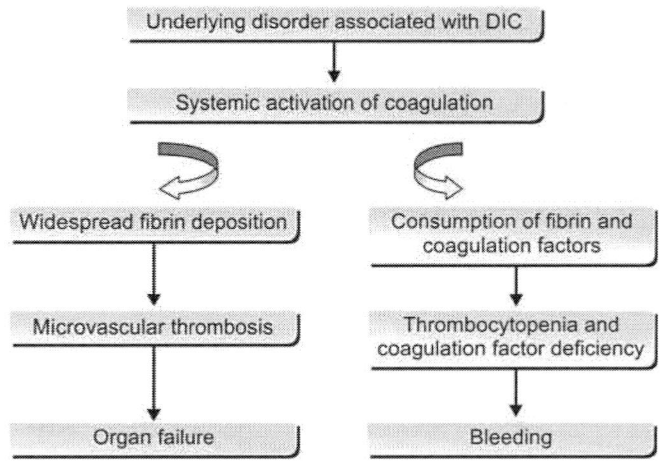

Fig. 28.1: Processes in DIC[2]

EPIDEMIOLOGY

Disseminated intravascular coagulation occurs in an estimated 1% of all hospitalized patients. Precise numbers on the occurrence of DIC are not known. The frequency of DIC should be seen in relation to the underlying disease. In virtually all patients with gram negative septicemia, overt, DIC can be found in 30 to 50% of patients. Severe trauma with inflammatory response may be associated with DIC in 50-70% of cases. This is closely related to the disease severity scores. Giant hemangiomas are associated with clinically significant DIC in up to 25% cases. Male and female sex is equally affected, besides no prediliction for any particular age group except the neonates who are more prone to DIC.[4]

Table 28.1: Various etiologies of DIC[5]

Causes	Acute DIC	Chronic DIC
Medical	Septicemia/Infections Fulminant hepatic failure Allergic reactions Transplantation Heat stroke Hypothermia Leukemia Homozygous protein C deficiency Snake bites	Solid tumors Liver cirrhosis Allergic reactions Vasculitis Kasabach-Merritt syndrome Adult respiratory distress syndrome Leukemia
Surgical	Poly-trauma Major operations Brain injury Extracorporeal circulation Thermal injury Fat embolism Cardiac bypass surgery Peritoneovenous shunt	Organ transplantation Aortic aneurysm Vascular tumors
Obstetrics and Gynecology	Amniotic fluid embolism Abruptio placentae Septic abortion Acute fatty liver Uterine rupture Toxemia of pregnancy Septicemia	Late gestation HELLP syndrome Retained dead fetus
Transfusion Medicine	Acute hemolytic transfusion reaction Massive transfusion Artificial surfaces	

ETIOLOGY

Disseminated intravascular coagulation occurs in a variety of clinical conditions (Table 28.1).[5] In older infants and children, the important causes of DIC include sepsis, trauma, and malignancies. In the neonate, DIC is caused primarily by sepsis and perinatal complications (e.g. birth asphyxia).

Older Infants and Children

Sepsis

This is the most common cause of DIC in older infants and children. DIC was classically recognized as a complication of endothelial damage produced by meningococcemia. Viral, rickettsial, fungal, parasitic, and other bacterial infections are also associated with DIC. Subsequently, the syndrome has been described with a variety of gram-negative and gram-positive organisms. As an example, overt DIC occurs in 30 to 50% of patients with Gram-negative sepsis.[6,7]

In animal models of endotoxin induced DIC, there is evidence that the pathogenesis involves both thrombin generation and suppression of normal antithrombotic mechanisms with down-regulation of the protein C/thrombomodulin system and perhaps impaired fibrinolysis. The balance between thrombin generation, clotting factor depletion, and thrombolysis determines the clinical presentation (i.e. bleeding or thrombosis).[8]

Shock is associated with reduced blood flow (which diminishes the beneficial effects of hemodilution) and tissue damage (which promotes further thrombin formation). Impaired hepatic perfusion or function causes inadequate hepatic removal of circulating activated procoagulants.

In sepsis-induced DIC, activation of the extrinsic pathway appears to be the primary activating pathway.[9] Endotoxemia also activates factor XII of the intrinsic pathway. This can lead to conversion of prekallikrein to kallikrein and kininogen into circulating kinins which can mediate increased vascular permeability, vasodilatation, and shock.[10] In experimental models of DIC, inhibition of intrinsic pathway activation ameliorates the hypotension but not the DIC.

Activation of coagulation is a consequence of endothelial damage and enhanced expression and release of granulocyte and macrophage procoagulant substances, such as tissue factor. Increased expression and release may be a direct action of endotoxin and other membrane lipopolysaccharides or it may be indirect with mediation via activation of cytokines, such as interleukin-6 and tumor necrosis factor alpha.[11] An additional mechanism may be involved in patients with meningococcal sepsis, which is associated with high levels of circulating microparticles, originating from platelets or granulocytes, and having procoagulant activity. In one report, the patients with the most severe manifestations had microparticles which, when added to normal plasma *in vitro*, generated a substantial amount of thrombin.[12]

Gram-positive bacteremias, including *Staphylococcus aureus, Streptococcus pneumoniae,* and *Clostridium perfringens,* also can be associated with DIC.[13-15] A variety of other infections, particularly viral infections (e.g. varicella, hepatitis) have rarely been associated with DIC.

Trauma and Tissue Injury

In children, DIC potentially is a serious complication of any major trauma or tissue injury. These include crush injury, massive burns, extensive surgery, severe hypothermia, heat exhaustion, and shock. In all these cases, release of tissue enzymes and phospholipids from damaged tissue into the systemic circulation triggers activation of the coagulation system. Brain tissue is a potent thromboplastin and patients who sustain severe brain injury are especially at risk for DIC.

Malignancy

In children with leukemia, laboratory abnormalities in the clotting system are common. DIC is rare in children with acute lymphocytic leukemia, although it has been reported in patients with the uncommon t(17;19) translocation. Patients with acute promyelocytic leukemia can present with acute hemorrhage due to DIC. In these patients, granules within the blast cells contain procoagulants that directly trigger the coagulation system.[16]

Miscellaneous

Acute hemolytic transfusion reactions: Release of adenosine diphosphate and phospholipids from the hemolyzed red cell activate platelet and the coagulation system respectively.

Kasabach Merritt (KM) syndrome: Patients with kaposiform hemangioendothelioma, an aggressive form of giant hemangioma, can develop KM syndrome, a localized form of DIC. The large hemangioma consumes fibrinogen and platelets resulting in thrombocytopenia and consumptive coagulopathy.

Snake and spider venoms: The venom of some snakes and spiders (e.g. rattlesnakes and Russell's viper) can directly activate the coagulation system and lead to DIC.

Liver disease: Disseminated intravascular coagulation (DIC) may be seen in patients with acute or chronic hepatocellular disease including Reye's syndrome.[17]

Neonates: Newborn infants, particularly preterm infants, are vulnerable to DIC because the anticoagulants, antithrombin, and protein C are normally low at this age. The main causes of DIC include sepsis, birth asphyxia, respiratory distress syndrome (RDS), and necrotizing enterocolitis (NEC). Neonatal viral infections (e.g. rubella, herpes, cytomegalovirus, and enterovirus), systemic candidiasis, and bacterial sepsis (e.g. Group B *Streptococcus* and gram-negative organisms) are causes of neonatal DIC.[18]

Perinatal conditions: Perinatal conditions associated with DIC include complications from pregnancy and delivery that lead to birth asphyxia, and diseases linked to prematurity.[19]

Obstetric complications: Fetal anoxia/birth asphyxia may cause neonatal DIC. These include abruptio placenta, preeclampsia, eclampsia, and fetal distress during labor.

Conditions associated with prematurity: Disseminated intravascular coagulation (DIC) is associated with necrotizing enterocolitis (NEC) and respiratory distress syndrome (RDS), both of which are seen more frequently in premature infants. In patients with NEC, ischemic bowel tissue releases tissue factor, which activates the coagulation system. Patients with severe RDS are also at risk for DIC presumably due to tissue damage from hypoxia. Autopsy studies in preterm infants with RDS have demonstrated fibrin deposition not only in the lungs but also the liver and kidney. Rare causes of neonatal DIC include hypothermia and massive hemolysis, such as seen in Rh incompatibility.

Congenital disorders: Congenital homozygous deficiency of protein C and S can present in the neonatal period with DIC and purpura fulminans, while neonates who have large hemangiomas can develop Kasabach Merritt syndrome.

GENETIC RISK FACTORS

It still remains a question whether genetic protein abnormalities contribute to the development of DIC. More studies are necessary to elucidate this subject. It may be that insight in the relationship between risk factors and DIC leads to adjustment of treatment to individual patients and, ultimately, to a better outcome of DIC. Inherited abnormalities of coagulation proteins that are essential for the pathophysiology of DIC, could contribute to the risk for DIC. Relatively few studies addressed this issue, in particular in meningococcal disease, which is often complicated by sepsis and DIC. Data from these studies suggest that inherited coagulation differences, PAI1 promoter polymorphisms and Factor V Leiden mutation, may affect the outcome in meningococcal disease. These data are very limited and controversial, Heterozygous protein C and S deficiencies could also be candidate risk factors for DIC because of the known relationship between homozygosity for protein C and S and development of spontaneous DIC in neonates. So far, there are only case reports but no controlled studies on this subject.[20,21]

PATHOPHYSIOLOGY

Disseminated intravascular coagulation is a complex disorder with variable pathophysiology highly dependent on the triggering event, the host response, and comorbid conditions. Our understanding of the pathogenesis of DIC comes from animal and human experimental models as well as from clinical experience in patients with sepsis.[22,23] Several reactions have been considered to play important role in the pathogenesis of DIC. These include: generation of a hyperthrombinemic state, alterations of physiologic anticoagulants, inhibition and impairment of the fibrinolytic mechanism, and activation of proinflammatory cytokines.

Generation of a Hyperthrombinemic State

It appears that the tissue factor (TF) pathway, rather than the contact factor pathway, plays the dominant role in the development of a hyperthrombinemic state in DIC, as suggested by experimental models of human endotoxemia.[24] In these models of endotoxin-induced DIC, increases in the mediator tumor necrosis factor (TNF) and release of interleukin IL-6 failed to show any change in the markers of activation of the contact system.[25] In contrast, blockage of the TF/factor VIIa pathway using monoclonal antibody directed against TF completely inhibited thrombin generation and prevented the onset of DIC.[26] The TF pathway can be activated by tissue injury, such as can occur in severe trauma, septicemia, or cancer. Severe trauma, inducing release of tissue phospholipids, can initiate activation of the clotting cascade. Once released, TF complexes with factor VII, which is activated by factor Xa to form the TF/VIIa complex. This complex activates factor IX and factor X, leading to the development of thrombin.[27] Thrombin plays an important role in conversion of fibrinogen into fibrin.[28] Thrombin can further activate factor V to Va and factor VIII to VIIIa, rapidly amplifying thrombin generation.

Alteration in Physiologic Anticoagulants

Normally, thrombin levels are regulated by the natural anticoagulants antithrombin, protein C, and TF pathway inhibitor (TFPI). Antithrombin and protein C have been shown to be markedly decreased in DIC. Antithrombin levels can be lowered as a result of consumption by the elaborated thrombin. In addition, interaction with elastase released from the neutrophils in septicemia, and anoxic liver impairment can cause decreased levels of antithrombin. Levels of protein C, another important inhibitor, can also fall due to capillary leakage, decreased synthesis from liver injury, and/or reductions in thrombomodulin expression on the vascular surface (downregulation). This occurs because of a release of TNF-α and other proinflammatory cytokines.[29-31]

Impaired Fibrinolysis in Onset of DIC

An experimental model of DIC in sepsis has shown increased fibrinolytic activity due to release of tissue plasminogen activator (TPA) from endothelial cells. This hyperfibrinolysis is followed by rapid release of plasminogen activator inhibitor 1 (PAI-1), which suppresses fibrinolysis, thus playing an important role in the pathogenesis of DIC. A functional mutation of the PAI-1 gene (4G/5G polymorphism) has also been demonstrated in DIC. This mutation induces increased plasma levels of PAI-1.[32,33]

Activation and Liberation of Inflammatory Cytokines in Pathogenesis of DIC

It is thought that activation of the clotting system concomitantly leads to activation of inflammatory cascades, which, in turn, induce endothelial cell synthesis of proinflammatory cytokines. These cytokines and other inflammatory mediators can lead to coagulation. The inflammatory cytokine thrombin and other serine proteases interact with protease-activated receptors on the cell surfaces, thereby inducing further inflammatory and clotting responses. Activated protein C (APC) has been considered to be a mediator of anti-inflammatory responses. This mediation occurs by its inhibition of endotoxin-induced production of TNF, IL-1β, IL-6, and IL-8. Therefore, depletion of protein C can induce and enhance a proinflammatory state, which can lead to activation of coagulation reactions.[34,35]

Excessive bleeding in patients with DIC has been reported after routine dental extractions, hip replacement, aortic aneurysm, leukemic states, and other disorders. Although the majority of elderly patients with DIC have the chronic form, severe acute bleeding can occur in this population.

DIC, therefore, can be considered to be a two-phase thrombohemorrhagic phenomenon, with thrombosis sometimes leading to bleeding. Clinical conditions underlying DIC can initiate hypercoagulability by activation of the clotting cascade along with depletion of natural anticoagulants, elaboration of proinflammatory cytokines, and abnormalities of the fibrinolytic pathway. This hypercoagulable state, if it continues to progress, can lead to depletion of clotting factors and platelets through utilization, and can sometimes lead to a bleeding diathesis (consumptive coagulopathy).[36,37]

CLINICAL PRESENTATION

The clinical presentation may vary in relationship to the primary condition. Clinical findings vary depending on the severity of DIC. In mild cases, bleeding may only be noted at venipuncture sites, but in other cases there may be severe hemorrhage and thrombosis with end-organ damage to the kidney, liver, lung, central nervous system (CNS), and extremities. Hemorrhage is the most common presentation followed by skin manifestations of purpura and acral gangrene (purpura fulminans). In neonates, the most common sites of bleeding are the gastrointestinal tract and venipuncture sites. In severe cases, intrapulmonary and intraventricular hemorrhages occur. Risk factors for DIC in neonates include prematurity, low birth weight, and low Apgar scores.[38]

Acute DIC

This is the most common form of DIC seen in clinical practice. Bleeding manifestations predominate and can be normally progressive. In some patients large acral cyanosis is seen due to thrombic occlusion of dermal vessels.

Chronic DIC

This occurs from a weak or intermittent activating stimulus. The destruction and production of clotting factors and platelets is balanced, so that the DIC is considered to be compensated. Chronic DIC is most commonly seen in patients with intrauterine fetal death, adenocarcinoma and other tumors, giant hemangiomas and certain types of vasculitis. Patients may have recurrent episodes of ecchymosis or mild bleeding and thrombophlebitis at unusual sites. Trousseau's sign is a form of chronic DIC.

LABORATORY EVALUATION

There is no single laboratory test that can establish or rule out the diagnosis of DIC. Thus, it is of utmost importance to assess the whole clinical picture, taking into account the clinical condition of the patient, the diagnosis, and all available laboratory results (Table 28.2).[39]

As such, a diagnosis of DIC should be made based on an appropriate clinical suspicion supported by relevant laboratory tests.[40] Because DIC is a continuously progressive process, it can be subdivided into three phases that might be helpful in making the diagnosis and in treating the patient.

Phase I: Compensated Activation of the Hemostatic System

During this phase, no clinical findings are observed, but the underlying disease may raise suspicion for the occurrence of DIC. Under these circumstances, tests

Table 28.2: Abnormalities of laboratory assays in DIC[39]

- Prolongation of prothrombin time
- Prolongation of activated partial thromboplastin time
- Decrease in platelet count
- Peripheral smear examination: schistocytes
- Decrease in fibrinogen
- Decrease in factor V
- Decrease in factor VIII
- Increase in fibrin split products (FSP)
- Increase in D-dimer
- Increase in prothrombin fragment 1+2
- Increase in soluble fibrin monomer
- Increase in plasmin
- Increase in fibrinopeptide A
- Increase in fibrinopeptide B
- Increase in thrombin-antithrombin complex

should be performed to demonstrate the activation of coagulation.

Phase II: Decompensated Activation of the Hemostatic System

In contrast to phase I, the prothrombin time (PT) and the activated partial thromboplastin time (aPTT) are prolonged. Under these circumstances, the thrombin time may still be normal, as the fibrinogen levels are still adequate and the level of fibrinogen degradation products (FDPs) is not very high. In this phase, frequent analyses are necessary to demonstrate the dynamics of the intravascular coagulation process. In phase II, repeated determinations will demonstrate a continuous drop in platelet count and in fibrinogen concentration and coagulation factor activities, especially factor V activity.

Phase III: Full-Blown DIC

Full-blown DIC is characterized by an extremely prolonged PT and aPTT. Frequently, the thrombin time is significantly prolonged. During this phase, the platelet count is very low, and the coagulation factor activities are less than 50% of normal. The continuous transition from phase I to phase II or even to phase III is typical for DIC. If, in the course of DIC, hemolysis and/or schistocytes are observed, this indicates that microclot formation is causing red blood cell damage.

Laboratory findings in DIC are classified based upon the pathologic process, i.e. consumption of coagulation factors and platelets, increased fibrin formation and increased fibrinolysis.

Consumption

Tests that show consumption of clotting factors and platelets include the following:

Platelet count: Thrombocytopenia (platelet count <100,000 per mm^3) usually is present in patient with DIC. On the peripheral smear, platelets are large, suggesting a destructive process.

Prothrombin time (PT): The PT is prolonged in 50 to 75% of cases. A prolonged PT reflects a reduction in the activity of the extrinsic and common coagulation pathways.

Activated partial thromboplastin time (aPTT): The aPTT is prolonged in 50 to 60% of cases. A prolonged aPTT reflects a reduction in the activity of the intrinsic and common coagulation pathways.

Factor V and VIII levels: Both Factor V (common coagulation pathway) and factor VIII (intrinsic pathway) are decreased. Some patients with DIC will have a normal PT and aPTT as noted above. This may be due to circulating activated clotting factors such as thrombin and factor Xa.[41]

Fibrin formation: Studies indicative of fibrin formation include:

Fibrinogen: When the fibrinogen concentration is low, it is consistent with a diagnosis of DIC due to its consumption in the formation of fibrin. However, fibrinogen is not a sensitive test for DIC because it is also an acute phase reactant. When the concentration is normal, it may represent a significant decrease in a patient whose fibrinogen level should be higher because of the inflammation from his/her underlying disease.

Thrombin time: Thrombin time is prolonged when the fibrinogen concentration is low. FDPs also impair fibrin formation, thereby prolonging the thrombin time.

Microangiopathic hemolytic anemia: Microangiopathic changes on the peripheral smear are suggestive of DIC and are due to mechanical shearing of red blood cells by intravascular fibrin strands.

Fibrinolysis: Disseminated intravascular coagulation (DIC) is unlikely if there is no evidence of fibrinolysis as indicated by the following:

Fibrin degradation products (FDPs): FDPs are products of plasmin degradation of fibrinogen and fibrin. They are present in 85 to 100% of patients with DIC. However, FDPs are not a specific test, since they are also present in patients who have systemic lupus erythematous, necrotizing enterocolitis, thrombotic events from causes other than DIC, and in some individuals taking oral contraceptives.

D-dimer: D-dimer is a neoantigen produced when cross-linked fibrin is degraded by plasmin. It is elevated in 90% of patients with DIC and is more specific than FDPs.[42]

Other Studies

Disseminated intravascular coagulation (DIC) is also characterized by decreased levels of antithrombin, and protein C and S, which lead to impairment of the anticoagulant pathway. Despite the decreased concentration of these anticoagulants, their measurement generally is not helpful in clinical management.

There are several other tests for DIC that may prove to be helpful but are not widely available or used.

Procoagulant Activation

Commercial assays are available to measure markers of procoagulant activation such as prothrombin fragment 1+2, fibrinopeptide A and fibrinopeptide B, and thrombin-antithrombin (TAT) complexes. Fibrinolysis can be detected by elevated levels of plasmin and plasmin-antiplasmin (PAP) complex. In neonates, establishing normal values for clotting factors and coagulation tests have been hampered by:

- Changes in concentration of coagulation factors and coagulation test values with gestational and postnatal age.
- Difficulties in obtaining adequate control groups of healthy preterm and term infants.

Normal ranges for coagulation tests and concentrations of specific clotting factors have been reported for full term infants and preterm infants (>30 weeks gestation) from birth to six months postnatal age.[43]

When interpreting coagulation tests, it is imperative to recognize the differences in the normal values of coagulation tests between the neonatal and adult patient. As an example, aPTT is normally prolonged in full term infants at birth compared to adults (mean values, 42.9 ± 11.6 versus 33.5 ± 6.8 sec, respectively).[44]

This difference is even greater in the preterm infant (mean value for infants 30 to 36 weeks gestation, 53.6 ± 26.1). The aPTT in both preterm and term infants decreases to adult values by six months of age.

Physiologic levels of factors V, VIII, and fibrinogen in full term infants are similar to those in adults and can serve as diagnostic markers for DIC in this age group. In preterm infants, fibrinogen concentration is low and D-dimer is commonly present without DIC, limiting their value in the diagnosis of DIC. In addition, neonates have relatively decreased amounts of plasma due to their higher hematocrit levels and, therefore, it is imperative that the correct anticoagulant to plasma ratio is obtained in the blood specimens to ensure accurate testing.

DIAGNOSIS

The diagnosis of overt DIC is based upon clinical findings of hemorrhage and microthrombi in patients with predisposing medical conditions and abnormal coagulation studies (Table 28.3).[45] Although laboratory studies are used to support the diagnosis, there is no single test that is sensitive or specific enough to assure a definite diagnosis. A reasonable panel of coagulation studies to establish the diagnosis includes:

- Complete blood count (CBC)
- Prothrombin time (PT)
- Activated partial thromboplastin time (aPTT)
- D-dimer level
- Fibrinogen level
- Factor V and VIII levels

Table 28.3: Reliability of laboratory tests in DIC (descending order of reliability)[45]

- Profragment 1+2
- D-dimer*
- Antithrombin III
- Thrombin precursor protein
- Fibrinopeptide A
- Platelet factor IV
- Fibrin degradation product*
- Platelet count*
- Protamine test
- Thrombin time
- Fibrinogen*
- Prothrombin time*
- Activated partial thromboplastin time*
- Reptilase time

*Tests that are used in common practice

Adding to the challenge of establishing the diagnosis, every patient with DIC does not have positive findings consistent with DIC in all laboratory studies. The most helpful tests clinically are those that indicate the presence of fibrinolysis (e.g. FDPs and D-dimers). D-dimer is a more specific test for DIC than FDPs. The latex agglutination assay for D-dimer is commonly used and is one of the more reliable tests. In addition, decreased levels of factors V and VIII help substantiate the diagnosis of DIC.

Serial measurements of coagulation parameters are more informative than laboratory measurements performed at a single time point. As an example, a prothrombin time, which is in the upper normal range but is significantly longer than an earlier measurement, reflects the consumptive process of DIC and not a normal hemostatic state. Serial measurements of platelet counts that document a downward trend are a sensitive but not specific sign for DIC.[46]

Neonatal Diagnosis

Similar to older patients, the diagnosis of DIC in the neonate relies on abnormal global coagulation tests in the appropriate clinical setting. However, it is more difficult to establish the diagnosis of DIC in these patients. Testing is limited because the volume of blood required may be difficult to attain in the neonate. In addition, the interpretation of these studies in the neonate is challenging as the hemostatic system is still in a state of flux at birth with physiologic alterations of coagulation and fibrinolysis. As a result, the diagnosis of DIC in the neonate may rely more heavily on the patient's clinical manifestations than on laboratory studies. The recognition of the underlying condition rather than establishing the diagnosis of DIC is more important as the most important therapeutic intervention is to treat the underlying disorder.

DIFFERENTIAL DIAGNOSIS

A number of clinical disorders not associated with DIC can result in an acquired bleeding diathesis and significant hemostatic laboratory abnormalities. A difficult clinical problem occurs in the patient with sepsis. Sepsis without DIC can be associated with a variable degree of thrombocytopenia; however, sepsis with platelet counts less than 50,000 is most often associated with DIC. Some other important differential diagnosis of DIC are depicted as following Table 28.4.[47]

SCORING SYSTEM

A scoring system to simplify the diagnosis of DIC has been developed by the DIC subcommittee of the International Society on Thrombosis and Hemostasis (ISTH).[48] This scoring system is based upon:

- Patients having a medical condition known to be associated with DIC.
- Readily available global coagulation tests that include platelet count, FDPs, PT, and fibrinogen concentration

Scores are dependent on the degree of abnormality measured by each test. As an example, a platelet count <50,000/μl is scored higher than one that is <100,000/μl Table 28.5.[2]

A preliminary study in critically ill adults with DIC reported 91% sensitivity and 97% specificity for the ISTH scoring system compared to clinical expert opinion. A review of the literature demonstrated several studies that have reported accurate prediction of mortality with the use of this scoring system. The system score also correlated with other markers of DIC including decreased antithrombin and protein C activity, and increased TAT complexes and soluble fibrin levels. The DIC subcommittee of the ISTH is developing a similar template for children and infants.

MANAGEMENT (ACUTE DISSEMINATED INTRAVASCULAR COAGULATION)

General

Key to the treatment of DIC is the specific and vigorous treatment of the underlying disorder. In many cases the DIC will spontaneously resolve when the underlying disorder is properly managed. Examples are the administration of antibiotics and/or surgical drainage in patients with DIC due to severe infection and sepsis. However, in some cases additional supportive treatment, specifically aimed at the coagulation abnormalities, may be required.

The overall approach is to restrain and eventually eliminate thrombin generation and replace blood components whose deficiency might either promote the hemorrhagic tendency or diminish the physiological anticoagulant response in endogenously regulating thrombin generation.

Table 28.4: Differential diagnosis of DIC[47]

Condition	*Similarities*	*Difference*
Liver disease	Bleeding common PT, APTT abnormal Platelet count low Fibrinogen low	D-dimer usually normal* FVIII levels not affected
Microangiopathic hemolytic anemia (e.g. HELLP, TTP)†	Microthrombi common Platelet count low	Bleeding uncommon Coagulation tests normal†
Hyperfibrinolysis	PT, APTT abnormal Fibrinogen low	Platelet count normal
Catastrophic antiphospholipid antibody syndrome	PT, APTT abnormal Platelet count low	Fibrinogen not low D-dimer normal‡
Massive transfusion	PT, APTT abnormal Fibrinogen low Platelet count low	D-dimer normal

*Unless additional disorders which increase the D-dimer coexist.
†Unless coexisting DIC.
‡ Some antibodies can affect the D-dimer results.
Abbreviations: HELLP: Hemolysis, elevated liver enzymes, low platelet count (syndrome); TTP: Thrombotic thrombocytopenic purpura

Table 28.5: ISTH diagnostic scoring system for DIC[2]

Scoring system in overt DIC

Risk assessment: Does the patient have an underlying disorder known to be associated with overt DIC?

If yes: Proceed

If no: Do not use this algorithm

Order global coagulation tests (PT, platelet count, fibrinogen, fibrin related marker)

Score the test results:

- *Platelet count* (>100 × 10^9/L = 0, <100 × 10^9/L = 1, <50 × 10^9/L = 2)
- *Elevated fibrin marker* (e.g. D-dimer, fibrin degradation products) (no increase = 0, moderate increase = 2, strong increase = 3)
- *Prolonged PT* (<3 s = 0, >3 but <6 s = 1, >6 s = 2)
- *Fibrinogen level* (>1 g/L = 0, <1 g/L = 1)

Calculate score

- ≥5 compatible with overt DIC: repeat score daily
- <5 suggestive for nonovert DIC: repeat next 1–2 day

Plasma and Platelets

Transfusion of platelets or plasma (components) in patients with DIC should not primarily be based on laboratory results and should in general be reserved for patients that present with bleeding. In patients with DIC and bleeding or at high-risk of bleeding (e.g. postoperative patients or patients due to undergo an invasive procedure) and a platelet count of <50 × 10^9/l, transfusion of platelets should be considered. In nonbleeding patients with DIC, prophylactic platelet transfusion is not given unless it is perceived that there is a high-risk of bleeding. In bleeding patients with DIC and prolonged PT and aPTT administration of FFP may be useful. There is no evidence that infusion of plasma stimulates the ongoing activation of coagulation. If transfusion of FFP is not possible in patients with bleeding because of fluid overload, consider using factor concentrates such as prothrombin complex concentrate, recognizing that these will only partially correct the defect because they contain only selected factors, whereas in DIC there is a global deficiency of coagulation factors. Severe hypofibrinogenemia (<1 g/L) that persists despite FFP replacement may be treated with fibrinogen concentrate or cryoprecipitate.[49]

Anticoagulants

In cases of DIC where thrombosis predominates, such as arterial or venous thromboembolism, severe purpura fulminans associated with acral ischemia or vascular skin infarction therapeutic doses of heparin should be considered. In those patients where there is perceived to be a coexisting high-risk of bleeding there may be benefits in using continuous infusion UFH due to its short half-life and reversibility. Weight adjusted doses (e.g. 10 U/kg/h) may be used without the intention of prolonging the aPTT ratio to 1.5-2.5 times the control. Monitoring the aPTT in these cases may be complicated and clinical observation for signs of bleeding is important. In critically ill, nonbleeding patients with DIC, prophylaxis for venous thromboembolism with prophylactic doses of heparin or low molecular weight heparin is recommended.[50,51]

Anticoagulant Factor Concentrates

Consider treating patients with severe sepsis and DIC with recombinant human activated protein C (continuous infusion, 24 μg/kg/h for 4 days). Patients at high-risk of bleeding should not be given recombinant human activated protein C. Current manufacturers guidance advises against using this product in patients with platelet counts of <30 × 10^9/L. In the event of invasive procedures, administration of recombinant human activated protein C should be discontinued shortly before the intervention (elimination half-life-20 min) and may be resumed a few hours later, dependent on the clinical situation. In the absence of further prospective evidence from randomized controlled trials confirming a beneficial effect of antithrombin concentrate on clinically relevant endpoints in patients with DIC and not receiving heparin, administration of antithrombin cannot be recommended.[52,53]

Antifibrinolytics

In general, patients with DIC should not be treated with antifibrinolytic agents. Patients with DIC that is characterized by a primary hyperfibrinolytic state and who present with severe bleeding could be treated with lysine analogues, such as tranexamic acid.[54]

Newer Strategies

Antithrombin (AT III): The circulating levels of AT are low in DIC, therefore supplementation should improve the outcome. However, studies are needed to confirm these findings.[55]

Tissue factor pathway inhibitor (TFPI): Since TF/ factor VIIa pathway plays a major role in coagulation activation in sepsis, TFPI substitution seems to be a reasonable option. It was tested in a phase III trial in patients with severe sepsis. Tifacogin (TFPI) was given in a dose of 0.025 mg/kg/hr for 96 hours. There was no effect on mortality and the risk of bleeding was increased.[56]

Protease Inhibitors

Gabexate mesylate is a synthetic inhibitor of serine proteases, including thrombin and plasmin. It would therefore seem to be a potentially useful agent for treating disseminated intravascular coagulation. In a limited number of patients, the drug (2 mg/kg/hr x 7 days) could not inhibit coagulation or fibrinolysis, improve the DIC score or reduce mortality in pre or mild DIC.[57]

C1-Inhibitor (C1-Inh)

Activation of factor XIa leads to a thrombin burst, therefore inhibition of factor XIa by C1-inhibitor might be beneficial. In a pilot study with limited number C1-inhibitor patients, C1-Inh was administered to patients with severe sepsis or septic shock. Organ dysfunction improved significantly but no effect on mortality was observed due to small number of patients.[4]

Synthetic Inhibitors

Heparin treatment may be ineffective because it requires antithrombin for anticoagulant activity and this is usually reduced in DIC. Direct thrombin inhibitors may be more effective as they do not require antithrombin. Recombinant hirudin reduces thrombin activity in DIC, but clinical benefit has not yet been evaluated. Novel antithrombin III—independent inhibitors of thrombin such as desirudin and related compounds, might be more effective than heparin, and experimental studies have had promising results. However, there have not yet been any controlled clinical trials of these drugs in patients with DIC and the relatively high-risk of bleeding associated with the use of these compounds may be the limiting factor.[4]

Chronic disseminated intravascular coagulation and Primary fibrinolysis: This condition is rarely if ever seen in the neonatal period.

CONCLUSION

DIC is not a clinical entity in itself. Instead, it always occurs secondary to a broad spectrum of various diseases. The generation of soluble fibrin in plasma is the prerequisite for microclot formation, which contributes to multiple organ failure. The massive and ongoing activation of coagulation may result in the depletion of platelets and coagulation factors. Activation of the fibrinolytic system may cause proteolysis of plasmatic coagulation factors, as well as generation of FDPs inhibiting fibrin polymerization and platelet aggregation. Thus, intravascular coagulation, as well as hyperfibrinolysis, result in a hemorrhagic diathesis (consumption coagulopathy). The diagnosis of DIC is based on the presence of an underlying disease and a combination of laboratory tests that indicate activation of the coagulation system, soluble fibrin formation, and consumption of platelets and coagulation factors. At present, no single laboratory test is available to definitively assess the presence or absence of DIC, but the combination of clinical findings and laboratory analysis allows one to make the diagnosis and differentiate three phases of DIC. There is a need to have a test available which specifically and quantitatively measures soluble fibrin, as the demonstration of soluble fibrin in plasma early in the disease process would allow prophylatic treatment of the patients in order to prevent microclot formation and bleeding complications.

REFERENCES

1. Taylor FB, Toh CH, Hoots WK, Wada M, Levi M. Towards a definition, clinical and laboratory criteria and a scoring system for disseminated intravascular coagulation. Thromb Haemost. 2000;86:1327-30.
2. Levi M, Toh CH, Thachil J, Watson HG. Guidelines for the diagnosis and management of disseminated intravascular coagulation. British Committee for standards in haematology. British Journal of Haematology. 2009;145:24-33.
3. Levi M. Disseminated intravascular coagulation. Crit Care Med. 2007;35:2191-5.
4. Matsuda T. Clinical aspects of DIC—disseminated intravascular coagulation. Pol J Pharmacol. 1996;48:73-5.
5. Kumar R, Gupta V. Disseminated intravascular coagulation: current concepts. Indian J Pediatr. 2008;75:733-8.
6. Thijs LG, de Boer JP, de Groot MC, Hack CE. Coagulation disorders in septic shock. Intensive Care Med. 1993;19: 8-15.
7. Gando S, Kameue T, Nanzaki S, Nakanishi Y. Disseminated intravascular coagulation is a frequent complication of systemic inflammatory response syndrome. Thromb Haemost. 1996;75:224-8.
8. Dempfle CE. Coagulopathy of sepsis. Thromb Haemost. 2004;91:213-24.
9. Levi M, ten Cate H, Bauer KA, van der Pol T, Edgington TS, Buller HR, et al. Inhibition of endotoxin-induced activation of coagulation and fibrinolysis by pentoxifylline or by a monoclonal anti-tissue factor antibody in chimpanzees. J Clin Invest. 1994;93:114-20.
10. Colman RW. Contact systems in infectious disease. Rev Infect Dis. 1989;4:689-99.

11. Jansen PM, Pixley RA, Brouwer M, de Jong IW, Chang AC, Hack CE, et al. Inhibition of factor XII in septic baboons attenuates the activation of complement and fibrinolytic systems and reduces the release of interleukin-6 and neutrophil elastase. Blood. 1996;87:2337-44.
12. Nieuwland R, Berckmans RJ, McGregor S, Boing AN, Romijn FP, Westendorp RG, et al. Cellular origin and procoagulant properties of microparticles in meningococcal sepsis. Blood. 2000;95:930-5.
13. Murray HW, Tuazon CU, Sheagren JN. Staphylococcal septicemia and disseminated intravascular coagulation. *Staphylococcus aureus* endocarditis mimicking meningococcemia. Arch Intern Med. 1977;137:844-7.
14. Stossel TP, Levy R. Intravascular coagulation associated with pneumococcal bacteremia and symmetrical peripheral gangrene. Arch Intern Med. 1970;125:876-8.
15. de Virgilio C, Klein S, Chang L, Klassen M, Bongard F. Clostridial bacteremia: implications for the surgeon. Am Surg. 1991;57:388-93.
16. Barbui T, Falanga A. Disseminated intravascular coagulation in acute leukemia. Semin Thromb Hemost. 2001; 27:593-604.
17. Pegelow C, Goldberg R, Turkel S, Powars D. Severe coagulation abnormalities in Reye syndrome. J Pediatr. 1977; 91:413-6.
18. Veldman A, Fischer D, Nold MF, Wong FY. Disseminated intravascular coagulation in term and preterm neonates. Semin Thromb Hemost. 2010;36:419-28.
19. Woods WG, Luban NL, Hilgartner MW, Miller DR. Disseminated intravascular coagulation in the newborn. Am J Dis Child. 1979;133:44-6.
20. Westendorp RG, Hottenga JJ, Slagboom PE. Variation in plasminogen-activator-inhibitor-1 gene and risk of meningococcal septic shock. Lancet. 1999;354:561-3.
21. Westendorp RG, Reitsma PH, Bertina RM. Inherited prethrombotic disorders and sinfectious purpura. Thromb Haemost. 1996;75:899-901.
22. Franchini M, Lippi G, Manzato F. Recent acquisitions in the pathophysiology, diagnosis and treatment of disseminated intravascular coagulation. Thrombosis J. 2006;4:4-9.
23. Levi M. Disseminated intravascular coagulation: what's new? Crit Care Clin. 2005;21:449-67.
24. Van Deventer SJ, Buller HR, ten Cate JW, Aarden LA, Lack CE, Sturk A. Experimental endotoxemia in humans: analysis of cytokine release and coagulation, fibrinolytic and complement pathways. Blood. 1990;76:2520-6.
25. Taylor FB Jr, Chang A, Ruf W, Morrissey JH, Hinshaw L, Catlett R, et al. Lethal *E. coli* septic shock is prevented by blocking tissue factor with monoclonal antibody. Circulatory Shock. 1991;33:127-34.
26. Levi M, ten Cate H, Bauer KA, van der Poll T, Edgington TS, Büller HR, et al. Inhibition of endotoxin-induced activation of coagulation and fibrinolysis by pentoxifylline or by monoclonal anti-tissue factor antibody in chimpanzees. Journal of Clin Invest. 1994;93:114-20.
27. Levi M, ten Cate H. Disseminated intravascular coagulation. New Engl J Med. 1999;341:586-92.
28. Berckmans RJ, Nieuwland R, Romijn FP, Hack CE, Sturk A. Cell-derived microparticles circulate in healthy humans and support low grade thrombin generation. Thromb Haemost. 2001;85:639-46.
29. Seitz R, Wolf M, Egbring R, Havemann K. The disturbance of hemostasis in septic shock: role of neutrophil elastase and thrombin, effects of antithrombin III and plasma substitution. Eur J Haematol. 1989;43:22-8.
30. Conway EM, Rosenberg RD. Tumor necrosis factor suppresses transcription of the thrombomodulin gene in endothelial cells. Molecular and Cellular Biol. 1988;8:5588-92.
31. Levi M, de Jonge E, van der Poll T. Rationale for restoration of physiological anticoagulant pathways in patients with sepsis and disseminated intravascular coagulation. Crit Care Med. 2001;29:590-4.
32. Mesters RM, Florke N, Ostermann H, Kienast J. Increase of plasminogen activator inhibitor levels predicts outcome of leukocytopenic patients with sepsis. Thromb Haemostas. 1996;75:902-7.
33. Westendorp RC, Hottenga JJ, Slagboon PE. Variation in plasminogen-acti-vator-inhibitor-1 gene and risk of meningococcal septic shock. Lancet. 1999;354:561-3.
34. Yuksel M, Okajima K, Uchiba M, Horiuchi S, Okabe H. Activated protein C inhibits lipopolysaccharide-induced tumor necrosis factor alpha production by inhibiting activation of both nuclear factor-kappa B and activator protein-1 in human monocytes. Thrombo Haemostas. 2002; 88:267-73.
35. Barbui T, Falanga A. Disseminated intravascular coagulation in acute leukemia. Semin Thromb Hemost. 2001; 27:593-604.
36. Karnad DR, Vasani J. Disseminated intravascular coagulation: A review with experience from an intensive care unit in India. J Postgrad Med. 1992;38:186-93.
37. Levi M, de Jonge E, van der Poll T, ten Cate H. Advances in the understanding of the pathogenetic pathways of disseminated intravascular coagulation result in more insight in the clinical picture and better management strategies. Semin Thrombo Hemost. 2001;27:569-75.
38. Buchanan GR. Coagulation disorders in the neonate. Pediatr Clin North Am. 1986;33:203-20.
39. Saba HI, Morelli GA.The pathogenesis and management of disseminated intravascular coagulation. Clin Adv Hematol Oncol. 2006;4:919-26.
40. Toh CH, Dennis M. Disseminated intravascular coagulation: old disease, new hope. BMJ. 2003;327:974-7.
41. Bick RL. Disseminated intravascular coagulation current concepts of etiology, pathophysiology, diagnosis, and treatment. Hematol Oncol Clin North Am. 2003;17:149-76.
42. Andrew M, Paes B, Milner R, Johnston M, Mitchell L, Tollefson DM, et al. Development of the human coagulation system in the healthy premature infant. Blood. 1988;72:1651-7.
43. Bick RL. Disseminated intravascular coagulation: a review of etiology, pathophysiology, diagnosis, and management: guidelines for care. Clin Appl Throm Hemost. 2002;8:1-31.
44. Andrew M. The relevance of developmental hemostasis to hemorrhagic disorders of newborns. Semin Perinatol. 1997; 21:70-85.
45. Favaloro EJ. Laboratory testing in disseminated intravascular coagulation. Semin Thromb Hemost. 2010;36:458-67.

46. Akca S, Haji-Michael P, de Mendonça A, Suter P, Levi M, Vincent JL, et al. Time course of platelet counts in critically ill patients. Crit Care Med. 2002;30:753-6.
47. Collins PW, Thachil J, Toh CH. Acquired bleeding disorders. In: Hoffbrand V, Catovsky D, Tuddenham Edward GD, Green AR (Eds). Postgraduate hematology, 6th ed. Wiley-Blackwell publishing; 2011. pp. 839-58.
48. Taylor FB Jr, Toh CH, Hoots WK, Wada H, Levi M. Towards definition, clinical and laboratory criteria, and a scoring system for disseminated intravascular coagulation. Thromb Haemost. 2001;86:1327-30.
49. Levi M, Opal SM. Coagulation abnormalities in critically ill patients. Critical Care. 2006;10:222.
50. Patel R, Cook DJ, Meade MO, Griffith LE, Mehta G, Rocker GM, et al. Burden of illness in venous thromboembolism in critical care: a multicenter observational study. Journal of Critical Care. 2005;20:341-7.
51. Samama MM, Cohen AT, Darmon JY, Desjardins L, Eldor A, Janbon C, et al. A comparison of enoxaparin with placebo for the prevention of venous thromboembolism in acutely ill medical patients. Prophylaxis in medical patients with enoxaparin study group. New England Journal of Medicine. 1999;341:793-800.
52. Abraham E, Laterre PF, Garg R, Levy H, Talwar D, Trzaskom BL, et al. Drotrecogin alfa (activated) for adults with severe sepsis and a low risk of death. New England Journal of Medicine. 2005;353:1332-41.
53. De Pont AC, Bakhtiari K, Hutten BA, de Jonge E, Vroom MB, Meijers JC, et al. Recombinant human activated protein C resets thrombin generation in patients with severe sepsis–a case control study. Critical Care. 2005;9:490-7.
54. Mannucci PM, Levi M. Prevention and treatment of major blood loss. New England Journal of Medicine. 2007;356: 2301-11.
55. Kienast J, Juers M, Wiedermann CJ, Hoffmann JN, Ostermann H, Strauss R, et al. Treatment effects of high-dose anti thrombin without concomitant heparin in patients with severe sepsis with or without disseminated intravascular coagulation. J Thromb Haemost. 2006;4:90-7.
56. Abraham E, Reinhart K, Opal S, Deineyer I, Daig C, Rodriguez AL, et al. OPTIMIST Trial study group. Efficacy and safety of tifacogin (recombinant tissue factor pathway inhibitor) in severe sepsis: a randomized controlled trial. JAMA. 2003;290:238-47.
57. Nishiyama T, Matsukawa T, Hanaoka K. Is protease inhibitor a choice for the treatment of pre or mild disseminated intravascular coagulation? Crit Care Med. 2000;27:657-66.

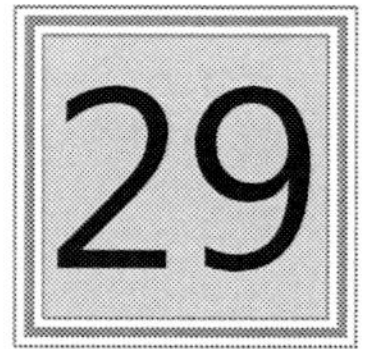

Disorders of White Blood Cells

AP Dubey

The white blood cells (leukocytes) comprise of neutrophils, eosinophils, lymphocytes, monocytes and basophils. The functions of the different types of leukocytes vary, but in general it can be said that their most important function is the defence of the body against infection. The white blood cell values for normal children vary with age as given in Table 29.1.[1] Normally the leukocytes undergo minor physiological and diurnal variations; it increases slightly in the afternoon (afternoon tide).

The disorders of white blood cells may be classified as per individual component of leukocytes. There can be an increase or decrease in the number of the white blood cells as a whole or it can affect only one or more individual components.

LEUKOCYTOSIS

An increase in the absolute number of leukocytes above the normal value is known as leukocytosis. This may be either physiological or pathological. The physiological causes include physical exercise, food intake and emotion. In majority of cases pathological leukocytosis is due to an increase in the neutrophil polymorphs. The various pathological causes of leukocytosis are described here.

Infections

This is the commonest cause of polymorphonuclear leukocytosis. The degree of cell increase depends upon the type and severity of infection. Bacterial infections with *pyogenic cocci (Staph, Strep, Pneumo)* and bacilli like *E. coli, Proteus, Pseudomonas* lead to a prompt and marked increase. Certain nonpyogenic conditions like acute rheumatic fever, scarlet fever, diphtheria, cholera and herpes zoster also give rise to leukocytosis. Septicemia is not only associated with pronounced leukocytosis but also bandemia. Severe infections are also accompanied by toxic and degenerative changes in the neutrophils.

Malignant Diseases

In children leukemias, lymphomas and Hodgkin's disease are characterized not only with a rise in total number of white blood cells but the peripheral blood may also show presence of a large number of immature cells (blasts).

Table 29.1: Normal white blood cell (WBC) values (thousands per mm^3)[1]

Age	*Total WBCs*	*Neutrophils*		*Lymphocytes*		*Monocytes*		*Eosinophils*	
	Mean	*Mean*	*%*	*Mean*	*%*	*Mean*	*%*	*Mean*	*%*
Birth	18.1	11.0	61	5.5	31	1.1	6	0.4	2
1 week	12.2	5.5	45	5.0	41	1.1	9	0.5	4
1 month	10.8	3.8	35	6.0	56	0.7	7	0.3	3
1 year	11.4	3.5	31	7.0	61	0.6	5	0.3	3
4 years	9.1	3.8	42	4.5	50	0.5	5	0.3	3
6 years	8.5	4.3	51	3.5	42	0.4	5	0.2	3
8 years	8.3	4.4	53	3.3	39	0.4	4	0.2	2
10 years	8.1	4.4	54	3.1	38	0.4	4	0.2	2
16 years	7.8	4.4	57	2.8	35	0.4	5	0.2	3

Hemorrhage

Severe hemorrhage usually leads to neutrophilic leukocytosis.

Trauma

The degree of cell increase depends upon the amount of tissue damage.

Collagen Diseases

Like juvenile rheumatoid arthritis, polyarteritis nodosa, disseminated lupus erythematosus.

Metabolic Disturbances

Like renal failure, diabetic coma, acute yellow atrophy of liver.

Miscellaneous Causes

Include intravascular hemolysis, acute anoxia, certain drugs and chemical poisoning.

LEUKOPENIA

Leukopenia is defined as a reduction in the number of leukocytes below the lower normal limit of 4 × 10/L. In majority of the cases leukopenia is due mainly to a reduction in neutrophils, the absolute lymphocyte count being normal or mildly reduced. The various causes of leukopenia are listed in Table 29.2.[2]

EOSINOPHILIA

The mean absolute eosinophil count of children and adults is 150 cells/mm^3, with a range up to 700 cells/mm^3. The lowest eosinophil counts are seen in the neonatal period after which the values are almost same in children and adults. The various causes of eosinophilia are given in Table 29.3.[3] The *Hypereosinophilic syndrome*, which is characterized by pulmonary infiltrates, cardiomegaly, congestive heart failure and elevated eosinophil count is a well known entity.[4] This includes disorders such as Loeffler's syndrome, eosinophilic leukemoid rection, pulmonary infiltrates with eosinophilia (PIE), disseminated eosinophilic collagen disease and eosinophilic leukemia.

Table 29.2: Causes of leukopenia[2]

1. Infections
   a. Bacterial—typhoid and paratyphoid fever, brucellosis
   b. Viral—influenza, measles, rubella, infective hepatitis
   c. Protozoal—malaria, kala-azar
   d. Rickettsial—typhus
2. Acute and subacute leukemia
3. Drug induced—selective or as a part of aplastic anemia
4. Aplastic anemia
5. Megaloblastic anemias
6. Hypersplenism
7. Idiopathic neutropenia—acute or chronic
8. Miscellaneous—myxedema, hypopituitarism, cirrhosis of liver

Table 29.3: Causes of eosinophilia[3]

1. *Allergic disorders*—asthma, urticaria, angioneurotic edema, drug sensitivity.
2. *Parasitic infections*—invasive helminth infections like toxocara, trichinosis, echinococcal infections and ascariasis, malaria.
3. *Skin disorders*—pemphigus, dermatitis herpetiformis.
4. *Hemato-oncologic disorders*—ALL, eosinophilic leukemia, Hodgkin's disease, pernicious anemia, postsplenectomy, immunodeficiency syndromes, polycythemia vera and other chronic myeloproliferative states.
5. *Infections*—scarlet fever, chorea, chlamydial infections, erythema multiforme.
6. *Inherited eosinophilia*
7. *Miscellaneous*—rheumatoid arthritis, radiation therapy, cirrhosis, Loffler's syndrome, peritoneal dialysis, sarcoidosis.

EOSINOPENIA

The causes of eosinopenia may be described as follows:

a. *Administration of hormones or drugs* like corticosteroids, adrenalin, ephedrine and insulin. It is usually transient.
b. *Endocrine disorders* like Cushing's disease and acromegaly.
c. *Response to stress* like acute infections, traumatic shock, burns, exposure to cold, severe exercise.
d. *Miscellaneous* like aplastic anemia, falciparum malaria, Down's syndrome.

MONOCYTOSIS

Monocytosis is defined as a count exceeding 0.8 × 10/L. The causes of monocytosis are listed in Table 29.4.[3] In most cases it is only moderate in degree.

BASOPHILIA

Basophilia is said to occur when the basophil count exceeds 100 to 150 cells/mm^3. Its various causes are given in Table 29.5.[3]

LYMPHOCYTOSIS

Except for pertussis, acute bacterial infections are rarely associated with lymphocytosis. However, chronic bacterial infections like tuberculosis may cause

Table 29.4: Causes of monocytosis[3]

1. *Bacterial infections*—tuberculosis, syphilis, subacute bacterial endocarditis, brucellosis.
2. *Nonbacterial infections*—malaria, kala-azar, typhus, trypanosomiasis.
3. *Hemato-oncologic disorders*—Hodgkin's disease, preleukemia, leukemia, non-Hodgkin's lymphoma, myeloproliferative disorders, congenital and acquired neutropenias, some hemolytic anemias, metastatic solid tumors, postsplenectomy
4. *Collagen vascular diseases*—SLE, rheumatoid arthritis, polyarteritis nodosa
5. *Miscellaneous*—ulcerative colitis, regional enteritis, tetrachlorethane poisoning, Hand-Schüller-Christian syndrome

Table 29.5: Causes of basophilia[3]

1. *Hemato-oncologic disorders*—some hemolytic anemias, Hodgkin's disease, chronic myeloproliferative disorders like CML and polycythemia vera
2. *Infections*—chronic sinusitis, varicella
3. *Endocrine*—hypothyroidism, ovulation, pregnancy
4. *Drugs*—estrogens, antithyroid medications
5. *Miscellaneous*—stress, nephrosis, radiations

sustained lymphocytosis. Although, most viral infections cause a mild lymphocytosis, infectious mononucleosis and CMV infections are the only likely causes of persistent atypical lymphocytosis. The various causes of lymphocytosis are given in Table 29.6.[3]

LYMPHOPENIA

Lymphopenia defined as the reduction in the number of lymphocytes below the normal value of 1.5 × 10/L

Table 29.6: Causes of lymphocytosis[3]

1. *Infections*—pertussis, infectious mononucleosis, infectious lymphocytosis, infective hepatitis, CMV, toxoplasmosis, syphillis, brucellosis, many common viral illnesses.
2. *Hematologic disorders*—lymphocytic leukemias, neutropenias (relative lymphocytosis)
3. *Miscellaneous*—thyrotoxicosis, Addison's disease

Table 29.7: Causes of lymphocytopenia[3]

1. *Infections*—active tuberculosis, malaria
2. *Collagen vascular disease*—SLE, regional enteritis
3. *Certain immunodeficiency syndromes*
4. *Endocrine disorders*—hyperadrenalism, adrenal corticosteroid administration
5. *Hemato-oncologic disorders*—Hodgkin's disease, aplastic anemia, solid tumors
6. *Excessive losses*—thoracic duct drainage, intestinal lymph-angiectasias

is usually seen with severe pancytopenia from any cause. Its causes have been listed in Table 29.7.[3]

REFERENCES

1. Dallman PR. In: Rudolph AM (Ed). Pediatrics, 16th edn. New York, Appleton-Century Crofts; 1977. p. 1178.
2. Penington D, Rush B, Castaldi P. The White cells. In: deGruchy (Ed). Clinical Haematology in medical practice. 4th edn, ELBS and Blackwell Scientific Publications, 1978. p. 399.
3. Nathan DG, Orkin SH. Hematologic manifestations of systemic diseases. In: Hematology of infancy and childhood. 5th edn, WB Saunders Co. 1998. pp. 1872-4.
4. Hardt WR, Anderson RE. The hyper-eosinophilic syndromes. Ann Intern Med. 1968;68:1120.

Hematological Changes in HIV Infection

Nitin K Shah

HEMATOLOGICAL CHANGES SEEN IN HIV

The main hematological manifestations in HIV include anemia, leukopenia, thrombocytopenia, bi/tri cytopenia, coagulation disorders, hematological malignancies, etc. There may be some bone marrow changes seen in HIV infection though none of them are specific to HIV. The various hematological changes seen in HIV are mediated by multiple etiological factors affecting the hematopoietic cells as well as the micro-environment. Hematological changes lead to increase in morbidity and mortality in HIV infected patients. Due to associated immune compromised state and use of multiple drugs, one cannot use optimal therapy, e.g. for cancers and there is suboptimal response to the therapy, again say for cancers.[1]

PATHOPHYSIOLOGY

The etiological factors for hematological changes seen in HIV include HIV *per se,* opportunistic infections, drugs used and associated cancers.

HIV itself can infect the stem cells, which are CD4 positive. This leads to decreased hematopoiesis. It also can expose certain antigens on the surface of the stem cells, which leads to immune damage to these cells. It also infects the accessory cells present in the marrow like T-cells, B-cells, endothelial cells, fibroblasts, monocytes and other stromal cells. These accessory cells secrete cytokines like colony stimulating factors, which stimulate the hematopoietic cells. They also secrete inflammatory cytokines like IL1, IL2, IL6, TNF-α, TGF-β, interferon, etc. which inhibit hematopoiesis. Infection of these cells leads to initial increase in colony stimulating factors leading to hyper cellular marrow and later to dysregulatuon of cytokines leading to ineffective hematopoiesis with peripheral cytopenia. Damage to the microenvironment leads to decreased support and homing into the stem cells. Lastly HIV can lead to huge splenomegaly, which can lead to hyper-splenism and peripheral destruction of cells.[1,2]

HIV infected patient suffers from multiple opportunistic infections, which can inhibit hematopoiesis. Infections like atypical mycobacterial infection or fungal infection can lead to direct infection of the marrow. HBV or HCV also can inhibit erythropoiesis. CMV can damage marrow and lead to anemia or aplasia. Parvovirus B19 can lead to chronic infection of marrow like in other immune compromised patient. It involves mainly the erythron leading to anemia.

Drugs like AZT, sulphas, antifungal, pyramethamine, pentamidine, gancyclovir, etc. are commonly used in HIV infected patients. They all are myelotoxic and cause cytopenia.

Lastly, HIV infected patient can develop different types of malignancies including non-Hodgkin's lymphoma, Kaposi's sarcoma, anorectal cancers, cervical cancers, Hodgkin's disease, leukemia and other soft tissue sarcoma. These cancers as well as their definitive therapy can lead to bone marrow toxicity.

ANEMIA IN HIV

Anemia is seen in 10-20% of HIV infected patients during early stage and in 70-80% during late stage of HIV infection. The incidence and the severity of anemia increase as the disease progresses. Most patients show picture like that seen in any other chronic infection. It shows normocytic normochromic picture with low retic count suggestive of bone marrow suppression. Serum iron and TS are low so also is TIBC. Serum ferritin levels are high. Patients may develop nutritional anemia due to poor intake. Serum B_{12} levels are low in some patients. Specific infections like CMV or Parvovirus B19 can depress erythropoiesis. Drug like AZT can lead to anemia when used in higher and prolonged dose schedule. Lastly 60-70% of patients in early symptomatic stage develop positive DCT and 80-85% during late symptomatic stage. In most cases it is weakly positive and rarely symptomatic with clinical hemolysis. It is usually due to adsorption of immune complexes on the surface of the red cells.[3]

The treatment of anemia includes improvement in the nutrition, iron and B_{12} therapy, avoidance of the offending drugs, optimizing the antiretroviral therapy especially NRTI group of drugs and effective and prompt treatment of opportunistic infections. Transfusion of packed red cells should be given only when strictly indicated as it can lead to many complications including plasma borne infections. Erythropoietin levels are low (<500 u/cumm) in 75% of patients and such patients can benefit by using injectable EPO. It is used in the dose of 200-400 units per kg body weight given IV or SC twice a week. This can obviate the need for transfusion.[4]

LEUKOPENIA IN HIV

As the disease progresses there is progressive decrease in lymphocyte counts especially CD4+ T-cells. This leads to progressive immunodeficiency. Ten to seventy five percent of patients develop neutropenia.[5] This is due to bone marrow suppression and rarely due to immune destruction of neutrophils. There may be associated dysmyelopoiesis showing decreased number of lobes and granules in the polymorphs. This is due to dysregulation of cytokines. Patients may have low levels of growth factors like G-CSF or GM-CSF. Such patients can benefit from the use of GM-CSF. It is used in the dose of 5-15 mcg per kg body weight given for 5-10 days. It may stimulate growth of HIV too. Hence it is always used along with antiretroviral therapy. There is increase in the polymorphic count as well as its function.

THROMBOCYTOPENIA IN HIV

Thirty to sixty percent of HIV infected patients develop thrombocytopenia.[6] It does not co-relate with the stage of HIV. Accordingly it can be seen at any stage of the disease. It may be the only presenting symptom of HIV. Some times it mimics like ITP. Clinical bleeding is uncommon as the patient may tolerate low levels of platelet counts like in chronic ITP. Patients can develop all types of bleeding like a patient with ITP. Intracranial bleeds can lead to diagnostic confusion with other intracranial diseases seen commonly in HIV infected patients.

It is caused by decreased production as well as increased destruction. Direct infection of marrow, immune destruction of megakaryocytes and cytokine dysregulation all lead to decreased production.[7] There is mimicry between gp 160 of HIV and gp IIb/IIIa of platelet. Accordingly the anti gp 160 antibodies cross react with gp IIb/IIIa complex of platelet leading to immune destruction of the platelets.[8] In most cases there is nonspecific adsorption of immune complexes on the platelet surface. Nonimmune destruction of platelets occurs due to repeated infections, fever, DIC, HUS, TTP and hypersplenism.

Ten to twenty percent of patients undergo spontaneous and long-term remission. Sudden rise in the platelet count indicates development of severe immune deficiency and grave prognosis. Treatment of thrombocytopenia is warranted only if the patient has clinical bleeding or when the counts are less than 5000-10000/cumm.

Use of AZT helps restore the platelet count in 30% patients. It may take up to 12 weeks for the response to occur. Steroids are used like in patient with ITP. Though 40-80% of patients may have acute response to steroids, only 10-20% maintain long-term remission.[9] Long-term use of high doses if steroids are not safe in HIV infected patients. Safer and better alternative is to use IVIG. This will also help fight infections. It is used in the same dose and schedule as in a patient with ITP. Though 70-90% patients develop acute response, less than 10% go into long-term remission.[10] Similarly anti-D globulin can be used in patients who are Rh positive and who do not have significant anemia. Acute response is seen in 75% of patients but only 10% maintain long-term response. Anti-D may take longer time than IVIG for the response to occur. Anti-D is much cheaper than IVIG.

Some patients who have significant bleeding in spite of all the previous modes of therapy may need splenectomy. Sixty to eighty percent of them develop immediate response whereas 40-60% go into permanent remission. Splenectomy does not increase the immunodeficiency. It may not be easy to get the required surgical expertise to perform splenectomy at all the centers. One may try splenic artery embolization to induce auto splenectomy. Low dose splenic irradiation can also be tried.[11] It is used in the dose of 900-1000 cGy over 4 weeks. This helps avoid major surgery as well as preserves some splenic function.

Other modes of therapy tried include use of dapsone; vincristine, anabolic steroids, interferon and high dose vitamin C. None of these are quite effective. Some of them are costly and even harmful.

BONE MARROW CHANGES

None of the changes seen in marrow are specific to HIV. Initially one sees hyper cellular marrow, which is seen in 90% of patients. This is not accompanied by increased peripheral counts indicating ineffective hematopoiesis. As the disease progresses one can see hypocellular marrow. This is seen in 5% of patients. One can see changes of dyshematopoiesis. Seventy percent show dysmyelopoiesis in the form of decreased lobes and granules in myeloid cells. Fifty percent show changes of dyserythropoiesis and 30% show dysmegakaryopoiesis. 20% of patients show lymphoid infiltration. Some may show increase in reticulin cells and fibers and some may show erythrophagocytosis.[3]

COAGULATION DISORDERS IN HIV

These changes are seen rarely and are not a common clinical problem. Besides thrombocytopenia as discussed before there may be associated platelet dysfunction. Infections can induce DIC in very sick patients. Anti phospholipid antibody syndrome can lead to presence of two types of autoantibodies i.e., Lupus Inhibitor and anticardiolipin antibody. Though Lupus inhibitor leads to prolonged APT time, clinically it leads to thromboembolism. Low levels of protein C and protein S due to antibodies against these proteins increase this risk.

HEMATOLOGICAL MALIGNANCIES IN HIV

HIV infected patient, like other immune compromised patients, is prone to develop many types of cancers. These include non-Hodgkin's lymphoma (NHL), Kaposi's sarcoma, cervical cancers, all of which are AIDS defining diseases. It also includes anorectal carcinoma, leukemia, soft tissue sarcomas, Hodgkin's disease, squamous cell carcinoma etc.[12,13] Multiple etiological factors lead to malignancies in immune compromised patients. This includes presence of opportunistic infections like CMV and EBV, which are carcinogenic, loss of immune surveillance and cytokine dysregulation.

The risk of NHL is increased by 100 times in HIV infected patients. It increases with length of survival and almost doubles every 2.4 years. Ten to twenty percent of all NHL seen in west are related to HIV infection. Three percent of patients with AIDS develop NHL in their lifetime if they live long enough. The risk is same irrespective of the mode of transmission of HIV. Cancers lead to decrease in longevity in 10% of the HIV infected patients. The chemotherapy that can be used is suboptimal due to toxicities of the drugs and associated serious diseases due to HIV. This also leads to poor long-term remissions.

NHL IN HIV

Non-Hodgkin's lymphoma (NHL) can be nodal or extra nodal in origin in HIV infected patients. In 30% of patients it is only extra nodal, in 30% only nodal and in 35% it is mixed in origin. The extra nodal sites include bone marrow (35%), GIT (27%), liver (9%), and CNS (15%). Ninety percent of NHL in HIV infected patients are B-cell in origin and show positive immune markers like CD 19, CD 20, CD 22, etc. Rest is other varieties including T-cell NHL. Sixty percent of the B-cell NHL are of large cell immunoblastic type, 20% are of small noncleaved cell type, i.e. Burkitt's type and 20% are large cell diffuse variety or low-grade NHL. Forty-two percent are polyclonal type, 38% are EBV associated and 23% are positive for MYC arrangements.

Primary NHL of brain is a AIDS defining disease. It can occur in the parenchyma of the brain or in the leptomeninges. Most of them are large immunoblastic variety and 100% of them are associated with EBV infection. The mean survival in spite of chemotherapy is only few months.

Therapy of NHL in HIV infected patients depends on various factors like stage of HIV, immune status, presence of associated infections and complications, side effects of the drugs, affordability and the survival goals. Aim of the therapy is to improve the quality of life. The regimens used include modified CHOP or mBACOP regimes. Only 17-50% survive for a median of 5 months in spite of chemotherapy.

REFERENCES

1. Doweiko JP, Groopman JE. Hematological complications of Human Immunodeficiency virus infection. In: Devita VT, Hellman S, Rosenberg SA (Eds). AIDS Etiology, Diagnosis, Treatment and Prevention. Published by Lippincott-Raven; 1997. pp. 429-43.
2. Mir N, Costello C, Luckitt J, et al. HIV disease and bone marrow changes: a study of 60 cases. Eur J Hematol. 1989; 80:3036.
3. Zon LI, Arkin C, Groopman GE. Hematological manifestations of the human immunodeficiency virus (HIV). Br J Hematol. 1987;66:251.
4. Spivak JL, Barnes DC, Fuch S, et al. Serum immunoreactive erythropoietin in HIV infected patients. JAMA. 1989; 261:3104.
5. Murphy MF, Metcalfe P, Waters AH, et al. Incidence and mechanism of Nutropenia and thrombocytopenia in patients with human immunodeficiency virus infection. Br J Hematol. 1987;66:337.
6. Stricker RB. Haemostatic abnormalities in HIV disease. Hematol Oncol Clin North Am. 1991;5:249.
7. Zauli G. Re MC, Gugliotta L, et al. Lack of compensatory megakaryopoiesis in HIV-1 seropositive thrombocytopenic individuals compared with immune thrombocytopenic purpura patients. AIDS. 1991;5:345.
8. Stanworth DR, Solder B, Lewin IV, et al. Related epitopes in HIV viral coat protein and human IgG. Lancet. 1989; 1:1458.

9. Karpatkin S. Immunological thombocytopenic purpura in HIV seropositive homosexuals, narcotic addicts and hemophiliacs. Semin Hematol. 1988;25:219.
10. Beard J, Savidge GF. High dose intravenous immunoglobulins and splenectomy for the treatment of HIV related immune thrombocytopenia in patients with severe hemophilia. Br J Hematol. 1988;68:303
11. Calverley DC, Jones GW, Kelton JG. Splenic radiation for corticosteroid resistant immune thrombocytopenia. Ann Intern Med. 1992;116:977.
12. Kristal AR, Nasca PC, Burnett WS, et al. Changes in the epidemiology of non-Hodgkin's lymphoma and selected malignancies in a population with a high incidence of acquired immunodeficiency syndrome (AIDS). Am J Epidemiol. 1988;128:711.
13. Tirrelli U, Errante D, Oksenhandler E, et al. Prospective study with combined low dose chemotherapy and zidovudine in 37 patients with poor prognosis AIDS related non-Hodgkin's lymphoma. Ann Oncol. 1992;3: 843.

Approach to a Patient with Splenomegaly and Lymphadenopathy

Sunil Narain, LS Arya

It is not uncommon in pediatric practice to encounter a child with physical findings including splenomegaly and lymphadenopathy. Since the myriad of possible underlying disorders can pose immense challenges in appropriate management of these children, a well organized approach can help reach a diagnosis expeditiously (Fig. 31.1).

The presence of generalized lymphadenopathy along with palpable spleen is usually a significant physical finding warranting further workup; a thorough history and physical examination remains the most important step while approaching such a patient. In the history, after ascertaining whether the illness is of acute or chronic nature, the focus should be on presence or recurrence of systemic symptoms. One should enquire about persistent or recurrent fever (infection, malignancy, collagen vascular disease), sore throat (infectious mononucleosis), cough (tuberculosis, fungal infection), epistaxis or easy bruising (leukemia), limp or limb pain (leukemia, juvenile rheumatoid arthritis [JRA], neuroblastoma). Besides noting the duration and severity of any systemic symptoms, it is also important to assess whether they are improving or progressing. One should also obtain details about any travel history and animal exposure (kala-azar, toxoplasmosis, cat scratch disease, brucellosis, leptospirosis) besides scrutinizing all past prescriptions. It is also important to inquire about possible exposure to tuberculosis and risk of infection with human immunodeficiency virus (HIV).[1]

A soft thin spleen may be palpable in 15% of newborns, 10% of children and 5% of adolescents.[2] However, in most instances, a palpable spleen, may be presumed to be enlarged since it has to grow to 2-3 times its size before it becomes palpable (Table 31.1). Hemolytic anemias including hemoglobinopathies, thalassemia, enzyme defects, hereditary spherocytosis and other autoimmune hemolytic anemias assume importance as underlying etiologies in a patient with splenomegaly, especially in absence of generalized lymphadenopathy (Fig. 31.2); congestive disorders as well as benign splenic lesions like cysts and hemangiomas should also be considered in the differential diagnosis of splenomegaly. Events in early infancy including umbilical sepsis, exchange transfusion, signs of hearing impairment, history of blood transfusions and jaundice can provide some important clues (extrahepatic portal hypertension, osteopetrosis).

Table 31.1: Causes of splenomegaly[3]

Hemolytic anemias	Hereditary spherocytosis, non-spherocytic hemolytic anemias, hemoglobinopathies, thalassemia major
Extramedullary hematopoiesis	Thalassemia, osteopetrosis, myelofibrosis
Neoplasms	Leukemia, lymphoma, metastatic malignancy, hemangioma, hamartoma
Storage and infiltrative diseases	Lipidosis, histiocytoses, mucopolysaccharidosis
Congestive disorders	Cirrhosis, hepatic fibrosis, cystic fibrosis, portal or systemic venous obstruction (Banti's syndrome), chronic congestive cardiac failure
Infectious and inflammatory responses	Bacterial (SABE), viral infection, (mononucleosis and others), protozoal (malaria), systemic lupus erythematosus (SLE) and sarcoidosis
Cysts	True and pseudocysts

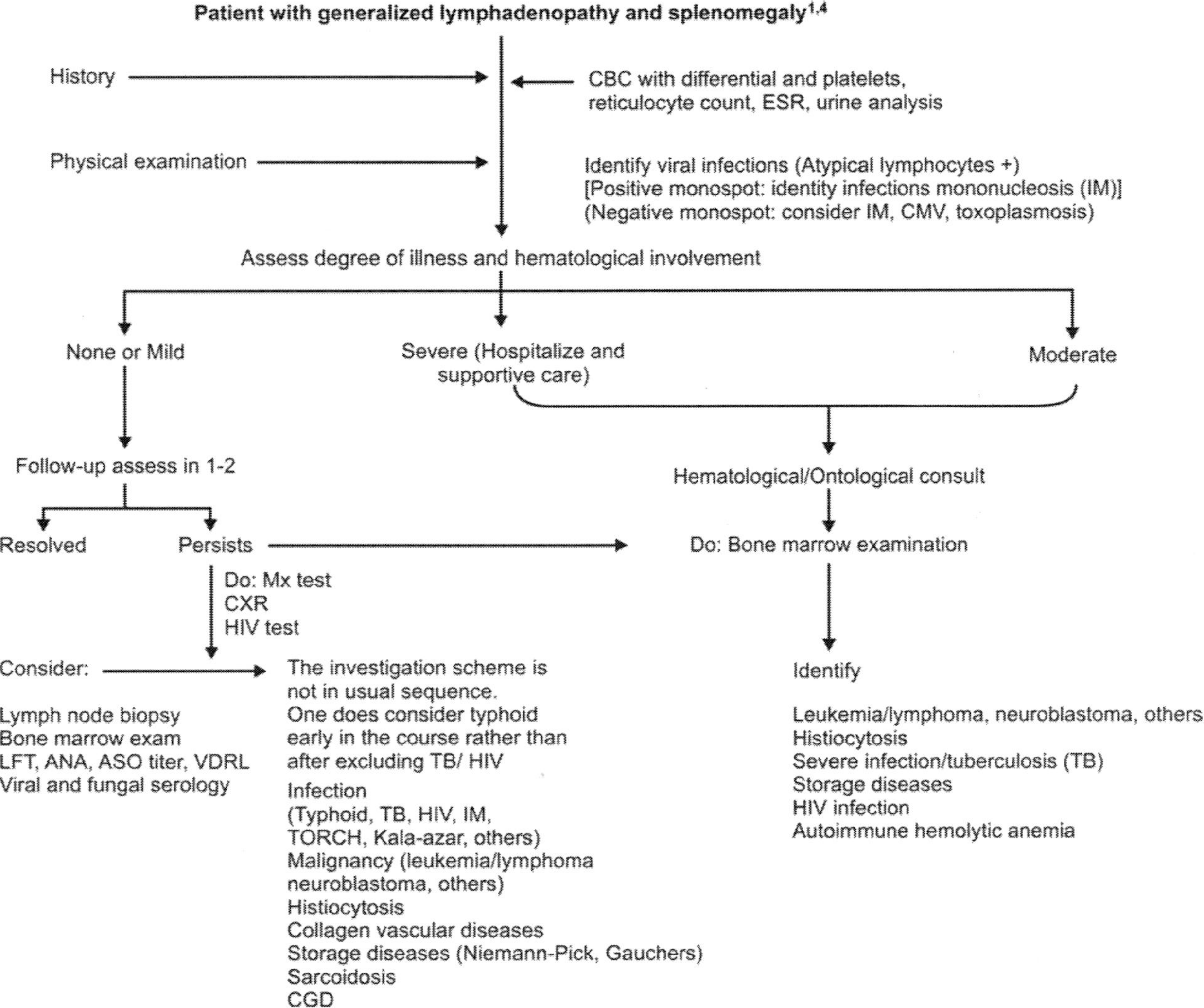

Fig. 31.1: Approach to a patient with generalized lymphadenopathy and splenomegaly[1,4]

A family history of hematologic disorders and possible food or drug exposure should also be ascertained. Enquiring about presence of systemic symptoms such as fever, jaundice, pallor, bleeding, tea colored urine is particularly useful in evaluating patients detected to have splenomegaly. Extramedullary hematopoiesis resulting in splenic enlargement is seen strikingly in thalassemia major, osteopetrosis and myelofibrosis. Although depression of formed elements is frequently seen in presence of large spleen, overt anemia and infection are unusual, suggesting that the cytopenias and anemia may be a consequence of excessive pooling and dilution rather than cell destruction.[3] The size and consistency of the spleen (massive in kala-azar, chronic myeloid leukemia (CML), Gaucher's disease, chronic hemolytic anemias like thalassemias and hard in storage disorders) should be noted. Percutaneous splenic aspiration may be both a useful and safe diagnostic procedure. If the spleen is huge, its edge may extend well down into the left lower quadrant. Palpation of the splenic notch is helpful in identification; however, ultrasonography, computed tomography or magnetic resonance imaging should be done to ascertain the nature of the left upper quadrant mass if there is any question.

Generalized lymphadenopathy (Table 31.2) is abnormal enlargement of more than 2 noncontiguous lymph node regions.[4] Evidence of recent infection in the region drained by the involved lymph nodes should be sought as early as possible. It is important to determine the need for a biopsy as early as possible in the workup of the patient; while investigations are generally guided

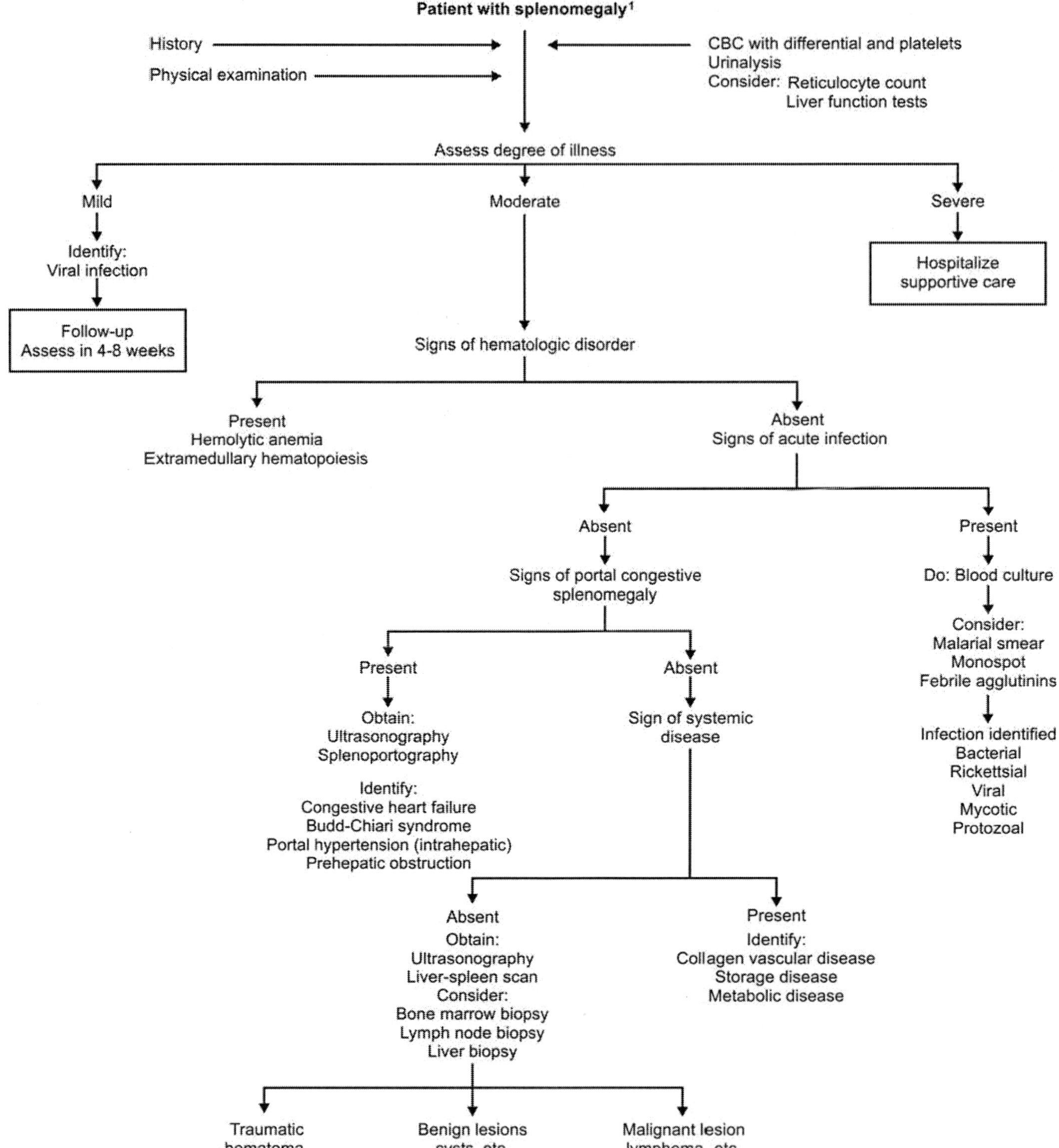

Fig. 31.2: Approach to a patient with splenomegaly[1]

by history and physical examination, lymph node biopsy should be considered in patients with persistent fever, weight loss, night sweats, hard nodes or increasing size of nodes (Fig. 31.3).[5,6] Involvement of supraclavicular nodes suggests mediastinal pathology mandating prompt work-up including a chest radiograph. In contrast, involvement of upper cervical lymph nodes is more likely to be the result of an upper respiratory tract infection. Signs of inflammation in the lymph nodes suggest an infectious etiology. In particular matted lymphadenitis with nodes fixed to the skin in the upper anterior cervical and preauricular areas are suggestive of atypical mycobacterial infection.[7] If no clues emerge following assessment of complete blood picture, blood culture, Mantoux testing, serologic testing and a chest radiograph, a lymph node biopsy is probably indicated. Nodes that are not enlarging but that have not diminished in size after 5-6 weeks or that do not return to normal size by 10-12 weeks, especially if associated with unexplained fever, weight loss or hepatosplenomegaly should also be biopsied. In general the largest node should be biopsied and the specimen sent for appropriate culture and supplemental studies as well as routine histopathology. Great care is required in biopsy procedure and the handling of specimen to maximize the yield. Errors in technique are the single most important cause of diagnostic difficulty. Unfortunately, the majority of lymph node biopsies fail to reveal a specific diagnosis.[5] A significant proportion (15-25%) of children with non-diagnostic lymph node biopsies are ultimately proven to have a significant specific disease.[5] Therefore, if the initial workup and biopsy fails to confirm a specific disease, a close follow-up is essential.

Work-up in the case of regional lymphadenopathy has to be tailored; however, children with probability of having serious disease can be selected for early biopsy. These include children with involvement of lower cervical and supraclavicular lymph nodes, children with constitutional symptoms such as weight loss, fever, bone pain. In asymptomatic children, an appropriate strategy may be to observe the child meticulously and possibly an empiric trail of antibiotics.

In the physical examination, a note of the degree and extent of lymphadenopathy should be made. Discrete, mobile, nontender lymph nodes are palpable in most normal children. Cervical or axillary nodes (1 cm of less) or inguinal nodes (less than 1.5 cm) should not be considered enlarged.[2] Also, small inguinal or high cervical (1 cm or <) and occipital, submandibular or axillary nodes (3 mm or <) are normal. Lymphadenopathy related to malignancy is often nontender and accompanied by fever, pallor and weight loss.[4] It is important to note the presence of hepatomegaly, especially massive hepatosplenomegaly (malignancy, storage disorders, infections), arthritis (leukemia, collagen vascular disease) or a characteristic rash/ conjunctivitis (viral exanthem, JRA-Still's disease, Kawasaki's disease, histiocytosis, leptospirosis). The presence of anemia, neutropenia or thrombocytopenia along with generalized lymphadenopathy suggests infiltration of bone marrow from malignant invasion or other infiltrative diseases or secondary to hypersplenism. A raised ESR may be seen in infectious as well as connective tissue disorders.

It is important to note that many viral infections can also manifest with lymphadenopathy and splenomegaly; atypical lymphocytes are commonly seen in such patients. A differential count with 10-20% atypical lymphocytes suggests infectious mononucleosis, cytomegalovirus (CMV) infection or toxoplasmosis. False negative monospot test frequently occurs early in

Table 31.2: Causes of lymphadenopathy in children[5]

1. Non-specific reactive lymphadenitis	
2. Infectious	Bacterial: streptococcal, staphylococcal, mycobacterial, brucellosis, syphilis
	Viral: Epstein-Barr virus, cytomegalovirus, HIV, rubella
	Fungal and protozoal (toxoplasmosis, malaria)
3. Autoimmune	Rheumatoid arthritis, SLE, serum sickness, autoimmune hemolytic anemia
4. Storage disorders	Niemann-Pick disease, Gaucher's disease
5. Drug reactions	Phenytoin and others
6. Malignancies	Leukemia and lymphomas, metastatic malignancies (neuroblastoma others)
7. Reactive lymphohistiocytosis	X-linked lymphoproliferative disorder (XLP), lymphomatoid granulomatosis, sinus histiocytosis with giant lymphadenopathy.
8. Miscellaneous	Angioimmunoblastic lymphadenopathy with dysproteinemia, giant lymph node hyperplasia, hyperthyroidism, sarcoidosis Kawasaki's disease, cat-scratch disease

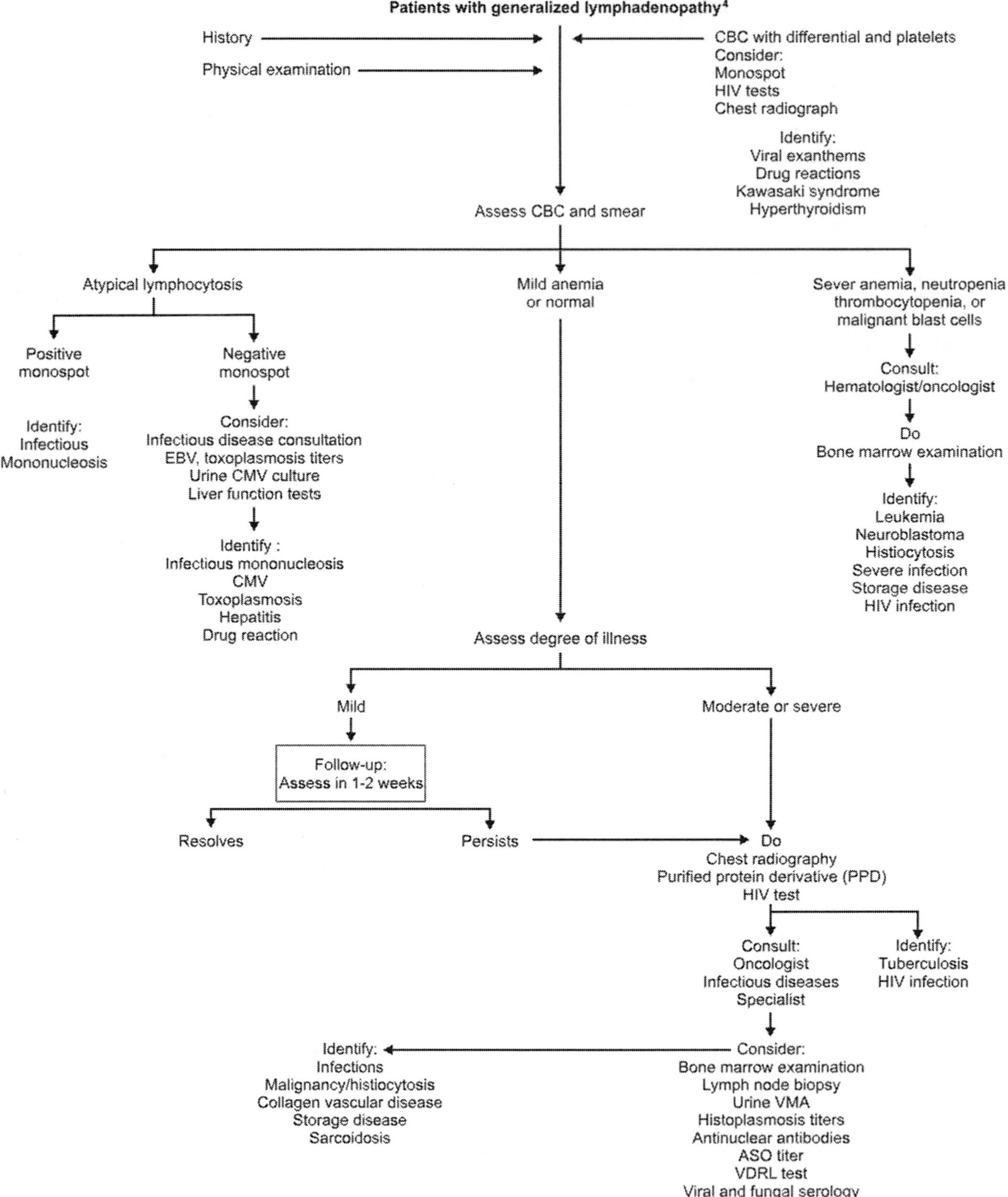

Fig. 31.3: Approach to a patient with generalized lymphadenopathy[4]

the course of infectious mononucleosis and are a common finding in very young children with Epstein-Barr virus (EBV) infection. Immune defects may be present in the child who has history of failure to thrive, recurrent infections and fever chronic granulomatous disease (CGD).[8]

In the older child with heart disease, bacterial endocarditis must be ruled out.[9] Signs pointing to severity of illness include persistent fever, extreme weight loss, severe hematological involvement, known exposure/ risk factors for tuberculosis and HIV or signs supporting toxicity.

To conclude a stepwise approach can be of immense help in managing patients detected to have splenomegaly and lymphadenopathy. While investigations are generally guided by history and physical examination, invasive tests such as lymph node biopsy and bone marrow aspiration/ biopsy can prove to be very informative. A bone marrow examination is especially useful in presence of involvement of the hematological system.

REFERENCES

1. Ocampo PS. Splenomegaly. In: Pediatric Decision Making. Ed. Berman S. 3rd edn. Mosby-Year Book, St. Louis; 1996. pp. 320–1.
2. Rock A, Camitta BM. The lymphatic system. In: Textbook of Pediatrics. Eds. Nelson WE, Behrman RE, Kliegman RM, Arvin AM. 15th edn, WB Saunders Company, Philadelphia; 1996.pp.1440-1.
3. Pearson HA. The spleen and disturbances of splenic function. In: Nathan DG, Orkin SH (Eds). Hematology of infancy and childhood. 5th edn. WB Saunders Company, Philadelphia; 1998.pp.1051–68.
4. Lane PA, Nuss R. Generalized lymphadenopathy. In: Berman S (Ed). Pediatric Decision Making. 3rd edn. Mosby-Year Book, St. Louis; 1996.pp.368–9.
5. Link MP, Donaldson SS. The lymphomas and lymphadenitis. In: Nathan DG, Orkin SH (Eds). Hematology of infancy and childhood. 5th edn WB Saunders Company, Philadelphia; 1998. pp. 1323-58.
6. Bedros AA, Mann JP. Lymphadenopathy in children. Adv Pediatr. 1981;28:341-76.
7. Knight PJ, Mulne AF, Vassy LE. When is lymph node biopsy indicated in children with enlarged peripheral nodes? Pediatrics. 1982;69:391-6.
8. Mascarenhas MR, Altschuler SM. Large spleen. In: Schwartz MW, Thomas AC, Sargent AJ, Bhim NJ, Fein JA (Eds). Pediatric Primary Care - A problem oriented approach. 3rd edn. Mosby-Year Book, St. Louis; 1997. pp. 308–12.
9. Cohen PS. Lymphadenopathy. In: Berkowitz CD (Ed). Pediatrics: A primary care approach. WB Saunders Company, Philadelphia; pp. 308-12.

Myelodysplastic Syndrome in Children

Gauri Kapoor, Anshul Gupta

DEFINITION

Myelodysplastic syndromes (MDS) are a heterogeneous group of hematological disorders, related to the transformation of a pluripotent hematopoietic stem cell, which acquires a proliferative advantage while its progeny retains its ability to differentiate. This results in a monoclonal population of mature cells resulting in peripheral cytopenias often in the presence of a cellular bone marrow. The explanation being probably an increased programmed cell death once the proliferating stem cells mature. The hematopoietic cells in the bone marrow and periphery are morphologically and functionally abnormal. Simply stated it is a case of ineffective hematopoiesis. The term '***Preleukemia***' was first used by Block et al,[1] in 1953 to describe patients with one or more refractory cytopenias whose natural history of disease included the potential for leukemic transformation.

Myelodysplastic syndrome was probably first described in 1900 by Leube as "leukanamie" (a macrocytic anemia progressing to acute leukemia). As the natural history is characterized by transformation to acute leukemia in 25-40%, MDS was considered a "preleukemic state".[2] Most studies in pediatric age group reveal that MDS constitute a significant portion of preleukemic states hence the term MDS is often used inter changeably with preleukemia although they are technically not synonymous. In the 1970's it was realized that, many such patients never developed acute leukemia but instead died of complications from the cytopenias hence, the "preleukemia" terminology faded away, and the term "myelodysplastic syndrome" became more widely accepted.

Myelodysplastic syndrome is very rare in children, constituting 1.1% to 8.7% of hematological malignancies.[3] There is a paucity of data from India. Singh et al report an incidence of 6% of all hematological malignancies in the age group 2-18 years from a single institution.[4] Interestingly another report from a single institutional study by Agarwal et al observes a higher incidence of MDS (16%) amongst all hematological malignancies and in over a third of AML patients.[5]

Myelodysplastic syndrome in children is different from adults because many children develop this disorder in association with genetic syndromes; and certain unique conditions observed in children and not seen in adults, i.e. JCML, JMML and infant monosomy.[7]

CURRENT APPROACH TO THE CLASSIFICATION OF CHILDHOOD MDS

Internationally consensus has been achieved on the classification of MDS in childhood.[6] Myelodysplastic and myeloproliferative disorders in children are separated into three main groups; MDS, JMML, and Down syndrome disease (Table 32.1).

Myelodysplastic syndrome is subdivided into refractory cytopenia (RC), refractory anemia with excess blasts (RAEB) and refractory anemia with excess blasts in transformation (RAEB-t). The classification is used for both *de novo* and secondary MDS. The change in nomenclature from refractory anemia (RA) to RC reflects that anemia is not a prerequisite for the diagnosis but only seen in about 50% and is less

Table 32.1: Diagnostic categories of myelodysplastic and myeloproliferative diseases in children[6]

Myelodysplastic/ Myeloproliferative disease	Juvenile myelomonocytic leukemia (JMML)
Down's syndrome (DS) disease	Transient abnormal myelopoiesis (TAM) Myeloid leukemia of DS
Myelodysplastic syndrome (MDS)	Refractory cytopenia (RC) (PB blasts <2% and BM blasts <5%) Refractory anemia with excess blasts (RAEB) (PB blasts 2-19% or BM blasts 5-19%) RAEB in transformation (RAEB-t) (PB or BM blasts 20-29%)

frequent than neutropenia, thrombocytopenia and macrocytosis.[7] It is suggested to retain the RAEB-t entity but to emphasize that the blast count is insufficient to differentiate AML from MDS. Myeloid leukemia in children with Down's syndrome has unique features and is kept separate as a distinct entity. The new pediatric modification of the classification[6] emphasizes the clinical relevant subtypes of pediatric MDS and eliminates adult subtypes that are rare or unseen. However, we will still face borderline cases that are difficult to fit into this classification. The myeloproliferative disorders include:

i. Chronic myeloid leukemia
ii. Polycythemia vera
iii. Primary thrombocythemia
iv. Myelofibrosis/agnogenic myeloid metaplasia.

In a retrospective study of 167 pediatric patients with myelodysplastic syndrome (MDS) and myeloproliferative disorders (MPS), Luna Fineman et al[8] observed Adult type MDS in 60%, juvenile myelomonocytic leukemia (JMML) in 36% and transient myeloproliferative syndrome (TMS) in 4% of the children. Adult type MDS was associated with Down's syndrome (n = 10), Familial myeloid disorder (n = 10), NF (n = 1), Fanconi's anemia (n = 12), Kostmann's syndrome (n = 11), JMML was associated with NF1 (n = 7), familial myeloid disorder (n = 1). Among TMS all 6/6 patients had Down's syndrome. Similar associations have been observed by other investigators. Interestingly, in the same study, 80% of patients had cytogenetic abnormalities, the most common being monosomy 7/del7q other abnormalities included monosomy 5/5 del and trisomy 21.[8] Most studies from different centers observe this pattern of cytogenetics, with the monosomy 7/del7q being the most frequent. Hence cytogenetic analysis is important for both prognostic and therapeutic reasons.

PRIMARY AND SECONDARY MDS

Myelodysplastic syndrome can arise in a previously healthy child and is conformingly named *de novo* or "primary". It may also develop in a child with a known predisposing condition and referred to as "secondary". Secondary MDS is seen in patients (a) after chemotherapy or radiation therapy (therapy related MDS), (b) with inherited BM failure disorders, c) with acquired aplastic anemia and d) with familial MDS (Table 32.2). It is to be recognized, however, that children with so-called "primary" MDS may have an underlying yet unknown genetic defect predisposing them to MDS at young age. Therefore, the distinction between primary and secondary disease may become arbitrary. Myeloid neoplasias in patients with predisposing conditions share the biological characteristics of MDS regardless of the presenting blast count. The prognosis appears to depend primarily on the cytogenetic profile.

DOWN'S SYNDROME

Children with Down's syndrome are characteristically known to present with abnormal myeloid proliferation at birth with transient abnormal myelopoiesis (TAM) which has an indolent course and resolves spontaneously.[9] They may show a clinical and morphological picture indistinguishable from AML. The blast cells often have cell surface antigens characteristic of megakaryoblasts.[9] Life-threatening complications may occur in a few patients, but spontaneous remission appears in the majority within 3 months. AML develops 1–3 years later in about one quarter of the children.[9] It is uncertain whether TAM should be considered a malignant disease.

After the neonatal period they may present with RAEB-t/ AML. Individuals with Down syndrome (DS) have a more than 50-fold increased risk of leukemia

Table 32.2: Abnormalities associated with JMML and MDS[6]

Associated with JMML	Constitutional conditions	Neurofibromatosis type 1 (NF1) Noonan's syndrome Trisomy 8 mosaicism
Associated with MDS	Constitutional conditions	Congenital bone marrow failure Fanconi's anemia Kostmann's syndrome Shwachman-Diamond syndrome Blackfan-Diamond anemia Trisomy 8 mosaicism Familial MDS (at least one first degree relative with MDS/AML)
	Acquired conditions	Prior chemotherapy/radiation Aplastic anemia

Table 32.3: Diagnostic guidelines for JMML[15]

Suggestive clinical features	Hepatosplenomegaly Lymphadenopathy Pallor Skin rash
Laboratorial criteria	
Minimal criteria (all 3 must be fulfilled)	No Ph chromosome, no BCR-ABL rearrangement PB monocyte count > 1 x 10^9/L Marrow blast count < 20%
Criteria for definite diagnosis (at least 2 must be fulfilled)	Hemoglobin F increased for age Myeloid precursors in blood smear White cell count >10 x 10^9/L Clonal abnormality GM-CSF hypersensitivity of myeloid progenitors

during the first five years of life.[10] They usually have a prolonged and indolent preleukemic phase and respond very well to chemotherapy. About half the leukemias in children with DS are myeloid often present with features of MDS. Amongst the AMLs, the M7 subtype (Acute megakaryotic leukemia) is more frequent.[11] The myeloid leukemia seen in young children with DS is unique and classified under the unifying term *myeloid leukemia of DS* (ML-DS).[6] ML-DS is preferred to acute megakaryoblastic leukemia because other phenotypes are observed sharing the same biologic and clinical characteristics. Myeloid leukemia in children with DS occurs characteristically at 1-4 years of age with an excess of megakaryoblasts and almost uniform presence of GATA1 mutation.[12] Myeloid leukemia in older DS children (3 years or older) behaves more like AML in patients without DS and has a poor prognosis.[13] Such patients may present as 'true *de novo*' AML[14] not fulfilling the criteria for myeloid leukemia of DS. It is no longer appropriate to use the terms MDS and AML in young children with DS.

JUVENILE MYELOMONOCYTIC LEUKEMIA

Juvenile myelomonocytic leukemia (JMML) is a unique pediatric disorder previously referred to as JCML or CMML. Diagnostic criteria for JMML are listed in Table 32.3.[15] Blood film appearance is characteristic and often more helpful in diagnostics than BM smear. Patients with JMML though may have up to 20% blasts in the blood the BM blast count at diagnosis is usually below 20%. Juvenile myelomonocytic leukemia includes patients with monosomy 7 previously considered to represent a distinct hematologic disorder described as the monosomy 7 syndrome.[16] There are no major clinical differences between JMML in children with and without monosomy 7.[17,18] The term CMML is included in the classification but is reserved for cases secondary to previous chemotherapy. BCR-ABL-negative chronic myeloid leukemia is extremely rare in children and most cases are probably JMML. When BCR-ABL-negative CML is diagnosed it should be included in the group of myelodysplastic/ myeloproliferative disorders. Mutations in the *Ras* gene is seen in 20%, in *PTPN11* 35%, *NF1* gene in 15% and clinical NF1 in another 15%, molecular genetics has, therefore, become very helpful in diagnosing JMML.[19]

MONOSOMY 7

Monosomy 7 is the most common cytogenetic abnormality among myeloid disorders during childhood.[20] It can be found in both preleukemic myelodysplastic syndrome (MDS) and acute myelogenous leukemia (AML). In patients with AML, monosomy suggests involvement of pluripotent hematopoietic stem cells in the leukemic process. The nonrandom association of monosomy 7 with myeloid leukemia is consistent with loss of function of a gene (or genes) located on chromosome 7 that regulates myeloid growth and differentiation.[21] The myeloid disorders associated with monosomy 7 develop in three contexts: (1) *De novo*, (2) Secondary, and (3) Constitutional. *De novo* cases arise without apparent predisposing factors. Secondary cases appear after cytotoxic chemotherapy for cancer, after occupational exposure to mutagens, and probably after immunosuppressive therapy for severe aplastic anemia (SAA). Constitutional cases arise in individuals with a genetic predisposition to leukemia like Fanconi anemia, severe congenital neutropenia, Neurofibromatosis type 1, Shwachman-Diamond syndrome.[22,23] A well defined myeloproliferative disorder with prominent bone marrow dysplasia and hepatosplenomeagly exists in young children and has been termed

Table 32.4: Clinical syndromes associated with Monosomy 7[8]

	JMML	*Monosomy 7 syndrome*
Age	<5 years	<5 years
Sex	M>F	M>F
Clinical finding	Hepatosplenomegaly, failure to thrive, skin rash, lung infiltrates	Hepatosplenomegaly, bacterial infections, skin rash
Laboratory finding	Leukocytosis, thrombocytopenia, anemia, monocytosis, increased HbF and vitamin B_{12}, decreased LAP	Leukocytosis, thrombocytopenia, anemia, monocytosis, normal or increased HbF
Bone marrow	Hypercellular, monocytosis, decreased megakaryocytes, dysplastic features less frequent, increased blasts but usually <30%	Hypercellular, dyserythropoiesis, monocytosis (vacuolated), increased blasts, Pelger-Huet
Progression to AML	If <6 months old, several years; if > 1-year-old, <2 years	If < 1-year-old, may smoulder several years; if > 1-year-old, in 1-2 years transform into M2, M4 or M6 FAB AML
Prognosis and survival	1-2 years, except in children <6 months at diagnosis	< 2 years

monosomy 7 syndrome.[16] This condition shares many clinical and epidemiologic features with juvenile chronic myelogenous leukemia (JCML). Distinguishing monosomy 7 syndrome from JCML is problematic, because both disorders predominantly affect young male patients and are characterized by thrombocytopenia, anemia, splenomegaly, and a poor prognosis (Table 32.4). Many children with monosomy 7 do not show the typical skin rash or increased fetal hemoglobin level that characterizes JCML, and 75 to 90% of patients with JCML do not have chromosome 7 deletions in their marrows at diagnosis.[24] However, patients with JCML may acquire monosomy 7 with disease acceleration. The relationship between the latter and JCML is perhaps as follows: The monosomy 7 syndrome is one of the number of distinct entities that are associated with chromosome 7 deletions, whereas JCML is a myeloproliferative disorder of infants and young children, 6 to 24% of whom show bone marrow monosomy 7 at diagnosis.[25] The epidemiologic and clinical similarities between monosomy 7 syndrome and JCML strongly suggests that these disorders share one or more pathogenic alterations in common. Children with monosomy 7 and MDS have an outcome similar to MDS patients without monosomy 7, whereas patients diagnosed as AML with monosomy 7 have a lower response rate to chemotherapy and a higher relapse rate compared with AML without -7.[24] Monosomy 7 may be regarded as a marker of an MDS-like disease.

Refractory Anemia with Excess of Blasts (RAEB) and RAEB in Transformation (RAEB-T)

RAEB as defined by FAB has a BM blast count between 5 and 20%. Auer rods are no longer a discriminator for classification. Patients with recurrent cytogenetic abnormalities typically associated with AML, e.g. t(15;17) (PML/RARalfa), t(8;21) (RUNX1/CBFA2T1), inv(16) (CBFB/MYH11), t(9;11) (MLL/MLLT3), should be diagnosed and treated as AML regardless of the blast count.[26] MDS and true de novo (TDN)-AML display significant differences in pathogenesis and natural course.[27] The cytogenetic differences predicting response to therapy in MDS/AML may reflect the underlying biological nature of the disease. TDN-AML is a chemo-sensitive disease characterized by specific recurring translocations, whereas MDS and secondary AML is characterized by numerical chromosomal abnormalities and are typically resistant to chemotherapy. Patients with adverse cytogenetics have a poor response to therapy irrespective of the proportion of blasts in the BM and have been described as MDS-related AML (MDR-AML).

The WHO classification[6] suggested abolition of the category of RAEB-t including most of these patients as AML with multilineage dysplasia. The cut-off point for diagnosis of AML was lowered from the traditional 30 to 20% blast cells. This distinction is clearly an arbitrary one and there must in practice be a continuum between RAEB and AML. There are no data to indicate whether a 20% blast cell cut off is useful in pediatrics. A British study[28] suggested a better outcome following AML therapy in patients with RAEB-t compared with RAEB, however, this was not found in an American study.[29] Until more data is available it is suggested maintaining the RAEB-t category in children. It is important to recognize that any threshold of blast percentage to separate MDS from AML is a surrogate marker for the underlying biological behavior of the disease. In patients with ambiguous blast count a more clinical relevant approach may be based upon clinical features, cytogenetics and serial assessment of the BM rather than predicting clinical behavior from a single examination.

Natural Course and Prognostic Factors in MDS

Children with RC or low-grade RAEB may show a long and stable clinical course without treatment. Blood transfusions are only required infrequently and severe infections are rarely seen. The condition may smolder with unchanged cytopenia for months or even years but will eventually progress in most patients. In a series of 67 children with primary RC, four died from complications of pancytopenia prior to therapy or progression and 20 progressed to more advanced MDS at a median of 1.7 years from presentation.[7] Although RC with monosomy 7 is associated with a higher risk of progression both RC and RAEB patients with monosomy 7 may show stable disease without treatment for several years.[24] Once progression has occurred the outcome is inferior even after stem cell transplant (SCT).[30] Spontaneous regression of MDS has occasionally been reported in the literature.[31] The International Prognostic Scoring System (IPSS) for MDS weighted data on BM blasts count, cytopenia and cytogenetics and separated patients into four prognostic groups.[32] The IPSS has been very useful in adults but is less informative in children.

It is interesting to note that in addition to the conditions described above there are certain well-described hematological conditions, which represent preleukemic states in a small percentage of children. These include Fanconi Anemia, severe aplastic anemia, paroxysmal nocturnal hemoglobinuria, therapy related leukemias particularly those secondary to alkylating agent therapy and radiation therapy. These patients present with a preleukemia syndrome which ultimately transforms to AML (M1 or M2 subtype), with an incubation period of about 5-year and an overall poor prognosis. BMT is recommended for them once they achieve remission.

FANCONI'S ANEMIA

This is an autosomal recessive condition that clinically presents with pancytopenia, associated with a variety of congenital anomalies and a high predisposition to malignancy. The incidence of AML in Fanconi's anemia (FA) patients is reported to be more than 15,000 times than that of the general population,[22] and this development has a very poor prognosis with death occurring by age 15 years. It is characterized by spontaneous chromosome breakage and hypersensitivity to DNA cross-linking agents. Diagnosis is confirmed by chromosomal fragility testing by diepoxybutane.[33] Monsomy 7 is the most frequently associated cytogenetic abnormality. Hence some workers consider Fanconi's anemia patients as a preleukemic condition.[22]

When to Suspect

Signs and symptoms are similar to those of leukemia, like prolonged fever of unknown origin; pallor not responding to hematinics, other features could variably include hepatosplenomegaly, lymphadenopathy, skin rash and stigmata of congenital syndromes. The course of illness is over months rather than weeks. Presence of cytopenias in this setting should bring to mind MDS as a possibility in the differential diagnosis.

A detailed family history and thorough physical exam to look for the described genetic syndromes is equally important as these will predict outcome and determine treatment strategy.

Investigative Work-up of a Patient with Myelodysplastic Syndrome

It is extremely important to confirm the diagnosis prior to embarking on treatment. The most essential ones include a complete hemogram with a well-stained peripheral blood smear examination followed by bone marrow aspiration and trephine biopsy (Figs 32.1A to E). Persistent cytopenias with bone marrow dysplasia affecting one or more cell lines are good clues to diagnosis. The diagnosis is often difficult and help of an experienced hematopathologist is recommended. In relevant cases a pretransfusion HbF, B_{12} and folic acid levels may be necessary. Once the bone marrow aspirate is done viral studies may also be required. In patients with MDS/MPS it is important to do iron stain and cytogenetic studies on the bone marrow (Table 32.5).

The two major diagnostic challenges are to distinguish MDS with a low blast count from aplastic anemia (AA) and other nonclonal BM disorders, and to differentiate MDS with excess of blasts from AML. The traditional classification has been based on morphology but a number of additional factors need to be considered. Myelodysplasia may occur in the BM in a variety of disorders of very different etiologies, e.g. infection,[34] drug therapy[35] and chronic disease.[36] Nonclonal disorders with dysplastic features, e.g. mitochondrial disorders like Pearson syndrome, should not be considered as MDS. It may be difficult to diagnose MDS in children who have a low blast cell count and no clonal marker. The proposed minimal diagnostic criteria may be helpful in this situation[6]

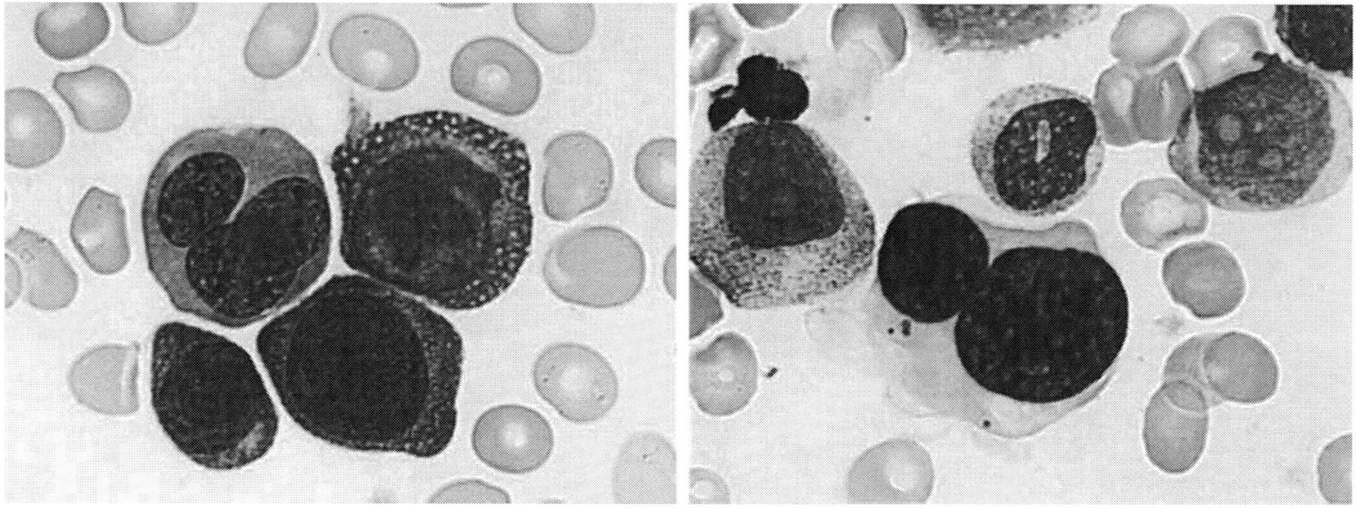

Fig. 32.1A: Dyserythropoiesis: BM *(For color version, see Plate 3)*

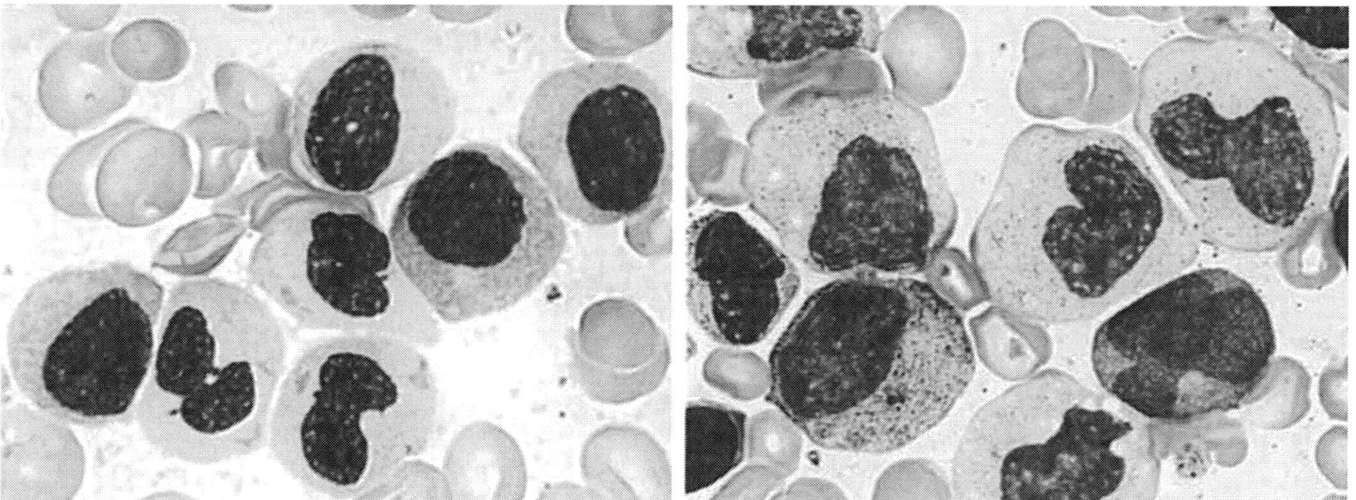

Fig. 32.1B: Dysgranulopoiesis: BM *(For color version, see Plate 3)*

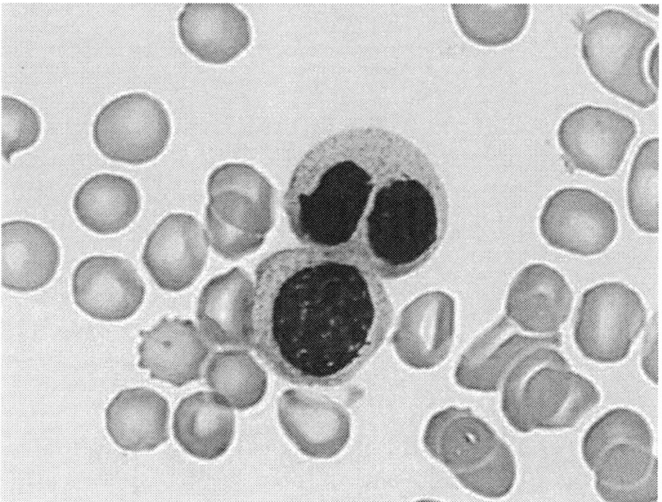

Fig. 32.1C: Dysgranulopoiesis: PB *(For color version, see Plate 3)*

(Table 32.6). Since hematopoiesis is often dysplastic in patients with congenital BM failure disorders, it is suggested diagnosing MDS in these patients only if the BM blast count is increased, a persistent clonal chromosomal abnormality is present or hypercellularity in the BM develops in the presence of persistent PB cytopenia. RARS is extremely rare in children. The finding of sideroblastic anemia should prompt investigation for possible mitochondrial cytopathy or disorders of heme synthesis.[37] A trephine biopsy of good quality is mandatory in the evaluation of a child with suspected AA or MDS. A careful search for morphological characteristics at diagnosis will often establish a distinction between the two entities. Hypoplastic MDS tends to show sparsely scattered granulopoietic cells, patchy islands of immature erythropoiesis and in most cases decreased megakaryo-

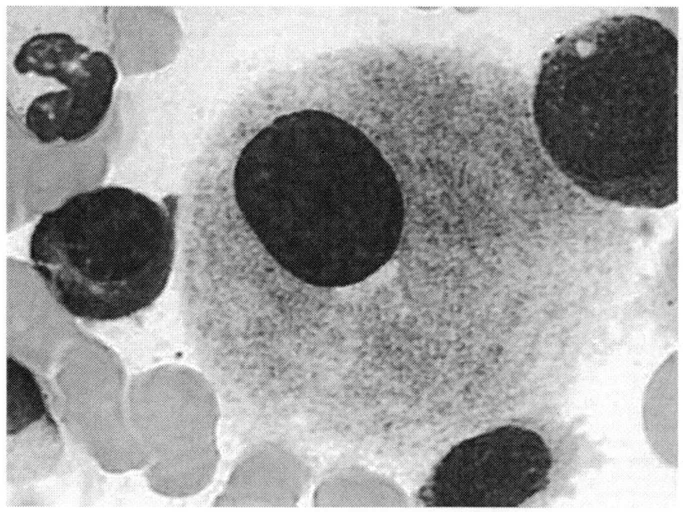
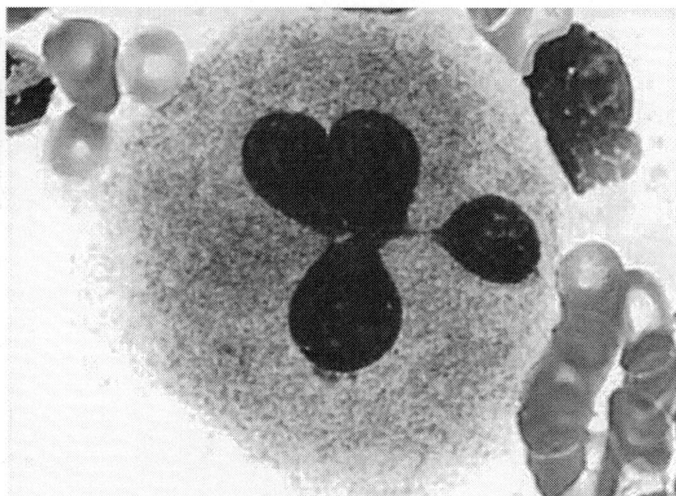

Fig. 32.1D: Dysmegakaryopoiesis: BM *(For color version, see Plate 4)*

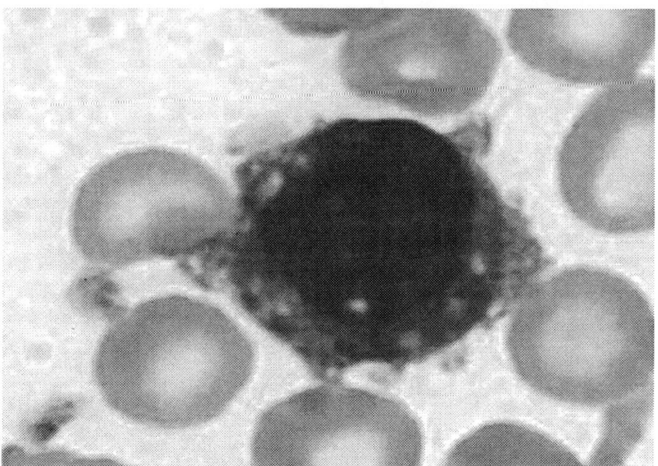

Fig. 32.1E: Micromegakaryocytes: BM *(For color version, see Plate 4)*

Table 32.5: Suggested diagnostic evaluation of pediatric myelodysplasia

History
- Family history of leukemia or genetic disorders
- History of previous cytotoxic therapy

Examination
- Look for congenital disorders, e.g. Fanconi's anemia, severe congenital neutropenia, Down's syndrome, Bloom's syndrome, Shwachmann syndrome, Kostmann's syndrome, Mitochondrial cytopathy, Neurofibromatosis 1

Laboratory
- Peripheral blood smear examination
- Full blood count (including indices, white count, differential and monocyte count)
- Bone marrow aspirate and biopsy (morphology, iron stain, cytogenetics)
- Folate and B_{12} levels in blood
- Hemoglobin F (pretransfusion)
- Viral studies—CMV and EBV

poiesis and in some micromegakaryocytes (Figs 32.1A to E). See algorithm in Flow chart 32.1 for approach to diagnosis.

Management

The three main approaches to treatment include:
1. Allogenic bone marrow transplantation (BMT)
2. AML—type chemotherapy
3. Conservative approach

It is essential to have a confirmed diagnosis prior to assigning treatment strategy. Patients with classical CML, and RAEB-t, mitochondral cytopathy (RARS), therapy related MDS respond to nothing short of BMT and this is the recommended strategy if a donor is available. In those where donor is not available AML-type treatment may be tried. Down's syndrome patients with MPS/AML do well with AML-type therapy and BMT is not indicated in them. Conservative approach is reserved for those patients where diagnosis is still uncertain, or if they have refractory anemia with normal cytogenetics and are not transfusion dependent. Patients with infantile monosomy 7 syndrome (age <1 year) may also do well with less intensive therapy like 6-mercaptopurine or 6-thioguanine. Neonates with myeloproliferative disorders should also be treated conservatively.

Allogenic SCT is the therapy of choice for virtually all forms of MDS in childhood. Studies specifically addressing the question of SCT in children have indicated a probability of disease-free survival (DFS)

Flow chart 32.1: Pancytopenia/bilineage or single lineage cytopenia

Pancytopenia/Bilineage or Single lineage cytopenia

↓

Red cell indices
PBS

Increased retic/
Evidence of hemolysis
(increased indirect bilirubin)

Direct Coomb's test +ve → Autoimmune Pancytopenia (Collagen vascular disease e.g. SLE)

Chronic Hemolysis + Hemoglobinuria → Flow cytometry CD55/CD59 → PNH

Blasts on PS → BMA/BMB → Leukemia, Lymphoma, Neuroblastoma, LCH, Osteopetrosis, Other solid tumors

Normal or decreased retic
No other evidence of hemolysis

Normal MCV → BMA/BMB

Marrow failure → Aplastic anemia

Fibrosis or dysplastic features → MDS, Myelofibrosis

Increased MCV
macro-ovalocytosis

N. B_{12}, N.folate → MDS, Methyl-malonic acidemia, Drugs (Zidovudine, Hydroxyurea, etc.)

Congenital malformation, increased HbF → Fanconi anemia, Dyskeratosis congenita

Hyper seg. polys, ↓ sed $S.B_{12}$, ↓ sed red cell folate → B_{12}/Folate deficiency anemia

Abbreviations: PBS: Peripheral blood smear; BMA/BMB: Bone marrow aspiration/bone marrow biopsy; MDS: Myelodysplastic syndrome; Retic: Reticulocyte count; HbF: Fetal hemaglobin; PNH: Paroxysmal nocturnal hemaglobinuria; SLE: System lupus erythematosus; LCH: Langerhan's cell histiocytosis

Table 32.6: Minimal diagnostic criteria for MDS[6]

At least two of the following:
• Sustained unexplained cytopenia (neutropenia, thrombocytopenia, or anemia)
• At least bilineage morphologic myelodysplasia
• Acquired clonal cytogenetic abnormality in hematopoietic cells
• Increased blasts (>5%)

following transplant with an HLA-matched family donor (MFD) of about 50%.[38,39] Children receiving a graft from an HLA-matched unrelated donor (MUD) have previously suffered a higher transplant-related mortality (TRM) and lower DFS but more recent studies have shown survival following MUD-SCT comparable to MFDSCT. A preparative regimen consisting of busulfan, cyclophosphamide and melphalan[40] has shown a high antileukemia effect.

REFERENCES

1. Block M, Hacobsen LO, Bethard WF. Preleukemic acute human leukemia. JAMA. 1953;152:1018-28.
2. Jackson GH, Carey PJ, Cant AJ, Bown NP, Reid MM. Myelodysplastic syndromes in children. Br J Haematal. 1993;84:185.
3. Arico M, Biondi A, Pui C. Juvenile myelomonocytic leukemia. Blood. 1997;90:479-88.
4. Singh ZN, Kashyap R, Pati HP, Choudhary VP. Myelodysplastic syndromes in childhood and adolescence: Clinical and hematological profile. Indian Pediatrics. 2001;38:72-5.
5. Agarwal BR, Currimbhoy ZE. Childhood myelodysplasia. Indian Pediatr. 1994;31:797-806.
6. Hasle H, Niemeyer CM, Chessells JM, et al. A pediatric approach to the WHO classification of myelodysplastic and myeloproliferative diseases. Leukemia. 2003;17:277-82.
7. Kardos G, Baumann I, Passmore SJ, et al. Refractory anemia in childhood: a retrospective analysis of 67 patients with particular reference to monosomy 7. Blood. 2003;102:1997-2003.

8. Luna-Fineman S, Shannon KM, Atwater SK, et al. Myelodysplastic and myeloproliferative disorders of childhood: A study of 167 patients. Blood. 1999;2:459-66.
9. Zipursky A, Brown E, Christensen H, Sutherland R, Doyle J. Leukemia and/ or myeloproliferative syndrome in neonates with Down syndrome. Semin Perinatol. 1997;21: 97-101.
10. Hasle H, Clemmensen IH, Mikkelsen M. Risks of leukaemia and solid tumours in individuals with Down's syndrome. Lancet. 2000;355:165-9.
11. Lange BJ, Kobrinsky N, Barnard DR, Arthur DC, Buckley JD, Howells WB, et al. Distinctive demography, biology, and outcome of acute myeloid leukemia and myelodysplastic syndrome in children with Down syndrome: Children's cancer group studies 2861 and 2891. Blood. 1998; 91:608-15.
12. Crispino JD. GATA1 mutations in Down syndrome: implications for biology and diagnosis of children with transient myeloproliferative disorder and acute megakaryoblastic leukemia. Pediatr Blood Cancer. 2005;44:40-4.
13. Gamis AS, Alonzo TE, Lange B, Woods WG, Smith FO. Acute myelogenous leukemia (AML) in Downs Syndrome (DS) patients: Outcome, toxicities, and prognostic factors from the CCG 2891 trial. Blood. 2001;98:720a.
14. Sato A, Imaizumi M, Koizumi Y, Obara Y, Nakai H, Noro T, et al. Acute myelogenous leukaemia with t(8;21) translocation of normal cell origin in mosaic Down's syndrome with isochromosome 21q. Br J Haematol. 1997;96:614-6.
15. Niemeyer CM, Fenu S, Hasle H, et al. Differentiating juvenile myelomonocytic leukemia from infectious disease. Blood. 1998;91:365-7.
16. Sieff CA, Chessells JM, Harvey BA, Pickthall VJ, Lawler SD. Monosomy 7 in childhood: a myeloproliferative disorder. Br J Haematol. 1981;49:235-49.
17. Niemeyer CM, Arico' M, Basso G, Cantu'-Rajnoldi A, Creutzig U, Haas OA, et al and members of the European Working Group on Myelodysplastic Syndromes in Childhood (EWOG-MDS). Chronic myelomonocytic leukemia in childhood: a retrospective analysis of 110 cases. Blood. 1997;89:3534-43.
18. Hasle H, Arico' M, Basso G, Biondi A, Cantu' -Rajnoldi A, Creutzig U, et al. Myelodysplastic syndrome, juvenile myelomonocytic leukemia, and acute myeloid leukemia associated with complete or partial monosomy 7. Leukemia. 1999;13:376-85.
19. Kratz CP, Niemeyer CM, Castleberry RP, et al. The mutational spectrum of PTPN11 in juvenile myelomonocytic leukemia and Noonan Syndrome/myeloproliferative disease. Blood. 2005;106:2183-5.
20. Evans JP, Czepulkowski B, Gibbons B, Swansbury GJ, Chessells JM. Childhood monosomy 7 revisited. Br J Haematol. 1988;69:41.
21. Weiss K, Stass S, Williams D, Kalwinsky D, Dahl GV, Wang W, et al. Childhood monosomy 7 syndrome: Clinical and in vitro studies. Leukemia. 1987;1:97.
22. Auerbach A. Fanconi anemia and leukemia: Tracking the genes. Leukemia. 1992;6:1.
23. Shannon KM, Watterson J, Johnson P, O'Connell P, Lange B, Shah N, et al. Monosomy 7 myeloproliferative disease in children with neurofibromatosis, type 1: Epidemiology and molecular analysis. Blood. 1992;79:1311.
24. Hasle H, Aricò M, Basso G, Biondi A, Cantù Rajnoldi A, Creutzig U, et al. Myelodysplastic syndrome, juvenile myelomonocytic leukemia, and acute myeloid leukemia associated with complete or partial monosomy 7. Leukemia. 1999;13:376-85.
25. Baranger L, Baruchel A, Leverger G, Schaison G, Berger R. Monosomy-7 in childhood hemopoietic disorders. Leukemia. 1990;4:345.
26. Chan GCF, Wang WC, Raimondi SC, et al. Myelodysplastic syndrome in children: differentiation from acute myeloid leukemia with a low blast count. Leukemia. 1997;11:206-11.
27. Head DR. Revised classification of acute myeloid leukemia. Leukemia. 1996;10:1826-31.
28. Webb DKH, Passmore SJ, Hann IM, et al. Results of treatment of children with refractory anaemia with excess blasts (RAEB) and RAEB in transformation (RAEB-t) in Great Britain 1990-99. Br J Haematol. 2002;117:33-9.
29. Woods WG, Barnard DR, Alonzo TA, et al. Prospective study of 90 children requiring treatment for juvenile myelomonocytic leukemia or myelodysplastic syndrome: A report from the Children's Cancer Group. J Clin Oncol. 2002;20:434-40.
30. Anderson JE, Gooley TA, Schoch G, et al. Stem cell transplantation for secondary acute myeloid leukemia: evaluation of transplantation as initial therapy or following induction chemotherapy. Blood. 1997;89:2578-85.
31. De Simone A, Cantù-Rajnoldi A, Sainati L, et al. Spontaneous remission from RAEB in a child. Leukemia. 2001; 15:856-7.
32. Greenberg P, Cox C, Le Beau MM, et al. International scoring system for evaluating prognosis in myelodysplastic syndromes. Blood. 1997;89:2079-88.
33. Young N, Alter B. Aplastic Anemia: Acquired and Inherited. Philadelphia, PA, Saunders; 1994.
34. Mueller BU, Tannenbaum S, Pizzo PA. Bone marrow aspirates and biopsies in children with human immunodeficiency virus infection. J Pediatr Hematol Oncol. 1996;18:266-71.
35. Brichard B, Vermylen C, Scheiff JM, et al. Haematological disturbances during long-term valproate therapy. Eur J Pediatr. 1994;153:378-80.
36. Yetgin S, Ozen S, Saatci U, et al. Myelodysplastic features in juvenile rheumatoid arthritis. Am J Hematol. 1997; 54:166-9.
37. Bader-Meunier B, Rötig A, Mielot F, et al. Refractory anaemia and mitochondrial cytopathy in childhood. Br J Haematol. 1994;87:381-5.
38. Locatelli F, Zecca M, Niemeyer C, et al. Role of allogeneic bone marrow transplantation for the treatment of myelodysplastic syndromes in childhood. The European Working Group on Childhood Myelodysplastic Syndrome (EWOG-MDS) and the Austria-Germany-Italy (AGI) Bone Marrow Transplantation Registry. Bone Marrow Transplant. 1996;18(Suppl 2):63-8.
39. Yusuf U, Frangoul HA, Gooley TA, et al. Allogeneic bone marrow transplantation in children with myelodysplastic syndrome or juvenile myelomonocytic leukemia: the Seattle experience. Bone Marrow Transplant. 2004;33:805-14.
40. Deeg HJ, Storer B, Slattery JT, et al. Conditioning with targeted busulfan and cyclophosphamide for hemopoietic stem cell transplantation from related and unrelated donors in patients with myelodysplastic syndrome. Blood. 2002; 100:1201-7.

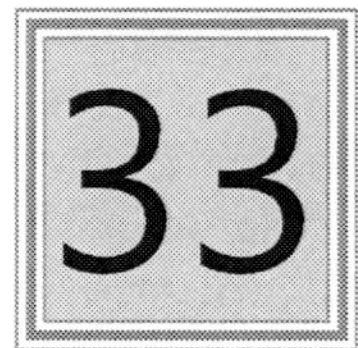

Storage Diseases of the Reticuloendothelial System

Nirmalya Roy Moulik, Archana Kumar

The lysosomal storage diseases (LSDs) comprise a heterogeneous group of almost 50 disorders that are caused by genetic defects resulting in lysosomal accumulation of substrates that are specific to each disorder. The progressive intracellular accumulation of substrates causes cellular dysfunction leading to tissue and eventually organ damage. These disorders involve multiple organs including the reticuloendothelial (RE) system, CNS, heart, bones and soft tissues. LSDs can produce significant changes in the peripheral blood as well as organs of the RE system causing cytopenias, vacuolization of mononuclear cells, accumulation of foam cells, hepatosplenomegaly and lymphadenopathy. The progressive pathogenesis leads to a slowly developing disease with variable degree of organ dysfunction, resulting in significant morbidity and reduction in lifespan of affected individuals.

INCIDENCE

Although each disorder is rare, LSDs as a group have a frequency of 1 in 7000-8000 live births.[1,2] They are more commonly encountered in populations like the Ashkenazi Jews. An unpublished Indian series estimates an annual incidence of 6000-8000 cases in India, but due to lack of suspicion and awareness, early detection of disease becomes difficult.

PATHOGENESIS

Lysosomes and their Function

Lysosomes are membrane-limited organelles found in all cells including leukocytes, erythrocytes and platelets in varying amounts. They contain acid hydrolases for the degradation of a variety of complex macromolecules at acid pH, which is provided in the lysosome by a hydrogen ion pump. These enzymes after synthesis in the Rough Endoplasmic Reticulum are modified with deletion and addition of residues at the Smooth Endoplasmic Reticulum and transported via the Golgi apparatus to be finally packaged into lysosomal vesicles. At least 50 enzymes acting on lipids, carbohydrates, proteins and nucleotides are present in lysosomes. The functions of lysosomes include catabolism of degenerated cellular products (autophagy), also ingested foreign materials (heterophagy).[3] The limiting membrane of lysosomes, under normal circumstances, prevents the cellular structures and organelles from autodigestion by these enzymes.

Mechanism of LSDs

Lysosomal storage diseases (LSDs) occur as a result of accumulation of substrates which would otherwise have been digested by lysosomal enzymes. This can be due to the following defects:

- The most frequent is the absence of an enzyme needed for degradation of substrates. This can be caused by mutations leading to either absent or defective protein, or defect in activator molecules needed for the degradation of sphingolipids, or defects of protective stabilizing proteins. The largest group of lysosomal disorders are due to deficiency of hydrolases involved in the degradation of heteroglycans, presenting as mucopolysaccharidoses, sphingolipidoses, glycoproteinoses and mucolipidosis (MPS I and IV).
- The second type results from defective synthesis of the specific carbohydrate recognition marker as in mucolipidosis II and III.
- The third group comprises transport defects through the lysosomal membrane as seen in cystinosis and in Salla disease (N-acetylneuraminic acid accumulation).

There are certain diseases which are likely to be caused by a lysosomal dysfunction with an as yet unidentified biochemical defect, like the large group of ceroid lipofuscinosis and Chédiak-Higashi syndrome.

GENETICS

All LSDs are inherited in an autosomal recessive fashion, except for Fabry, Hunter (mucopolysaccharidosis type II) and Danon diseases, which are X-linked. Some disorders are more prevalent in certain geographic areas or among particular population groups, (e.g. Gaucher, Tay-Sachs, Niemann-Pick type A, and mucolipidosis IV are more common in Ashkenazi Jews), largely as a result of ancestral founder mutations.[4-6] In many diseases, such as Fabry, most Kindred's have private mutations.

Genotype-Phenotype Correlation

A single clinically defined disorder may be caused by more than one enzymatic defect, such as Sanfilippo disease (MPS III), which can be caused by a deficiency in any one of four hydrolases. On the other hand, a single enzyme deficiency may give rise to a wide range of clinical manifestations depending on the amount of residual enzyme activity. This may lead to variations in age of onset, severity of symptoms, organ systems affected, and degree of CNS manifestations, which can vary markedly, sometimes even within families.[7] Although specific mutations or types of mutations can be associated with certain outcomes, genotype-phenotype correlations are typically not strong as with Gaucher's disease (GD), where patients with the same mutations may present in childhood or remain asymptomatic throughout adulthood.[8] Knowledge of patient's family history is often helpful to determine a diagnosis.

CLINICAL FEATURES

The deposition of macromolecules is not uniform throughout all the organs of the body. Substrates are preferentially deposited in organs where they are actively metabolized or utilized as structural components. The involvement of specific tissues and organs thus determine the manner of clinical presentation in various storage disorders. The severity of LSDs may depend on the degree of organ involvement and age at presentation. Dysmorphic facial features, hepatosplenomegaly, evidence of connective tissue infiltration such as joint contractures, skeletal dysplasia, and corneal clouding are some of the common presenting features. Signs of central nervous system dysfunction such as slowed development, regression of previously acquired developmental milestones, hypotonia and excessive startle response, may suggest gangliosidosis. Seizures, macrocephaly, and blindness may occur later in the course of ganglioside storage disease. Regression in neurologic functioning may also occur in mucopolysaccharidoses and Niemann-Pick disease. Generally the later the onset of clinical signs, the slower is the progression and lesser the severity of the disease. The detailed discussion of clinical features of individual LSD's is not the purpose of this chapter and the interested reader is referred to standard textbooks.[3,9,10] A brief account of the relatively common LSDs has been provided in Tables 33.1 to 33.3.

The reticulo-endothelial involvement in LSDs manifests as hepatosplenomegaly, lymphadenopathy and pancytopenia. Some degree of liver enlargement occurs in most of these disorders including Gaucher's disease, Niemann-Pick disease, Sialidosis type II and Wolman's disease. Splenomegaly is also a common presenting sign in Gaucher, Niemann-Pick and Wolman diseases. Lymphadenopathy may be found in Farber disease. There are many reports of LSDs presenting as non-immune hydrops in fetus and neonates.[11]

In a series from India (n=21), common clinical signs observed in all LSDs were regression in milestones (78%) followed by dysmorphic features (75%), organomegaly (60%), macrocephaly (43%), hypotonia (52.17%) and seizures (21%).[12]

While evaluating a child with suspected LSD special importance should be given to the onset and progression of the disease as well as family history. Also, a careful assessment of the neurological, reticuloendothelial and musculoskeletal systems is essential. However, because of considerable genetic heterogeneity the physical signs and severity of the LSDs vary considerably making clinical diagnosis often difficult. Laboratory studies, therefore, become indispensible for establishing a definitive diagnosis.[3]

LABORATORY DIAGNOSIS

Principles of Laboratory Diagnosis

Probands are typically ascertained because of clinical signs and symptoms, often after the disease is advanced and interventions less efficacious. Pre-symptomatic individuals may be diagnosed by screening of family members of the proband, carrier screening, prenatal testing, screening of populations at risk for a genetic disorder, or newborn screening (NBS).

MORPHOLOGICAL DIAGNOSIS[3]

By the specific staining characteristics and ultrastructure of the storage products which form inclusions in the cells of peripheral blood, bone marrow, lymph nodes, skin, liver or spleen.

Table 33.1: Salient features of common mucopolysaccharidosis

Disease	*Inheritance/Genes*	*Enzyme deficiency/Substrate accumulating*	*RE system manifestations*	*Distinguishing clinical features*	*Specific treatment available*
MPS I (Hurler)	AR / 4p16.3	a-L-Iduronidase/Dermatan sulfate, Heparan sulfate	Vacuolated lymphocytes, hepatosplenomegaly	Coarse facies, joint stiffness, corneal clouding, CVS involvement	ET, BMT
MPS II (Hunter)	XLR / Xq27–q28	Iduronate sulfatase/Dermatan sulfate, Heparan sulfate	Granulated lymphocytes, hepatosplenomegaly	Retinal degeneration, no corneal clouding, coarse facies, mental retardation	ET
MPS III (San Fillipo)	AR/Varies with type of disease	Heparan-N-sulfatase/ Heparan sulfate	Granulated lymphocytes, variable hepatosplenomegaly	Severe mental retardation, mild coarse facies	—
MPS IV (Morquio)	AR/16q24	N-acetylgalactosamine-6-sulfate sulfatase/Keratan sulfate, Chondroitin-6 sulfate	Granulated neutrophils, variable hepatosplenomegaly	Distinctive skeletal deformity, odontoid hypoplasia, aortic valve disease, corneal clouding	—
MPS VI (Maroteaux-Lamy)	AR/5q13-q14	Arylsulfatase B/Dermatan sulfate	Granulated neutrophils and lymphocytes, hepatosplenomegaly	Coarse facies, valvular heart disease, corneal clouding	ET, BMT
MPS VII	AR/7q21.1-q22	Glucuronidase/Dermatan sulfate, Heparan sulfate	Granulated neutrophils, hepatosplenomegaly	Coarse facies, vascular involvement, hydrops fetalis in neonatal form, corneal clouding	—

Table 33.2: Salient features of common sphingolipidosis

Disease	*Inheritance*	*Enzyme deficiency/ Substrate accumulating*	*RE system manifestations*	*Distinguishing clinical features*	*Specific treatment available*
Tay-Sachs disease	AR/15q23-q24	Hexosaminidase A/GM_2 gangliosides	None	Cherry red spots, seizures, mental retardation	—
Sandhoff's disease	AR/5q13	Hexosaminidases A and B/ GM_2 gangliosides	Variable hepatosplenomegaly	Cherry red spots, Macrocephaly, hyperacusis	—
Fabry's disease	XLR/Xq22	Galactosidase A/ Globotriaosylceramide	None	Painful acroparesthesias, cutaneous angiokeratomas, hypohydrosis, corneal dystrophy	ET
Gaucher's disease	AR/17q23	Acid glucosidase/ Glucosylceramide	Gaucher cells in bone marrow, cytopenias, hepatosplenomegaly	Skeletal dysplasias	ET, SRT
Niemann-Pick disease A (neuronopathic) and B (non-neuronopathic)	AR/11p15.1-p15.4	Sphingomyelinase/ Sphingomyelin	Foam cells in bone marrow, hepatospleno-megaly	Mental retardation and seizures, macular degeneration, pulmonary infiltrates	—

Table 33.3: Salient features of other common LSDs

Disease	*Inheritance*	*Enzyme deficiency/ Substrate accumulating*	*RE system manifestations*	*Distinguishing clinical features*	*Specific treatment available*
Mucolipidosis-II, I-cell disease	AR/4q21-q23	UDP-*N*-Acetylglucosamine-1-phosphotransferase/ Glycoprotein, glycolipid	Vacuolated and granulated neutrophils, variable hepatospleno-megaly	Mild mental retardation, corneal clouding, coarse facies	—
Mucolipidosis-III, pseudo-Hurler polydystrophy	AR/-	UDP-*N*-Acetylglucosamine-1-phosphotransferase/ Glycoprotein, glycolipid	None	Mild mental retardation, corneal clouding, retinopathy, coarse facies	—
Krabbe's disease	AR/14q31	Galactosylceramidase/ Galactosylceramide	None	Mental retardation	BMT
Metachromatic leukodystrophy	AR/22q13	Arylsulfatase/ Cerebroside sulfate	None	Mental retardation, dementia, psychosis, optic atrophy	—
Multiple sulfatase deficiency	AR/-	Active site cysteine to C_a-formylglycine-converting enzyme/Sulfatides, mucopolysaccharides	Vacuolated and granulated cells, variable hepatosplenomegaly	Mental retardation, retinal degeneration	—
Wolman's disease	AR/10q23.2-q23.3	Acid lysosomal lipase/ Cholesterol esters, triglycerides	Hepatosplenomegaly	Mild mental retardation, adrenal calcification	BMT

Peripheral Blood

a. *Vacuolated lymphocytes*: These are commonly found in storage diseases and contain PAS positive granules in Sandhoff's disease and sialidoses. The vacuoles are utrastructurally dense cytoplasmic bodies or lamellar arrays surrounded by a single limiting membrane. Both intracytoplasmic and intranuclear vacuoles may be seen in Wolman's disease. Vacuoles may also be seen in other types of circulating monocytes in sialidoses and mucolipidosis II.
b. *Hypergranulated neutrophils*: Excessive granulation of neutrophils may be noted in several storage diseases. Metachromatic granules (Alder-Reilly bodies) may be present in the mucopolysaccharidoses and in mucosufatidosis. Azurophilic hypergranulation of neutrophils is a feature of neuronal ceroid lipofuscinoses.

Bone Marrow

Demonstration of cells with special morphological pattern in bone marrow or tissue sections are often helpful in the diagnosis of LSDs, however, they are non-specific and are not diagnostic of any disease entity in particular. A brief description of few such cells follows:

a. *Foam cell*: It is a lipid laden macrophage, easily recognized in unstained preparations as an oval cell 20-90 μm in diameter, with usually a single eccentric nucleus and a prominent nucleolus. Foam cells appear as large glistening cells with cytoplasmic droplets under phase contrast microscopy. The droplets are fairly uniform in size and often bi-refringent when viewed under polarization microscopy. In stained preparations foam cells are found to have a finely reticulated cytoplasmic web. The staining properties of foam cells may differ in different storage diseases. When sudanophilic material is present they stain red with oil-red-O and black with Sudan black B, with a weakly positive PAS reaction. Auto fluorescence under ultraviolet light is observed when lipofuscin is present. Since histochemical reactions may be lost if alcohol or other lipid solvents are used as fixatives of bone marrow smears, only formalin fixed tissues should be used.
b. *Sea-blue histiocytes:* These are large cells (up to 60 μm in diameter) containing large homogeneous granules that stain blue or blue-green with Giemsa or Wright's stains. These are seen in many systemic lipidosis including Niemann-Pick disease. Ultrastructurally these granules consist of lamellar as well as amorphous and granular cytosomes.
c. *Gaucher's cell:* It is a large histiocyte (20-100 μm in diameter) containing striated rod-shaped inclusion bodies in its cytoplasm that give it a tissue paper or crumpled silk appearance. Gaucher's cell stain pale pink with hematoxylin and eosin and stains only slightly with oil-red-O and Sudan back B. The inclusions are PAS positive and autofluorescent.

   Gaucher's cell is unique to the Gaucher form of inherited lipidosis but can occasionally be found in the bone marrow of patients with chronic myelogenous leukemia and thalassemia. They are probably formed by inability of macrophages to metabolize excessive lipids released from increased breakdown of RBC's.
d. Other abnormal structures can also be detected in some storage diseases such as Alder-Reilly bodies in Hurler's disease and vacuolated plasma cells in mucolipidosis II and IV.

Liver

Though cellular changes in the liver may be similar to those in the bone marrow, a needle liver biopsy also provides additional tissue for biochemical and other analyses. Due consideration should, therefore, be given to appropriate collection and storage of different pieces of the biopsy specimen. Presence of Gaucher cell in liver specimens is specific for the diagnosis of Gaucher disease and the presence of both intralysosomal and cytoplasmic glycogen for Pompe disease. However, other histologic changes are not distinctive enough to permit the diagnosis of a specific storage disease. Some of these changes include enlargement and vacuolation of Kupffer's cells, infiltration of the sinuses with vacuolated histiocytes, and a variable hepatic parenchymal cell involvement ranging from mild vacuolar change to more extensive foamy metamorphosis. Inclusions may also be seen in the hepatic vascular endothelial cells and in some cases the lobular architecture of the liver may be disturbed.

Skin

Skin biopsy can be useful for the histologic diagnosis of storage diseases. Vacuoles may be found in secretory coils of sweat glands, bulbs of hair follicles, fibroblasts, and Schwann's cells in a number of diseases. Complex osmophilic lipid deposits in axons, Schwann's cells and nerve changes in ceroid-lipofuscinosis may be of particular diagnostic value as they reflect the same pattern of inclusions as seen in the nervous system.

Cultured skin fibroblasts are less informative, but ultrastructural changes have also been noted in these cells. However, not all storage diseases produce histologic changes in the skin.

BIOCHEMICAL DIAGNOSIS[3]

Detection of storage materials in body fluids forms the basis of many screening tests for LSDs. However, specific tests involve demonstration of decreased levels of enzyme implicated for a specific disease and forms the current investigation of choice for LSDs.

Storage Substances

A number of laboratory techniques have been developed to facilitate the screening of storage substances in readily available tissue and fluid specimens. However, characterization of these compounds is more difficult than assaying the relevant enzyme for diagnostic purposes.

a. **Urine:** It is a rich source of storage material in patients with sphingolipidoses, mucopolysaccharidoses, mucolipidoses, and other oligosaccharidosis. The sphingolipids can be quantitated by a combination of thin-layer and gas liquid chromatography in a filter paper urinary specimen of 24 hours. An excess of mucopolysaccharides in urine can be identified by a positive Berry spot test. Simple thin layer chromatography methods in desalted urine have been employed to diagnose fucosidosis, mannosidosis, GM1-gangliosidosis, and sialidosis.
b. **Plasma:** Sphingolipids present in plasma can be quantitated by high performance liquid chromatography.
c. **Cultured skin fibroblasts:** High performance liquid chromatography has also been used to demonstrate elevated sphingomyelin levels in cultured skin fibroblasts in Type A Niemann-Pick disease. The storage phenomenon can be documented by cultured skin fibroblasts in other storage diseases as well.

Deficiency of Enzyme Activity

Enzymatic assays, using readily accessible material such as serum, plasma, leukocytes, lymphocytes, cultured skin fibroblasts, and tears, are convincing means for confirming the diagnosis of a storage disorder. Recently developed methods for the determination of enzymatic activities are based on elution of the enzyme using dried blood spot, which is further assessed by using fluorescent or radiolabeled substrates. Immune capture of the enzyme before the determination of enzyme activity is an alternative approach. Monoclonal and polyclonal antibodies can also be used for the immune quantification of specific lysosomal proteins from biological samples. These assays provide a convenient and economical means for diagnosis of these disorders.[13,14]

Tandem mass spectrometry has been used effectively to investigate stored substrates in many of the LSDs and may also help in monitoring of responses to therapy.[15,16]

GENETIC DIAGNOSIS

Molecular characterization of a defect by PCR is confirmatory for diagnosis, however, it is rarely used for primary diagnosis of LSDs.[11] Molecular testing is the preferred technique for prenatal diagnosis, provided the genotype of the proband is known. This approach is useful not only for carrier testing and prenatal diagnosis but can also be extended to retrospective diagnosis for an affected family member who died without a specific biochemical diagnosis. This can be done through PCR amplification of genomic DNA wherever a previously obtained biopsy or autopsy specimen is available.[7]

NEWBORN SCREENING FOR LYSOSOMAL STORAGE DISORDERS

Early detection of LSDs by newborn screening can be important for patients and their families as for several disorders earlier initiation of therapy can make a substantial difference in outcome. Rarity of LSDs prevents early diagnosis due unawareness of signs and symptoms on the part of practitioners.[7] Irreversible damage may therefore have occurred by the time a diagnosis is made. Also, many patients may remain undiagnosed, often resulting in birth of a second affected child before the first is diagnosed.

Ethical and economic considerations influence the decision regarding the advisability of newborn screening. Population screening for this group of disorders in the Indian set-up is currently debatable due to financial constraints and inadequate prevalence data.

APPROACH TO DIAGNOSIS

As discussed earlier, LSDs are multisystem disorders with significant phenotypic variability making clinical suspicion all the more difficult. LSDs should be suspected in children presenting with skeletal deformities, neuroregression, seizure and organomegaly with abnormal facial features. A child referred to a hematologist with anemia, thrombocytopenia, hepatosplenomegaly or lymphadenopathy should be suspected to have a storage disorder after common causes are ruled out. Patients may present at any age from infancy to adulthood depending on the severity of involvement. A definitive diagnosis may be difficult to obtain clinically and needs laboratory support. Diagnosis in presymptomatic individuals can be ascertained only by laboratory tests.

PRINCIPLES OF TREATMENT OF LYSOSOMAL STORAGE DISORDERS

Because of their wide-ranging medical and psychosocial problems, LSDs require a multidisciplinary team approach to treatment. Comprehensive management generally combines disease-specific therapy (if available) with symptom specific measures.

Goals of Therapy

1. *Quality-of-life:* To restore daily activities and improve quality-of-life scores.
2. *Promoting growth:* To achieve normal growth rate and puberty.
3. *Halt progression of disease:* By specific therapy
4. *Reverse established organ damage:* By specific therapy.

Symptomatic Treatment

Treatment should be focused on alleviating or ameliorating existing signs and symptoms and often forms the cornerstone of care in less affluent countries in absence of specific therapy.

- **Nutrition:** Adequate caloric and nutrient intake should be ensured by making appropriate changes in the consistency of feeds and techniques of feeding, particularly in children with neurological involvement.
- **Physiotherapy:** It is important to ensure adequate joint mobility and prevent contractures.
- **Seizures:** Occurring in the course of gray matter storage disorders should be managed by combinations of anticonvulsant drugs including carbamazepine, valproic acid, diazepam and clonazepam.
- **Orthopedic corrective procedures** and other types of operative interventions aimed at providing symptomatic relief or improving nursing care should not be with-held.
- **Schooling of mentally and physically challenged** children should be attempted in special schools.

Specific Treatment

Intermittent Therapy

Mostly comprises of enzyme replacement therapy (ERT). With rapid expansion in the field of biotechnology specific treatments for LSDs are evolving rapidly. ERT involves supplying the missing enzyme exogenously through repeated intravenous infusions. ERT can achieve higher levels of deficient enzyme as compared to stem cell transplant; however, the blood-brain barrier (BBB) cannot be crossed, precluding its use for CNS disease. To circumvent this problem of BBB intrathecal ERT is being tried for certain diseases like MPS types I and II. ERT is currently commercially available for Gaucher, Fabry, MPS I, II, VI, and Pompe diseases, but is prohibitively expensive.

Continuous Therapy

Hematopoietic stem cell transplantation (HSCT) has been used successfully in the management of some LSDs. The rationale for its use is reconstitution of the hematopoietic system from a healthy, matched donor, containing stem cells capable of producing the missing enzyme. The advantage of HSCT is that cells can integrate into many tissues, including the CNS. The major drawback of HSCT is its high morbidity and mortality although both have improved over time, particularly with the use of refined conditioning regimens and cord blood as a stem cell source. Other drawbacks are low level of correction and long time required for integration of the cells into other tissues, factors that currently preclude HSCT from being curative.

Miscellaneous Therapies

Substrate reduction therapy (SRT)[17,18] and Gene Therapy are being tried in various LSDs with limited success till now, detailed description of these are beyond the scope of this chapter.

To date there is no cure for LSDs, therefore early diagnosis and treatment is essential for optimal treatment.[19,20]

REFERENCES

1. Meikle PJ, Hopwood JJ, Clague AE, Carey WF. Prevalence of lysosomal storage disorders. JAMA. 1999;281:249-54.
2. Poorthuis BJ, Wevers RA, Kleijer WJ, et al. The frequency of lysosomal storage diseases in The Netherlands. Hum Genet. 1999;105:151-6.
3. Kolodny EH, Charria- Ortiz G. Storage Diseases of the Reticuloendothelial System. In: Nathan DG, Orkin SH, Ginsburg D, Look AT, (Eds). Nathan and Oski's Hematology of Infancy and Childhood, 6th edn; Saunders 2003;2: 1399-454.
4. Mistry PK. Gaucher's disease: a model for modern management of a genetic disease. J Hepatol. 1999;30(Suppl 1):1-5.
5. Natowicz MR, Prence EM. Heterozygote screening for Tay-Sachs disease: past successes and future challenges. Curr Opin Pediatr. 1996;8:625-9.

6. Schuchman EH, Miranda SR. Niemann-Pick disease: mutation update, genotype/phenotype correlations, and prospects for genetic testing. Genet Test. 1997;1:13-9.
7. Wang RY, Bodamer OA, Watson MS, Wilcox WR. ACMG Work Group on Diagnostic Confirmation of Lysosomal Storage Diseases. Lysosomal storage diseases: diagnostic confirmation and management of presymptomatic individuals. Genet Med. 2011;13(5):457-84.
8. Beutler E, Grabowski GA. Gaucher disease. In: Scriver CR, Beaudet AL, Sly WS, Valle D (Eds). The metabolic and molecular bases of inherited diseases, 8th edn. New York: McGraw-Hill. 2001;2:3635-68.
9. Scriver CR, Beaudet AL, Sly WS, Valle D (Eds). The metabolic and molecular bases of inherited diseases, 8th ed. New York: McGraw-Hill, 2001.
10. Spranger J. Mucopolysaccharidoses. In: Kleigman RM, Behrman RE, Jenson HB, Stanton BF (Eds). Nelson Textbook of Pediatrics, 18th edn; Philadelphia Saunders 2007;2:604-5.
11. Staretz-Chacham O, Lang TC, LaMarca ME, Krasnewich D, Sidransky E. Lysosomal storage disorders in the newborn. Pediatrics. 2009;123(4):1191-207.
12. Sheth J, Patel P, Sheth F, Shah R. Lysosomal storage disorders. Indian Pediatr. 2004;41(3):260-5.
13. Brooks DA, McCourt PA, Gibson GJ, Ashton LJ, Shutter M, Hopwood JJ. Analysis of N-acetylgalactosamine-4-sulfatase protein and kinetics in mucopolysaccharidosis type VI patients. Am J Hum Genet. 1991;48(4):710-9.
14. Umapathysivam K, Hopwood JJ, Meikle PJ. Determination of acid alpha-glucosidase activity in blood spots as a diagnostic test for Pompe disease. Clin Chem. 2001;47(8): 1378-83.
15. Carpenter KH, Wiley V. Application of tandem mass spectrometry to biochemical genetics and newborn screening. Clin Chim Acta. 2002;322(1–2):1-10.
16. Chace DH, Kalas TA, Naylor EW. The application of tandem mass spectrometry to neonatal screening for inherited disorders of intermediary metabolism. Annu Rev Genomics Hum Genet. 2002;3:17-45.
17. Cox T, Lachmann R, Hollak C, et al. Novel oral treatment of Gaucher's disease with N-butyldeoxynojirimycin (OGT 918) to decrease substrate biosynthesis. Lancet 2000;355: 1481-5.
18. Elstein D, Hollak C, Aerts JM, et al. Sustained therapeutic effects of oral miglustat (Zavesca, N-butyldeoxyno-jirimycin, OGT 918) in type I Gaucher disease. J Inherit Metab Dis. 2004;27:757-66.
19. Heese BA. Current strategies in the management of lysosomal storage diseases. Semin Pediatr Neurol. 2008; 15(3):119-26.
20. Hopkin RJ, Grabowski GA. Lysosomal Storage Diseases. In: Fauci AS, Braunwald E, Kasper DL, Hanser SL, Longo DL, Jameson JL,Localzo J (Eds). Harrisons Principles of Internal Medicine; 17th edn, Mc Graw Hill. 20082: 2452-6.

Molecular Biology Revolution in Hemato-oncology—From Bench to the Bedside

IC Verma, Vaishnavi Reddy

These are exciting times for molecular biology, genetics and hemato-oncology. The revolution was set in motion by the completion of the Human Genome Project in 2003, and the publication of the total sequence of the human genome. An improved understanding of the molecular mechanisms in hemato-oncologic disorders followed, resulting in the development of precise diagnostic tests, prognostic indicators, rational therapies, and markers for predicting response to therapy. These innovations are evolving towards personalized therapy for various disorders. A perfect example of this is the use of STI571 (signal transduction inhibitors) in the treatment of chronic myeloid leukemia. It is now apparent that molecular biology is no longer an esoteric science confined to the bench, but has found application in everyday clinical practice of hematology/oncology.

Knowledge of molecular mechanisms of disease has benefited all sections of hematology. In this chapter we will provide brief information on structure of genes, how they function and tools of the molecular trade. We will describe applications of molecular biology in thalassemia, hemophilia, telomere disorders, leukemias, neuroblastoma, mention briefly about rapid diagnosis of infections, and emphasize the prerequisites for prenatal diagnosis of hematological disorders.

PRIMER OF MOLECULAR BIOLOGY

The complete set of instructions for making an organism is called its genome. It contains the master blueprint for all cellular structures and activities for the lifetime of the cell or the organism. Found in every nucleus of a person's trillions of cells, the human genome consists of tightly coiled threads of deoxyribonucleic acid (DNA) and associated protein molecules, organized into structures called chromosomes.

Deoxyribonucleic Acid

Deoxyribonucleic acid (DNA) molecule consists of two strands resembling a ladder whose sides, made of sugar and phosphate molecules, are connected by rungs of nitrogen-containing chemicals called bases. Each strand is a linear arrangement of repeating similar units called nucleotides, which are each composed of one sugar, one phosphate, and a nitrogenous base. Four different bases are present in DNA: adenine (A), thymine (T), cytosine (C), and guanine (G). The particular order of the bases arranged along the sugar-phosphate backbone is called the DNA sequence. The nucleotides in one strand pair with those in a complementary strand. Adenine will only pair only with thymine (an A-T pair) and cytosine with guanine (a C-G pair). These are depicted in Figure 34.1.

Genes

Each chromosome contains many genes. The specific sequence of nucleotide bases in the gene carry the information required for constructing proteins, which provide the structural components of cells and tissues as well as enzymes for essential biochemical reactions. The human genome is estimated to be comprised of about 25,000 genes.

Human genes vary widely in length, often extending over thousands of bases, but only about 10% of the genome is known to include the protein-coding sequences (exons) of genes. Interspersed within many genes are intron sequences, which have no coding function. The balance of the genome consists of other noncoding regions (such as control sequences and intergenic regions), whose functions are obscure. The structure of a typical gene is depicted in Figure 34.2.

Humans can synthesize at least 100,000 different kinds of proteins that are large, complex molecules

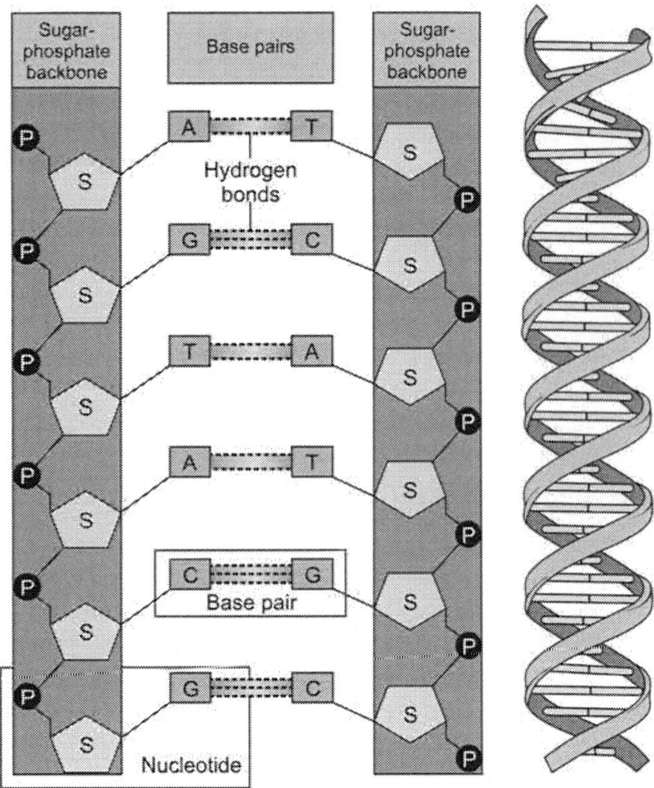

Fig. 34.1: Helical structure of DNA: The backbone of the helix consists of a sugar phosphate, while the inside comprises of the four nitrogenous bases, showing hydrogen bonds between base pairs. Note that thymine (T) always pairs with adenine (A) and guanine (G) with cytosine (C)

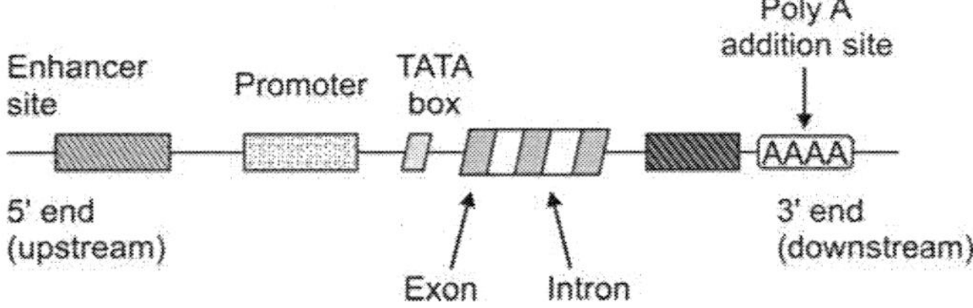

Fig. 34.2: Organization of a gene: Details of gene structure, showing promoter and upstream regulation (enhancer), introns, exons and poly A addition site

made up of long chains of subunits called amino acids. Twenty different kinds of amino acids are usually found in proteins. Within the gene, each specific sequence of three DNA bases (codons) directs the cells protein-synthesizing machinery to add specific amino acids. For example, the base sequence ATG codes for the amino acid methionine. The genetic code is thus a series of codons that specify which amino acids are required to make up specific proteins. The dogma used to be that one gene codes for one protein but we know now that this is untrue, as one gene is known to code for many proteins due to alternate splicing.

Genes occur in clusters, with genes of similar function located near each other—for example, alpha and beta globin gene clusters on chromosome 16 and 11 respectively. Control of gene expression is carried out through locus control regions (LCR), enhancer and promoter regions. Enhancers are DNA sequences that increase transcription from a nearby gene. The promoter is defined as the sequence elements immediately 5′ to the gene that interact with RNA polymerase and other components of transcription machinery. The important promoter regions are generally located in the region 100-200 bp 5′ to the gene. Most human genes have a TATA box sequence, which is located 25-30 bp 5′ to the start of transcription, and seems to be involved in the precise localization of the start. Further upstream there is often a CCAAT box sequence located 75-80 bp 5′ to the start site. It seems to be required for quantitatively efficient transcription. Housekeeping genes that are present in all cells often lack these two boxes.

Genes have a precise organization: At the beginning of the gene is a sequence, which remains untranslated into RNA, while the part to be translated always has the base ATG, as the first base. Introns which intervene between exons have to be removed, a process called splicing. The intron always begins with a GT (the splice donor), and ends with an AG (splice acceptor). The adjacent bases tend to follow a certain sequence, referred to as the consensus sequence (Fig. 34.2). Most messenger RNAs are characterized by the addition of a string of about 200 adenosine residues at their 3′ end (polyadenylation). 18-20 bases downstream of this a hexa nucleotide signal AAUAAA is attached. The poly A sequence stabilizes the RNA molecule during its exit from the nucleus into the cytoplasm.

The protein-coding instructions from the genes are transmitted indirectly through messenger ribonucleic acid (mRNA), a transient intermediary molecule similar to a single strand of DNA. For the information within a gene to be expressed, a complementary RNA strand is produced (a process called transcription) from the DNA template in the nucleus. This mRNA is moved from the nucleus to the cellular cytoplasm, where it serves as the template for protein synthesis. The cells protein-synthesizing machinery (the ribosomes) then translates the codons into a string of amino acids that will constitute the protein molecule for which it codes. In the laboratory, the mRNA molecule can be isolated

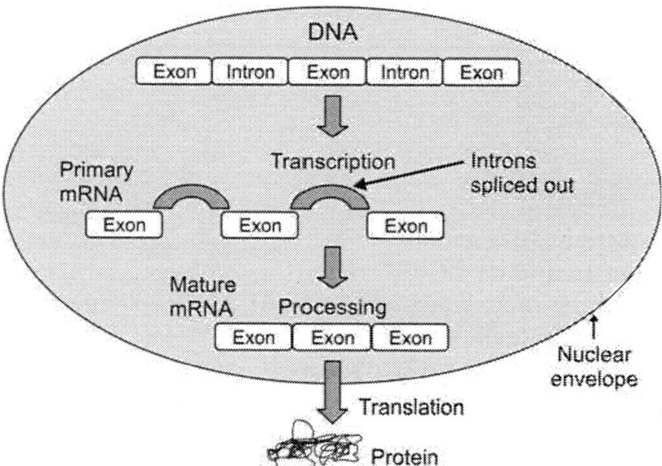

Fig. 34.3: Translation of DNA to protein: Summary of the steps leading from DNA to proteins. Replication and transcription occur in the cell nucleus. The mRNA is then transported to the cytoplasm, where translation of the mRNA into amino acid sequences composing a protein occurs

and used as a template to synthesize a complementary DNA (cDNA) strand. This sequence of events is illustrated in Figure 34.3.

Chromosomes

The human genome is organized into 24 distinct, physically separate microscopic units called chromosomes. The genes are arranged linearly along the chromosomes. The nucleus of most human cells contains 2 sets of chromosomes, one set contributed by each parent. Each set has 23 single chromosomes - 22 autosomes and an X or Y sex chromosome. A normal female will have a pair of X chromosomes; a male will have an X and Y pair.

Chromosomes can be seen under a light microscope and, when stained with certain dyes, reveal a pattern of light and dark bands reflecting regional variations in the amounts of A and T vs G and C. Differences in size and banding pattern allow the 24 chromosomes to be distinguished from each other, an analysis called a karyotype. A few types of major chromosomal abnormalities, including missing or extra copies of a chromosome or gross breaks and rejoinings (translocations), can be detected by microscopic examination; Down's syndrome, in which an individual's cells contain a third copy of chromosome 21, is diagnosed by karyotype analysis. Similarly chromosomal studies in the bone marrow have become an essential investigation in cases of leukemias.

TOOLS OF THE TRADE

1. *Restriction enzymes (RE):* These are the scissors that cut the DNA into smaller pieces, so that they can be studied. REs are derived from bacteria.
2. *Oligonucleotides:* An oligonucleotide is a small sequence of DNA that is synthesized by the machine. It has the propensity to pair with its complementary strand, thus allowing a method to identify that particular sequence in a mixture of DNAs.
3. *Polymerase chain reaction (PCR):* Polymerase chain reaction is a method to amplify segments of DNA in a short time. The number of copies increases exponentially—doubling with each cycle. In 30 cycles about one billion copies are generated. While single or few copies of a gene cannot be visualized on ordinary gels, when million copies exist, these can be seen as a band on the gel, after electrophoresis. Figure 34.4 shows the sequence of a PCR reaction. For performing a PCR reaction one requires oligonucleotides that attach to their complementary sequence, and grow towards the 5′ end by addition of more nucleotides that exist in the solution, in the presence of an enzyme-Taq polymerase. PCR has been a very fundamental advance, for which a Nobel Prize was granted to Mullis, the discoverer of the technique.
4. *Southern blot:* This is named after Ed Southern. In this technique the DNA to be studied is cut into smaller fragments by restriction enzymes, electrophoresed to separate the fragments according to size, and then transferred to a membrane. A probe with an appropriate label is then used to identify the gene of interest among the various fragments of DNA on the membrane. This was an essential technique before but now is replaced by simpler techniques.
5. *Genome wide association studies (GWAS):* In many common disorders discovery of new associations with markers and genes is being achieved by carrying our GWAS studies. A large number of SNPs (single polymorphic nucleotides) spread throughout the genome are loaded on microarrays and the DNA of interest is hybridized to these SNPs, A comparison is made of the pattern in cases with controls, and SNPs uniquely associated with the disease are identified. The area around the associated SNPs is searched for genes that may be related to the disorder. This is a powerful technique and often yields expected associations. However, large number of samples is required in cases of common disorders. A smaller sample size is needed

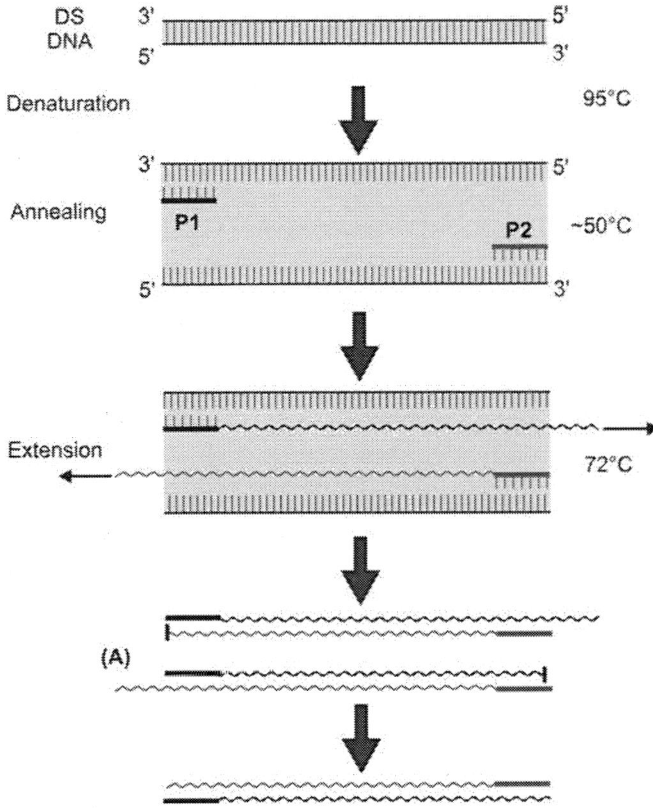

Fig. 34.4: Polymerase chain reaction: This is a schematic representation of the steps involved in PCR. STEP 1 is to first unzip the DS-DNA, also called denaturation, into two complementary single strands of DNA by heating the reaction mix to 95 degrees Celsius. STEP 2 isolates the target region of the genomic DNA by landing 2 primers (P1 and P2) which exactly match two 20-30 unique base pair regions that bookend the target region. This is called annealing. Once time is allowed for the primers to land on the sites, STEP 3 invloves heating the mix to 72 degrees at which point a special polymerase builds the DNA strand starting at the primers and continuing in the 5 prime direction. This is called extension. These three steps are repeated 25-40 times to produce millions of exact copies of the target region of DNA

for single gene disorders. The technique can also be used to map areas of homozygosity and this is often of great use in identifying new genes in consanguineous couples having children with unidentified disorders.

6. *Exon sequencing:* This technique involves sequencing of all the exons in the human genome. This is an ideal and very useful technique to obtain the sequence of all the coded part of the gene and is invaluable for discovering new genes.

APPLICATIONS OF MOLECULAR BIOLOGY

Molecular biology has advanced knowledge in all hematological fields. This chapter will briefly describe some of the applications of this new knowledge.

β-Thalassemia

This is the most common single gene disorder in India. Carrier frequency of this gene is as high as 5-10% in many states, with a mean of 3.3%. About 10,000 infants affected with thalassemia major and about 6000 affected with sickle cell disease are born every year. Application of molecular biology to thalassemia has provided means of precise diagnosis, improved therapy, prenatal diagnosis, and a way to prevent and control this burdensome disease.

The β-globin gene is a small gene, being only 1.2-kilo bases in length. Many of the general features of eukaryotic genes were first defined through study of β-globin gene. The promoter region contains a TATA box, but the sequence is actually just ATA. There is also a CCAAT box, and somewhat further upstream a sequence CACCC, which is repeated once, and is present in many other globin genes. Some distance away from β-globin gene is another critical regulator, called the locus control region, which is important for regulation of all genes within β-globin gene cluster.

The gene has three exons and two introns, with the second intron considerably larger than the first. There are short 5′ and 3′ untranslated regions and capping, polyadenylation and splicing all proceed in the usual fashion. Five mutations account for almost 90% of the cases, while IVS1-5 G to C is the most common Indian mutation, although almost 61 mutations in the beta globin gene have been described among Indian subjects (Verma et al, 2011). The various techniques used for identification of mutations are ARMS, reverse dot blot, DGGE and SSCP.

The mutations in the β-globin gene can be divided into those causing qualitative abnormalities (such as sickle cell anemia), or those causing quantitative abnormalities (such as thalassemias). The qualitative abnormalities are due to mis-sense mutations that alter the amino acid sequence encoded by a particular 3-base codon. Many such changes do not cause any disease. Quantitative changes in production of β-globin messenger RNA cause β-thalassemia. The mutations are distributed throughout the β-globin gene. Point mutations in the promoter region of the gene make about 10% of the normal amount of mRNA, and lead to mild thalassemia. A number of mutations interfere with the efficient translation of the β-globin mRNA into protein, including mutations in the translation initiation codon itself. Chain terminator mutations resulting from non-sense mutations or frame-shift mutations early in the coding region result in protein that is totally non-functional. A number of abnormalities occur in splicing signals that lead to beta zero thalassemia, IVS1-5 G to C, or A, and IVS1-1 G to T are the commonly observed mutations in India. Mutations in the third exon often lead to thalassemia that is inherited as autosomal dominant.

The Thalassemia International Federation Manual on the management of thalassemia recommends that following molecular studies be done at the time of first diagnosis in every case of beta thalassemia:

a. Mutation in the β-globin gene to see if they are β^0 or β^{+}. The former refers to a mutation which results in almost absent β-globin synthesis, while the later refers to where the β-α-globin synthesis is reduced.
b. Study of the α-globin gene, as any deletion in this gene would ameliorate the clinical picture, while triplication of the gene would worsen the clinical condition.
c. Study of the γ-globin gene, essentially analysis of Xmnl1 polymorphism. The presence of this polymorphism (Xmnl1+ve) leads to synthesis of a greater amount of fetal hemoglobin, thus resulting in milder clinical features.

The importance of analysis of mutations is threefold. Firstly, knowing the mutations one can predict whether clinical behavior of the disorder would be mild or severe. If there are favorable features in all the three genes then it is likely that the thalassemia would behave as intermedia and could be managed without blood transfusions, with/without treatment with hydroxyurea. Studies in UK, and India show that about 10% of thalassemia patients of Indian origin belong to this category. Secondly this information is crucial for prenatal diagnosis in a future pregnancy. Thirdly, it is of great help in establishing a diagnosis of β-thalassemia major in the first year of life, as the amount of fetal hemoglobin is raised even in normal infants.

Gene Therapy

In β-thalassemia an allogenically matched bone marrow transplant is curative, although it is restricted to those with matched donors. Gene therapy holds the promise of "fixing" one's own bone marrow cells by transferring the normal β-globin gene into hematopoietic stem cells (HSCs) to permanently produce normal red blood cells. Requirements for effective gene transfer for the treatment of β-thalassemia are regulated, erythroid-specific, consistent, and high-level β-globin expression. Lentivirus vectors have been shown in several studies to correct mouse and animal models of thalassemia. The immediate challenges of the field as it moves toward clinical trials are to optimize gene transfer and engraftment of a high proportion of genetically modified HSCs and to minimize the adverse consequences that can result from random integration of vectors into the genome by improving current vector design or developing novel vectors. The current state of the art in gene therapy for β-thalassemia and some of the challenges it faces in human trials have been well discussed by Arugum and Malik (2010).

Abnormal Hemoglobins

In the eastern states Hb E is fairly common and when combined with a β-thalassemia mutation behaves as â-thalassemia major, although there is a considerable variability in the clinical manifestations. This is due to the interaction among the different globin genes. Homozygous Hb E is fairly innocuous. Sickle cell disease is prevalent mostly in tribal communities in central India, Maharashtra, Gujarat, Rajasthan, Nilgiri hills and Wynad district of Kerala. Sickle cell/β-Hb combination occurs to a small extent. Among Punjabis Hb D Punjab is observed in about 1-2% of cases. It is also most often asymptomatic, and does not cause problems even in combination with a β-thalassemia mutation. Now that the HPLC system (Biorad) is being used extensively many other hemoglobins are being recognized. It is good to know about them and their significance. For example, Hb Q India (an alpha globin gene variant) and Hb D Iran (a β-globin variant) are asymptomatic even when occurring with a β-thalassemia mutation. However, these should be confirmed by molecular studies, before ignoring them.

Hemophilia

Hemophilia A (HA), caused by defects in the F8 gene on the X-chromosome, is a common coagulation disorder with an incidence of about 1–2 in 10,000 men worldwide and is with no significant racial difference. In a recent review Howard et al (2011) assert that in hemophilia management it is the time to get personal. In those on factor VIII therapy, the possibility of allo-immunization depends mainly on three risk factors. The first is the degree of structural difference between the therapeutic protein and the patient's own endogenous protein. Such differences depend on the nature of the disease mutation and the premutation endogenous protein structure as well as on post-translational changes and sequence-engineered alterations in the therapeutic protein. The second set of risk determinants are genetic variations in the recipient's immune systems that may lead to deleterious immune responses. The third variable is the presence or absence of immunologic danger signals during the display of foreign-peptide/ MHC-complexes on APCs. A choice between existing therapeutic products or the manufacture of new proteins, which may be less immunogenic in some patients or patient populations, may require prior definition of the first two of these variables. This leads then to the possibility of developing personalized therapies for disorders due to genetic deficiencies in endogenous proteins, such as hemophilia A and B.

Unlike thalassemia where five mutations are responsible for about 90% of the cases, disorders like hemophilia A and B have mostly different mutations in each family. Diagnosis by direct detection of the mutation is thus costly and time-consuming. It has to depend upon coagulation and factor assays, and not on mutation analysis.

The treatment of the disease is expensive and lack of appropriate treatment often leads to disabilities. Therefore there is a demand for prenatal diagnosis and carrier screening. The technique used for this purpose varies with the severity of hemophilia:

It has been discovered that almost half of the subjects with severe hemophilia and some with moderate hemophilia have an inversion of intron 22, which results in a malfunctioning of the gene. A lower level (1-5%) of inversion is also observed in intron 1 of the gene. Therefore, in such cases one examines for this mutation directly, and if present it provides an easy and accurate method of prenatal diagnosis and carrier screening.

All remaining cases result from numerous point mutations and small insertions/deletions, one-third of these being *de novo* mutations. Ideally mutation screening by direct DNA sequencing would be the best means for identifying genetic defects in these cases. However, the strategy is time consuming and relatively expensive for F8 gene owing to its large size (186 kb) with 26 exons. In these cases, carrier screening and prenatal diagnosis has to be undertaken by linkage studies. However this analysis requires that the blood (or DNA) of the affected boy should be available to permit linkage studies, and the mother should be heterozygous for that particular marker being studied.

Fortunately enough data has been generated on the polymorphisms useful in the Indian population. Recently Saha et al (2011) recommended that a set of five microsatellite markers, namely, DSX9897, DSX1073, intron 1 (GT)n, intron 22 (CA)n and intron 25 (CA)n, in and around the F8 gene be used to achieve better sensitivity for carrier detection.

Thrombophilias

One mechanism for increased predisposition to thrombosis is the protein C activation pathway. Thrombin efficiently generates fibrin clot from fibrinogen, but when it is bound to thrombomodulin it cleaves protein C to generate activated protein C (APC). APC proteolytically inactivates factor Va and factor VIIIa aided by its cofactor protein S. A mutation in factor V (R506Q) renders FV resistant to inactivation by APC, resulting in a mild thrombotic disorder. All cases of venous thrombosis at an early age require analysis for this mutation. The frequency in most of India is 2-4%, but a high frequency has been reported in Parsees and South Indians.

In cases of arterial thrombosis, such as stroke in the young, it has recently become evident that one should check serum homocysteine level. A raised level often results from C378T polymorphism of 3′5′methylene tetra hydrofolate reductase enzyme. This raised homocysteine can be reduced by administration of folic acid, pyridoxine and viatmin B_{12}.

A polymorphism in prothrombin molecule (G20210A) has also been associated with thrombophilia. This polymorphism is very rare in India, and routine testing for this polymorphism in cases of thrombophilia in India is questionable (Tripathi et al, 2010).

Telomeres and Disease

Telomeres are at the ends of linear chromosomes and are composed of many (500 to 2000 in human cells) tandem repeats of a hexanucleotide (TTAGGG) in the leading 5′-strand of DNA and associated proteins, collectively termed the shelterin complex. The single-stranded 3′ overhang folds back to anneal with the C-rich strand of the double helix, forming the T loop. The associated shelterin proteins bind to the telomere, providing molecular signals that prevent the DNA repair machinery from mistaking the chromosome end for a double-stranded break. Telomere length in cells provides a mitotic clock, a measure of the cell's replicative history; 50 to 100 base pairs are lost with each human cell division. Telomeres of leukocytes and some other tissues also shorten with aging of the organism, but there is considerable overlap of telomere length of the very young and the very old.

The recent recognition of genetic defects in telomeres and telomere repair in multiple human diseases has practical implications for hematologists and oncologists and their patients; consequences for future clinical research in hematology and other subspecialties; and even importance in the interpretation of animal experiments involving cell propagation. Telomere diseases include the syndrome constitutional marrow failure dyskeratosis congenita, some apparently acquired aplastic anemia, myelodysplasia and acute myeloid leukemia; pulmonary fibrosis; and hepatic nodular regenerative hyperplasia and cirrhosis. Accelerated telomere attrition is a likely pathophysiology of cancer arising from chronic inflammation. Telomerase can be modulated by sex hormones, which may explain the activity of androgens in marrow failure. Measurement of telomere length of peripheral blood leukocytes is a simple screening clinical assay. Detection of a mutation in a patient has implications for therapy, prognosis, monitoring, and genetic counseling (Kelland 2001; Blanche et al 2007; Young, 2010).

Leukemias and Lymphomas (Table 34.1)

The process of malignant transformation in pediatric acute leukemias is complex, requiring at least two leukemogenic hits that result in DNA damage, ranging from point-mutations to double-strand DNA breaks. This leads to chromosomal translocations, deletions, duplications, or inversions. Investigations with single nucleotide polymorphism arrays have confirmed that leukemic blasts have multiple copy-number aberrations. The exception seems to be leukemias with translocations involving the mixed lineage leukemia gene, *MLL*, which are rarely accompanied by other genetic lesions. This suggests that *MLL* rearrangements are oncogenic events with the potential to induce leukemia in a single hit (Szczepański, 2010).

Chromosomal translocations are typically primary leukemogenic events with two main outcomes. In BCR-ALL, the translocation breakpoints disrupt two genes that lead to fusion of the coding regions of both genes, at least one of which is a transcription factor or a signaling molecule. The fusion (chimeric) gene encodes a chimeric protein that provides the affected hematopoietic cell with leukemogenic potential. Many of these transformed preleukemic cells are characterized by stem-cell features with the ability to proliferate continuously with little or no further differentiation. Becoming independent and resistant to normal apoptosis, the cells are predisposed to subsequent genetic abnormalities. An example of oncogene activation by chromosome translocation is the Philadelphia chromosome. This translocation fuses the ABL proto-oncogene, located at 9q to BCR gene on chromosome 22q. The resulting chimeric BCR-ABL protein retains the protein kinase activity of ABL gene, but this becomes aberrant because of the nearby BCR gene. And this is a causative factor in the development of CML. STI571 is a novel anticancer agent that selectively inhibits the BCR-ABL tyrosine kinase. The use of this drug has revolutionized the therapy of CML. Studies have also shown that the simultaneous administration of STI571 with other chemotherapeutic agents except methotrexate, would be advantageous for cytotoxic effects against Ph (+) leukemias.

In about 40% of T-cell acute lymphoblastic leukemia (T-ALL) the aberration affects the T-cell receptor (TCR) gene. In less than 5% of B-cell precursor ALL (BCP-ALL)

Table 34.1: Structural rearrangements in malignant myeloid and lymphoid disease

Disease	*Chromosome abn*	*Involved gene*
Chronic myeloid leukemia	t(9;22)	ABL-BCR
CML in blast phase	t(9;22) with +8, + Ph,	
Myeloid leukemias	+19, or i (17q)	
AML with *incr.* basophils	t(6;9)	DEK-CAN
AML-M2	t(8;21)	ETO-AML1
Promyelocytic (APL-M3)	t(15;17)	PML-RARA
Myelomonocytic (AMMoL-M4)	inv (16), 16q-	MYH11-CBFB
Monoblast (AMoL-M4/5)	t involving chm 11	MLL
AML	t(9;11)(p22;q23)	MLLT3-MLL
AML	inv(3), or t 3;3	RPN1-EVI1
Acute lymphatic leukemia:		
Pre-B	t(12;21)	TEL-AML1
B or B myeloid	t(9;22)	BCR-ABL
	t(5;14)	IL3 –IGH
	t(1;19)	E2A – TCF3
Burkitt's lymphoma	t(14;18)	MYC-IGH-IGK-IGL

the aberration affects immunoglobulin antigen-receptor genes. In these translocations, the strong promoters of the genes or the removal of negative regulatory elements upregulate the expression of the juxtaposed translocation partner gene (oncogene).

Retrospective investigation of newborn peripheral blood from patients who developed childhood leukemia has shown that chromosomal translocations are the primary preleukemic events, with a substantial proportion of translocations arising *in utero*. However, studies of cord blood showed that less than 1% of children with detectable translocations develop leukemia. Therefore, neonatal screening for evidence of predisposition to acute leukemia is unlikely to be useful. The secondary leukemogenic events leading to overt leukemia are heterogeneous and include activating mutations of transcription factors or kinases, inactivating mutations, and deletions of tumor suppressor genes.

Burkitt's lymphoma: In this there is a balanced translocation between chromosomes 8 and 14. As a result, Myc proto-oncogene on chromosome 8q24 is brought next to immunoglobulin heavy chain locus on chromosome 14q32. This leads to MYC activation resulting in lymphomatous transformation.

Genetic Aberrations at Diagnosis

One of the most studied aberrations in BCP-ALL is the translocation t(9;22)(q34;q11.1). This results in the *BCR–ABL1* fusion gene, which encodes a chimeric tyrosine kinase. This translocation is associated with an unfavorable outcome and is usually stratified as high-risk in most current ALL treatment protocols. Similarly, the presence of t(4;11)(q21;q23) results in *MLL–AFF1* fusion and is linked to a poor outcome in childhood ALL, particularly for those patients less than 2 years of age. For many patients with t(9;22) or young children with t(4;11) positive ALL, allogeneic hematopoietic stem-cell transplantation from a matched related donor is the only curative option.

The prognostic significance of other *MLL* gene rearrangements is inconclusive, except in infant ALL, where all *MLL* rearrangements are significantly associated with an aggressive disease and worse outcome. In several treatment protocols, hypodiploidy with fewer than 45 chromosomes is a factor associated with high-risk of poor outcome, although only 1% of patients with BCP-ALL have this abnormality. Prognosis seems to worsen with decreasing chromosome number, and patients with fewer than 44 chromosomes have a very poor outcome. By contrast, several abnormalities are associated with an improved outcome in BCP-ALL and include high hyperdiploidy (51–65 chromosomes) and the presence of t(12;21)(p13;q22) with the *ETV6–RUNX1* fusion. The Children's Oncology Group (COG) identified that high hyperdiploidy with the triple trisomies of chromosomes 4, 10, and 17 was associated with a good prognosis and have applied these findings to risk stratification for treatment. Trisomy 18 is the most informative marker of a favorable outcome.

AML with recurrent genetic aberrations is now officially recognized in the World Health Organization (WHO) classification of tumors of hematopoietic and lymphoid tissues. Three recurrent chromosomal aberrations are recognized as favorable risk features: t(8;21)(q22;q22) with *RUNX1-RUNX1T1* fusion, t(15;17)(q22;q21) with *PML-RARA* fusion, and inv(16)(p13;q22), t(16;16)(p13;q22) with *CBFM-MYH11* fusion (Estey, 2010; Grimwade and Mrozek, 2011). Almost all children with AML characterized by these translocations are cured with current chemotherapy regimens (5-year overall survival of 85–90%). In about 20% of patients, various *MLL* translocations occur, with t(9;11)(p21;q23) characterized by *MLL–MLLT3* fusion being the most common. The t(9;11) rearrangement is associated with good outcome on some treatment protocols. However, meta-analysis of more than 750 patients with AML associated with *MLL* showed heterogeneity, and cumulative event-free survival below 50%. Only t(1;11)(q21;q23) was a marker of favorable outcome, whereas the risk of treatment failure was significantly increased in patients with t(6;11)(q27;q23), t(10;11)(p12;q23), and t(11;19)(q23;p13).

Among the numerical chromosomal aberrations in AML, monosomy 7 is a predictor of poor outcome, with AML preceded by a myelodysplastic phase in some of these patients. Meta-analysis showed that the prognosis of patients with AML with 7q deletions is significantly better than for those with AML with monosomy 7. About 10% of patients with *de novo* AML have constitutional trisomy-21 and Down's syndrome. These patients usually have AML of megakaryocytic lineage associated with acquired inactivating *GATA1* mutations and can be cured with standard chemotherapy.

Neuroblastoma

Neuroblastoma is the most common extra-cranial solid tumor in children with 7.5% cases for every 100,000 infants. Furthermore, there are 1.3% new cases per 100,000 children under the age of 15 years every year, which accounts for 9.0% of all childhood cancers. 90% of children with the disease are diagnosed in the first 5 years of life. Its incidence peaks in infancy with a median age at diagnosis of 17 months. Derived from postganglionic sympathetic neuroblasts, neuroblastoma may arise anywhere within the sympathetic nervous system. The majority of primary tumors arise within the abdomen and classically involve the adrenal medulla.

Neuroblastoma is often described as enigmatic and unpredictable because it is associated with contrasting patterns of clinical behavior: life threatening progression, maturation to ganglioneuroblastoma or ganglioneuroma, and spontaneous regression. However, a significant proportion of tumors (>10%) undergo complete spontaneous regression in the absence of or with minimum therapeutic intervention. The incidence of spontaneous regression in neuroblastoma is between 10 and 100 times greater than that for any other human cancer.

Tumor-specific genomic information has increasingly been used for risk stratification to predict outcome and guide optimal therapy. A recently proposed International Neuroblastoma Risk Group (INRG) staging system utilizes both clinical characteristics and tumor biology to identify clinical risk groups with statistically different event-free survival rates. Independently prognostic baseline characteristics included in this system are patient age, tumor stage, histology, grade of differentiation, DNA index, MYCN oncogene amplification status, and the presence of copy number aberrations at chromosome arm 11q. The identification of other segmental chromosome aberrations, such as loss of heterozygosity at 1p and gain at 17q, have also been found to have prognostic significance. Gene expression profiling has been used to define prognostic signatures in neuroblastoma and may provide insight into the molecular basis of the observed clinical heterogeneity (Schwab et al, 2003; Deyell and Attiyeh, 2011).

Although only 1-2% of neuroblastoma is familial the genetic predisposition in these rare pedigrees is now understood for the majority of affected individuals. Familial cases occur at a younger median age than sporadic cases, are associated with multifocal primary tumors, and follow an autosomal dominant pattern of inheritance with incomplete penetrance. Heritable germline mutations in ALK and PHOX2B account for approximately 90% of hereditary neuroblastoma. Genetic testing should be considered for patients with a family history of neuroblastoma or other disorders of neural crest origin, or for patients with evidence of multifocal primary neuroblastomas. This may facilitate the identification of unaffected siblings who carry highly penetrant germline mutations and would justify screening in an attempt to ensure early detection of neuroblastoma.

Diagnosing Infections in Leukemias

Using PCR many opportunistic infections in hematologic malignancies can be diagnosed rapidly - CMV, toxoplasmosis, tuberculosis, herpes simplex, chickenpox, and *P. carinii*.

CONCLUSION

It must feel good to be young and have the whole field of molecular hemato-oncology to work on to identify new genes, their mutations and functions and echo the words of the Nobel laureate Max Perutz, who unraveled the structure of hemoglobin and found his wife too while working for it, "to make a discovery is like reaching the top of Mount Everest and falling in love at the same time."

BIBLIOGRAPHY

1. Arumugam P, Malik P. Genetic therapy for b-thalassemia: from the bench to the bedside. Hematology; 2010. p. 445. Amer Soc Hematology.
2. Blanche P Alter, Gabriela M Baerlocher, Sharon A Savage, Stephen J Chanock, Babette B. Very short telomere length by flow fluorescence *in situ* hybridization identifies patients with dyskeratosis congenita. Blood. 2007;110:1439-47.
3. Deyell RJ, Attiyeh EF. Advances in the understanding of constitutional and somatic genomic alterations in neuroblastoma. Cancer Genet. 2011;204(3):113-21.
4. Estey E. High Cytogenetic or Molecular Genetic Risk Acute Myeloid Leukemia Hematology; 2010. p. 474.
5. Grimwade D, Mrózek K. Diagnostic and prognostic value of cytogenetics in acute myeloid leukemia. Hematol Oncol Clin N Am. 2011;25:1135-61.
6. Howard TE, Yanover C, Mahlangu J, Krause A,Viel KR, Kasper CK, Pratt KP. Hemophilia management: time to get personal? Hemophilia. 2011;17:721-8.
7. Kelland LR. Telomerase: biology and phase I trials. The Lancet Oncology Lancet Oncol. 2001;2:95-102.
8. Saha A, Nayak S, Mani KR, Chandak GR, Ray K, Mukhopadhyay A. Indian genome variation consortium. A set of five microsatellite markers linked to F8 gene can detect hemophilia A carriers across India. Hemophilia. 2011;17(5):e928-35.
9. Schwab M, Westermann F, Hero B, Berthold F. Neuroblastoma: biology and molecular and chromosomal pathology. Lancet Oncol. 2003;4:472-80.
10. Szczepański T, Harrison CJ, van Dongen JJM. Genetic aberrations in pediatric acute leukemias and implications for management of patients. Lancet Oncol 2010;11:880-9.
11. Tripathi G, Sankhwar SN, Sharma RK, Baburaj VP, Agrawal S. Role of thrombotic risk factors in end-stage renal disease. Clin Appl Thromb Hemost. 2010;16(2):132-40.
12. Verma IC, Saxena S, Kohli S. Past, present and future scenario of thalassemic care and control in India. Indian J Med Res. 2011;134:507-21.
13. Young NS. Telomere biology and telomere diseases: implications for practice and research. Hematology, American Society of Hematology; 2010. p. 35.

Hematopoietic Stem Cell Transplantation

Mammen Chandy, Biju George, Leni Mathew

INTRODUCTION

Hematopoietic stem cell transplantation (HSCT) is widely used to treat various malignancies and a number of hematologic, immune and genetic diseases. The annual rate of allogeneic HSCT now exceeds 40,000. Hematopoietic stem cell transplantation is an effective treatment for acute leukemias and bone marrow failure syndromes such as aplastic anemia and myelodysplastic syndromes. In thalassemia major, HSCT now provides a cost-effective alternative to transfusion/chelation therapy. Graft versus host disease, interstitial pneumonia, leukemic relapse and infection remain the major complications. HSCT can be:

1. *Allogeneic:* Where the donor is a histocompatible sibling or family member (related) or from a donor registry (unrelated). Another source can be umbilical cord blood, which is a rich source of hematopoietic stem cells.
2. *Syngeneic:* Where the donor is an identical sibling. These transplants are easier to perform because engraftment is faster and GVHD is rare and if present mild. However, relapse is much higher in syngeneic transplants for leukemia because there is no graft versus leukemia effect.
3. *Autologous:* Here, the patient acts as his own donor. Usually done in diseases where the marrow is free of tumor and the dose limiting toxicity of chemotherapy is marrow suppression. The patient's own marrow can be harvested, cryopreserved and then returned back after ablative chemotherapy. In some situations, the marrow will be treated (purging) with either drugs or monoclonal antibodies to remove any minimal tumor in the harvest.

Graft Source

Bone marrow has traditionally been the graft source but increasing number of transplants are being done with mobilized peripheral blood stem cells [PBSCT], however, because of the larger number of T-cells there is a significant increase in chronic graft versus host disease. For the patients who do not have a matched sibling donor, there are three alternatives:

- Haplo-identical transplant
- Matched unrelated cord blood transplants
- Matched unrelated transplant.

Allogeneic Transplant

Indications for allogeneic transplantation are lited in Table 35.1.

The Donor

Once the decision to have a bone marrow transplant has been made, the next step is to perform HLA typing on the patient, sibling and parents. Most centers would perform a transplant only if there is a full six antigen HLA A, B and DR matched related donor available. Bone marrow transplantation can be done even if the

Table 35.1: Indications for allogeneic transplantation

1. **Malignant diseases**
   i. Acute myeloid leukemia presence of >15% blasts after 1st course of chemotherapy, absence of favorable genetic abnormalities, presence of adverse genetic abnormalities e.g. –5, –7, del (5q).
   ii. Acute lymphoblastic leukemia—high-risk ALL in CR1 especially if MRD positive, relapsed ALL in CR2.
   iii. Juvenile chronic myeloid leukemia (JCML).
2. **Bone marrow failure:** Severe aplastic anemia, diamond blackfan anemia (DBA), Fanconi's anemia, myelodysplastic syndromes.
3. **Genetic disorders**
   i. *Immune:* SCID, X-linked agammaglobulinemia.
   ii. *Granulocyte disorders:* Kostman's syndrome, CGD, Chédiak-Higashi.
   iii. *Platelet disorders:* Wiskott-Aldrich, Glanzman's thrombasthenia.
   iv. *Red cell disorders:* Thalassemia major, sickle cell disease.
   v. *Enzyme deficiency disorders:* Gaucher's, Leukodystrophies, Lesch-Nyhan, etc.
   vi. Osteopetrosis.

donor and recipient are not ABO blood group matched unlike solid organ transplants. If there are no matched siblings who can serve as a donor then an extended family search can be done in which parents or cousins are tested. The probability of finding a donor is small except where the parents are consanguineous. If there is only one child then the family can plan to have another child and HLA typing can be performed on the DNA sample that has been obtained from a chorionic villous sample. When this child is born either a cord blood transplant can be done or a regular transplant can be done when the baby is 2 years old.

Transplant Procedure

At the time of transplant the patient and donor undergo a series of tests after which the patient is admitted to the ward. The patient is then taken to the operating room where a dual lumen Hickman catheter is inserted under anesthesia. This catheter is used thereafter for blood tests, transfusions and administration of medication and fluids. It is removed when the patient is ready to go home. The catheter is dressed twice weekly and flushed with heparin saline when not in use. The patient is transferred to the bone marrow transplant unit prior to initiation of the conditioning regimen and is kept in the positive pressure high efficiency particulate air (HEPA) filtered unit till engraftment has occurred and the absolute neutrophil count is over 500/cumm. The HEPA filters are high efficiency filters with a size of 0.3 microns with a trapping efficiency of 99.97%.

Conditioning

This refers to the treatment given to the patient, which permits engraftment of donor marrow and involves the creation of space by destroying the patient's own marrow (cytoreduction) and immunosuppression to prevent rejection. The choice of conditioning regimen for a given patient is dictated by the underlying disease and donor characteristics. Most transplant centers use chemotherapeutic agents alone for conditioning; busulphan orally at a dose of 16 mg/kg over 4 days is administered followed by cyclophosphamide 50 mg/kg for 2-4 days. Treosulphan based conditioning has lower toxicity and is being used for transplants for genetic disorders. Total body irradiation 12 Gy over 3 days is often used for transplant conditioning in patients with acute lymphatic leukemia. In patients with a high-risk of rejection such as thalassemia, antilymphocyte globulin may be added to the conditioning regime. In older patients who need a transplant, nonmyeloablative or reduced intensity conditioning transplants are being increasingly used. Here drugs such as fludarabine are used to suppress the patient's immune system enough to allow engraftment of donor cells.

Bone Marrow Harvest

The donor is admitted a day or two before the harvest. Under general anesthesia marrow is aspirated from the iliac bone using either a harvest needle or as is done in our center a sternal aspirate needle. There is no surgical incision. The volume of marrow harvested is dependent on the weight of the patient: a nucleated cell dose of 300 million-marrow cells/kg (3×10^8) of the recipient is required. If the donor is over 25 kg, 8 ml/kg of blood can be collected pretransplant and used as an autologous transfusion during the harvest. If autologous transfusion is not feasible, then if blood needs to be transfused during the harvest, a directed donor is used and the blood is irradiated and leuko-depleted. The donor is discharged the day after the harvest.

Stem cells can also be collected from the donor using an apheresis machine after administration of G-CSF for 4-5 days and this is called a peripheral blood stem cell transplant (PBSCT). Engraftment is faster following a PBSCT as compared to BMT but the incidence of chronic graft versus host disease (GVHD) is also greater with PBSCT.[1] In certain situations such as high-risk leukemia, chronic GVHD is often associated with graft versus leukemia translating to higher cure rates with PBSC than with bone marrow transplant.[2]

The harvested cells are usually not treated and are directly infused into the patient like a blood transfusion. If the patient and donor have different blood groups, the product may need to be red cell depleted either using hydroxy-ethyl starch or using a red cell separator.

Transplant

The harvested marrow looks just like blood and is infused to the donor like a blood transfusion. Following the infusion of donor marrow the stem cells home in to the patient's marrow and a rising white cell count over the next 15 days is evidence of engraftment. One may use colony stimulating factors (G-CSF, GM-CSF) to hasten engraftment in sick patients. Red cell genotyping, cytogenetics or DNA fingerprinting will be used post BMT to document engraftment and to look for residual disease. Prior to transplant, the patient and donor DNA is tested using a set of VNTR's to look for specific DNA patterns and this is used post-transplant to see if the hematopoietic cells being produced belong to the donor. The patient is considered to be a full chimera if all the cells in the blood are donor in origin and a mixed chimera if residual host cells are present. Usually patients achieve full donor chimerism 30-45 days following BMT if a myeloablative conditioning protocol is used. The patient is transferred out of the BMT unit when his neutrophil count is over 500/cumm and discharged when there are no IV medications to be administered.

COMPLICATIONS (TABLE 35.2)

Graft versus host disease (GVHD), infection and regimen related toxicity are the major acute complications of BMT. The late complications include relapse, sterility, cataract and second malignancies.

Table 35.2: Complications following hematopoietic stem cell transplantation

- Acute complications
  - Acute graft versus host disease
  - Infections
  - Graft rejection
  - Veno-occlusive disease
  - Hemorrhagic cystitis
  - Interstitial pneumonia
- Chronic complications
  - Chronic graft versus host disease
  - Relapse
  - Sterility
  - Cataract
  - Second malignancy

GRAFT VERSUS HOST DISEASE

This is one of the most devastating complications of BMT and is termed acute if it occurs in the first 100 days following transplantation and chronic if it continues or develops after this period. Despite a six-antigen HLA match, the donor T. lymphocytes on entry into the patient may recognize minor differences in the recipient's cells, recognizing them as foreign and attack the recipient. Any organ in the body may be affected but the skin, intestine and liver usually bear the brunt of the attack by the donor lymphocytes in acute GVHD. Generalized erythema, maculopapular rash involving palms and soles and in severe cases toxic epidermal necrolysis (TEN) are the main cutaneous manifestations. Intestinal involvement usually manifests as diarrhea while upper gastrointestinal involvement may manifest with vomiting and loss of appetite. Progressive jaundice with minimal elevation of enzymes is seen in hepatic GVHD. Severe GVHD is associated with delayed engraftment and increased propensity to infections particularly with cytomegalovirus (CMV). Acute GVHD develops in 30-60% of patients transplanted with HLA identical marrow and may be an indirect cause of death in 20-30% of affected individuals. Acute GVHD is graded 1 to IV based on the degree of target organ involvement. Increased host age and transplants from female donors to male recipients particularly if the female is multiparous or has been transfused greatly increases the risk of GVHD.

Chronic GVHD produces a picture similar to scleroderma. In the skin, manifestations range from dry patches or areas of variegated pigmentation to extensive dermal scarring that produces thickened atrophic skin. The GI tract involvement may result in lichenoid lesions in the oral mucosa, xerostomia, dysphagia, diarrhea or malabsorption. Chronic GVHD of the liver usually presents as a cholestatic process, which can progress to a syndrome similar to primary biliary cirrhosis. The other manifestations include sicca syndrome, pulmonary dysfunction and development of auto-antibodies. Chronic GVHD is graded as either limited or extensive.

Methotrexate and cyclosporine are used as prophylaxis for GVHD. Methotrexate is given as an intravenous push in 3-4 doses over the first 10 days following BMT. Cyclosporine is continued for a period of 6-12 months depending upon the disease and the presence of GVHD. This is unlike solid organ transplantation where the drug has to be continued life long. Once GVHD develops the main stay of treatment is with corticosteroids. In refractory cases, antithymocyte globulin (ATG), OKT3, mycophenolate, sirolimus and IL2 antibody may be used. Chronic GVHD is managed with prednisolone along with cyclosporine.

Infection

In the initial period following transplantation, profound neutropenia, disruption of anatomic barriers secondary to mucositis and presence of central venous catheters are the most important risk factors resulting in bacterial and disseminated fungal infections with *Aspergillus* and *Candida*. At the earliest sign of infection or fever the patient is started on intravenous antibiotics usually a third or fourth generation cephalosporin. If there is persistent fever, carbepenems such as imipenem or meropenem and glycopeptides such as vancomycin or teicoplanin are added. Antifungals like fluconazole and amphotericin are routinely administered even if fungal infection is not documented if there is persistent fever beyond 72-96 hours.

Viral infections with herpes, CMV and adenoviruses contribute to the morbidity and mortality of transplantation after engraftment. The presence of GVHD, high intensity of immunosuppression, manipulations of the graft (T-cell depletion) and use of fludarabine/

campath (Anti-CD52 monclonal antibody) as part of conditioning are the risk factors for CMV and adenovirus infections. CMV infection commonly targets lungs, liver and intestine. Rapid early detection tests using PCR or antigenemia assays and prophylactic administration of ganciclovir or acyclovir on prophylactic basis to high-risk patients reduces the incidence of CMV. The most common manifestation of adenovirus infections is hemorrhagic cystitis, gastroenteritis, pneumonia and liver cell failure. Treatment options are limited with anecdotal reports of success using cidofivir. Patients with chronic GVHD are immunosuppressed and remains at risk for infections with encapsulated organisms such as *Pneumococcus* and *Meningococcus* and viruses. Prophylactic penicillin or trimethoprim sulpha in the first year post-transplant is useful in reducing the incidence of bacterial sepsis.

Interstitial Pneumonia

This complication is observed in 30% of patients where radiation is used for the conditioning and can be crippling. In transplants where radiotherapy is seldom used, busulphan related lung damage, GVHD, CMV and *Pneumocystis carinii* are other etiologic agents that have to be considered.

Regimen Related Toxicity (RRT)

Veno-occlusive disease of the liver (VOD) is a major problem with conditioning regimens containing busulphan and cyclophosphamide. It is characterized by weight gain, ascites and tender hepatomegaly, which appears within the first week after transplant and usually resolves by the third week. If severe, it can progress to hepatic failure and death. Treatment is supportive with careful fluid management.

Hemorrhagic cystitis is a well-known complication of cyclophophamide but can also arise from infection with adeno or BK virus. This is prevented by hydration and MESNA. Severe cases may require continuous bladder irrigation, cystoscopy and clot evacuation.

Graft Failure

Graft failure is defined as failure to achieve neutrophil recovery (ANC>500) by day +30 after transplant. Risk factors include inadequate conditioning, inadequate cell dose, T-cell depletion of the donor cells and HLA disparity between donor and recipient. With appropriate conditioning regimens graft failure is rare.

ABO Mismatched Transplants

ABO identity is not essential for BMT unlike solid organ transplants since stem cells do not carry ABO antigens. Removal of red cells from the harvested marrow with cell separators or gravity sedimentation with hydroxyethyl starch is all that is necessary in order to prevent hemolysis during infusion of the marrow in a group-mismatched transplant. Delayed red cell engraftment [PRCA] can occur in about 20% of major ABO mismatched transplants but most patients recover as the recipient's immune system is replace by the donors.

Blood Support

Aggressive blood and blood component support is crucial during the mandatory period of aplasia, while awaiting marrow recovery. Red cell transfusions are given to keep the hemoglobin levels above 9 g% (PCV 27%) and platelets transfusions given to maintain a platelet count above 10×10^9/L. All blood products are irradiated to prevent transfusion associated GVHD.

Post-transplant Care

Following a bone marrow transplant for a patient who has no graft versus host disease cyclosporine is given at full doses for six months after which it is tapered and stopped one-year post-transplant. *Pneumocystis carinii* prophylaxis and supplemental folic acid is given for one year. The child or adult can return to normal activities within 6 months after a transplant and the quality of life is excellent. Most patients do not require any special treatment or care one-year post-transplant unlike solid organ transplants, where they are on life long immunosuppression with its associated complications and high cost (Table 35.3).

Table 35.3: Post-HSCT immunization schedule

Mandatory 1 year			
1. Tetanus toxoid 0.5 ml IM	0 month	2 months	4 months
2. Inactivated Polio vaccine 0.5 ml IM	0 month	2 months	4 months
3. *Haemophilus influenzae* B	one dose		
4. Pneumococcal vaccine (23 valent)	one dose		

Tetanus and polio to be given simultaneously. *Haemophilus influenzae* and pneumococcal vaccine to be given one month apart starting one month after initiation of the tetanus and polio vaccination.

2 years
No graft versus host disease/not on immunosuppression
1. Measles/Mumps/Rubella — one dose

Optional after 1 year
1. Hepatitis B
2. Typhoid
3. Cholera
4. Rabies (if indicated)

Immunization

All children who have received allogeneic HSCT should be reimmunized. It should commence 12 months after a HLA-identical sibling donor transplant. The child should be off all immunosuppressive treatment including steroids and cyclosporine and should not have evidence of active chronic GVHD.

Autologous Transplantation

Megatherapy with stem cell reinfusion (MGT/STR) is widely used in pediatric malignancies. The rationale for this treatment is that dose intensification of chemotherapeutic agents increases response rate of chemo sensitive tumors. However, hematopoietic toxicity is a limiting factor, therefore, harvesting HSC, cryopreserving and reinfusing after intensive chemotherapy and radiotherapy would allow the procedure to be done with faster recovery of blood counts. MGT is usually given as consolidation therapy after a full course of standard chemotherapy. The out come of MGT is closely correlated with tumor burden at the time of transplant (Table 35.4).

Table 35.4: Diseases treated with MGT/HSC

Neuroblastoma	Stage 2-4, at any age with MYCN amplified tumor Stage 4 disease in children over 1 year of age. Relapse
Soft tissue sarcoma	Primary refractory disease Stage 4 disease at diagnosis
Ewing's tumor	>10% viable tumor in the resected tumor after induction therapy. Relapse
Wilms' tumor	Primary refractory disease Relapse in case of unfavorable histology 2 or more relapses
Brain tumor	Medulloblastoma in CR2 PNET in CR2

ALTERNATE DONOR TRANSPLANTATION

Allogeneic transplantation requires the presence of a 6 antigen matched HLA-identical donor. The chance that a sibling will be 6 antigens identical will be around 25% if there is only one sibling and this improves to 30-40% using an extended family search. This means that a large number of patients who require a transplant will not find a HLA identical donor within the family. In this situation, the options of transplant and donor source include:

- Matched unrelated donor (MUD)
- Cord blood transplants (CBT)
- Haplo-identical transplants.

These transplants may be associated with slower engraftment, higher rejection rates and higher incidence of GVHD and hence necessary modifications in conditioning protocols and manipulation of stem cells may be required to make the transplant a successful one.

Matched unrelated donor (MUD) transplants: The absence of a HLA identical sibling donor and the necessity for BMT has led to the formation of a number of bone marrow donor registries around the world. These registries maintain detailed HLA records of donors who are immediately accessible on request. It is estimated that approximately 17 million donors are registered in marrow donor registries around the world thus forming a large donor pool. Once a donor search is initiated, the initial reports of donors identified all over the world may be available within 5-7 days and a single donor is identified subsequently after high resolution HLA molecular typing is done. The average time from initiation of a donor search to transplant can vary between 3 and 6 months depending upon the country and the marrow registry. The bone marrow is usually harvested in the country where the donor is a resident (usually in a hospital recognized by the NMDP) and then transported to the country/place where the patient has been conditioned for transplant. Though the HLA typing identifies a 10 antigen matched donor, minor mismatches are more disparate than HLA identical sibling and hence the risk of graft rejection and GVHD are higher as compared to transplants using HLA identical siblings. With recent improvements in conditioning regimens and manipulation of the graft, MUD transplants in acute leukemias offer as good a chance of cure as with HLA identical sibling transplants.

Cord blood transplant: Hematopoietic stem cells from an unrelated cord blood (UCB) transplant can restore hematopoiesis and immune function after a myeloablative conditioning regimen, even if the graft is not perfectly HLA identical to the recipient. Umbilical cord is a rich source of stem cells that have a high pluripotent potential and are immunologically naive and hence these transplants are associated with a decreased risk of GVHD. This has led to the generation of both public and private cord blood banks (UCB) where cord blood units are stored for use in related and unrelated patients. UCB offers the advantage of significantly faster availability of banked cryopreserved UCB units compared with the availability of unrelated bone marrow grafts.

In children with acute leukemia, cord blood has potential advantages compared with bone marrow hematopoietic stem cells, namely, the rapid availability of cells and less stringent requirements for HLA identity between donor and recipient because of the lower risk of acute and chronic graft-versus-host disease (GVHD). In addition, CIBMTR and eurocord data show that UCBT in children with AL gives results comparable to those reported with other sources of stem cells. For diseases like aplastic anemia and thalassemia UCBT may be associated with higher rejection rates than peripheral blood or bone marrow transplantation.

Haplo-identical transplant: The broader application of stem cell transplantation (SCT) for pediatric diseases has been limited by a lack of human leukocyte antigen (HLA)-matched donors. Virtually all children, however, have at least one haploidentical parent who could serve as a donor. The product (either bone marrow or PBSC) is manipulated to obtain maximum stem cells (CD34 positive cells) with minimal lymphocytes (CD3 positive cells). The high number of CD34 cells ensures adequate engraftment thus reducing the risk of rejection while low numbers of CD3 positive cells will reduce the risk of grade IV acute GVHD. This manipulation is done using monoclonal antibodies (either CD34 positive selection or CD 3 depletion) in a MACS (Magnet activated cell sorting) system. These technological advances appear to have overcome the historical problems of graft rejection and severe graft versus host disease in the haploidentical setting, however immune reconstitution and infection are still a problem but being overcome by changing the immune cell depletion strategy.

BMT for India

For a developing country like India, it would seem irrational to develop such high technology medical treatment that is likely to benefit only a few when there are more urgent health priorities competing for scarce resources. The current cost of bone marrow transplantation in the United States is about $150,000 (75 lakh rupees). It is possible to transplant patients in India at a cost of about Rs 6-8 lakhs. The costs involved in alternate donor transplantation will be much higher and can vary between Rs 20 and 25 lakhs depending on the type of transplant. These costs will still be much lower than if the patient traveled abroad for a transplant. There are approximately 12-14 transplant centers in Indian performing allogeneic and autologous transplants with a cumulative number of 1000 transplants between 2001 and 2010. Approximately 30% of these transplants will be for children.

SUMMARY

Hematopoietic stem cell transplant offers curative therapy for a number of malignancies and hematological diseases in children. Based on the donor, it is classified into allogeneic, syngeneic and autologous. The source of stem cell could be from the bone marrow, peripheral blood or cord blood. Complications of HSCT fall into three main categories, namely, GVHD, infections and regimen related toxicity. Improvement in supportive care and better understanding of transplant immunology have led to dramatic improvement in transplant related morbidity and mortality.

BIBLIOGRAPHY

1. Alonzo TA, Wells RJ, Woods WG, et al. Postremission therapy for children with acute myeloid leukemia: the children's cancer group experience in the transplant era. Leukemia. 2005;19(6):965-70.
2. Badell I, Munoz A, Ortega JJ, et al. Spanish Working Party for BMT in Children (GETMON). Long-term outcome of allogeneic or autologous haemopoietic cell transplantation for acute lymphoblastic leukaemia in second remission in children. GETMON experience 1983-1998. Bone Marrow Transplant. 2005;35(9):895-901.
3. Bearman SI, Lee JL, Baron AE. Treatment of hepatic veno occlusive disease with recombinant human tissue plasminogen activator, and heparin in 42 marrow transplant patients. Blood. 1997;89:1501-6.
4. Chandy M, Srivastava A, George B, et al. Allogeneic bone marrow transplantation in the developing world: experience from a center in India. Bone Marrow Transplant. 2001;27(8):785-90.
5. Dini G, Cancedda R, Locatelli F, Bacigalupo A, et al. Italian Bone Marrow Transplant Group (GITMO). Unrelated donor marrow transplantation: an update of the experience of the Italian Bone Marrow Group (GITMO). Haematologica. 2001;86(5):451-6.
6. Gluckman E, Rocha V. Cord blood transplantation for children with acute leukaemia: a Eurocord registry analysis. Blood Cells Mol Dis. 2004;33(3):271-3.
7. Hale GA, Rochester RI, Heslop, HE, et al. Haemorrhagic cystitis after allogeneic bone marrow transplantation in children: Clinical characteristics and outcome. Biol Blood Marrow Transplant. 2003;9:698-705.
8. Lang P, Greil J, Bader P, Handgretinger R, et al. Long-term outcome after haploidentical stem cell transplantation in children. Blood Cells Mol Dis. 2004;33(3):281-7.
9. Meisel R, Enczmann J, Balzer S, et al. Similar survival following HLA-identical sibling transplantation for standard indication in children with haematologic malignancies: a single center comparison of mobilized peripheral blood stem cell with bone marrow transplantation. Klin Padiatr. 2005;217(3):135-41.
10. Nemecek ER, Gooley TA, Woolfrey AE, et al. Outcome of allogeneic bone marrow transplantation for children with advanced acute myeloid leukemia. Bone Marrow Transplant. 2004;34(9):799-806.

11. Pan L, Teshima T, Hill GR, et al. Granulocyte colony-stimulating factor-mobilized allogeneic stem cell transplantation maintains graft-versus-leukemia effects through a perforin-dependent pathway while preventing graft-versus-host disease. Blood. 1999;15;93(12):4071-8.
12. Ravindranath Y, Chang M, Steuber, CP et al. Pediatric Oncology Group. Pediatric Oncology Group (POG) studies of acute myeloid leukemia (AML): a review of four consecutive childhood AML trials conducted between 1981 and 2000. Leukemia. 2005;19(12):2101-16.
13. Richardson P, Guinan E. The pathology, diagnosis and treatment of hepatic veno occlusive disease; current status and novel approaches. Br J Haematol. 1999;107:485-93.
14. Sakata N, Kawa K, Kato K, et al. Unrelated donor marrow transplantation for congenital immunodeficiency and metabolic disease: an update of the experience of the Japan Marrow Donor Program. Int J Hematol. 2004;80(2):174-82.
15. Shah AJ, Lenarsky C, Kapoor N, et al. Busulfan and cyclophosphamide as a conditioning regimen for pediatric acute lymphoblastic leukemia patients undergoing bone marrow transplantation. J Pediatr Hematol Oncol. 2004; 26(2):91-7.
16. Sharathkumar A, Saunders EF, Dror Y, et al. Allogeneic bone marrow transplantation vs chemotherapy for children with Philadelphia chromosome-positive acute lymphoblastic leukemia. Bone Marrow Transplant. 2004;33(1):39-45.
17. Styczynski J, Cheung YK, Garvin J, et al. Outcomes of unrelated cord blood transplantation in pediatric recipients. Bone Marrow Transplant. 2004;34(2):129-36.
18. Veys P, Amrolia P, Rao K. The role of haploidentical stem cell transplantation in the management of children with haematological disorders. Br J Haematol. 2003;123(2):193-206.
19. Wall DA, Carter SL, Kernan NA, et al. COBLT Steering Committee. Busulfan/melphalan/antithymocyte globulin followed by unrelated donor cord blood transplantation for treatment of infant leukemia and leukemia in young children: the Cord Blood Transplantation study (COBLT) experience. Biol Blood Marrow Transplant. 2005;11(8):637-46.
20. Yumura-Yagi K, Inoue M, Sakata N, et al. Unrelated donor bone marrow transplantation for 100 pediatric patients: a single institute's experience. Bone Marrow Transplant. 2005;36(4):307-13.
21. Yusuf U, Frangoul HA, Gooley TA, et al. Allogeneic bone marrow transplantation in children with myelodysplastic syndrome or juvenile myelomonocytic leukemia: the Seattle experience. Bone Marrow Transplant. 2004;33(8):805-14.

Psychological Support of Chronic Blood Disorders

Roma Kumar, Ushma Singh, Anupam Sachdeva

The diagnosis of chronic disease in children sets the stage for a total change in the way of life experienced by patients and family. Implications are far reaching, affecting everyday routines, hopes and ambitions, and the relationships both between family members and with the outside world. On diagnosis, few families realize the extent to which chronic disease will change every aspect of their lives. Chronic blood disorders create a variety of difficulties with both practical and emotional implications. Some of the more routine aspects of childcare become more complicated time consuming and emotionally laden. A commonly experienced aspect of child rearing becomes a major family crisis. Treatments may disrupt family life. It may be necessary for the child to have medications at specified times and this may result in interruption in play or family activities. Some families become more cohesive, developing increased strength and a positive redefinition of values.[1,2]

Parent's perceptions and attitudes towards the child can also be affected. Marital relationships may be strained by increased care taking and sometimes by anxiety and guilt about the child's disease. Social life may be compromised, especially if parents feel that no competent childcare facility is available. Child and parents spend more time with the sick child with the result that time for other members of the family reduces. Family activities also can be more difficult to organize and consequently everybody comes to lead a restricted life.

Chronic blood disorders are conditions that affect children for extended periods of time, often for life. These disorders can be managed to the extent that a degree of pain control or reduction in attack, bleeding episodes or maintenance of normal hemoglobin levels can be achieved.

WHY IS PSYCHOLOGICAL SUPPORT SO IMPORTANT?

The way the diagnosis is conveyed to the child and the family, significantly influences initial response to medical treatment. It also has long-term bearing on continuing treatment, compliance and cooperation with treating team.[3] Chronic blood disorders have important psychological implications. The way in which the family and the patients come to term with the disease and its treatment will have a critical effect on the patient's survival. Without understanding and acceptance of the disease and its implications by patients and family, there is increased risk of disease complications and poor survival. A key role for doctors and other health care professionals is to help patients and families face up to the difficult demands of treatment. It is important to promote the patient's physical, emotional and social development. Chronic illness is a strong front of emotional problems that intensify at each significant development stage of the patient's life. Patients can feel that they are different, limited or isolated. Their state of mind may shift rapidly from depression to anger and vice versa. The doctor must be prepared to accept this shift and to help them deal with these feelings.

COMMUNICATION BY DOCTORS AND HEALTHCARE PROFESSIONALS WITH PATIENTS

This should include as far as possible:

Listening: To be interested in the patients emotional and real experiences.

Accepting: Both respecting the patient's point of view and being sensitive in the timing of personal communication.

Sharing: Being consistently close to the patient's positive and negative feelings as human being.

Understanding: Not simply at an intellectual level but at the emotional one.

Empathy: To compassionately feel the patient's and their family's emotions and then rendering them tender loving care.

Maintaining boundaries: Giving help and relief, but keeping in mind his/her role as a physician.

This type of interaction can be extremely beneficial for the patient, helping him/her to cope better with the disease and to maintain a sense of balance. It can also be extremely rewarding for the physician both in medical and emotional terms. If the doctor manages to maintain a constant dialogue, she/he can often find in people with chronic diseases skills greatly surpassing those of their peers when facing the great challenges of life such as birth/death, love/loneliness and possibilities/limits.

COMING TO TERMS WITH THE DIAGNOSIS

The day of the diagnosis is usually recalled by parents as shocking and overwhelming. To assist them in coping with this distressing information, communication about the diagnosis has to be done within a specific setting.

1. The room and time should be chosen to provide an atmosphere that will sustain hopes without deluding or depressing.
2. The doctor should discuss the diagnosis with both parents together allowing ample time to listen to their concerns and respond to questions.
3. Information must be sincere, complete and repeated as often as needed. The weight of negative emotions may be so great that parents may appear confused even after complete information has been given more than once.
4. In the months following diagnosis the discussion must be renewed, with the same attention to the setting and preferably with the same doctor to preserve continuity.

The child has to be included as soon as possible. From as early as three to five years of age, young patients begin to ask crucial questions about duration of care and possibilities of recovery. These should be dealt with sensitively and honestly.

How and whether feelings, worries and concerns about the disease are expressed, is of immense importance. Very often, however we do not express ourselves because we are afraid we may be rejected or not liked by others. Fear of death, anxiety anger and depression are common and say nothing about the mental health of the individual. The presence of a chronic blood disorder is a very demanding condition that will unavoidably cause a number of intense emotional reactions. The accurate perception of the implications of such illness cannot but create feeling of anger and depression, fears and worries. Understanding that these feelings are normal and that it is all right to express them greatly reduces their impetus. The presence of a chronic illness can be growth promoting if it is not viewed as "God's verdict" for a miserable existence. It is a threat needing urgent attention but also an opportunity for growth.

INFORMED CONSENT

Careful explanations of the disease and its treatment are to be explained to the parents and the child. Tailoring the explanations according to understanding of each family significantly improves compliance. When the family asks a lot of questions, expresses concern, actively participates in discussion, it is a positive sign. It increases their understanding of the disease and treatment.[4]

PSYCHOLOGICAL IMPACT OF ADMISSIONS TO HOSPITAL

Admission to a hospital can be a traumatic experience. Children can have quite distorted views about what goes on in hospitals, what doctors do and what medical treatment involves. As they grow up, children become more knowledgeable about what happens in hospital their knowledge may not always be entirely accurate however, it is a place where things "hurt". Parents and medical staff like to assure children that treatment does not hurt, but in fact it often does, and it may be more honest to say so. Older children become increasingly adult-like in their understanding of what happens in hospitals, but even adolescents have needs quite distinct from those of adult. Adolescents do not want to be treated like babies; they do not altogether fit in well on the adult ward either. Children can come to believe that doctors and nurses deliberately inflict pain and even enjoy doing it. Many children grow to resent the medical profession due to these reasons. Children need to be prepared. They should be provided proper information, encourage emotional expression and establish a trusting relationship with medical and hospital staff.

ADJUSTMENT IN THE CHILD WITH CHRONIC BLOOD DISORDERS

Caring for a chronically sick child is extremely demanding both physically and emotionally. Parents are taught to undertake much of the routine care. They must ensure that appropriate medication is taken. The emotional problems for families are no less daunting. Parents must come to terms with the fact that the ambitions they had for the child may never materialize. Illness can compromise achievement by limiting experience and the acquisition of skills. These diseases are associated with periods of stability followed by periods of relapse and illness. Even when the child is well, families may feel uneasy and anxious that the child will relapse. Parents have to cope with a great deal of uncertainty about child's health and future.

The way in which the family handles these difficulties is likely to determine the child's response to the disease. For the child, chronic disorders may be particularly important in compromising school achievement and academic success. Repeated absences and periods of ill health can naturally limit achievements. Absences also interrupt social relationship. In addition changes in physical appearance can result in children with chronic disease being rejected by peers and becoming unpopular figures in school. Restrictions imposed by treatment schedules can be especially difficult for adolescents resulting in limited social and emotional lives.

Some children with chronic disorders show an increased risk of maladjustment, but many children show up measurable deficits.

ADJUSTMENT IN THE FAMILY

Having a child diagnosed with a catastrophic disease challenges the coping resources of the entire family. Parents must meet the physical and emotional need of their child while attempting to juggle the demands of work and normal household responsibilities. Research has demonstrated that their adjustment can be similar to that of families without a chronically ill child. They need to plan in issues related to family relationships financial stresses and need to remain in close proximity to a major medical facility.

As with children themselves, chronic illness imposes a risk of maladjustment on parents. Although the etiology, symptoms treatments and prognoses vary significantly between different chronic blood disorders the resultant stresses on parents are very similar, e.g. financial burden, changing in parenting roles, sibling resentment, risk for psychosocial adjustment, difficulties in the ill child and healthy siblings, social isolation, frequent hospitalization and grief. Mobilization of materialistic and human resources needs to be considered for optimization.

At times, clinical observations suggest that the stresses of illness alone may lead to deterioration in marital relationships. More often, it is observed that marriages already suffering may succumb under the stresses of the illness. There are instances in which parents report improvement both in their relationship and in other family relationships as well. Close cooperation is necessary between husband and wife to meet the many demands of caring for their ill child.

Children are inevitably affected when a brother or sister becomes seriously ill. Some may feel anxious that they are responsible for the onset of the disease, or even worry that they themselves will also develop the condition. Siblings may feel neglected by parents or other family members.

Children cope not only with stresses associated with their disease but also with a host of others. These stresses stem from situations at school, at home and with friends or strangers. The strategies that children rely on to deal with their disease are based on those that they have learned to use successfully in other contexts. The psychological repercussions of chronic disease are intimately bound up with development in this wider context.

WHEN TREATMENT FAILS

Although now the survival is much better than it used to be in the past, the course of disease for some children remains a series of treatment relapses and responses leading to a time when all curative treatment has been exhausted. A few patients remain refractory to all treatments. Recent developments have happened in providing care to children towards end of life. It should include psychosocial factors from earlier in the disease process also.[5]

PAIN CONTROL

Proper pain control enhances the child's capacity to respond to all treatments, improve self care, and to engage with care givers, family members and school.[6] Analgesics should be administered in the context with other medications maintaining a regular blood level for optimum pain control.

SELF-HELP GROUPS

- Education resource information
- Disease management, daily care activities, finances, physical activity, touching, sharing experiences, discussing problems and giving a practical solution and help
- Stress management training.

Individual patients and families react differently to the disorder thus affecting the family atmosphere and outcome. Anxiety disorders, cognitive impairment and depression are one of the most common psychological complications of chronic blood disorders, recognition and correction of these help patients and families to cope with the problem and get better quality of life and better health. Specialized workers like dedicated social worker, psychiatrist, counselors, nursing staff, all having knowledge of disease and associated problems are a great help for these patients and families. Patients and families should undergo regular surveillance, especially at the time of treatment failure of suicide, drug abuse, etc. to offer them support and assistance in coping with the situation.

REFERENCES

1. Futterman EH, Hoffman J. Crisis and adaptation in the families of fatally ill children. In: Anthony EJ, Koupernik E (Eds): The child and his family. New York: Willy and Sons; 1973. p.127.
2. Spinetta JJ, Swarner JA, Sheposh JP. Effective parental coping following the death of a child from cancer. J Pediatr Psychol. 1981;6:251-63.
3. Grossman H, Simmons JE, Dyer AR. The physician and the mental health of the child. Assessing development and treating disorders within a family context. Monroe WI American Medical Association 1979;1:52.
4. Prugh DG. The psychosocial aspects of pediatrics. Philadelphia: Lea and Febiger, 1983;92:483.
5. American Academy of Pediatrics Committee on Bioethics and Committee on Hospital care. Palliative care for children. Pediatrics 2000;106:351-7.
6. Greenham DE, Lohman RA. Children facing death: recurring patterns of adaptation. Health Soc Work 1982; 7:89-94.

37 Vascular Access and Specialized Techniques of Drug Delivery

R Parakh

INTRODUCTION

The use of chronic indwelling venous access catheters has translated into a marked improvement in safety and quality of life for patients undergoing prolonged intravenous therapy. For physicians, the availability of continuous, reliable intravenous catheterization has provided an opportunity to design and develop more complex, potentially more effective, multidrug delivery systems. Because of the increasing popularity of chronic indwelling venous access catheters since their introduction into clinical practice almost 20 years ago, it is essential for all health personnel involved with their use to have understanding of appropriate catheter selection, routine maintenance procedures, and treatment related complications.

INDICATIONS

- Chemotherapy
- Long-term intravenous alimentation
- Intravenous antibiotics.

Implantable ports were introduced into clinical practice almost 15 years ago. Port housing are generally constructed of titanium or plastic and have a thick, compressed silicone diaphragm designed to withstand repeated punctures with the non-coring Huber needle and provide needle stability when accessed. Port housings are also designed to provide minimal distortion artifact on magnetic resonance imaging or CT scans and are available as single or double lumen ports. A low profile port housing is available for pediatric or asthenic adult patients. Ports are placed in subcutaneous pockets adjacent to the venous insertion site and are anchored to the underlying fascia.

TYPES OF DEVICES

Traditional central lines: The Seldinger technique is now used to place most central lines, with flow-Doppler ultrasonography, and fluoroscopy used to improve accuracy in patients with access difficulties, and a history of prior lines.

Silastic surgically implanted lines: Least irritating material, but requires an increased catheter size.

Implanted infusion ports: It requires the use of a smaller gauge needle; the close proximity of the skin puncture to the vein puncture increases chance of infection; therefore, this device is not recommended for use in neutropenic patients.

Long-line central access: Although some types are associated with thrombosis and phlebitis, they are easy to insert, making them appropriate for use in outpatient setting.

PURPOSE OF ACCESS

Intravenous drug delivery: Allows administration of drug into large blood vessel, lessening the negative effects of vesicant drugs.

Blood sampling: Many factors negatively affect the ability to aspirate blood.

CATHETER AND PORT INSERTION TECHNIQUES

- Seldinger closed insertion most common
- A learning curve exists to achieve a high success rate and low incidence of complication.

CATHETER INSERTION COMPLICATIONS

- Any procedure that involves placement of a catheter inside a blood vessel carries certain risks. These risks include damage to the blood vessel, bruising or bleeding at the puncture site, and infection.
- Bleeding or hemorrhaging may occur. This risk can be minimized through a blood test in advance to be sure that the blood clots normally. If the blood is too

thin, the procedure may be postponed and medication or blood products to improve blood clotting may have to be given.

- Very rarely a patient may develop a condition called a pneumothorax, a collection of air in the chest that may cause one of the lungs to collapse. This may occur during placement of a catheter or port using a vein in the chest or neck, but not when an arm vein is used. The risk is lessened when catheter placement is guided by ultrasound or fluoroscopy. Placement of these catheters by interventionalists using appropriate imaging guidance significantly decreases the risk of pneumothorax.
- The normal heart rhythm may be disturbed while the catheter is inserted, but this is usually only temporary. The problem is easily recognized during the procedure and eliminated by adjusting the catheter position.
- Rarely, the catheter will enter an artery rather than a vein. If this happens, the catheter will have to be removed. Most often the artery then heals by itself, but occasionally it has to be surgically repaired.

Delayed Risk

- A hole or break in the catheter may lead to leakage of fluid. Breaks may be avoided by never using too much force when flushing it.
- Catheters rarely fracture inside the body, but if this does happen, a chest X-ray will show the problem. The broken fragment can usually be removed without open surgery by snaring the free portion of the catheter through a retrieving catheter.

CATHETER MAINTENANCE

Wound dressings: Gauze, transparent membranes (semipermanent: Tegaderm; permeable: Opsite 3000), Vigilon, Tegasorb, Primapore.

Antibacterial ointments: Betadine, Tribiotic, Sivadine.

Catheter patency: Low-dose coumadin to high-dose heparin; Thrombolytic agents such as streptokinase, urokinase and tissue plasminogen activator (t-PA) may be needed for intraluminal clots.

Alternate routes for long-term access, if the superior vena cava cannot be used include the transfemoral venous or translumber routes to the inferior vena cava, or on rare occasions, the percutaneous transphepatic route.

TECHNIQUE OF CATHETER INSERTION

Most procedures can be performed safely on an outpatient basis, typically in an operating suite, to maximize sterile conditions although an increasing number of external catheters are being inserted in an interventional radiology suite. Fluoroscopy is used to confirm appropriate catheter placement. Catheters can be inserted using a local anesthetic with monitored anesthesia sedation. The preferred technique and most accessible site of insertion is the percutaneous method of Seldinger using the subclavian vein, which can be performed more quickly and with comparable safety to an open venous cut down. The precordium is prepared sterile and a local anesthetic is infiltrated infraclavicularly. With the patient in Trendelenburg position, a needle is advanced into the vein with the bevel up while gently aspirating on the attached 5 ml syringe. Entry into the vein is confirmed by flow of venous blood into the syringe, at which time the needle is rotated 90 degrees, the syringe is disconnected, taking care not to allow air to be entrained into the vein through the needle, and a flexible guide wire is advanced through the needle. If pulsatile backflow of blood is observed through the needle, the subclavian artery has been cannulated and, after removal of the needle, direct pressure for several minutes should produce adequate hemostasis. If resistance is encountered after the flexible wire has been advanced 2-3 cm, the needle is most likely not in the vein. In this situation the needle should be withdrawn with the wire to avoid the possibility of shearing the wire. At this point a site on the precordium is selected as exit site and infiltrated with anesthetic, and the catheter is tunneled through the subcutaneous tissue to the insertion site so that the Dacron cuff is situated subcutaneously just above the exit site. The skin adjacent to the wire insertion is then incised slightly and a peel away sheath/vessel dilator is gently advanced over the wire. It is very important to ensure that the sheath dilator is threading over the wire by intermittently advancing it and withdrawing the wire slightly and checking for resistance. The advance of the dilator can also be controlled by fluoroscopy. It is possible for the sheath dilator to bend the wire and for the surgeon to advance the dilator through the mediastinal structures; one episode has been fatal. Ideally, the catheter tip should lie at the superior vena cava-right atrial junction or just inside the right atrium. A higher rate of catheter occlusion or thrombotic complication has been noted when the catheter tip was higher in the superior vena cava or subclavian vein compared with catheters with tip located in the right atrium. The catheter is cut to its estimated desired length, which is determined from external bony landmarks. Typically, the right superior vena cava-right atrial junction will lie approximately 4-6 cm inferior to the angle of Louis.

PROBLEM SOLVING IN CATHETER USE

If a catheter does not have a blood return or will not infuse solution, before proceeding with the declotting procedure perform these troubleshootings techniques to diagnose the problem:

1. Connect a flush bag of NSS of D5W to the catheter and open the roller clamp to allow the fluid to flow by gravity.
2. Have the patient change position, take deep breaths, and cough while observing the drip rate.
3. When the fluid infuses at a faster rate, lower the bag and observe for a blood return.
4. If a blood return is observed, use the catheter as indicated, making a note that it is positional.
5. If no blood return is observed in any position, if gravity flows freely in all positions, and if the lateral chest radiograph verifies catheter tip in the SVC, proceed to declot the catheter with a known clot busting agent (catheter has a fibrin sheath).
6. If the radiograph shows that the catheter tip position is questionable, obtain a dye study. Dye study is contrast injected through the lumen of the catheter to verify exact location of the tip, integrity of the catheter and flow of solution.

Before urokinase can be instilled, a dye study must be done if the radiograph shows the catheter tip position to be questionable.

Declotting Procedure

See guidelines above before proceeding to declot as follows:

1. Using a 1 ml syringe, create a vacuum by aspirating back on the plunger (at the hub) can clamp. Repeat once.
2. Instill 2 ml 1:1000 U heparin solution (in each lumen) and let dwell for 1 hour. Assess for a blood return.
3. If line remains clotted, instil the appropriate amount of urokinase and normal saline solution (listed in Table 37.1) using the same technique as with the heparin.
4. Let dwell for 30 minutes to 1 hour and then assess for a blood return. May repeat the procedure as long as the recommendation of 30,000 U/d is not exceeded. Complete aspiration of the solution may not be possible and systemic urokinase may be harmful.

Table 37.1: Urokinase and normal saline solutions

Catheter type (ml)	*Urokinase (ml)*	*Normal saline (ml)*
Central line, 14 gauge	0.7	0
Central line, 16 gauge	0.5	0
Hickman, 12 F	1	0.6
Hickman, 10 F	1	0.3
PIC	0.5	0
Groshong	1	0.6
Plasmapheresis	1	0.4

COMPLICATIONS

The inability to infuse fluids or withdraw blood from long-term indwelling venous access catheters can be a result of catheter tip malposition, catheter kinking, fibrin sheath around the catheter, luminal occlusion due to blood clot or precipitation of drug solutions, or catheter tip abutment against the venous wall. A chest radiograph should be obtained to rule out catheter malposition or kinking. One should consider the possibility of a fractured catheter, if the patient experiences pain when the catheter is irrigated. If there is no catheter migration, then the etiology is likely to be catheter lumen occlusion. If one can infuse but not aspirate from the catheter this is termed withdrawal occlusion and has been attributed to the development of a fibrin sheath around the tip of the catheter acting as a flap valve, which will not interfere with infusion but does prevent aspiration. The incidence of fibrin sheath in subclavian venous catheters has been reported to occur in up to 80% of patients. After the appropriate location of the catheter is confirmed on chest radiograph, attempts to restore patency of occluded catheters or manage persistent withdrawal occlusions can be undertaken with a variety of thrombolytic agents, which have been very successful. Although there is some possibility of embolising a small luminal clot into the lungs, the clinical consequences are unknown but do not appear significant.

CATHETER-RELATED VENOUS THROMBOSIS

The presence of chronic indwelling catheter in the subclavian vein and the associated intimal injury at the insertion site predispose patients to the development of subclavian vein thrombosis and have been reported to occur in up to 40% of patients by clinical assessment or autopsy. Once a diagnosis of subclavian vein thrombosis is made, particularly if symptoms are present, prompt treatment is indicated. Initial supportive measures include arm elevation and analgesia for pain. In the past, systemic anticoagulation with heparin, catheter removal, and subsequent coumadin has been fairly standard approach for catheter related thrombosis. Several reports have demonstrated highly successful treatment outcomes with anticoagulation or thrombolytic agents while the catheter remains *in situ*. One approach is to infuse thrombolytic agent directly into the site of subclavian vein thrombosis through an ipsilateral vein. Local infusion of urokinase has resulted in dissolution in 25 of 30 thrombi within four days with minimal morbidity.

CATHETER-RELATED INFECTIONS

Catheter-related infections are mainly exit site infections, which are localized at the point where an external device exits the skin and are manifested by localized erythema and induration without systemic signs of infection. Most exit site infections are secondary to *Staphylococcus epidermis* and initial management with local wound care and appropriate oral antibiotics without removing the catheter is indicated and frequently successful. However, if there is evidence of developing bacteremia associated with an exit site infection, particularly, if the isolated pathogen is *S. aureus*, catheter removal may be necessary in up to 90% of cases. The difficulty in deciding exactly when a catheter should be removed is difficult to know, as many reports on this topic do not have standardized criteria for catheter removal.

Limitations of Vascular Access Procedures

- Although some types of central venous catheter may remain in place for months or even years, most catheters require replacement after certain time frame because of poor function. The reservoir septum of most types of implanted ports has a useful lifetime of about 1,000 punctures and so is not suitable for patients who require IV access on a daily basis
- Some patients have very poor veins that are not well suited for catheter placement. This usually happens when these access veins have been used for a long period of time (years of intravenous feeding, etc.). It may be very difficult to find a suitable vein to place a catheter in these patients, and may require unusual venous entry sites (e.g. through the back or through the liver).

Index

Page numbers followed by *f* refer to figure and *t* refer to table

B

C

G

H

Q

R

S

T

U

V

W

X

Z